Second Edition

Review of GENERAL INTERNAL MEDICINE

A SELF-ASSESSMENT MANUAL

Edited by

LLOYD H. SMITH, JR., M.D.

Professor and Chairman, Department of Medicine
University of California, San Francisco

JAMES B. WYNGAARDEN, M.D.

Frederic M. Hanes Professor and Chairman,
Department of Medicine
Duke University Medical Center

1982

W. B. SAUNDERS COMPANY **Philadelphia London Toronto**
Mexico City Rio de Janeiro Sydney Tokyo

W. B. Saunders Company: West Washington Square
Philadelphia, PA 19105

1 St. Anne's Road
Eastbourne, East Sussex BN21 3UN, England

1 Goldthorne Avenue
Toronto, Ontario M8Z 5T9, Canada

Apartado 26370—Cedro 512
Mexico 4, D.F., Mexico

Rua Coronel Cabrita, 8
Sao Cristovao Caixa Postal 21176
Rio de Janeiro, Brazil

9 Waltham Street
Artarmon, N.S.W. 2064, Australia

Ichibancho, Central Bldg., 22-1 Ichibancho
Chiyoda-Ku, Tokyo 102, Japan

Library of Congress Cataloging in Publication Data

Main entry under title:

Review of general internal medicine.

Includes bibliographies.

1. Internal medicine—Examinations, questions, etc. I. Smith, Lloyd Holly, 1924– II. Wyngaarden, James B. [DNLM: 1. Internal medicine—Examination questions. WB 18 R454]

RC58.R48 1982 616′.0076 81–48529

ISBN 0–7216–8429–7 AACR2

Review of General Internal Medicine: A Self-Assessment Manual ISBN 0-7216-8429-7

Last digit is the print number: 9 8 7 6 5 4 3 2 1

CONTRIBUTORS

HOMER A. BOUSHEY, M.D.

Respiratory Disease

Associate Professor of Medicine, University of California, San Francisco, California.

JOHN P. CELLO, M.D.

Gastrointestinal Disease

Assistant Professor of Medicine, University of California, San Francisco. Chief, Gastroenterology, San Francisco General Hospital, San Francisco, California.

PETER M. ELIAS, M.D.

Dermatology

Vice-Chairman and Associate Professor, School of Medicine, Department of Dermatology, University of California, San Francisco, California. Chief, Dermatology Service, Veterans Administration Medical Center, San Francisco.

GEORGE J. ELLIS, M.D.

Endocrinology and Diabetes Mellitus

Associate Professor of Medicine, Duke University School of Medicine, Durham. Attending Physician, Duke University Medical Center, Durham, North Carolina.

JAMES H. GRENDELL, M.D.

Gastrointestinal Disease

Assistant Professor of Medicine and Physiology, University of California, San Francisco. Attending Physician, San Francisco General Hospital, San Francisco, California.

BARRIE J. HURWITZ, M.B., M.R.C.P., F.C.P. (SA)

Neurologic Disease

Assistant Professor of Medicine, Neurology, Duke University School of Medicine, Durham. Neurologist, Duke University Medical Center, Durham, North Carolina.

RICHARD A. JACOBS, M.D., Ph.D.

Infectious Diseases

Assistant Clinical Professor of Medicine, University of California, San Francisco, California.

GERALD LOGUE, M.D.

Hematology and Oncology

Associate Professor of Medicine, Duke University School of Medicine, Durham. Chief of Hematology and Medical Oncology, Durham Veterans Administration Medical Center, Durham, North Carolina.

J. SCOTT LUTHER, M.D.

Neurologic Disease

Associate in Medicine, Neurology, Duke University School of Medicine, Durham. Neurologist, Duke University Medical Center, Durham, North Carolina.

FRANCIS A. NEELON, M.D.

Endocrinology and Diabetes Mellitus

Associate Professor of Medicine, Duke University School of Medicine, Durham. Attending Physician, Duke University Medical Center, Durham, North Carolina.

DAVID S. PISETSKY, M.D., Ph.D.

Clinical Immunology and Rheumatology

Assistant Professor of Medicine and Immunology, Duke University Medical Center, Durham. Chief of Rheumatology, Durham Veterans Administration Hospital, Durham, North Carolina.

VINCENT G. PONS, M.D.

Infectious Diseases

Assistant Clinical Professor of Medicine and Neurosurgery, University of California, San Francisco, California.

JOHN R. RICE, M.D.

Clinical Immunology and Rheumatology

Assistant Professor of Medicine, Division of Rheumatic and Genetic Disease, Duke University Medical Center, Durham, North Carolina.

BRUCE F. SCHARSCHMIDT, M.D.

Gastrointestinal Disease

Associate Professor of Medicine, University of California, San Francisco. Attending Physician, University of California Hospitals and San Francisco General Hospital, San Francisco, California.

REBECCA W. VAN DYKE, M.D.

Gastrointestinal Disease

Research Fellow in Medicine, University of California, San Francisco, California.

DAVID G. WARNOCK, M.D.

Renal Disease

Associate Professor of Medicine, Division of Nephrology, Department of Medicine, University of California, San Francisco. Attending Physician, University of California Hospitals, San Francisco, California.

ROBERT A. WAUGH, M.D.

Cardiovascular Diseases

Assistant Professor of Medicine, Duke University Medical Center, Durham, North Carolina.

GUY WEINBERG, M.D.

Genetics and Metabolic Disease

Medical Staff Fellow, National Heart, Lung, and Blood Institute, National Institutes of Health, Bethesda, Maryland. Formerly Fellow in Medical Genetics, University of California Hospitals, San Francisco, California.

PREFACE

The scope of medicine, much like Einsteinian space, has no discrete boundaries. To the student this open-ended nature of the discipline evokes anxiety, for there are no limits—no margins that define when clinical medicine has been successfully mastered. During the years devoted to basic science, such an open-ended commitment does not appear to pertain, for there are lecture notes, syllabi, and standard textbooks that collectively encompass that portion of biochemistry or of histology that the student is expected to know. The clinical years, however, dispel any sense of certainty. How much should we know about hypertension, for example? As much as can be learned within the limits of the time, energy, and resourcefulness that one can devote to the demanding profession of medicine. To understand this single pathologic condition we must be knowledgeable of selective elements of epidemiology, physiology, biochemistry, pathology, pharmacology, and many of the specialties of internal medicine (cardiology, nephrology, endocrinology, neurology, etc.). The subject carries us further into preventive medicine, public health, and public policy. Similar ramifications spread out endlessly from all clinical problems. The physician must be primarily concerned with the unique individuality of the patient, whose welfare cannot be defined as the simple integral of these formidable disciplines into which biomedical science has been conveniently but arbitrarily segregated. It has been said that M.D. stands for "moderately done," in contrast to Ph.D., which stands for "phenomenally done." It is this continuing sense of incompletion that is the main defense against complacency, the dry rot of our profession.

There are many ways in which to learn medicine. Each student or physician will differ in the methods by which he or she learns most easily and effectively. Education has been defined as what you have left when you have forgotten the facts. "The facts" are nowhere more transient than in medicine, so that a premium must be placed on education as defined above. This includes the ability to reason effectively from data that are often incomplete. This manual has been developed as a series of questions that test both knowledge and the ability to utilize it effectively in clinical medicine. As such it is designed to reinforce the use of knowledge already obtained from other sources or of skills already obtained through experience. The form of a question is a challenge that requires that we assess what we know or, more important, what we do not know about the topic at hand. It crystallizes a problem set and demands that we take a position. Answers are supplied not only to indicate what is correct or incorrect but also to offer a rational explanation for these choices. This book has been constructed primarily to assist in the education or continuing education of medical students in advanced clerkships, house staff, internists, family physicians, or anyone who wishes to maintain competency in internal medicine. Both its content and form make it useful also to physicians preparing for certification or recertification by the American Board of Internal Medicine.

The *Cecil Textbook of Medicine* has been the standard definitive textbook of medicine in the United States since its introduction more than fifty years ago (1927). For convenience most of the references in the answer section have been directed to the sixteenth edition of *Cecil*, of which this is a companion book. Other useful general references are included as well. Through these references each topic can be pursued in much more depth than allowed within the confines of this book.

This is the second edition of *Review of General Internal Medicine*. It has been extensively revised since the first edition, with 11 new contributors and approximately 1000 new questions. The supporting references have been updated as well, both those relating to the sixteenth edition of *Cecil* and those relating to other standard sources. We would like to express special gratitude to our colleagues at the Duke University Medical Center and at the University of California, San Francisco, for their excellent contributions in preparing these self-assessment exercises in the respective disciplines of internal medicine.

In all phases of revising this book Ms. Carolyn Strecker has been an invaluable colleague. Her expertise, gained while associated with the American Board of Internal Medicine, has shaped the presentation of this question-answer format throughout the book. We are indebted to her for the skill and resourcefulness that she has brought to this enterprise.

LLOYD H. SMITH, JR., M.D.
JAMES B. WYNGAARDEN, M.D.

CONTENTS

INSTRUCTIONS

This book is designed to provide a comprehensive review of internal medicine in the form of a self-assessment examination. The format enables you to answer the questions, to quickly determine which ones you got right and wrong, and then to review those questions you answered incorrectly. The examination is divided into 11 Parts. These Parts may be taken individually, in any order. To take advantage of this book's special features, we suggest the following steps:

1. Tear out the answer sheet (located on perforated pages at the end of the book) for the Part you want to use.

2. Take the test, recording your answers on the answer sheet. Note that there are three different question types used; be sure to read and follow the directions for each of them.

3. To quickly determine how many questions you answered correctly, compare your answers with the answer key (pp. 319–326). On your answer sheet, circle any questions you may have missed.

4. For a detailed discussion of questions answered incorrectly, refer to the Answers following the questions in each Part. References to Wyngaarden and Smith: *Cecil Textbook of Medicine* (16th ed.) and to other sources are provided for more extensive review. As time permits, reading the discussions of questions you answered correctly should also prove beneficial.

No criteria for deciding "how well" you did are provided because we believe that in a self-assessment examination you are the best judge. Read the discussions of the questions you missed and decide for yourself why you answered incorrectly, whether you should have known the answer, and whether the material deserves further study.

No time limits have been set, and no harm will be done by taking a Part over several days. We recommend that you do not look up any answers until you have completed the entire Part. In order to get maximal benefit from this style of review, it is essential that you treat the questions as you would questions in a "real" examination. Don't just "take a stab" at a question because you know the answer is easy to look up. Reading the answers is not an adequate substitute for taking as much time as you need and doing your best on each question.

An index to the questions is on pages 299–318. The purpose of the index is to lead you to questions about subjects in which you may have an interest. In particular, you may find it useful when, while preparing for an examination, you wonder "what they might ask about ______." It is important to note, however, that the index attempts to list only the general thrust of each question and thereby facilitate very directed review.

There is considerably more information present in the questions and discussions than is indexed. Because the index is by subject, it tends to provide clues to some correct answers. Therefore, for self-assessment, use of the index should be delayed until after you have taken the examination.

PART 1

CARDIOVASCULAR DISEASES

DIRECTIONS: For questions 1 to 46, choose the ONE BEST answer to each question.

1. Most deaths in hypertensive individuals in the United States are due to which one of the following?

A. Stroke
B. Renal failure
C. Congestive heart failure
D. Myocardial infarction
E. Dissecting aneurysm

2. In which one of the following conditions does pulmonary angiography carry the highest risk for death?

A. Multiple pulmonary emboli
B. Primary pulmonary hypertension
C. Mitral stenosis
D. Eisenmenger ventricular septal defect
E. Peripheral pulmonic stenosis

3. What accounts for most of the resistance across the pulmonary vascular bed?

A. The pulmonary arterioles
B. The pulmonary capillaries
C. The pulmonary venules
D. The pulmonary veins
E. The left atrium

4. In which one of the following conditions would the symptoms of congestive heart failure carry the most ominous prognostic significance?

A. Muscular subvalvular aortic stenosis
B. Valvular aortic stenosis
C. Mitral regurgitation
D. Aortic regurgitation
E. Mitral stenosis

5. In which one of the following conditions would a normal time-motion echocardiographic study be most likely?

A. Mitral valve prolapse
B. Mild rheumatic mitral stenosis
C. Acquired aortic stenosis
D. Muscular subvalvular aortic stenosis
E. Moderate aortic regurgitation

6. Auscultation during the continued strain phase of the Valsalva maneuver will help to differentiate which one of the following sets of conditions?

A. Rheumatic mitral regurgitation from valvular aortic stenosis
B. Muscular subvalvular aortic stenosis from membranous subvalvular aortic stenosis
C. Aortic regurgitation from pulmonary regurgitation
D. Mitral stenosis from tricuspid stenosis
E. Pulmonary stenosis from aortic stenosis

7. Which one of the following drugs is most likely to be of immediate benefit in the treatment of shock secondary to gram-negative sepsis?

A. Digitalis
B. Phentolamine
C. Nitroprusside
D. Corticosteroids
E. Norepinephrine

8. In which one of the following conditions is atrial fibrillation most likely to occur at some point in the course of the disease?

A. Aortic stenosis
B. Muscular subvalvular aortic stenosis (IHSS)
C. Mitral regurgitation
D. Mitral stenosis
E. Aortic regurgitation

9. The total number of myocardial infarctions occurring in the United States in 1978 was

A. less than 500,000
B. 500,000–750,000
C. 750,000–1,000,000
D. greater than 1,000,000

10. Which of the following is most important in increasing cardiac output during exercise?

A. Constriction of the systemic veins
B. Arteriolar dilatation
C. An increase in stroke volume
D. An increase in heart rate
E. An increase in central venous pressure

11. Which of the following statements concerning heart failure is the most accurate?

A. It is present when there is ventricular dilatation
B. It is defined as the inability of the heart to match its output to the metabolic needs of the body
C. It is present when the left ventricular end-diastolic pressure is elevated
D. It is frequently preceded by defects in the manufacture of high-energy phosphate stores
E. It is frequently associated with defective myocardial cell protein synthesis

12. In the treatment of a patient with severe hemorrhagic shock, what is the most important *initial* step?

A. Start prophylactic antibiotics
B. Administer lidocaine for premature ventricular contractions
C. Give large doses of steroids
D. Begin volume replacement
E. Start vasoconstrictors

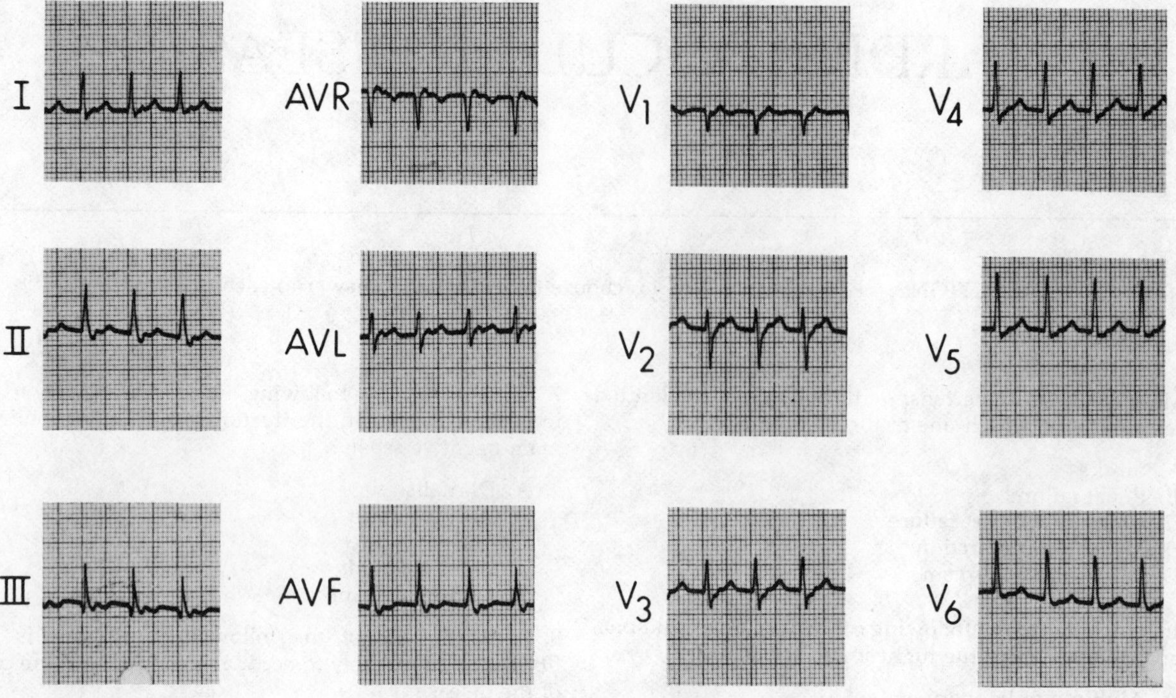

13. A patient with dyspnea and acute anterior myocardial infarction should be treated routinely with all of the following EXCEPT

A. oxygen
B. small doses of furosemide, orally
C. morphine as required for pain relief
D. low doses of heparin
E. prophylactic lidocaine

QUESTIONS 14–15

14. The electrocardiogram illustrated above is from a 29-year-old man who complains of palpitations. The patient's rhythm is

A. atrial flutter with 2:1 atrioventricular (AV) block
B. sinus tachycardia with first-degree AV block
C. an accelerated junctional (His) pacemaker
D. AV junctional re-entry tachycardia
E. ectopic atrial tachycardia

15. The treatment of choice to terminate this arrhythmia is

A. direct current cardioversion
B. diazepam, intravenously
C. digitalization
D. verapamil, intravenously
E. propranolol, intravenously

---

16. The auscultatory findings illustrated on p. 3 are best explained by which one of the following?

A. Rheumatic mitral valve disease
B. Pulmonary hypertension
C. Muscular subvalvular aortic stenosis
D. Mitral valve prolapse
E. Aortic valve stenosis

17. Which of the following is LEAST likely to precipitate an attack of angina pectoris?

A. A rise in carboxyhemoglobin level
B. An increase in myocardial contractility
C. A drop in hemoglobin
D. An increase in blood pressure
E. A decrease in preload
F. Vasospasm

18. Which of the following is LEAST likely with type I second-degree AV block?

A. Progressive lengthening of the P-R interval, culminating in a dropped beat
B. Prior administration of digoxin, 1.0 mg intravenously, for 2 doses 4 hours apart
C. Progressive shortening of the R-R interval, culminating in a dropped beat
D. A preceding acute diaphragmatic myocardial infarction
E. Progression to permanent, complete heart block

19. Which of the following patients is the most suitable candidate for direct current cardioversion?

A. One who has had atrial fibrillation for approximately 16 months
B. One with atrial fibrillation and an echocardiographic left atrial diameter of 6.7 cm
C. A dyspneic hyperthyroid patient in atrial fibrillation with a very rapid ventricular response
D. One with frequent, paroxysmal atrial fibrillation
E. One with an acute anterior myocardial infarction and atrial fibrillation with a rapid ventricular response
F. One in atrial fibrillation who is suspected of having digitalis toxicity

20. Which one of the following would be LEAST expected in a patient with atrial fibrillation?

A. Systemic embolization

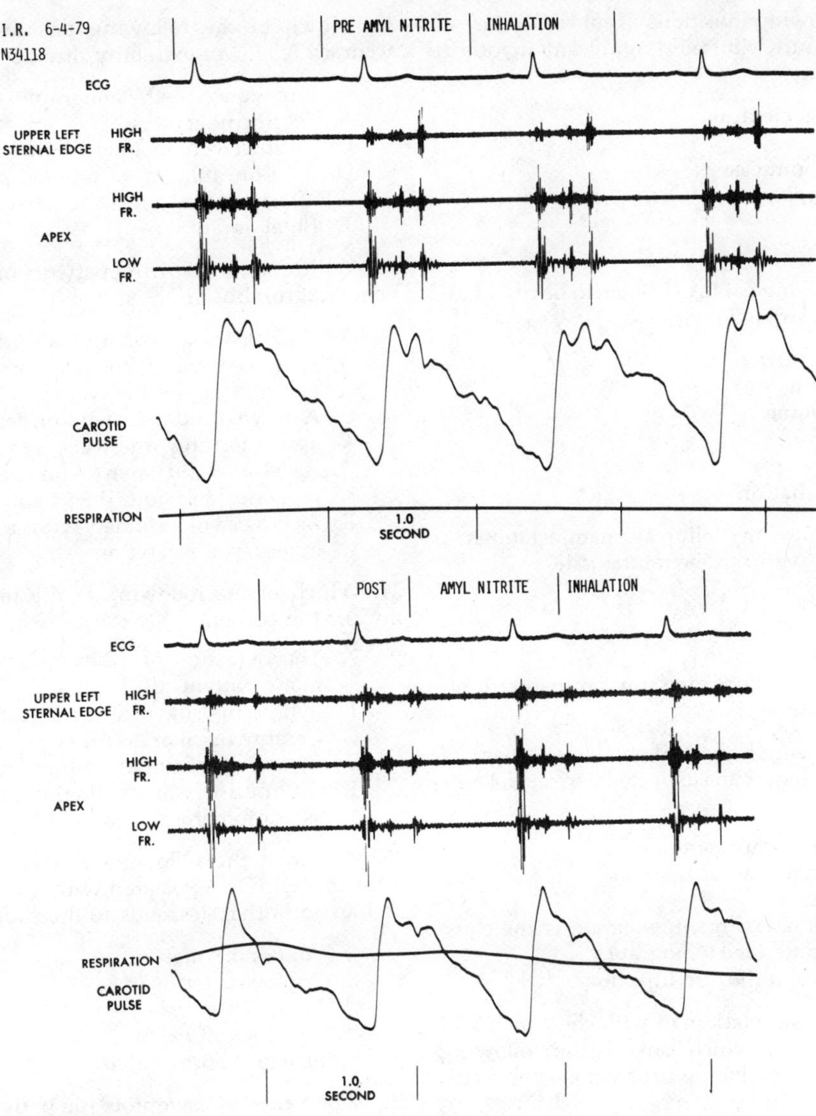

B. A ventricular response greater than 200 per minute in the setting of accessory conduction (Wolff-Parkinson-White syndrome)
C. Cardioversion to sinus rhythm by 10 joules
D. Embolization after cardioversion despite three weeks of preceding anticoagulation
E. Conversion to sinus rhythm with quinidine

21. Which of the following arrhythmias is LEAST likely to be the result of digitalis toxicity?

A. Ectopic atrial tachycardia (atrial rate 150 per minute) with a 2:1 ventricular response
B. Normal sinus rhythm with ventricular bigeminy
C. Normal sinus rhythm with junctional premature beats
D. Atrial fibrillation with a ventricular response that is regular at 48 per minute; narrow QRS
E. AV dissociation secondary to an accelerated junctional rhythm at 80 per minute
F. Ventricular tachycardia
G. Type II second-degree AV block

22. A decrease in the gradient and loudness of the murmur in asymmetric septal hypertrophy with obstruction (hypertrophic obstructive cardiomyopathy) would be LEAST expected with which one of the following interventions?

A. Prompt squatting
B. Phenylephrine infusion
C. Volume infusion
D. Isoproterenol infusion
E. Intravenous propranolol
F. Lying down

23. Which of the following symptoms of obstructive hypertrophic cardiomyopathy (ASH with obstruction or IHSS) is LEAST likely to respond to surgical myectomy?

A. Angina
B. Dyspnea
C. Paroxysmal arrhythmia
D. Orthopnea
E. Syncope

24. Myocardial involvement is LEAST likely in which one of the following heredofamilial neuromyopathic diseases?

A. Myotonic muscular dystrophy
B. Friedreich's ataxia
C. Duchenne's muscular dystrophy
D. Facioscapulohumeral dystrophy of Déjerine and Landouzy
E. Erb's limb-girdle dystrophy

25. Which of the following infectious agents or diseases is LEAST likely to produce clinically significant myocarditis?

A. Group A coxsackievirus
B. Poliomyelitis
C. Infectious mononucleosis
D. *Toxoplasma gondii*
E. Trichinosis
F. *Trypanosoma cruzi*

26. Which of the following is LEAST likely to be associated with pericarditis/pericardial effusion?

A. Rheumatoid arthritis
B. Hypothyroidism
C. Blunt chest trauma
D. Tuberculosis
E. Scleroderma
F. Mediastinal radiation

27. Which of the following clinical manifestations is LEAST likely to occur with cardiac tamponade?

A. Kussmaul's sign
B. Dyspnea
C. Tachycardia
D. Decreased arterial blood pressure on inspiration
E. Venous distention

28. Which of the following is most likely to yield diagnostic information in a patient with suspected pericardial effusion?

A. Time-motion echocardiogram
B. Two-dimensional echocardiogram
C. Heart-liver scan
D. Overpenetrated lateral roentgenogram of the chest
E. Enhanced computerized tomography
F. Intravenous carbon dioxide injection

29. In a febrile 44-year-old black man with chest pain and a pericardial friction rub, which one of the following would be most helpful in excluding tuberculous pericarditis?

A. Clear lung fields on chest film
B. A negative tuberculin skin test
C. Diffuse S-T segment elevation on the electrocardiogram
D. Lack of significant effusion on the echocardiogram
E. A negative acid-fast stain of aspirated pericardial fluid

30. Which of the following is the LEAST likely manifestation of constrictive pericarditis?

A. An increased pre-ejection period to left ventricular ejection time (PEP–LVET) ratio
B. A prominent "Y" descent in the jugular venous pulse
C. Kussmaul's sign
D. An early diastolic sound at the lower left sternal edge that increases with inspiration
E. Calcification of the pericardium on chest film

31. The most predictive sign of calf vein thrombophlebitis is

A. edema
B. a tender cord
C. calf pain on exertion
D. Homans' sign
E. venous distention

32. Which of the following has the highest diagnostic accuracy for lower extremity thrombophlebitis?

A. Impedance plethysmography
B. ^{125}I fibrinogen test
C. Doppler venous blood flow studies
D. Pain on inflation of a blood pressure cuff over the affected area to less than 160 mm Hg
E. Phlebography

33. Which of the following patients has the highest risk for venous thrombosis?

A. A 22-year-old woman taking birth control pills
B. A 46-year-old man who has had pneumococcal pneumonia for one week
C. A 36-year-old man who underwent uncomplicated appendectomy one week ago
D. A 59-year-old man who underwent retropubic prostatectomy four days ago
E. A 39-year-old woman with a small anterior lateral myocardial infarction

34. Which of the following is the most likely way for a myxoma to present?

A. The detection of a heart murmur in an asymptomatic patient
B. Symptoms suggesting congestive heart failure
C. Cerebrovascular accident
D. As a fever of undetermined origin
E. On routine echocardiographic examination of an asymptomatic patient

35. Which of the following congenital heart diseases is most likely to be associated with a right-sided aortic arch and an aorta that descends to the right of the esophagus?

A. Pulmonary atresia
B. Truncus arteriosus
C. Tricuspid atresia
D. Tetralogy of Fallot
E. Bicuspid aortic valve

36. A 68-year-old asymptomatic patient with mild hypertension (blood pressure 170/98 mm Hg) is noted to have a pulsatile abdominal mass. Ultrasound examination shows this to be an abdominal aortic aneurysm that arises below the renal arteries and has a diameter of 8.0 cm. Which of the following is most appropriate at this time?

A. Antihypertensive therapy and close medical follow-up
B. Operative resection and repair of the aneurysm
C. Close medical follow-up with frequent abdominal ultrasound examinations
D. No drugs or studies, but have the patient return at the first hint of abdominal pain
E. Abdominal aortography to define the aneurysm more precisely

QUESTIONS 37–38

37. A 70-year-old man has exertional chest pain and a pulsatile mass in the second right intercostal space. The patient tells you that he was treated in 1938 for "bad blood" with a series of injections. Blood pressure is normal, and no diastolic aortic murmur is noted. Roentgenogram of the chest reveals calcification in a dilated aortic root. Serologic test for syphilis is negative. What is the most likely diagnosis?

A. Aortic dissection
B. Congenital aneurysm of the sinus of Valsalva
C. Syphilitic aortitis (VDRL)
D. Marfan's syndrome
E. Traumatic aortic aneurysm

38. Which test is most likely to provide additional etiologic information in this patient?

A. *Treponema pallidum* immobilization test (TPI)
B. Fluorescent treponemal antibody-absorbed test (FTA-ABS)
C. Measurement of urinary amino acids
D. Echocardiography of the aortic and mitral valves
E. Aortography

---

39. With arteriosclerosis obliterans, which of the following has the most serious implications?

A. Intermittent claudication
B. A cool, pale foot
C. Pain while at rest
D. A venous filling time greater than 30 seconds
E. Vascular calcification on roentgenogram

40. A 56-year-old man with a cardiomyopathy has suspected digoxin toxicity as manifested by frequent unifocal premature ventricular contractions. Serum electrolytes and renal function studies are all normal. Which one of the following would be CONTRAINDICATED in this patient?

A. Potassium chloride, orally or intravenously
B. Lidocaine, 1 mg/kg by intravenous bolus followed by a continuous intravenous infusion at 1–4 mg/minute
C. Quinidine sulfate, 200 mg orally four times daily
D. Discontinuing the digitalis preparation
E. Phenytoin, 5–10 mg/kg given slowly intravenously

41. The principal adverse side effect of rapid intravenous administration of procainamide is

A. seizure
B. atrial fibrillation
C. hypotension
D. complete heart block
E. sinus bradycardia

42. Which one of the following would be most helpful in differentiating *primary* from *secondary* pulmonary hypertension?

A. Wide splitting of the second heart sound
B. A pulmonary ejection sound
C. Absence of the typical murmurs ordinarily associated with congenital left-to-right shunts
D. A dilated pulmonary artery on roentgenogram
E. Left ventricular enlargement

QUESTIONS 43–44

43. The electrocardiogram illustrated below is from a 63-year-old man with anterior chest pain. An ECG obtained six weeks ago was normal. What is the most likely diagnosis?

A. Prinzmetal's variant angina
B. An acute anterior myocardial infarction
C. Acute pericarditis
D. Right heart strain compatible with pulmonary embolism
E. Left bundle branch block

44. Which of the following is indicated for this patient?

A. Anticoagulation
B. Temporary transvenous pacemaker
C. Indomethacin
D. Pulmonary angiography
E. Exercise stress testing

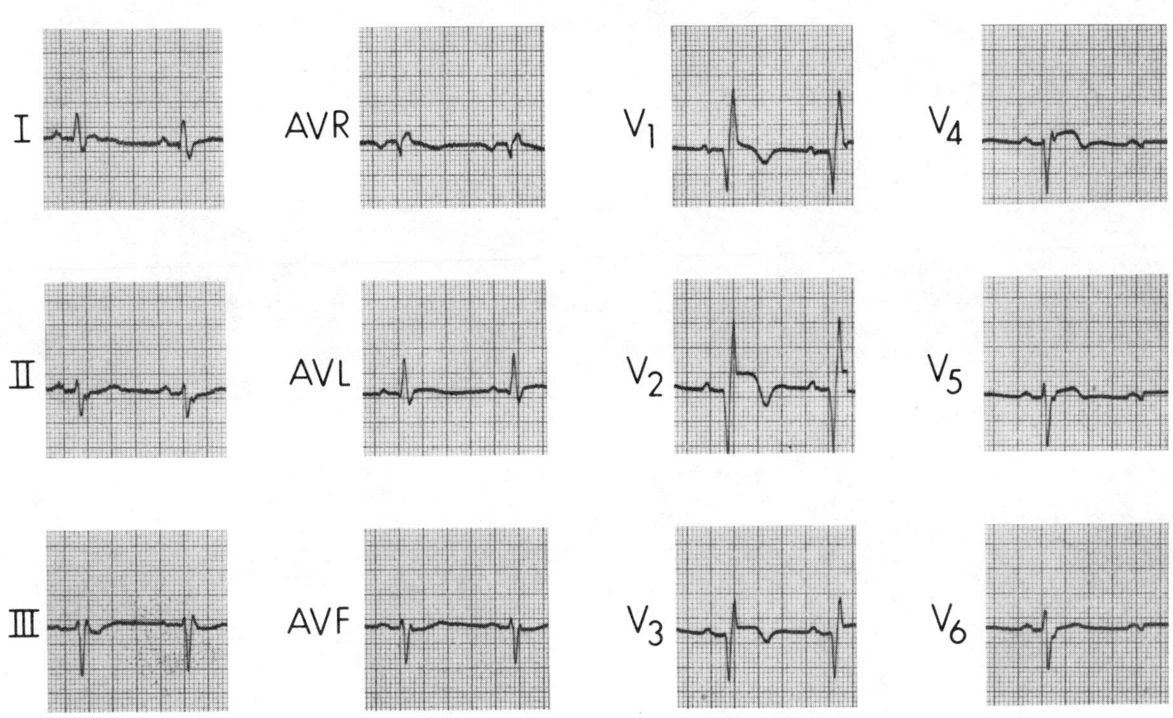

45. Central nervous system symptoms related specifically to hypertension may be due to any of the following EXCEPT

A. rupture of a berry aneurysm
B. rupture of a Charcot-Bouchard aneurysm
C. cerebral edema
D. embolization from an atheroma in the carotid arteries
E. embolization from the heart

46. A 45-year-old man who had an acute myocardial infarction is under your care on the coronary care unit. Several episodes of ventricular tachycardia have been treated with intravenous lidocaine. The blood lidocaine level is currently 3.4 μg/ml, and the patient is lethargic. Which of the following is most appropriate to prevent ventricular tachycardia if it continues to recur?

A. Double the lidocaine infusion rate
B. Continue lidocaine and begin digoxin, intravenously
C. Continue lidocaine and begin phenytoin sodium, intravenously
D. Continue lidocaine and begin quinidine sulfate, intravenously
E. Discontinue lidocaine and begin procainamide, intravenously

DIRECTIONS: For questions 47 to 109, you are to decide whether EACH choice is true or false. Any combination of answers, from all true to all false, may be present. Mark the answer sheet "T" or "F" in the space provided.

47. Risk factors related to developing rheumatic fever include

A. upper respiratory infection with group A beta-hemolytic streptococci
B. evidence of glomerulonephritis
C. socioeconomic status
D. rheumatoid arthritis
E. climate

48. Which of the following statements concerning the decline in the age-adjusted cardiovascular death rate in the United States is/are true?

A. The decrease in mortality from rheumatic heart disease began with the introduction of antibiotics.
B. Cardiovascular disease accounted for one half of all deaths in the United States in 1978
C. The downward trend has also occurred in other industrialized nations (e.g., Sweden, France, Denmark, Austria)
D. The rate of decline has been sharper since about 1970
E. The decline can be attributed primarily to risk factor modification

49. Which of the following factors is/are important in determining blood levels for orally administered drugs?

A. Rate of absorption
B. Gastrointestinal motility
C. Hepatic metabolism
D. Renal clearance rate
E. Tissue distribution

50. The *major* risk factors for coronary artery disease include

A. hypertension
B. diabetes
C. type A personality
D. cigarette smoking
E. low plasma HDL cholesterol levels
F. increasing age
G. obesity

51. Plasma LDL cholesterol levels

A. are directly related to the risk of coronary artery disease in younger patients
B. rise with age
C. fall with exercise
D. rise with ingestion of 2–3 oz of alcohol daily
E. are increased by diets rich in cholesterol and saturated fats

52. Important factors determining the heart's performance as a pump include which of the following?

A. Preload
B. Pericardial compliance
C. Afterload
D. Contractility
E. Heart rate
F. Carotid chemoreceptors
G. Ventricular wall tension

53. Compensatory mechanisms that aid the failing heart include which of the following?

A. Ectopic ventricular rhythms
B. Increased sympathetic nervous system activity
C. Ventricular dilatation
D. Ventricular hypertrophy
E. Increased central venous pressure
F. Decreased renal blood flow

54. Important determinants of myocardial oxygen consumption include

A. ventricular wall tension
B. extent of fiber shortening
C. metabolism of the sarcoplasmic reticulum
D. heart rate
E. contractility
F. ventricular diastolic compliance

55. Which of the following statements concerning digitalis therapy is/are true?

A. Beginning therapy with the recommended maintenance dose is a safe and effective way to achieve digitalization
B. Digoxin frequently lessens the severity of angina pectoris in patients with coronary artery disease and normal heart size
C. In a patient with chronic atrial fibrillation, a regular pulse at 70 per minute following an increase in the daily digoxin dose to 0.375 mg probably means that the patient has converted to normal sinus rhythm
D. The combination of atrioventricular block and enhanced ectopy is highly suggestive of digitalis toxicity
E. Diuretics increase the likelihood of digitalis toxicity

56. Reliable indicators of cardiovascular shock in a patient with chest pain include which of the following?

A. Hypotension (arterial systolic blood pressure less than 90 mm Hg)
B. The absence of neck vein distention
C. Cyanotic, cool, diaphoretic skin
D. Urinary output of less than 20 ml per hour
E. Confusion

57. Findings indicating stage III shock include

A. cellular death owing to vasoconstriction and diminished blood flow
B. diminished blood flow to vital organs
C. absorption of bacterial toxins from the gastrointestinal tract
D. sinus tachycardia
E. increased peripheral vascular resistance

58. Which of the following statements concerning the interpretation of plasma drug concentrations is/are true?

A. Plasma drug levels should be measured during the distribution phase shortly after drug administration
B. Variations in binding to plasma proteins are an important source of pharmacodynamic variation in patient response to drug therapy

C. Metabolites of the drug, if pharmacologically active, must be measured to interpret properly the relationship between plasma concentration and drug effect.
D. The tissue response for some plasma drug levels must be interpreted within the context of concomitant serum electrolyte levels
E. In the presence of renal insufficiency, the average drug dose (even for those drugs eliminated primarily by renal tubular secretion) is proportional to the reduction in the creatinine clearance

59. Which of the following is/are important in controlling vascular smooth muscle tone during shock?

A. Renin-angiotensin
B. Vasopressin
C. Bradykinin
D. Acetylcholine
E. Beta-endorphin

60. Which of the following factors contribute(s) to the accumulation of fluid in the extracellular space in hypovolemic shock?

A. A decrease in plasma oncotic pressure
B. An increase in the vascular tone of postcapillary venules
C. A decrease in the vascular tone of precapillary resistance vessels
D. A decrease in capillary permeability
E. A rise in left atrial pressure

61. Appropriate procedures for following patients in severe shock secondary to myocardial infarction should include which of the following?

A. Urinary catheterization for hourly measurement of urinary output
B. Monitoring of intra-arterial pressure
C. Monitoring of central venous pressure
D. Monitoring of arterial blood gases
E. Monitoring of pulmonary artery oxygen saturations

62. The natural history of functionally normal bicuspid aortic valves includes which of the following?

A. They remain functionally normal
B. They become calcified and stenotic
C. Progressive aortic regurgitation develops
D. Bacterial endocarditis supervenes

63. Which of the following statements concerning adverse drug reactions is/are true?

A. In the hospital, the incidence of adverse drug reactions is about 5%
B. Less than 5% of adverse drug reactions in outpatients are serious enough to warrant hospitalization
C. Fatal adverse drug reactions commonly involve heparin, potassium chloride, and insulin
D. The majority of fatal drug reactions occur in patients with advanced cancer or liver disease
E. The fatality rate in patients suffering adverse drug reactions is less than 3%

64. Which of the following congenital heart diseases is/are associated with an increased incidence of aortic valve disease?

A. Supravalvular aortic stenosis
B. Membranous ventricular septal defect
C. Muscular subvalvular aortic stenosis (IHSS)
D. Membranous subvalvular aortic stenosis
E. Coarctation of the aorta

65. Which of the following statements is/are true regarding the evaluation of a 32-year-old woman with a suspected atrial septal defect?

A. V waves in the jugular venous pulse equal to the height of the A wave suggest concomitant tricuspid regurgitation
B. A normal time motion echocardiogram makes the possibility of atrial septal defect very unlikely
C. A systolic thrill at the second left intercostal space is best explained by concomitant valvular pulmonic stenosis
D. Left axis deviation on electrocardiogram suggests an ostium primum type of defect
E. Atrial fibrillation would be an unusual complication

66. Significant risk factors for adverse drug reactions include

A. increasing age
B. male sex
C. cirrhosis
D. uremia
E. hypertension

67. A significant risk for infective endocarditis is present in which of the following conditions?

A. Ventricular septal defect with 1.5:1 left-to-right shunt
B. Patent ductus arteriosus with a 1.7:1 left-to-right shunt
C. Coronary atrioventricular fistula that was ligated two years ago
D. Uncorrected secundum atrial septal defect
E. Tetralogy of Fallot

68. Which of the following would help to distinguish Ebstein's anomaly of the tricuspid valve from an ostium secundum atrial defect in a 50-year-old woman?

A. Accentuation of the tricuspid valve closure sound
B. Splitting of the first heart sound by more than 0.06 seconds
C. Paradoxical interventricular septal wall motion on echocardiogram
D. A Wolff-Parkinson-White type of accessory conduction
E. Increased pulmonary blood flow on chest film
F. A mid-diastolic rumble along the lower left sternal edge

69. The differential diagnosis of a cyanotic child with increased pulmonary blood flow on roentgenogram of the chest includes

A. complete transposition of the great vessels
B. total anomalous pulmonary venous return
C. truncus arteriosus
D. Ebstein's anomaly of the tricuspid valve
E. Lutembacher's syndrome
F. Taussig-Bing anomaly (double-outlet right ventricle)

70. Valid situations to justify cardiac catheterization include which of the following?

A. To measure the aortic valve gradient in a 46-year-old man with a murmur of aortic stenosis; he is

asymptomatic but has a sustained, enlarged, nondisplaced left ventricular impulse
B. To evaluate the status of the aortic valve and coronary arteries in a 68-year-old man with a prominent systolic crescendo-decrescendo murmur at the second right intercostal space and exertional substernal aching
C. To measure outflow gradient in a 26-year-old man with prominent septal thickening and systolic anterior motion of the mitral valve on echocardiogram; he had exertional substernal chest pain that disappeared with propranolol therapy
D. To assess the status of valve function in a 36-year-old patient with class III congestive heart failure who has murmurs of mitral stenosis and regurgitation and an early diastolic blowing murmur at the fourth left intercostal space
E. To assess the status of left ventricular function in a patient with class III congestive heart failure who has a grade 3/6 apical holosystolic, plateau-shaped blowing murmur that radiates to the left axilla

71. The differential diagnosis of a patient with pulmonary hypertension includes

A. left heart failure
B. tricuspid regurgitation
C. mitral stenosis
D. pulmonary regurgitation
E. hepatic cirrhosis
F. chronic obstructive pulmonary disease

72. Which of the following patients should definitely receive chronic anticoagulant therapy?

A. One in normal sinus rhythm following an open commissurotomy for mitral stenosis
B. One in atrial fibrillation who underwent porcine heterograft replacement of the mitral valve one month ago
C. One who underwent aortic valve replacement with a Starr-Edwards prosthesis two months ago
D. One with pulmonary embolic disease who has tricuspid valve endocarditis
E. One without neurologic symptoms who has idiopathic atrial fibrillation

73. A 46-year-old man comes to your office with a chief complaint of heart pounding, sweating, and dizziness but no overt syncope. Further history reveals that he was being treated for a depressed mood and hypertension, but he stopped both medications the day before his visit to you. He has no idea what the medications were and cannot identify them from pictures in the *Physicians' Desk Reference.* He began taking Tuss-Ornade, a cold remedy containing phenylpropanolamine hydrochloride, six hours ago. Family history reveals that his mother had hypertension. On physical examination blood pressure in the right arm is 196/116 mm Hg supine and 130/70 mm Hg standing. Pulse rate is 110 per minute and regular. The heart is not enlarged and there are no abnormalities on auscultation. The pulse in the legs is not delayed. The remainder of the examination, electrocardiogram, roentgenogram of the chest, and urinalysis are normal. The differential diagnosis includes which of the following?

A. Interaction of the cold preparation with the antidepressant drug
B. Clonidine withdrawal
C. Pheochromocytoma
D. Coarctation of the aorta
E. Essential hypertension

74. Which of the following is/are likely to cause significant hemolysis in a G6PD-deficient patient?

A. Sulfanilamide
B. Primaquine
C. Penicillin
D. Vitamin K
E. Propranolol

75. Which of the following has/have been proposed as the pathophysiologic mechanism(s) of essential hypertension?

A. Resetting of the arterial baroreceptor reflex arc
B. Excessive CNS-mediated stimulation of the adrenergic nervous system
C. Increased intravascular fluid volume
D. Elevated angiotensin II levels
E. Elevated plasma renin levels

76. Which of the following adverse reactions occurs with penicillin?

A. Urticaria
B. Anaphylaxis
C. Angioneurotic edema
D. Serum sickness
E. Nephritis

77. Hypertension in pregnancy is associated with which of the following?

A. Small birth weight
B. An increased incidence of intrauterine death
C. Prematurity
D. Hydrops fetalis
E. The development of eclampsia

78. Patients with malignant hypertension typically have which of the following findings?

A. Diastolic blood pressure in the range of 130–170 mm Hg
B. Left ventricular hypertrophy and/or failure
C. Retinal papilledema with hemorrhages and exudates
D. Morning headaches
E. Fibrinoid necrosis of arterioles

79. Important risk factors for the subsequent development of coronary artery disease include which of the following?

A. Hypertriglyceridemia
B. Inactivity
C. Family history of sudden death of an elderly parent
D. Male sex
E. High-cholesterol diet

80. Factors that are associated with increasing blood pressure levels in the United States include

A. increasing age
B. heredity
C. body weight
D. increasing salt intake
E. increasing saturated fat intake

81. Which of the following findings would help to differentiate *primary* from *secondary* pulmonary hypertension?

A. Pulmonary artery dilatation with cephalization of pulmonary venous blood flow on roentgenogram

B. Cough and sputum production 11 months of the year
C. A diastolic rumbling murmur at the apex
D. A high-frequency decrescendo murmur at the fourth left intercostal space
E. Peripheral edema

82. Particular care should be taken to avoid which of the following in patients with primary pulmonary hypertension?

A. Volume depletion with diuretics
B. Elective surgery involving general anesthetics
C. Pneumothorax
D. Lung biopsy
E. Digoxin therapy

83. Which of the following statements concerning steroid therapy is/are true?

A. ACTH is superior to glucocorticosteroids in the treatment of ulcerative colitis
B. Dexamethasone is the most potent commonly used glucocorticosteroid
C. Glucocorticosteroids are teratogenic
D. Peptic ulcer disease is a contraindication for glucocorticosteroid use
E. Hypertension is typically exacerbated by glucocorticosteroids

84. The natural history of primary pulmonary hypertension typically includes which of the following events?

A. Sudden death
B. Spontaneous remission
C. Pulmonary hemorrhage
D. Syncope
E. Angina-type chest pain

85. Which of the following statements concerning patients with primary pulmonary hypertension is/are true?

A. Women are more likely to be affected than men
B. The pathologic picture is distinct from that of other causes of pulmonary hypertension
C. Differentiation from multiple pulmonary emboli is difficult even with pulmonary angiography
D. Cyanosis and clubbing are a prominent part of the clinical presentation
E. Significant palliation with hydralazine has been reported

86. High-altitude pulmonary edema responds readily to which of the following?

A. Diuretics
B. Returning to sea level
C. Oxygen administration
D. Digitalization

87. Which of the following statements concerning the control of pulmonary vascular resistance is/are true?

A. The fall in pulmonary vascular resistance with exercise is augmented by a more negative intrapleural pressure
B. With upright exercise, the size of the pulmonary vascular bed is increased
C. The venoconstrictor response to hypoxia is blunted by alkalosis
D. Autonomic control of pulmonary vascular resistance is a well-documented fact
E. The effect of hypoxia on pulmonary vascular resistance is mediated by histamine

88. In which of the following conditions will auscultation during inhalation of amyl nitrite help to refine the differential diagnosis?

A. The murmur of mitral stenosis from an Austin-Flint murmur
B. The murmur of mitral regurgitation from the murmur of aortic stenosis
C. The murmur of tricuspid regurgitation from the murmur of mitral regurgitation
D. The murmur of aortic regurgitation from the murmur of an AV fistula
E. The murmur of pulmonic stenosis from the murmur of aortic stenosis

89. Which of the following physical findings favor(s) acute mitral regurgitation rather than chronic mitral regurgitation?

A. Atrial fibrillation
B. A loud atrial gallop
C. A left ventricular third heart sound
D. A mid-diastolic apical rumble
E. Pulmonary hypertension
F. Wide splitting of the second heart sound

QUESTIONS 90–92

A 52-year-old man consults you because he wishes to undertake an exercise program. For six years he has had nonradiating, vague substernal pressing sensation without associated diaphoresis or dyspnea that occurs only with exertion, such as walking rapidly in his job as a tobacco buyer. He learned to avoid such situations so that his symptoms have remained stable and have not interfered with his 40-hour work week. The chest discomfort is always relieved within five minutes by rest and has never occurred at night or at rest. Four years ago the patient's physician prescribed hydrochlorothiazide, 50 mg daily, and propranolol, 20 mg orally four times daily for high blood pressure. The frequency of the episodes decreased from four per week to the current one to two per week. There is a 15-year history of palpitations with exercise, but the patient has never had dizziness or syncope. There is no history of a heart murmur, myocardial infarction, or symptoms of congestive heart failure. There are no other risk factors for coronary artery disease and the remainder of the history is unremarkable. On physical examination the blood pressure in the right arm is 150/90 mm Hg seated. Pulse rate is 64 per minute and regular. The remainder of the physical examination is within normal limits. Complete blood count, blood urea nitrogen, serum potassium, and urinalysis are within normal limits.

90. Which of the following additional tests is/are indicated to evaluate this patient's symptoms further?

A. Electrocardiogram
B. Roentgenogram of the chest
C. Holter monitoring
D. Rest and exercise radionuclide angiography
E. Treadmill exercise testing
F. Cardiac catheterization

91. Treadmill exercise testing is performed and the results are illustrated on p. 11 (top). Which of the following statements regarding these results is/are correct?

A. They confirm the diagnosis of coronary artery disease

I.R. 6-4-79
N34118

STANDING CONTROL ECG

BP 130/90

HR 68/MIN

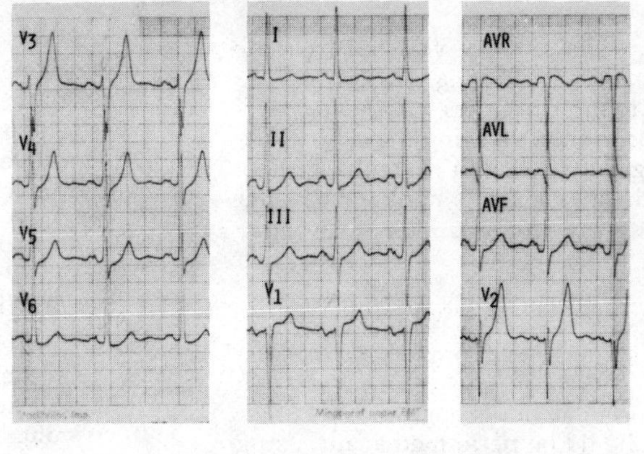

STANDARDIZATION = 1 MV/20 MM

PEAK EXERCISE ECG
(BRUCE PROTOCOL)

1.0 MIN 20 SEC.
OF STAGE I

BP 160/90
HR 122/MIN
NO PAIN

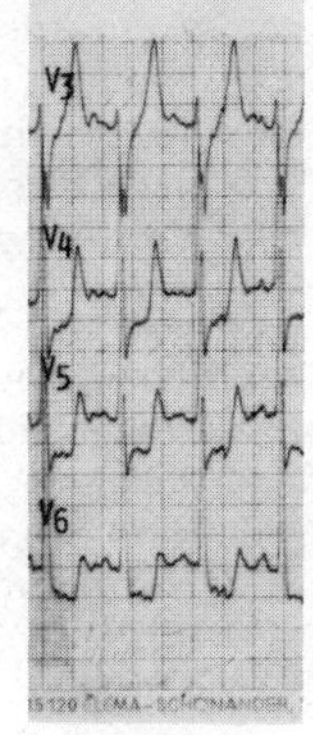

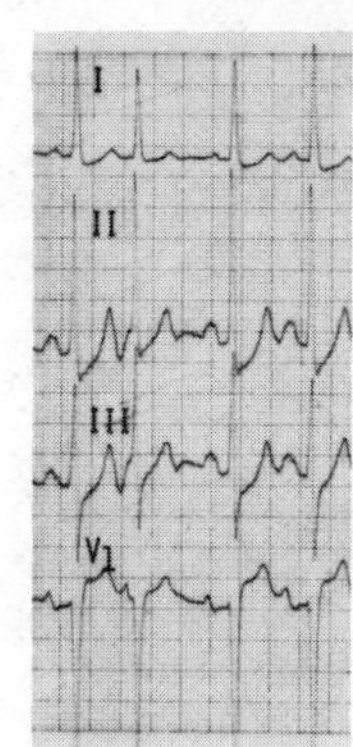

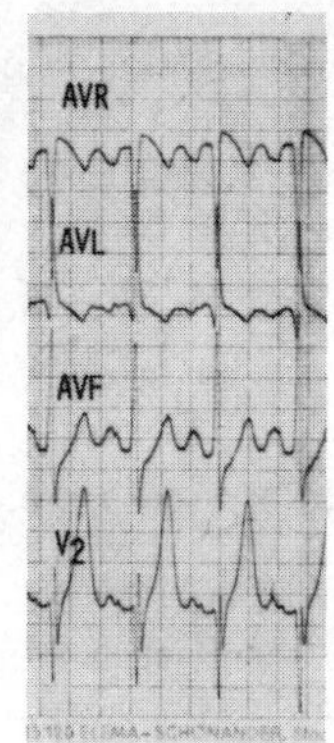

B. The absence of chest pain connotes a poor prognosis
C. There is an increased likelihood of main left or three-vessel coronary artery disease
D. The likelihood of this test being falsely positive is less than 10%
E. The patient should undergo emergency cardiac catheterization

92. In the post-exercise period, the rhythm strip shown below was obtained. Which of the following statements regarding this arrhythmia is/are true?

A. It predicts that sudden death is likely
B. It can be used as a criterion to interpret the exercise test as positive
C. Antiarrhythmic therapy is indicated
D. An exercise program for this patient is contraindicated
E. The arrhythmia is probably related to the degree of left ventricular dysfunction

---

93. Atherosclerotic plaques contain which of the following?

A. Smooth muscle cells
B. Elastin
C. Glycosaminoglycans
D. Intracellular and extracellular lipid deposits
E. Calcium
F. Blood

I.R. 6-4-79
N34118

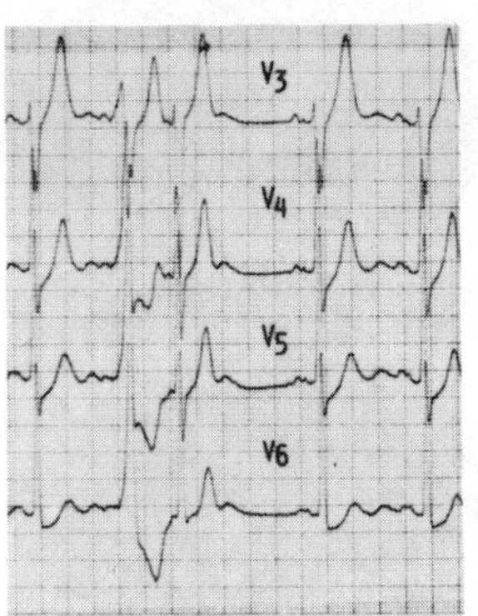

1 MIN. POST EXERCISE

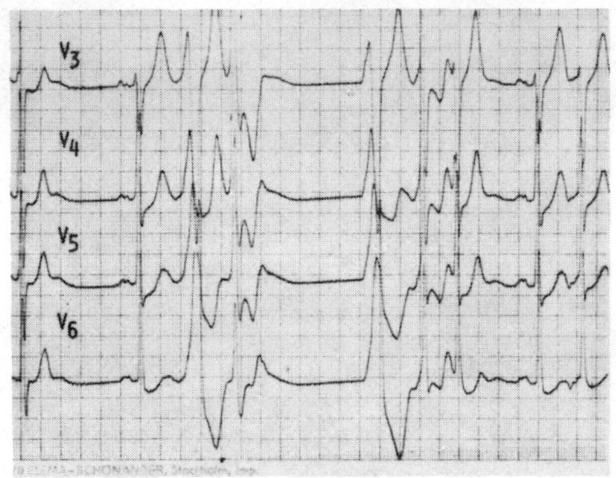

2 MIN. POST EXERCISE

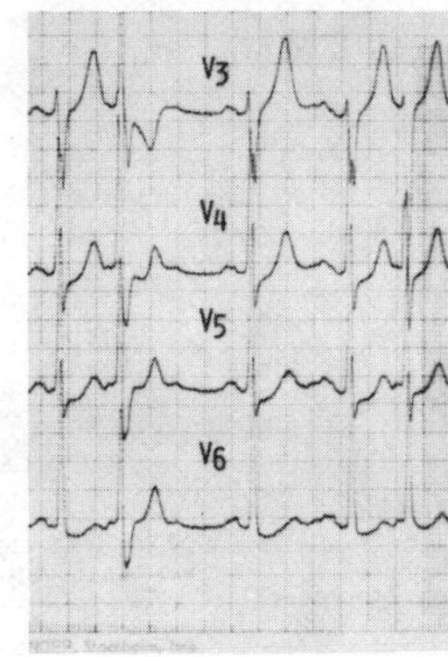

4 MIN. POST EXERCISE

QUESTIONS 94–95

A 49-year-old man complains of three years of sporadic nocturnal chest pain, typically awakening him at 3 or 4 AM and relieved within two to three minutes with nitroglycerin. He has no exercise intolerance during the day and is able to jog and play singles tennis with no problem. Rest and exercise radionuclide angiogram is normal. A Holter monitor recording during symptoms is illustrated below and on p. 13.

94. Which of the following statements is/are true?

A. The patient has three-vessel coronary artery disease
B. The patient has preinfarctional angina
C. Exercise testing should be performed again, using thallium perfusion scanning
D. The patient has Prinzmetal's variant angina
E. The presence of underlying atherosclerotic coronary artery disease cannot be excluded
F. These changes also occur in the absence of symptoms

95. Which of the following is/are indicated for this patient?

A. Nitrates, as required
B. High doses of beta-adrenergic blocking agents
C. Nifedipine
D. Coronary artery surgery
E. Percutaneous transluminal angioplasty

96. Which of the following is/are likely with atrial flutter?

A. To be the result of digitalis toxicity
B. Cardioversion to sinus rhythm with 20 joules
C. An increase in the ventricular rate with quinidine
D. Cardioversion to sinus rhythm by atrial pacing
E. Cardioversion to sinus rhythm by carotid sinus massage

97. Which of the following statements concerning asymmetric septal hypertrophy (hypertrophic cardiomyopathy) is/are true?

A. It is inherited as an autosomal dominant trait with a high degree of penetrance
B. Systolic anterior motion of the mitral valve correlates well with the presence of a gradient
C. The abnormal initial forces on the electrocardiogram are due to the depolarization of the abnormally thickened septum
D. Myocardial fiber disarray localized in the septum is pathognomonic
E. Mitral regurgitation typically regresses after myectomy

98. Which of the following is/are capable of producing a congestive cardiomyopathy?
A. Alcohol
B. Radiation
C. Doxorubicin
D. Emetine
E. Cobalt

H.S. 3-16-79

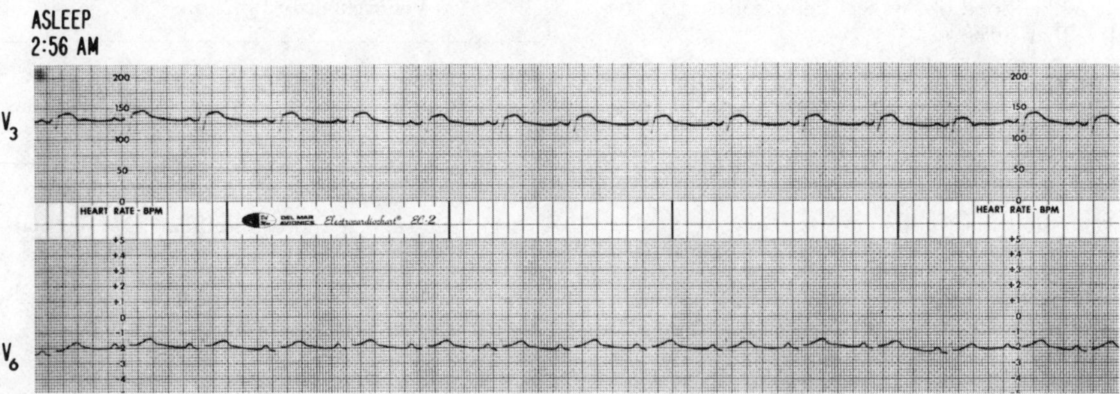

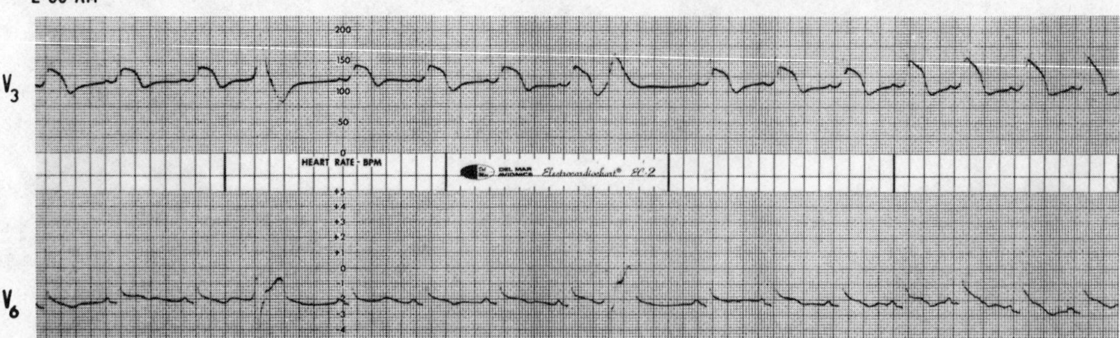

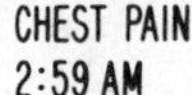

CHEST PAIN
2:59 AM

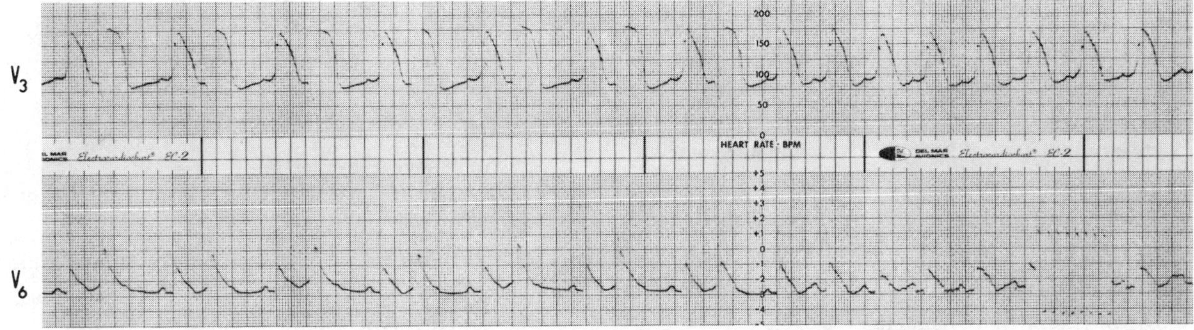

3:00 AM

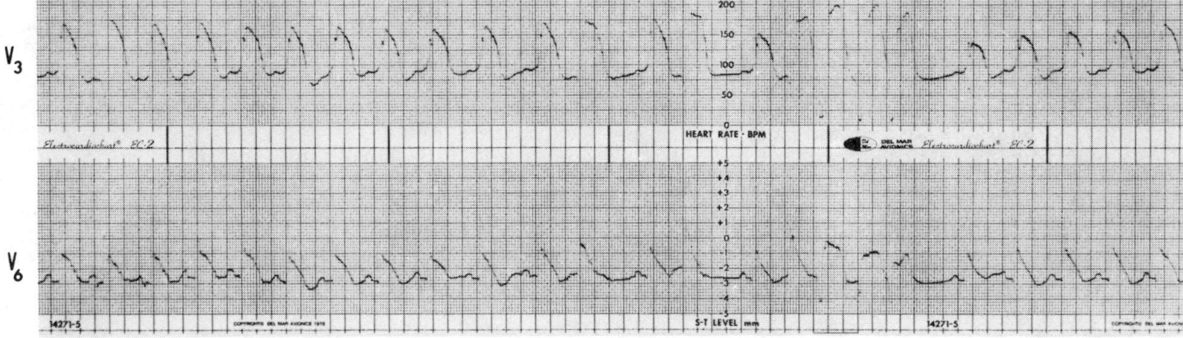

99. In aortic coarctation, collateral blood supply develops via which of the following routes?

A. Internal mammary to anterior intercostal arteries
B. Internal mammary to superior epigastric arteries
C. Vertebral to gastroepiploic arteries
D. Subclavian to posterior intercostal arteries
E. Innominate to bronchial arteries

100. Which of the following statements concerning immersion foot and frostbite is/are true?

A. Vasoconstriction is an important pathophysiologic factor
B. The affected extremity becomes numb and anesthetized
C. The affected part should be rewarmed with massage and exercise
D. Sympathectomy is of proved efficacy
E. A conservative operative approach is indicated

101. Which of the following statements concerning heparin is/are correct?

A. Minidose heparin is an effective method of preventing thrombosis in patients with fractures
B. Continuous intravenous infusion is the safest method for full heparin anticoagulation
C. The aim of heparin therapy in patients with deep vein thrombophlebitis is to prolong the activated partial thromboplastin time to 2.0–2.5 times control
D. Immunologically mediated thrombocytopenia should be treated by changing brands of heparin
E. Protamine reverses the effects of heparin on 1 mg = 100 units basis

102. Which of the following statements concerning superficial calf vein thrombophlebitis is/are true?

A. Anticoagulation therapy is usually necessary
B. The risk of pulmonary embolism is low
C. Ambulation is allowable
D. Indomethacin attenuates inflammation and pain
E. Broad-spectrum antibiotics facilitate resolution

103. The natural history of a patient with coarctation of the aorta who undergoes repair with a tubular prosthesis at age 16 includes

A. continuing hypertension
B. formation of an aneurysm at the repair site
C. aortic stenosis
D. paraplegia
E. aortic regurgitation
F. normal longevity

104. In aortic dissection, acute operative intervention is indicated in which of the following situations?

A. When the dissection originates distal to the aortic arch
B. When the dissection is leaking
C. When the pain and blood pressure cannot be controlled medically
D. When the dissection occurs in the absence of hypertension
E. When there is congestive heart failure from associated aortic regurgitation

105. Reasonable therapeutic measures in arteriosclerosis obliterans include which of the following?

A. Percutaneous transluminal angioplasty
B. Preganglionic lumbar sympathectomy
C. Amputation
D. Femoropopliteal bypass grafting
E. Vasodilator drugs
F. Exercise rehabilitation program

106. Causes of peripheral vascular arterial insufficiency include

A. thromboangiitis obliterans
B. cauda equina disease
C. arteriosclerosis obliterans
D. arterial embolism
E. ingestion of methysergide
F. vasospasm

107. Which of the following statements about Raynaud's disease is/are true?

A. There is a frequent history of exposure to polyvinyl chloride
B. The affected digits are cold and pale, and may be cyanotic during an attack
C. Increased erythrocyte sedimentation rate and arthralgias are common
D. The symptoms typically respond well to vasodilator therapy
E. Lumbar sympathectomy usually relieves lower extremity symptoms

108. Which of the following statements concerning heart failure is/are true?

A. A pleural effusion is more likely when there is biventricular failure
B. Rusty sputum production usually indicates concomitant pulmonary infarction
C. An early clue to left heart failure is a rise in central venous pressure (CVP)
D. Intravascular blood volume is doubled in moderately severe congestive failure
E. Fatigue and weakness usually indicate biventricular failure

109. Which of the following statements concerning sudden death is/are true?

A. When death occurs in young athletes, coronary artery disease is usually the explanation
B. Most adults who are resuscitated from near sudden death will evolve a myocardial infarction
C. Mitral valve prolapse is a common etiologic factor
D. Resuscitated victims who do not evolve a myocardial infarction have a better long-term survival than those who do
E. Antiarrhythmic therapy typically prevents another episode in patients resuscitated from near sudden death

DIRECTIONS: Questions 110 to 231 are matching questions. For each numbered item, choose the most likely associated lettered item from those provided. Each numbered item has ONLY ONE answer. Within each group, each lettered item may be the answer to one, more than one, or none of the numbered items.

QUESTIONS 110–112

For each of the following statements concerning the recording of blood pressure using indirect sphygmomanometry, select the appropriate Korotkoff phase.

A. Phase 1
B. Phase 2
C. Phase 3
D. Phase 4
E. Phase 5

110. Corresponds most closely to systolic arterial blood pressure

111. Corresponds to the muffling of Korotkoff sounds

112. Corresponds most closely to the true diastolic blood pressure

QUESTIONS 113–117

For each of the following antihypertensive agents, choose the most likely of the listed side effects.

A. Hyperuricemia
B. Hypocalcemia
C. Worsening of claudication
D. Sedation
E. Depression
F. Inhibition of ejaculation

113. Reserpine

114. Guanethidine

115. Methyldopa

116. Propranolol

117. Hydrochlorothiazide

QUESTIONS 118–122

For each of the following clinical conditions, select the most likely associated valvular heart lesion.

A. Aortic regurgitation
B. Aortic stenosis
C. Mitral regurgitation
D. Mitral stenosis
E. Tricuspid regurgitation
F. Tricuspid stenosis

118. Hurler's syndrome

119. Ankylosing spondylitis

120. Left ventricular aneurysm

121. Drug addiction

122. Carcinoid syndrome

QUESTIONS 123–127

For each of the following statements, select the most likely type of adult valvular heart disease.

A. Mitral stenosis/mitral regurgitation
B. Aortic stenosis
C. Tricuspid regurgitation
D. Mitral regurgitation
E. Aortic regurgitation

123. Most likely to be due to previous rheumatic fever

124. Most likely in Eisenmenger's syndrome

125. Compatible with the longest latent period between onset and the development of symptoms

126. Most likely to be associated with symptomatic premature ventricular contractions

127. Most likely to produce symptomatic neck pulsations

QUESTIONS 128–131

For each of the following congenital shunt lesions, select the most likely clinical findings.

A. A mimic of a continuous murmur
B. Continuous murmur over the right lower sternal edge
C. A history of maternal rubella in the first trimester of pregnancy
D. A lateral myocardial infarction pattern on electrocardiogram
E. Clubbing of the fingers but not the toes

128. Patent ductus arteriosus with a 2.5:1 left-to-right shunt

129. Ventricular septal defect with aortic regurgitation

130. Coronary atrioventricular fistula

131. Anomalous origin of the left coronary artery

QUESTIONS 132–137

For each of the following clinical situations, select the most likely description of the second heart sound. Assume in each case that the patient is a 14-year-old girl.

A. A second heart sound that is split by 0.06 seconds on inspiration with A2 louder than P2 at the second left intercostal space; the second heart sound on expiration is single
B. A second heart sound that is split by 0.07 seconds on expiration with A2 equal to P2 at the second left intercostal space; respiratory variation is less than 0.02 seconds
C. A second heart sound that is split by 0.045 seconds on expiration and becomes single on inspiration

D. A second heart sound that is split by 0.09 seconds on expiration with little respiratory variation and a soft pulmonic component
E. A second heart sound that is single and shows little or no respiratory variation and a markedly accentuated P2
F. A second heart sound that is split by 0.03 seconds on expiration and by 0.07 seconds on inspiration; the pulmonic component is of normal intensity

132. An atrial septal defect with a 2.5:1 left-to-right shunt and normal pulmonary artery pressures

133. An innocent pulmonary flow murmur

134. An Eisenmenger atrial septal defect

135. Mild valvular pulmonic stenosis

136. Moderate-to-severe infundibular pulmonic stenosis

137. Moderate supravalvular pulmonic stenosis

QUESTIONS 138–142

For each of the following causes of left ventricular outflow tract obstruction, select the most likely clinical finding

A. A rapid carotid upstroke with a normal pulse pressure
B. A prominent aortic ejection sound
C. Associated aortic regurgitation
D. A diminished or absent left brachial pulse
E. Prominent radiation of the systolic murmur to the right carotid pulse

138. Supravalvular aortic stenosis

139. Membranous subvalvular aortic stenosis

140. Valvular aortic stenosis

141. Muscular subvalvular aortic stenosis

142. Isolated coarctation of the aorta

QUESTIONS 143–147

For each of the following clinical conditions, choose the most likely radiographic appearance of the thoracic aorta.

A. A dilated aortic root with a normal arch and descending aorta
B. A dilated aortic root, arch, and descending aorta
C. No aortic dilatation in any of its portions
D. A dilated aortic root, arch, and left subclavian artery with localized dilatation of the descending thoracic aorta

143. Membranous subvalvular aortic stenosis

144. Valvular aortic regurgitation

145. Valvular aortic stenosis

146. Coarctation of the aorta

147. Muscular subvalvular aortic stenosis

QUESTIONS 148–152

For each of the following causes of hypertension, select the most likely physical, laboratory, or historical finding.

A. Continuous murmur over the posterior lung fields
B. Epigastric bruit
C. Weight loss
D. Abdominal striae
E. Hypernatremia
F. Enlarged kidneys

148. Renal artery stenosis

149. Pheochromocytoma

150. Cushing's syndrome

151. Coarctation of the aorta

152. Hyperaldosteronism

QUESTIONS 153–157

For each of the following drug combinations, select the most likely resulting interaction that influences the resulting drug levels.

A. Induction of hepatic enzymes
B. Inhibition of hepatic enzymes
C. Chemical bonding and inactivation
D. Alteration in absorption
E. Displacement of protein-bound drug

153. Oral warfarin–chloramphenicol

154. Intravenous 10% calcium chloride–sodium bicarbonate

155. Oral warfarin–phenylbutazone

156. Oral phenothiazine–antacids

157. Oral warfarin–phenobarbital

QUESTIONS 158–161

For each of the following antihypertensive drugs, select its main mechanism of action.

A. Inhibition of renin release
B. Natriuresis
C. Reduction of cardiac output
D. Centrally mediated decrease in sympathetic activity
E. Vasodilatation
F. Blocking of postganglionic alpha-receptors

158. Hydrochlorothiazide

159. Propranolol

160. Methyldopa

161. Hydralazine

QUESTIONS 162–167

For each of the following clinical situations, select the dominant resulting hemodynamic change.

A. An increase in afterload
B. An increase in preload
C. An increase in contractility
D. A decrease in afterload
E. A decrease in preload
F. A decrease in contractility

162. Intravenous administration of propranolol to a normotensive patient with no heart disease

163. Nitroprusside infusion in a patient with a normal pulmonary capillary wedge pressure

164. Digoxin therapy in a patient without heart failure

165. Paroxysmal atrial tachycardia (heart rate 165/minute) in an otherwise healthy 18-year-old woman

166. Sublingual nitroglycerin during an attack of angina pectoris

167. Nitrol paste in a patient with congestive heart failure secondary to chronic aortic regurgitation

QUESTIONS 168–173

For each of the following physiologic events, choose the appropriate effector receptor system.

A. $Beta_1$-adrenergic receptor
B. $Beta_2$-adrenergic receptor
C. $Alpha_1$-adrenergic receptor
D. $Alpha_2$-adrenergic receptor
E. Dopaminergic receptor

168. Platelet aggregation

169. Increased inotropy

170. Renal arteriolar dilatation

171. Bronchial dilatation

172. Systemic arteriolar dilatation

173. Systemic arteriolar constriction

QUESTIONS 174–177

For each of the following clinical situations, select the most likely finding on roentgenography of the chest.

A. Cardiothoracic ratio greater than 55%
B. Kerley's B lines
C. Cephalization of pulmonary blood flow
D. Inward displacement of the subepicardial fat line on the lateral view
E. A calcified mitral valve
F. Large central pulmonary arteries with attenuation of the peripheral vessels

174. Significant chronic pulmonary venous hypertension

175. Moderate-to-severe chronic aortic regurgitation without congestive heart failure

176. Detected best by cardiac fluoroscopy

177. Early congestive heart failure

QUESTIONS 178–183

This diagram shows 3 different starting points on a ventricular function curve and 9 potential responses (A–I) to different hemodynamic interventions. For each of the following patients, select the most likely shift in ventricular function.

178. A 36-year-old woman given furosemide for premenstrual abdominal discomfort

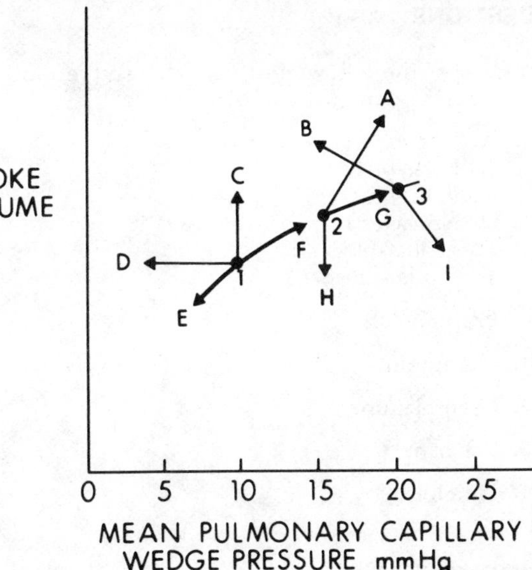

179. A 46-year-old normotensive man given excessive plasma and whole blood following a nephrectomy

180. A 21-year-old woman with postoperative septic shock; no volume replacement has been given

181. A 52-year-old man with a large diaphragmatic myocardial infarction and no clinical evidence of failure who is given 2 liters of plasma intravenously

182. A 46-year-old dyspneic woman with a cardiomyopathy (ejection fraction = 31%) who is given hydralazine

183. A 51-year-old dyspneic man with an acute anterior myocardial infarction and a third heart sound who is given phenylephrine for hypotension

QUESTIONS 184–189

For each of the following patients, choose the laboratory evaluation that is most likely to be immediately helpful in terms of diagnosis and therapy.

A. Phonocardiography
B. Electrocardiography
C. Rest and exercise radionuclide angiography
D. Cardiac catheterization
E. Echocardiography
F. Holter monitoring
G. Vector cardiography

184. A patient with chest pain and a rapid irregular pulse

185. A 52-year-old man with left bundle branch block and disabling chest pain that is atypical for angina

186. A patient with changing murmurs

187. A patient with an extra sound regarding which there is controversy over whether it is early or midsystolic in the cardiac cycle

188. A patient with catheterization-documented coronary artery disease, syncope, and a normal bedside examination

189. A 42-year-old man with class IV angina pectoris who is receiving propranolol and vasodilators

QUESTIONS 190–194

For each of the following drugs, choose the most appropriate description of receptor activity.

A. Nonselective beta-blocker
B. $Beta_1$-blocker
C. $Beta_2$-blocker
D. Nonselective alpha-blocker
E. $Alpha_1$-blocker
F. $Alpha_2$-blocker

190. Propranolol

191. Metoprolol

192. Phentolamine

193. Prazosin

194. Timolol

QUESTIONS 195–201

For each of the following complications of diuretic therapy, select the class of diuretics most likely to be responsible.

A. Ethacrynic acid/furosemide
B. Thiazides
C. Organomercurials
D. Triamterene
E. Carbonic anhydrase inhibitors
F. Aldosterone antagonists

195. Severe electrolyte imbalance

196. Agranulocytosis

197. Hypercalcemia

198. Hyperkalemia

199. Hypercalciuria

200. Deafness

201. Gynecomastia

QUESTIONS 202–207

For each of the following congenital heart conditions, select the most likely associated clinical feature.

A. Premature birth
B. Down's syndrome (trisomy 21)
C. Turner's syndrome
D. Trisomy 18
E. Holt-Oram syndrome
F. Male predominance

202. Atrial septal defect

203. Isolated ventricular septal defect

204. Patent ductus arteriosus

205. Bicuspid aortic valve

206. Coarctation of the aorta

207. Endocardial cushion defect

QUESTIONS 208–211

For each of the following congenital heart defects, select the most likely associated clinical finding.

A. Stomach bubble in the right upper quadrant
B. Loud P2, a pulmonary ejection sound, and a right ventricular lift
C. Loud S2 and regurgitation of the systemic atrioventricular valve
D. Cannon A waves in the jugular venous pulse with variable diastolic gallops
E. Midsystolic click and late systolic murmur

208. Congenitally corrected transposition of the great vessels

209. Congenital complete heart block

210. Situs inversus

211. Cor triatriatum

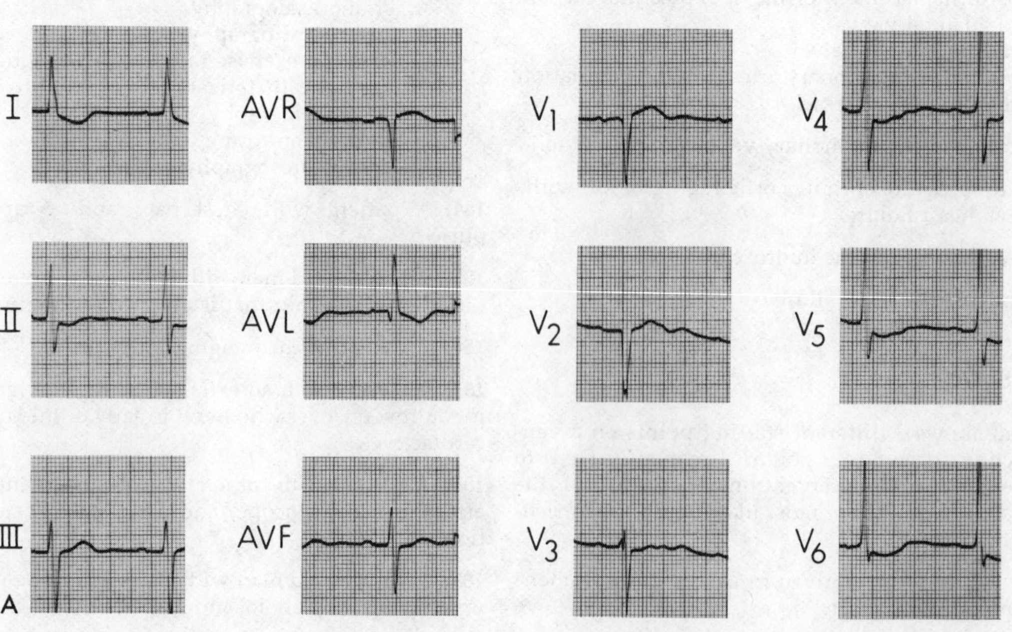

QUESTIONS 212–216

For each of the following patients, select the most likely electrocardiogram (A–E) illustrated on pp. 18–20.

212. A 56-year-old man with eight hours of epigastric discomfort and nausea partially relieved by belching and antacids

213. A digitalized 52-year-old woman who is receiving hydrochlorothiazide, 100 mg daily, for high blood pressure; she is poorly compliant to her low-salt diet

214. A 49-year-old man who has just experienced 20 minutes of precordial burning after rushing to your office in order not to be late for his appointment; he was asymptomatic when the ECG was recorded

215. An asymptomatic octogenarian

216. A 22-year-old woman who is asymptomatic except for infrequent 10- to 20-minute bouts of palpitations characterized by the sudden onset and offset of a rapid regular heart beat

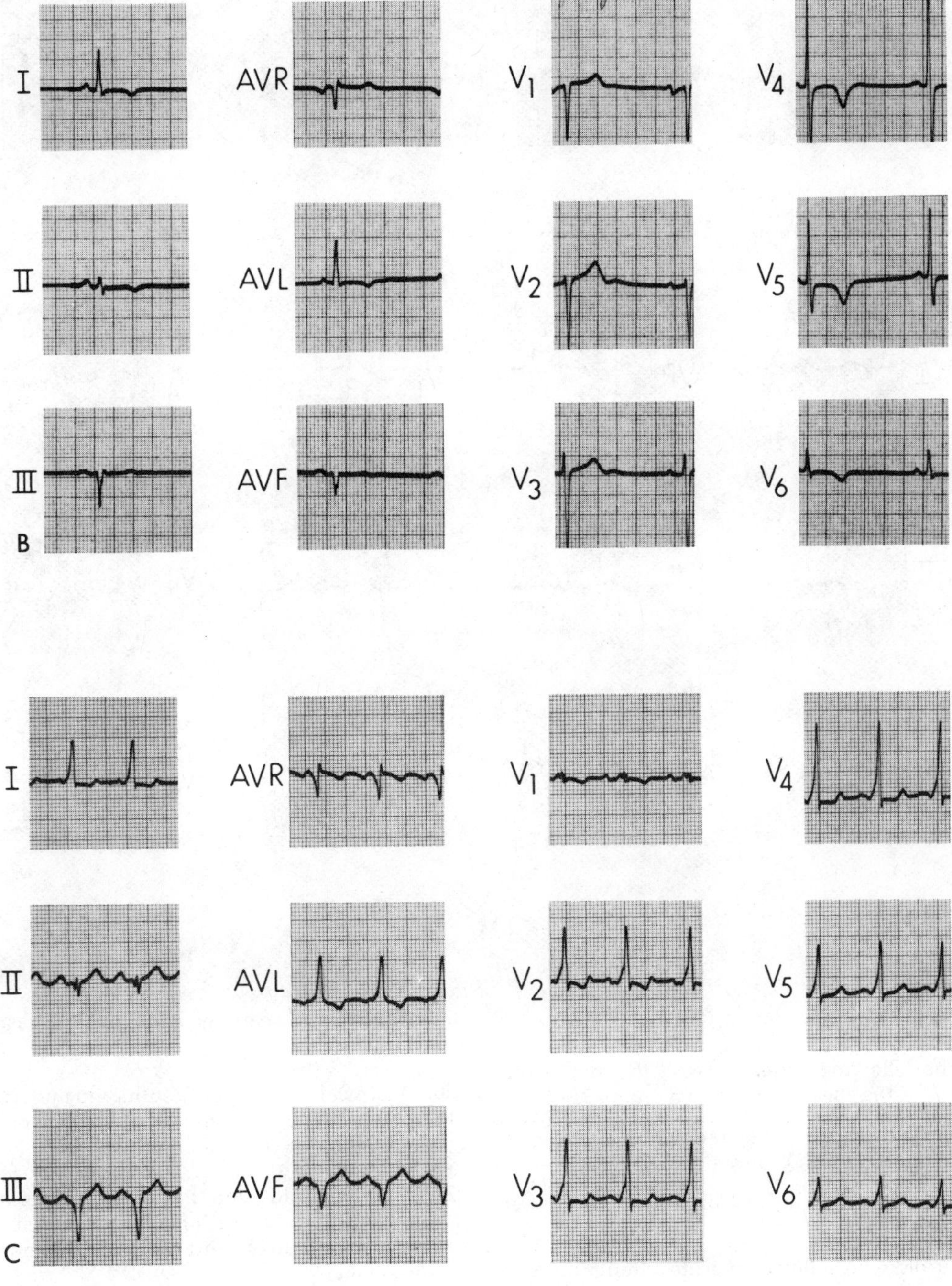

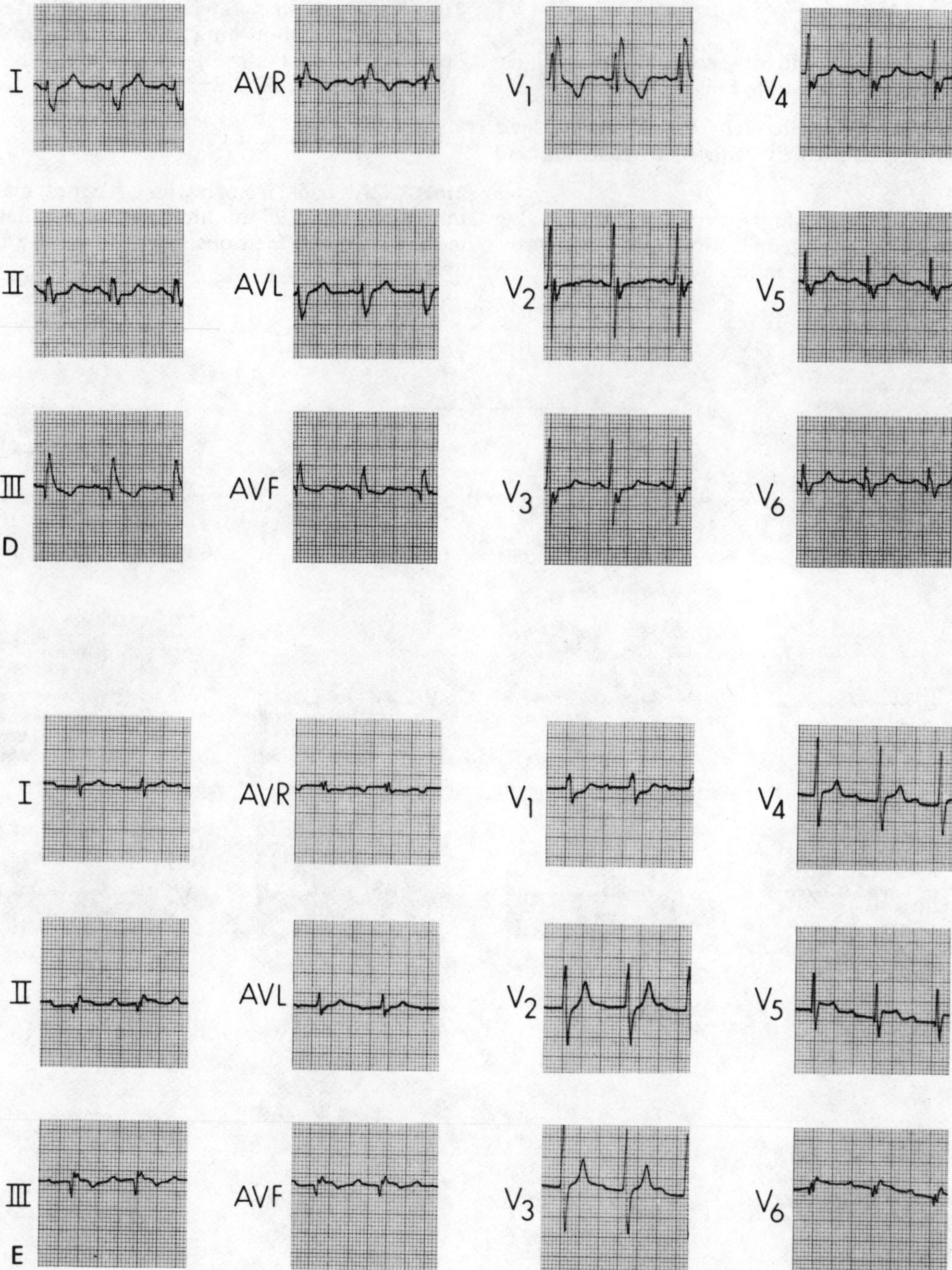

QUESTIONS 217–221

For each of the following patients, select the most likely roentgenogram of the chest (A–E) shown on pp. 21–23.

217. A 45-year-old jogger who fainted during a 15-kilometer race on the fourth of July

218. A 39-year-old with a history of arthritis of the left knee and ankle at age 13

219. A 52-year-old who suffered an acute anterior myocardial infarction six years ago and who now has dyspnea and palpitations.

220. A 42-year-old who 12 months ago underwent a course of radiation therapy for lymphoma with involvement of the hilar and anterior cervical lymph nodes

221. A 52-year-old who has had progressive dyspnea, fatigue, and peripheral edema for the past six months; the patient awoke acutely short of breath six hours before this film was taken

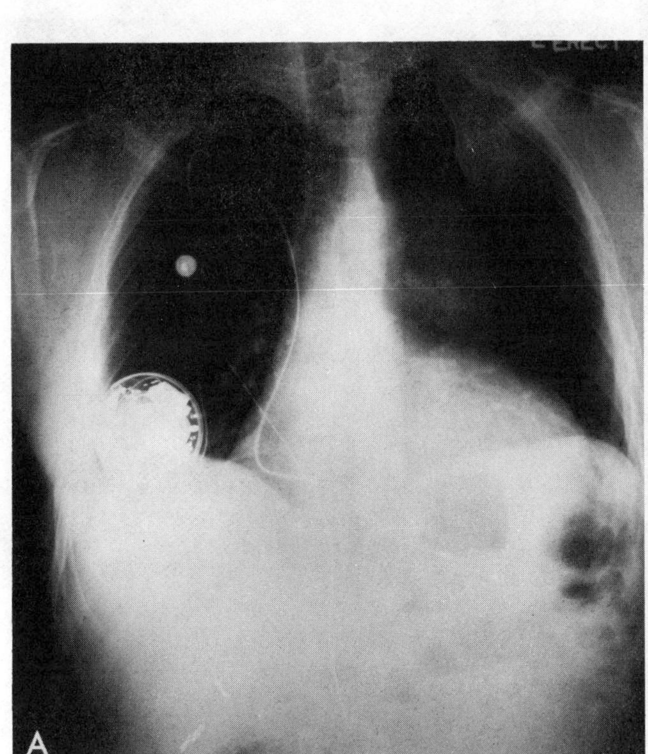

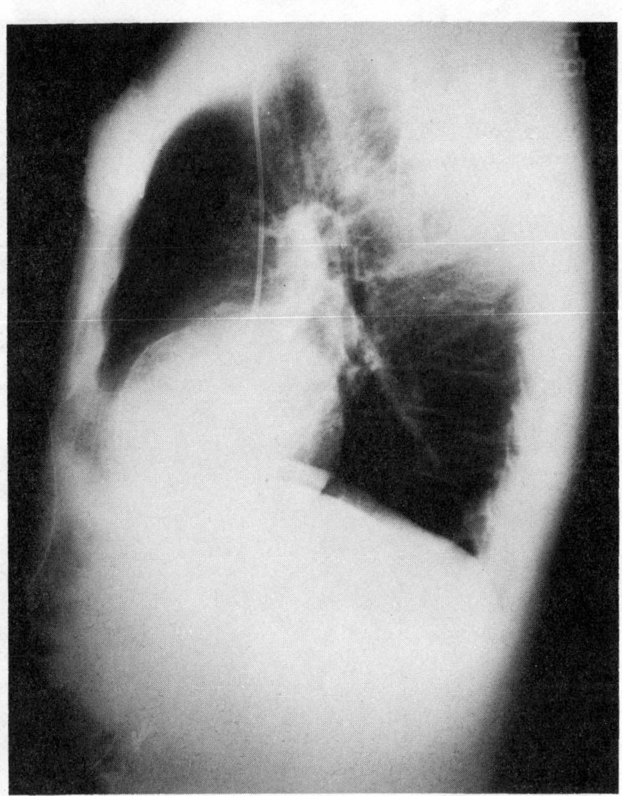

A, Left, PA view; *right,* lateral view.

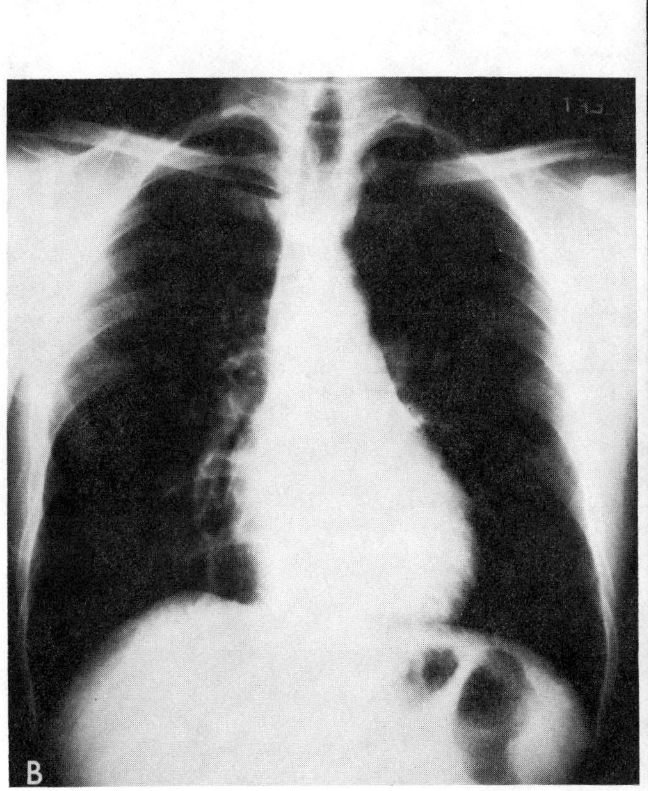

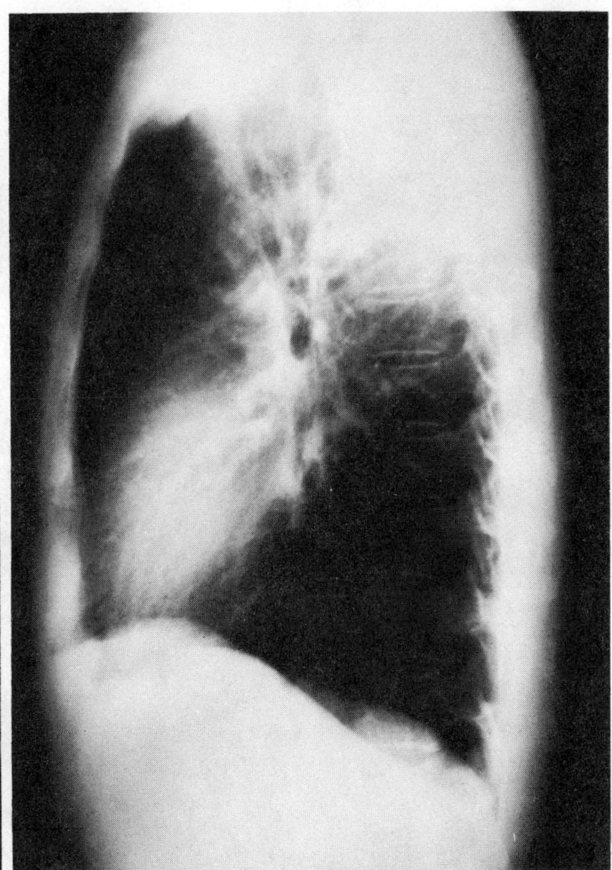

B, Left, PA view; *right,* lateral view.

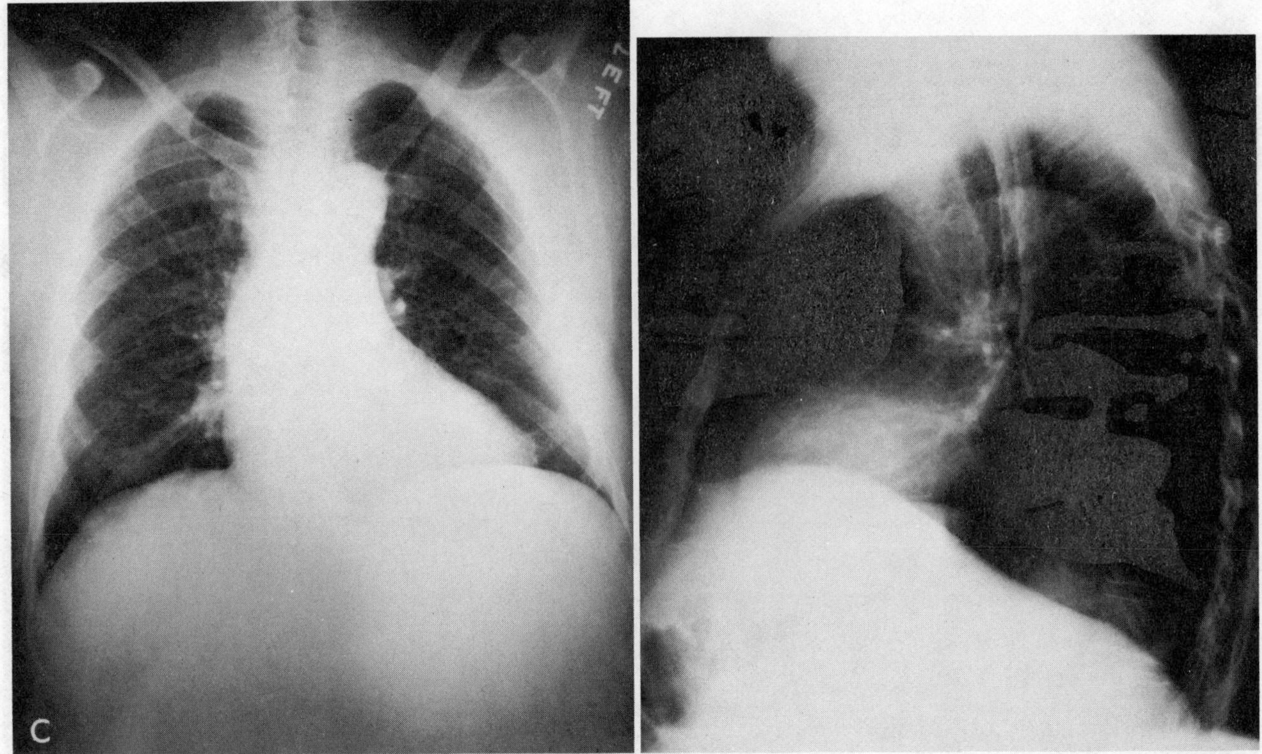

C, Left, PA view; *right,* lateral view.

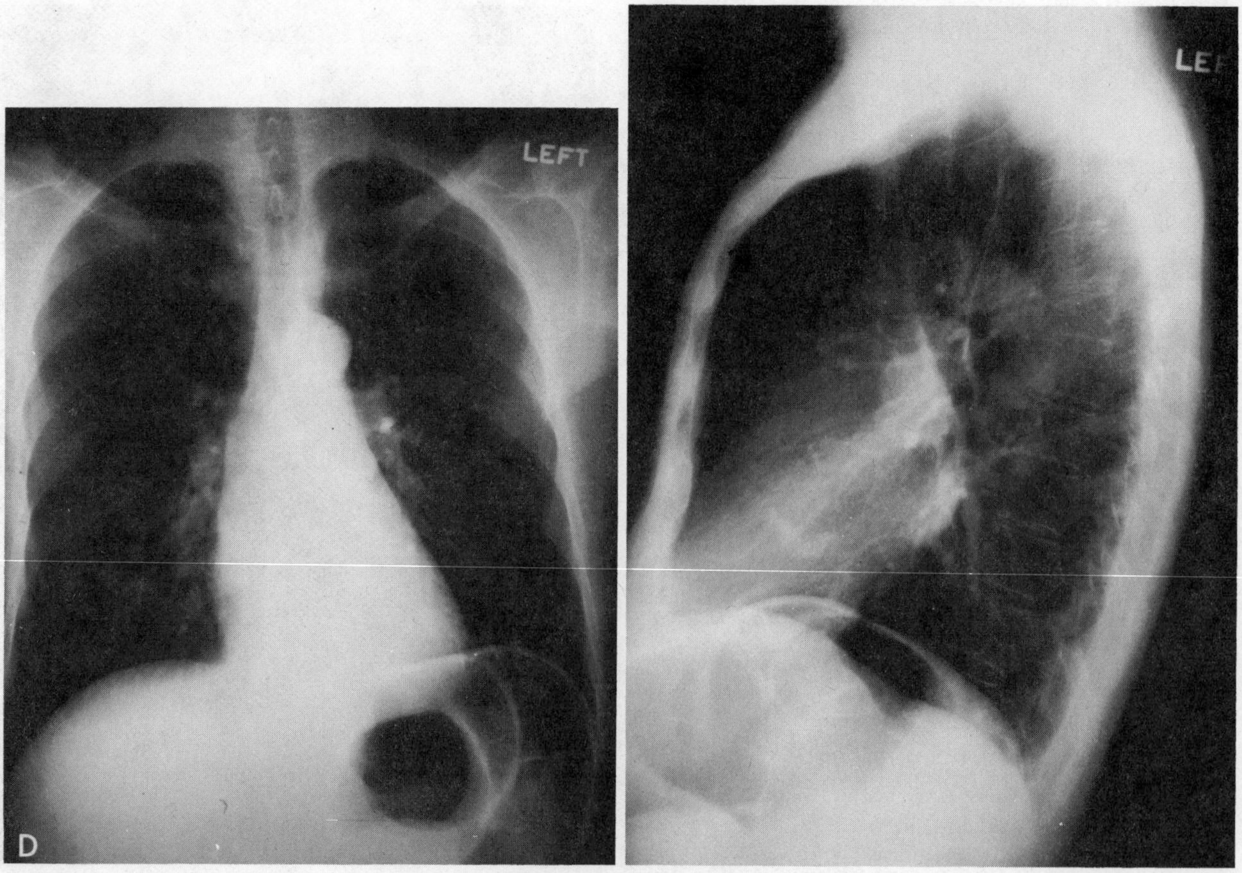

D, Left, PA view; *right,* lateral view.

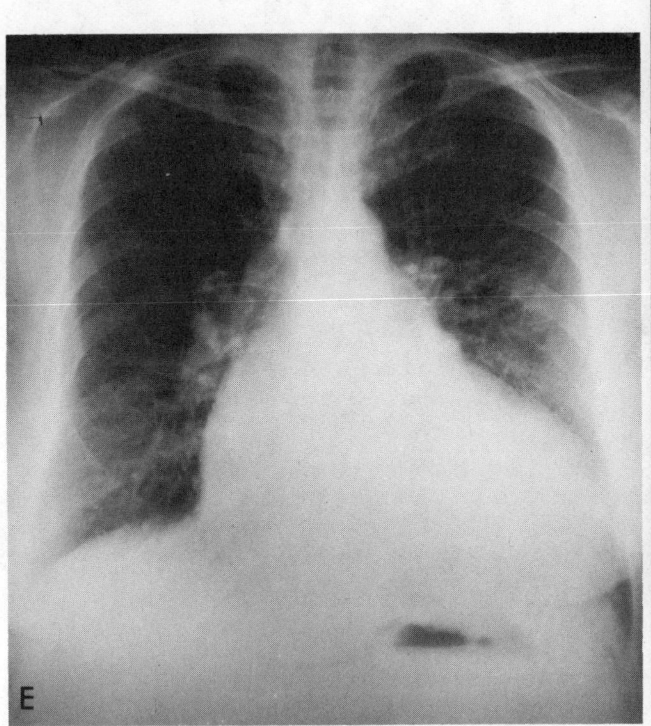

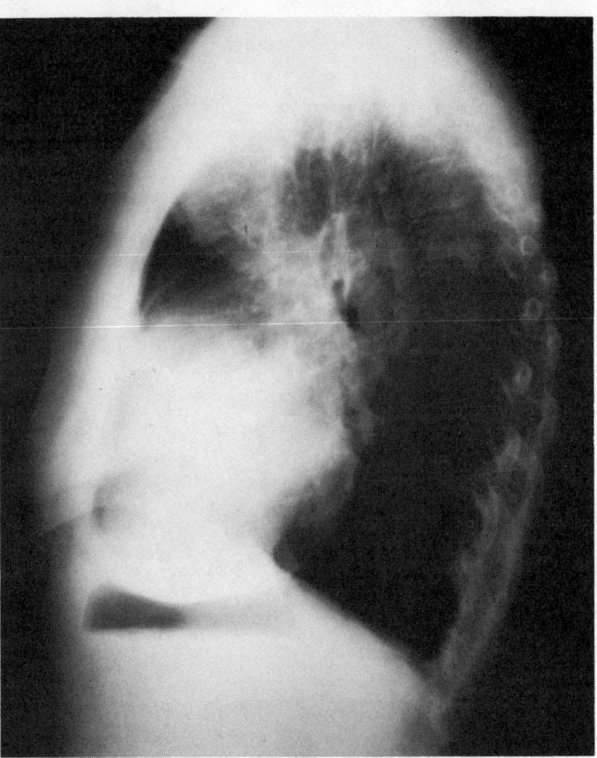

E, Left, PA view; *right,* lateral view.

QUESTIONS 222–226

For each of the following patients, select the most likely time-motion echocardiogram (A–E) shown on pp. 23–25.

222. A 36-year-old woman with an ejection sound at the second left intercostal space, a loud pulmonary closure sound, and a lower left parasternal lift with no discernible apical impulse

223. An asymptomatic 17-year-old boy with a bifid arterial pulse; a laterally displaced, hyperdynamic apical impulse; an ejection sound at the apex; and a diastolic murmur

224. A 36-year-old man with chills, arthralgias, dyspnea, and a blood pressure of 140/76 mm Hg; the first heart sound is soft, and there is a short diastolic murmur at the fourth left intercostal space

225. A 22-year-old man with a brisk upstroke of the carotid pulse, a triple apical impulse, and paradoxical splitting of the second heart sound

226. A 68-year-old man with a small carotid pulse, a palpable fourth heart sound, a sustained apical impulse, a systolic murmur, and a soft second heart sound

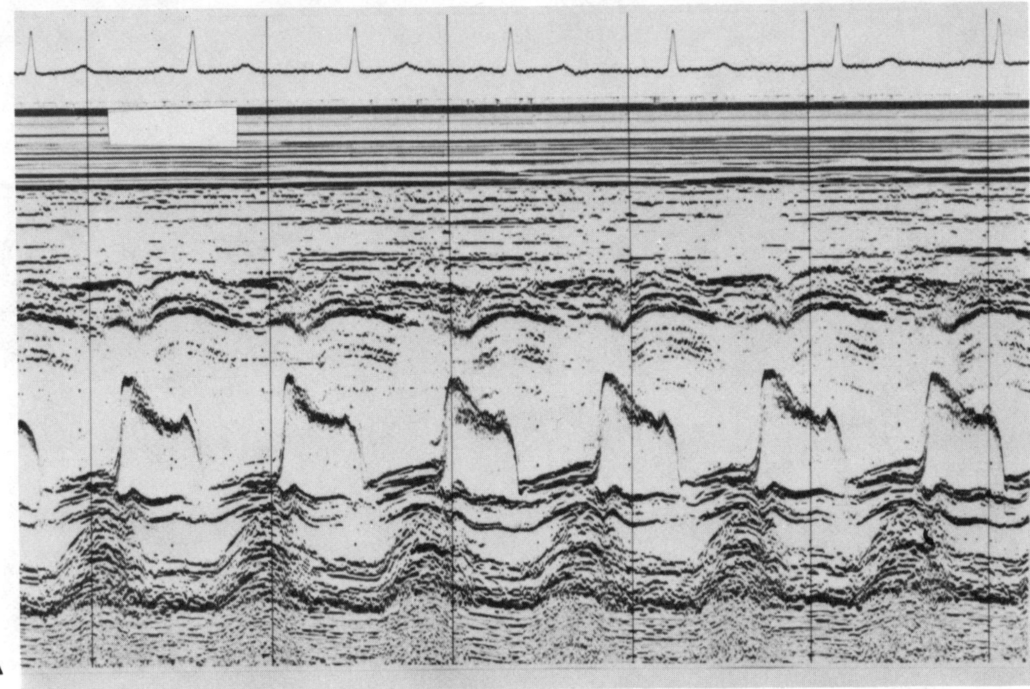

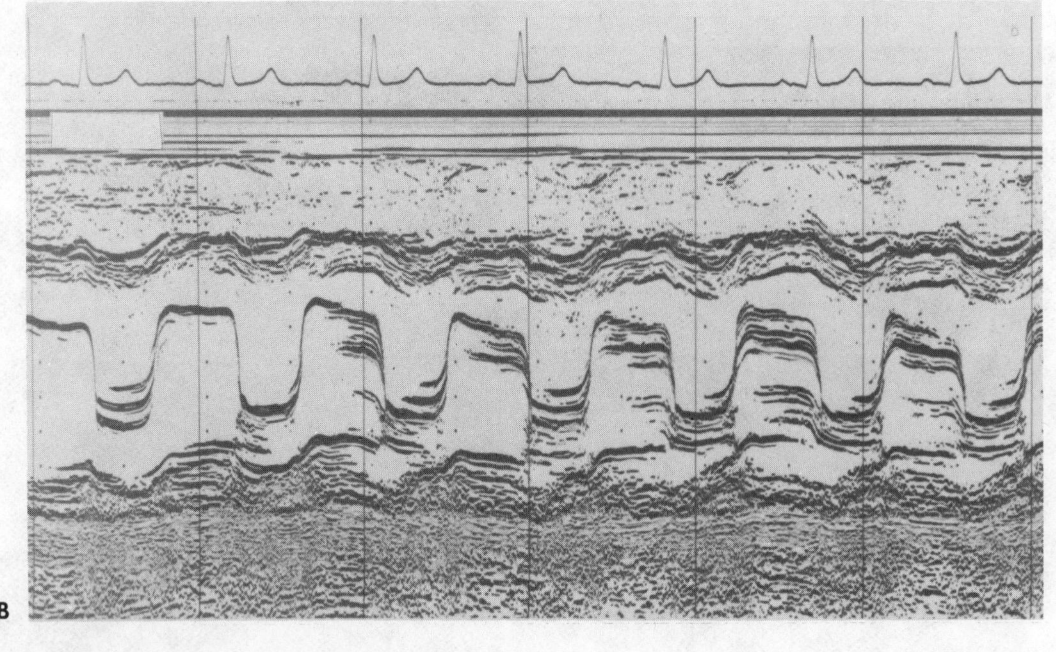
B

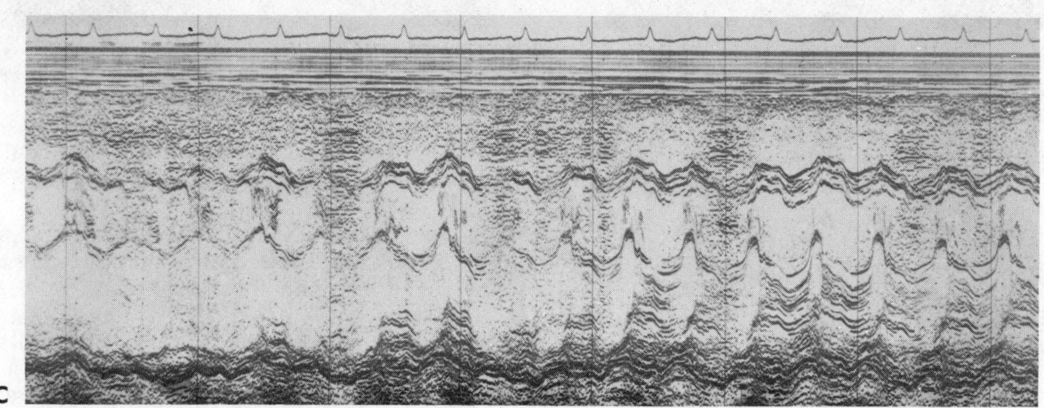
C

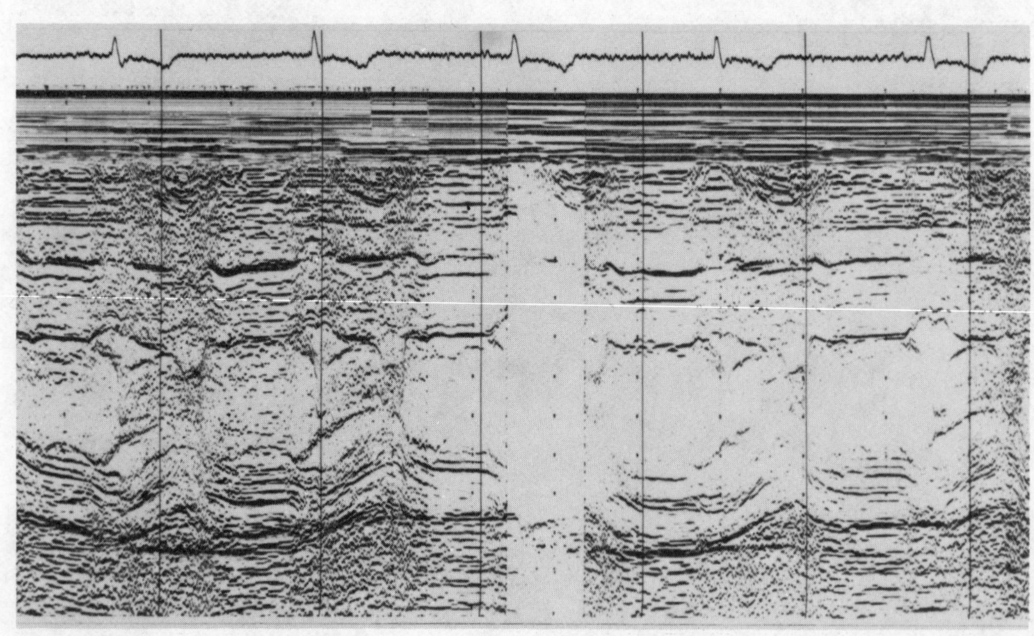
D

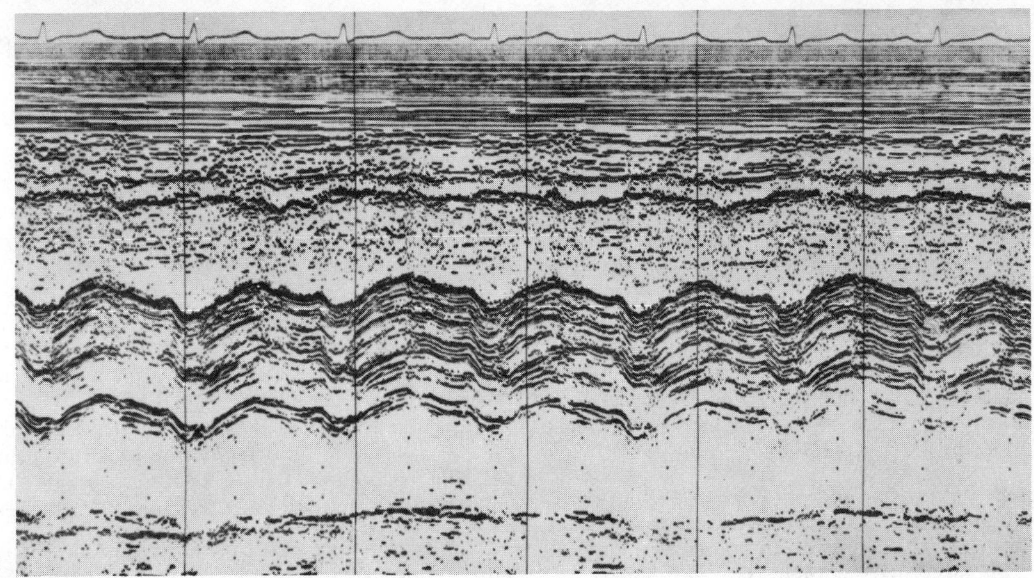

QUESTIONS 227–231

For each of the following diseases, select the most likely site of aortic involvement.

A. Proximal and ascending thoracic aorta
B. Thoracic aortic arch
C. Descending thoracic aorta
D. Abdominal aorta

227. Marfan's syndrome

228. Osteogenesis imperfecta

229. Pseudoxanthoma elasticum

230. Arteriosclerosis

231. Syphilis

PART 1

CARDIOVASCULAR DISEASES

ANSWERS

1. **(D)** In the United States, the overwhelming majority of patients with hypertension die of myocardial infarction, although the other listed complications do contribute to the total mortality. In Japan, however, where hypertension is very prominent, the incidence of coronary artery disease is much less than in the United States. *(Cecil, p. 226)*

2. **(B)** Although pulmonary angiography in patients with pulmonary hypertension of any cause carries a risk, it appears to be the most dangerous in primary pulmonary hypertension. If pulmonary angiography is needed, it is best to use manual injections of small amounts of dye into segments of the lung rather than use large amounts of dye and a pressure injector. *(Cecil, p. 216)*

3. **(A)** The pulmonary arterioles account for some 40–50% of the resistance drop across the pulmonary vascular bed. The pulmonary capillaries and venules account for the remaining drop in pressure. The left atrium may contribute to total pulmonary resistance but not directly to the pulmonary vascular resistance. *(Cecil, p. 212)*

4. **(B)** Symptoms of congestive heart failure in valvular aortic stenosis carry dire prognostic significance. *(Cecil, pp. 203, 208–209)*

5. **(A)** An echocardiogram may be falsely positive because of overinterpretation, a likely explanation for many of the "acoustically silent prolapses" that are diagnosed by echo. A time-motion echocardiographic study may be completely normal, however, despite unequivocal bedside findings. This is more likely when there is an isolated click than when there is a late systolic or holosystolic murmur. A completely normal echo would be most unusual with the other listed conditions. *(Cecil, pp. 196, 202, 204–205, 208, 291)*

6. **(B)** The only murmur that typically increases during the Valsalva strain phase is muscular subvalvular aortic stenosis (IHSS). The other conditions have murmurs that would diminish. The murmur of mitral valve prolapse typically lengthens, but unless a "whoop" is induced its intensity does not increase. *(Cecil, pp. 200, 201, 202–205)*

7. **(E)** Since the prımary hemodynamic abnormality in septic shock is a marked decrease in peripheral vascular resistance, norepinephrine may be quite effective in restoring the blood pressure without diminishing cardiac output. Although steroids are almost always part of the treatment of septic shock, the evidence that they are effective is not convincing. Unless there is concomitant myocardial disease, digitalis has no role in the treatment of gram-negative sepsis. Nitroprusside, an arteriolar vasodilator, would compound the problem. *(Cecil, pp. 165–167)*

8. **(C)** Mitral valve disease is, far and away, the most likely to be associated with atrial fibrillation, and mitral regurgitation is even more likely than mitral stenosis. The incidence in both is well over 50%. In the elderly, aortic stenosis and/or aortic regurgitation may be associated with atrial fibrillation, presumably owing to the rise in left ventricular end-diastolic pressure associated with chronic heart failure in these entities. A small percentage of patients with IHSS also have atrial fibrillation, presumably related to the marked decrease in left ventricular compliance as well as the associated mitral regurgitation. The loss of atrial systole may have disastrous hemodynamic consequences in these patients. *(Cecil, pp. 195, 197, 199–200, 291)*

9. **(D)** Despite encouraging trends in morbidity and mortality, coronary artery disease remains very much with us and is a leading cause of disability, hospital utilization, lost wages, and decreased productivity. *(Cecil, p. 98)*

10. **(D)** Most of the increase in cardiac output with exercise is mediated by an increasing heart rate. The increase in preload is counterbalanced by the increased sympathetic tone that prevents cardiac dilatation. Thus, stroke volume remains fairly constant until near maximal workloads are reached, when it may increase slightly. *(Cecil, pp. 106–107)*

11. **(B)** Both ventricular dilatation and elevation of the left ventricular end-diastolic pressure may be present without heart failure: e.g., the patient with well-compensated aortic regurgitation who has ventricular dilatation but normal ventricular function, and the patient with aortic stenosis who has an increased left ventricular end-diastolic pressure but normal ventricular function. Extensive biochemical research has failed to reveal a consistent defect either in energy metabolism or in protein synthesis. *(Cecil, pp. 133–136, 139)*

12. **(D)** Although all these choices may be appropriate for treatment of shock at or sometime during its course, the most important initial step is to begin volume replacement. Depending on availability, O-negative blood may be given pending typing and cross matching. *(Cecil, pp 163–165)*

13. **(B)** Routine use of oral furosemide in this setting is to be discouraged. Although the dyspnea may reflect an elevated left ventricular end-diastolic pressure, lowering this pressure with diuretics may result in reduced cardiac output and hypotension. Treatment with vasoactive agents may be best monitored by measuring pulmonary artery pressure and oxygen saturation. *(Cecil, p. 254)*

14. **(D)** The patient's ventricular rate is approximately 150 per minute but the atrial rate is also approximately 150 per minute excluding atrial flutter with 2:1 conduction. The P waves are inverted in leads II, III, and AVF, suggesting retrograde activation of the atria. Sinus tachycardia, therefore, is eliminated from consideration. An accelerated junctional pacemaker is a possibility but the rate is extremely fast. At this atrial rate, one would expect higher degrees of AV block if this were due to an accelerated or ectopic atrial pacemaker. This arrhythmia is typical of AV junctional re-entry tachycardia (so-called PAT). *(Cecil, pp. 269–273, 275–277)*

15. (D) Many patients learn how to terminate such arrhythmias themselves with the Valsalva maneuver, squatting, carotid sinus massage, hand stands, or immersing the face or hands in ice-cold water. For paroxysmal atrial tachycardia unresponsive to such maneuvers, intravenous verapamil has recently been approved and is the treatment of choice for acutely terminating such arrhythmias. Unless there is significant hemodynamic deterioration, cardioversion as an initial treatment is not indicated. Digitalization, propranolol, and sedation (e.g., with Valium) have also been used to treat this arrhythmia, but they are not as effective as verapamil. Long-term management involves either trying to suppress the premature beats that typically initiate the tachycardia or altering the electrophysiologic characteristics of part of the pathway. Digitalis, quinidine, and propranolol have all been used with varying degrees of success. Several centers are now studying the efficacy of long-term orally administered verapamil for suppressing paroxysmal atrial tachycardia. *(Cecil, pp. 276–278, 286)*

16. (D) The phonocardiogram shows two or more mid-to-late systolic clicks superimposed on a late systolic murmur. Following amyl nitrite inhalation, the late systolic murmur is softer and the clicks move earlier in the cardiac cycle. These findings are classic for mitral valve prolapse. *(Cecil, pp. 201–202)*

17. (E) A decrease in preload or left ventricular diastolic filling will decrease heart size and should diminish myocardial oxygen consumption. This may indeed be the mechanism for the salutary effects of nitroglycerin on angina pectoris. The other factors increase myocardial oxygen consumption and therefore should worsen or precipitate angina pectoris. *(Cecil, pp. 243–244)*

18. (E) Type I second-degree AV block (Wenckebach) is usually transient, and progression to complete heart block and/or a need for a permanent pacemaker is unusual. Progressive P-R interval lengthening and R-R interval shortening (the latter because of the decremental increase in the P-R interval) are typical. Type I second-degree AV block is particularly likely to be seen with diaphragmatic myocardial infarction and after large intravenous doses of digitalis. *(Cecil, pp. 280–281)*

19. (E) Heart rate is an important determinant of oxygen consumption, and in a patient with acute anterior myocardial infarction, efforts to decrease the ventricular rate as quickly as possible are warranted. Digoxin therapy takes time and may not work. Many of the other antiarrhythmic therapies may have untoward myocardial depressant effects. Cardioversion is rapid and usually very effective at reverting the patient to normal sinus rhythm. The most common underlying cause of atrial fibrillation in acute myocardial infarction is left ventricular failure with atrial distention. Such patients should always be carefully evaluated for the presence or absence of congestive heart failure, and appropriate therapy undertaken. Procainamide and/or quinidine may be indicated following reversion to sinus rhythm in order to prevent recurrent atrial fibrillation. A patient with an echocardiographic left atrial diameter of 6.7 cm or one in whom atrial fibrillation has persisted for more than a year would be unlikely to maintain sinus rhythm following cardioversion. A hyperthyroid patient is also unlikely to remain in sinus rhythm even if cardioversion is achieved in the first place. Beta-blockers and correction of the underlying hyperthyroidism would be much more appropriate. Cardioversion has no role in paroxysmal atrial fibrillation except to acutely correct an arrhythmia having disastrous hemodynamic consequences or unless it is applied in combination with other antiarrhythmic measures. Direct current discharges in the setting of digitalis toxicity are one way to convert a bothersome but nonlethal arrhythmia into ventricular tachycardia/ventricular fibrillation, which may be extremely difficult to deal with. *(Cecil, p. 288)*

20. (C) Atrial fibrillation is due to generalized atrial reentry, and most patients can be successfully cardioverted using direct current discharge. In general, however, higher energies are required than for atrial flutter and most laboratories would begin with at least 50–100 joules. Systemic embolization, either spontaneously or following cardioversion (and even with preceding anticoagulation) is a consequence of the arrhythmia. Quinidine therapy causes reversion to sinus rhythm in approximately 15–20% of patients. Ventricular responses above 150–160 per minute suggest that there has been a loss of the protective effects of the AV node and should raise the suspicion of concomitant Wolff-Parkinson-White syndrome. *(Cecil, pp. 270–272, 277, 284, 288)*

21. (G) Type II second-degree AV block is located in the His-Purkinje system and is not a manifestation of digitalis toxicity. An ectopic atrial tachycardia with 2:1 AV block is classic for digitalis toxicity. This is sometimes called "paroxysmal atrial tachycardia with block." This is a misnomer because the arrhythmia is due to an accelerated pacemaker, and therefore is not paroxysmal and not amenable to cardioversion. Premature beats, whether ventricular or junctional, should always raise the suspicion of digitalis toxicity, as should an accelerated junctional rhythm (another example of an accelerated pacemaker). Ventricular tachycardia may also be due to digitalis intoxication. *(Cecil, pp. 269–272, 273–274, 279–280)*

22. (D) Isoproterenol causes arteriolar vasodilatation, tachycardia, and increased contractility. All these responses would worsen the obstruction, augment the gradient, and cause the murmur to increase. Squatting and phenylephrine infusion would increase afterload and the distending pressure of the left ventricular outflow tract, and therefore lessen the gradient. Volume infusion and lying down would both augment left ventricular volume and lessen the severity of the obstruction in late systole. Propranolol is a negative inotropic agent that would decrease end-systolic dimension and, therefore, the severity of the gradient. *(Cecil, p. 292)*

23. (C) With the exception of paroxysmal arrhythmia, all these symptoms are likely to respond to surgical myectomy. Whether or not sudden death, a possible correlate of syncope, is also favorably influenced by myectomy is more controversial. *(Cecil, p. 292)*

24. (D) The cardiomyopathy associated with these diseases occasionally may be the initial mode of presentation. In Duchenne's dystrophy and Friedreich's ataxia, clinical cardiac involvement occurs in up to 50% of patients. *(Cecil, p. 293)*

25. (C) All these agents may be associated with an inflammatory myocardial reaction, but infectious mononucleosis is the least likely to be clinically significant. *(Cecil, pp. 293–295)*

26. (E) The association of pericardial disease with scleroderma is distinctly unusual and should cause a diligent search for other causes. *(Cecil, pp. 301–303)*

27. (A) With the exception of Kussmaul's sign, these are all classic manifestations of cardiac tamponade. Despite the high venous pressure and compromised cardiac function in cardiac tamponade, inspiration continues to be associated with a drop in venous pressure; therefore, Kussmaul's sign is unusual, although it *has* been reported. It is much more typical of constrictive pericarditis. *(Cecil, p. 304)*

28. (B) All these studies have been used to evaluate the presence or absence of pericardial effusion. Echocardiography is the most sensitive technique, and two-dimensional echocardiography has the added advantage of being able to localize loculated pericardial effusions that may not be within the time-motion echo's "ice pick" view of the heart. Intravenous carbon dioxide injection was a technique used to outline the right atrium and to allow the distance between the right atrial endocardial surface and heart border to be measured. If increased, pericardial effusion or thickening was the usual cause. *(Cecil, p. 304)*

29. (D) Tuberculous pericarditis is particularly likely to be associated with pericardial effusion, and the absence of effusion by echo is a highly significant negative finding. A negative skin test is also unusual, although it is possible with overwhelming infection. Clear lung fields are not at all unusual. It also is not unusual to have a negative stain and even a negative culture of pericardial fluid in the presence of documented tuberculous pericarditis. S-T segment elevation is a nonspecific finding. *(Cecil, pp. 301–303)*

30. (A) Systolic time intervals showing an increased PEP-LVET ratio are compatible with left ventricular dysfunction. The ratio is typically normal with constrictive pericarditis. The early diastolic sound is usually a pericardial knock, and an inspiratory rise in venous pressure (Kussmaul's sign) is seen in 40–50% of cases. *(Cecil, pp. 137, 305–306)*

31. (B) Although highly predictive of underlying thrombophlebitis, the presence of a tender cord is not a very sensitive sign (less than 20% of cases). Over 50% of patients with calf vein thrombophlebitis are asymptomatic. *(Cecil, p. 328)*

32. (E) Although all these noninvasive methods have helped in the evaluation of patients with suspected thrombophlebitis, none has achieved the diagnostic accuracy of venous angiography. Unfortunately, angiography itself may cause thrombophlebitis and it therefore is not a screening procedure. *(Cecil, pp. 328–329)*

33. (D) Patients undergoing retropubic prostatectomy and those with hip fractures or strokes have a 50% or greater incidence of venous thrombosis. The remaining patients are at increased risk for venous thrombosis in comparison with the rest of the population, but their risk is not as high as that of patient D. *(Cecil, pp. 328–329)*

34. (B) The hemodynamic consequences of a cardiac myxoma are the most frequent mode of presentation. For patients who are clinically symptomatic, vague systemic symptoms (e.g., fever, arthralgias, anemia) are the least likely method of presentation. Since "routine echos" should not be done on asymptomatic patients, this would be an unlikely way for a myxoma to present. *(Cecil, pp. 333–334)*

35. (D) Tetralogy of Fallot is the most common cyanotic congenital heart disease, and approximately 25% of such patients will have a right-sided aortic arch and descending aorta. *(Cecil, p. 308)*

36. (B) What to do with an asymptomatic abdominal aneurysm is sometimes a difficult decision. An aneurysm of this dimension, particularly in the absence of associated disease that would place the patient at a higher operative risk, should probably be repaired electively even though the patient is asymptomatic. The larger the aneurysm, the greater the wall tension and the more likely it is to rupture. Sometimes, impending rupture may be heralded by abdominal pain, but frequently the first evidence of rupture is severe pain and cardiovascular collapse. Close medical follow-up or simply awaiting symptoms may not be in the patient's best interest. Because of clot lining the aneurysm, abdominal aortography may be misleading, and the role of this technique, particularly with the availability of enhanced computerized tomography and/or ultrasound, has become controversial. *(Cecil, p. 310)*

37. (C) "Bad blood" is a lay term highly suggestive of syphilis. Pencillin was not available in 1938, and the injections were undoubtedly a series of heavy metals. This history plus the location of calcification in the aortic root is highly suggestive of syphilitic aortitis. The exertional chest pain may be from ostial involvement of the coronary arteries or concomitant coronary artery disease. *(Cecil, pp. 312–313)*

38. (B) The VDRL is positive in a high percentage of patients with syphilitic aortitis (98–99%), but it may be negative in older patients. Either the older TPI test or the more readily available FTA-ABS test are more likely to be positive in this clinical setting. Since there is no evidence of Marfan's syndrome, neither the measurement of urinary amino acids nor echocardiography of the mitral valve is likely to be helpful in diagnosis. Echocardiography of the aortic root may show the dilatation, as may aortography, but neither is likely to provide additional etiologic information. *(Cecil, p. 312)*

39. (C) Pain at rest is an ominous sign indicating that arterial blood supply is marginal even for the small metabolic demands of the skin. *(Cecil, pp. 316–317)*

40. (C) Quinidine, presumably by displacing digoxin from binding sites in body tissue and by reducing its renal clearance, has the potential of increasing the digoxin level, and would be contraindicated in this situation. The remaining therapies are all valid depending on the clinical situation. Life-threatening arrhythmias may be controlled with either lidocaine, phenytoin, or propranolol. Lidocaine is easiest to give, as phenytoin is dissolved in an alkaline vehicle and has to be given very slowly in a large-caliber vein, and propranolol may have an undesirable negative inotropic effect. *(Cecil, pp. 145–148, 149, 283–284; Doering)*

41. (C) Hypotension commonly occurs during the rapid intravenous administration of procainamide. Procainamide should be given in divided doses, and the blood pressure should be monitored frequently during administration. Procainamide slows conduction velocity in the Purkinje system and myocardium, and therefore may prolong the duration of the QRS complex. Complete heart block is a rare complication of procainamide administration, occurring in patients with advanced conduction system disease. *(Cecil, pp. 284–285)*

42. (E) With the exception of left ventricular enlargement, all these physical and laboratory findings can be found in both primary and secondary pulmonary hypertension. The presence of left ventricular enlargement would suggest that the pulmonary hypertension is due either to left-sided heart disease or a left-to-right shunt that, at one time, involved the left ventricle (e.g., PDA-VSD — patent ductus arteriosus-ventricular septal defect). Left ventricular enlargement, however, may resolve with the development of pulmonary vascular disease and therefore be absent later in the patient's course. *(Cecil, p. 217)*

43. (B); 44. (B) The electrocardiogram shows right bundle branch block with left anterior hemiblock along with Q waves in the anterior precordial leads and S-T segment elevation with T-wave inversions. These changes are compatible with an acute anterior myocardial infarction. The normal ECG six weeks ago indicates that the conduction disturbance is a result of the infarction and places the patient at high risk for complete heart block. Progression to higher degrees of AV block is typically sudden and may be catastrophic in that a stable ventricular escape rhythm may not supervene. A prophylactic transvenous pacemaker is indicated. If higher degrees of AV block do occur, even if normal conduction returns by the time of discharge, there are some data to suggest that a permanent transvenous pacemaker is indicated. *(Cecil, pp. 251–252)*

45. (E) Although embolization from the heart is not unexpected because of the associated incidence of coronary artery disease, such an event is not a complication of hypertension, per se. Hypertension does, however, speed the atherosclerotic process in the carotid arteries, and an ulcerated plaque is a very common cause of CNS embolization. *(Cecil, p. 229)*

46. (E) The patient is receiving an adequate dose of lidocaine, and lethargy is most likely a manifestation of lidocaine toxicity. Therefore, the lidocaine rate should not be increased. Intravenous digoxin may aggravate ventricular tachycardia and therefore should not be given. Intravenous phenytoin sodium is less effective than procainamide. Intravenous quinidine sulfate is associated with marked hypotension and is used only rarely in clinical practice. *(Cecil, pp. 273, 284–285)*

47. (A — True; B — False; C — True; D — False; E — True) The most important risk factor for rheumatic fever is a previous upper respiratory infection due to group A beta-hemolytic streptococci. The incidence of rheumatic fever and rheumatic heart disease is decreasing in the United States but continues at near-epidemic rates in developing countries. Crowded living conditions and poor nutrition (correlates of poor socioeconomic status) and a temperate climate are also important risk factors. Although glomerulonephritis may result from a prior group A beta-hemolytic streptoccal infection (most commonly of the pharynx but also of skin), the nephritogenic strains (mainly M type 12) do not appear to be rheumatogenic. Susceptibility to rheumatoid arthritis is unrelated to rheumatic fever. *(Cecil, p. 1452)*

48. (A — False; B — True; C— False; D — True; E — False) The mortality rate for cardiovascular disease emphasizes its importance as a continuing health problem. Although the decline in rheumatic heart disease became more precipitous after the introduction of antibiotics, it began before these drugs were available. The decline in cardiovascular mortality in the United States has been even more precipitous since 1970 and is in sharp contrast to the increasing mortality rates of other developed countries. There have been many favorable changes in the American lifestyle in the past 15 years (decrease in smoking, reduction in saturated fat consumption, increase in exercise, more widespread treatment of hypertension). Although all these changes in lifestyle have occurred in the setting of a decreasing cardiovascular mortality rate, it is difficult to prove a cause-effect relationship. *(Cecil, pp. 98, 101)*

49. (All are True) All these factors may be important in determining the blood levels resulting from the oral administration of a drug. For slowly absorbed drugs, gastrointestinal motility may become very important. For rapidly absorbed drugs, GI motility is less important. Hepatic removal or "first pass" elimination of orally administered drugs can sometimes be overcome by giving very large doses. The volume in which the drug is distributed is, of course, a very important factor determining the blood level. The two major mechanisms of drug clearance are hepatic metabolism (biliary excretion) and renal filtration (urinary secretion). The rate of these processes, which is usually proportional to the plasma concentration of the drug, may become important in determining drug blood levels. *(Cecil, pp. 48–51)*

50. (A — True; B — True; C — False; D — True; E — True; F — True; G — False) Type A personality has not yet been shown to be a *major* risk factor for coronary artery disease. Similarly, obesity does not have independent significance once associated diabetes, hypertension, and cholesterol levels are controlled. *(Cecil, pp. 100–101, 240–242)*

51. (A — True; B — False; C — False; D — False; E — True) Plasma LDL cholesterol levels appear to be primarily genetically determined, although diet can significantly alter them. In contrast, plasma HDL cholesterol levels are *inversely* related to the risk of coronary artery disease; they rise with modest alcohol ingestion, exercise, and weight loss. *(Cecil, pp. 100–101, 241–242)*

52. (A — True; B — False; C — True; D — True; E — True; F — False; G — False) The left ventricular filling pressure (preload), impedance to left ventricular emptying (afterload), the vigor of contraction (contractility), and the heart rate are the most important determinants of cardiac pump performance. The pericardium appears to play little role in normal ventricular function. Wall tension is determined by LV pressure and radius. Attempts by the heart to normalize wall tension may be an important stimulus to hypertrophy but they are not an important determinant of cardiac performance, per se. *(Cecil, pp. 102–103)*

53. (A — False; B — True; C — True; D — True; E — False; F — False) Dilatation and hypertrophy are interrelated compensatory mechanisms. A pure volume overload (e.g., aortic regurgitation) increases mass and chamber size. Total wall thickness changes little even though individual myocardial cells are hypertrophied. This is termed eccentric hypertrophy. In chronic pressure overload (e.g., aortic stenosis) a normal diastolic chamber dimension is maintained, whereas the wall thickens. This is termed concentric hypertrophy. Increased sympathetic nervous system activity is an early compensatory response that increases contractility and heart rate. Unfortunately, peripheral vascular resistance also increases and this usually counterbalances the beneficial effect of any increased inotropy. The reflex increase in heart rate is much more supportive of the cardiac output. Increased sympathetic nervous system activity may also cause ventricular ectopy and decreased renal blood flow, but these are deleterious side effects. The rise in central venous pressure is the result of congestive heart failure rather than a compensatory mechanism. *(Cecil, pp. 137–139)*

54. (A — True; B — False; C — False; D — True; E — True; F — False) Early ventricular diastolic compliance is, at least partially, an active process, but it is not an important determinant of oxygen consumption. Similarly, the metabolism of the sarcoplasmic reticulum, although important in cardiac function, is a minor determinant of oxygen consumption. Fiber shortening is dependent on preload, afterload, and the status of contractility, but is not a direct determinant of myocardial oxygen consumption. Heart rate, the status of contractility, and developed ventricular wall tension are important determinants of myocardial oxygen consumption; the last-named is the most important. *(Cecil, p. 139)*

55. (A — True; B — False; C — False; D — True; E — True) Patients placed on a normal maintenance dose (e.g., digoxin, 0.25 mg per day) will reach a steady state in approximately one week, and most patients can be safely and effectively "digitalized" by this method. The combination of angina, normal heart size, and digitalis therapy, by increasing myocardial oxygen consumption, may increase the severity of angina. A regularization of the ventricular response in a patient in chronic atrial fibrillation is not likely to be due to conversion to sinus rhythm. A more likely possibility is increased AV block and a regular escape (or, in this case, accelerated junctional) rhythm. When AV block and ectopy occur in a patient receiving digitalis, toxicity should be presumed until it is proved otherwise. Diuretics, by diminishing potassium stores, potentiate the effects of digitalis and enhance the likelihood of toxicity. *(Cecil, pp. 146–148, 283–284)*

56. (A — False; B — False; C — True; D — True; E — True) Although an arterial systolic blood pressure less than 90 mm Hg should alert one to the possibility of shock, it does not invariably identify the patient in shock; patients with pre-existent hypertension may be in shock with an even higher blood pressure. The absence of neck vein distention, particularly in a patient with acute coronary artery disease, is of no help. The other choices clearly identify a patient as having inadequate perfusion. *(Cecil, p. 155)*

57. (A — True; B — True; C — True; D — True; E — False) During this last stage of shock, the absorption of bacterial toxins causes the release of vasodilator polypeptides that cause a fall in peripheral vascular resistance. *(Cecil, p. 156)*

58. (A — False; B — True; C — True; D — True; E — True) Data on therapeutic windows are determined by trough or minimal concentrations, and it is therefore best to measure plasma levels just prior to the next dose or during a steady-state infusion. If the free, or unbound, drug is primarily responsible for the drug effects, variations in plasma protein binding may be very important sources of apparent differences in patient responses to therapy. Similarly, if metabolites of the drug exert a similar pharmacologic effect, they must be recognized and measured in order to interpret the response to drug therapy. Concomitant changes in serum electrolytes may be very important modifying factors in certain drug responses. A classic example is the development of digitalis toxicity with the advent of hypokalemia. For drugs that have an important renal clearance mechanism, the average daily maintenance dose may be calculated in proportion to the reduction in creatinine clearance. This holds true even for compounds that have an active tubular secretion elimination mechanism. *(Cecil, pp. 54–55)*

59. (A — True; B — True; C — True; D — False; E — False) In response to hypotension, renin is released from the kidney. The resulting formation of angiotensin causes arteriolar vasoconstriction and increased secretion of aldosterone, which promotes sodium and water retention. The role of vasopressin in shock is less clear, but it is a vasoconstrictor, and blood levels of vasopressin rise with hypotension. Bradykinin may have a role in the vasodilation associated with sepsis and anaphylaxis. Beta-endorphins may have a potent direct myocardial depressant effect in shock states, but do not affect vascular smooth muscle. *(Cecil, pp. 158–159)*

60. (A — True; B — True; C — True; D — False; E — False) Since the colloid osmotic pressure is the main determinant of intravascular volume, any decrease (a frequent finding in shock) facilitates the accumulation of fluids in the extracellular space. The combination of a decrease in the resistance of precapillary vessels with an increase in the resistance of the postcapillary venules (with or without a differential responsiveness of the two to catecholamines) contributes to transudation of fluid into the extracellular space. Vasoactive polypeptides released during shock contribute to increased vascular permeability. A rise in left atrial pressure would not occur with hypovolemia and has no role in extracellular fluid accumulation. *(Cecil, pp. 159–160)*

61. (A — True; B — True; C — False; D — True; E — True) The measurement of urinary output by catheter drainage provides a valid index of renal perfusion and the adequacy of response to therapy. Intra-arterial pressure monitoring also facilitates the assessment of blood pressure and its response to therapy. A central venous pressure monitor may be misleading in this setting as it does not provide a valid index of left ventricular filling pressure. A Swan-Ganz catheter, on the other hand, provides a valid index of left atrial filling (the pulmonary artery diastolic pressure is roughly equivalent to the pulmonary capillary wedge pressure, which in turn reflects the mean left atrial pressure). In the absence of associated mitral stenosis, any of these pressures reflect left ventricular filling pressure. A Swan-Ganz catheter may also be used to follow pulmonary artery oxygen saturations, and in combination with arterial blood gases, allows the calculation of cardiac output. Either O_2 saturations or blood gases would provide a sensitive index of the adequacy of the cardiac output and the patient's response to therapy. *(Cecil, p. 163)*

62. (All are True) All these choices are possible, although the unfavorable courses indicated by the latter three are more likely. *(Cecil, p. 174; Roberts)*

63. (All are True) These data are taken from the Boston Collaborative Drug Surveillance Program. Most drug reactions were self-limited and of little consequence in the course of primary illness. The patients at highest risk for serious drug reactions were those most severely ill. *(Cecil, p. 62)*

64. (A — False; B — True; C — False; D — True; E — True) Approximately 4–10% of patients with ventricular septal defects have associated aortic regurgitation due to loss of support for the aortic valve cusp whose base lies in close proximity to the defect in the membranous septum. About 10% of membranous subvalvular aortic stenoses are associated with aortic regurgitation — presumably because of a jet lesion distorting the aortic valve. The risk of developing aortic regurgitation is one rationale for surgical correction of this lesion when it is identified. Coarctation of the aorta has about a 25% incidence of associated bicuspid aortic valves. Such valves may be either stenotic or regurgitant. *(Cecil, pp. 175–176, 182; Perloff, pp. 112–113; 421–428)*

65. (A — False; B — True; C — False; D — True; E — False) Dominant V waves in the jugular venous pulse are typical of an atrial septal defect and are probably due to augmented right atrial filling. Since the atria form a common chamber, the accentuated V wave may also be due to transmission of the normally much higher left atrial V wave to the systemic venous pulse. In the Mayo clinic series, only two of 120 patients (2%) had a normal right ventricular dimension index. Eighty-seven per cent had abnormal septal wall motion. Thus, a completely normal echocardiogram is distinctly unusual with atrial septal defect. Although a systolic thrill at the upper left sternal edge might suggest concomitant valvular pulmonic stenosis, about one third of patients with atrial septal defects may have such a thrill owing to increased flow alone. Electrocardiographic left axis deviation is so much to be expected in ostium primum atrial septal defects that its absence is reason enough to discard the diagnosis. The incidence of atrial fibrillation begins to rise in the fourth decade. *(Cecil, p. 180; Radtke et al.)*

66. (A — True; B — False; C — True; D — True; E — False) The elderly, presumably because of diminished drug inactivation and clearance and changes in drug distribution, have an increased incidence of adverse drug reactions. Cirrhosis, particularly if severe, can impair drug clearance, resulting in prolonged and more severe adverse drug reactions. Hepatic disease also may result in hypoalbuminemia that in turn decreases plasma protein binding of some drugs, with a resultant potentiation of their effects. Renal insufficiency is perhaps the most common cause for decreased drug clearance. Many drugs also are nephrotoxic and contribute to a further depression of renal function. For reasons not clearly understood, women have a greater incidence of adverse drug reactions. Hypertension is not a risk factor. *(Cecil, pp. 62–63)*

67. (A — True; B — True; C — False; D — False; E — True) Endocarditis is extremely unusual in secundum atrial defects unless there is associated mitral valve disease. Similarly, a patient who has had a coronary AV fistula corrected should not be at risk for endocarditis. *(Cecil, pp. 180, 182, 185, 187)*

68. (A — False; B — True; C — False; D — True; E — True; F — False) Both Ebstein's anomaly and secundum atrial septal defect may be associated with accentuated tricuspid valve closure, paradoxical septal wall motion, and a mid-diastolic rumble along the lower left sternal edge. Atrial septal defects occasionally result in wide splitting of the first heart sound, but the split is rarely more than 0.06 seconds. In the adult, such splitting should raise the possibility of Ebstein's anomaly. Wolff-Parkinson-White (type B) patterns on electrocardiogram are much more common in Ebstein's anomaly than in atrial septal defect. A chest film showing increased pulmonary blood flow would be much more compatible with an atrial septal defect than with Ebstein's anomaly, where the problem may be obstruction to blood flow into either the right ventricle or the pulmonary outflow tract. When shunting occurs in Ebstein's anomaly, it is typically right-to-left, although an occasional patient with minimal hemodynamic dysfunction of the tricuspid valve may show increased pulmonary blood flow. *(Cecil, pp. 177, 180)*

69. (A — True; B — True; C — True; D — False; E — False; F—False) Ebstein's anomaly of the tricuspid valve is classically associated with normal or decreased pulmonary vascularity. Lutembacher's syndrome occurs when mitral stenosis combines with atrial septal defect; although there is increased pulmonary blood flow, such patients are not cyanotic. A double-outlet right ventricle is associated with cyanosis, but the pulmonary blood flow appears normal on chest film. *(Cecil, pp. 185–186)*

70. (A — False; B — True; C — False; D — True; E — True) In a patient with angina and a murmur suggestive of aortic stenosis (patient B) catheterization is indicated as a preliminary to surgery. In a patient of this age the study would also define the status of the coronary arteries. A patient with class III heart failure and rheumatic mitral valve disease (patient D) is a candidate for mitral valve replacement. The diastolic murmur may represent pulmonary hypertension or associated aortic regurgitation, and these possibilities must be evaluated. A patient with mitral regurgitation and class III congestive heart failure (patient E) is also a candidate for operative intervention. Although the status of left ventricular function appears to be an important prognostic variable, the relationship between preoperative ejection fraction and postoperative hemodynamic benefit is not "tight." Patients with clinical findings of aortic stenosis (patient A) usually are not candidates for catheterization until they develop symptoms or unless there is a dramatic change in heart size on chest film or echocardiogram. Current research is aimed at testing the utility of various noninvasive measurements of left ventricular function in helping to time surgical intervention appropriately for patients with aortic or mitral regurgitation. A patient with idiopathic hypertrophic subaortic stenosis, and particularly one who has responded to propranolol (patient C), does not need cardiac catheterization. Echocardiography can define the diagnosis, and there are even echocardiographic indices that roughly correlate with the degree of left ventricular output tract obstruction. Symptoms refractory to medical therapy might constitute an indication to proceed to perform cardiac catheterization in such a patient. *(Cecil, pp. 126–127)*

71. (A — True; B — False; C — True; D — False; E — True; F — True) Left heart failure is the most common cause of pulmonary hypertension. Tricuspid and pulmonary regurgitation are frequently the result of, rather than the cause of, pulmonary hypertension. Mitral stenosis, hepatic cirrhosis, and chronic obstructive pulmonary disease are all well-recognized causes of pulmonary hypertension. *(Cecil, pp. 196–197, 218–219)*

72. (A — False; B — False; C — True; D — False; E — False) A patient who has had an open commissurotomy and is in sinus rhythm is not a candidate for anticoagulation in the absence of documented embolic events. It is likely that the left atrial appendage, a common location for clots, would have been removed during surgery, thus adding further caution to the theoretic need for anticoagulant therapy. Porcine valves are associated with mild stenosis. Such patients therefore have a hemodynamic situation that is equivalent to mild mitral stenosis with atrial fibrillation. There is controversy concerning whether such patients, in the absence of documented previous embolic events, should be anticoagulated. Patients with Starr-Edwards prosthetic valves are at high risk for embolic events and should receive anticoagulants regardless of the valve model. Patients with pulmonary embolic disease in the setting of tricuspid valve endocarditis will most likely have septic emboli and are not candidates for anticoagulation therapy. Embolic events occur in patients with atrial fibrillation regardless of its etiology, but atrial fibrillation is such a common arrhythmia and the risk of embolism is so low that a universal recommendation to anticoagulate all patients with atrial fibrillation is not thought to be indicated. Patients with paroxysmal atrial fibrillation are more likely to have embolic events than those with chronic atrial fibrillation. *(Cecil, pp. 194, 197–198)*

73. (A — True; B — True; C — True; D — False; E — True) These symptoms are classic for pheochromocytoma, but the history should lead to a diligent search for prior treatment with MAO inhibitors and the possibility of clonidine withdrawal. MAO inhibitors potentiate the vasoconstrictor effects of α-adrenergic agents contained in typical cold preparations. Coarctation of the aorta is excluded by the normal examination. The patient may simply have essential hypertension, of course, although the postural drop in blood pressure is unusual. *(Cecil, pp. 231–232, 238)*

74. (A — True; B — True; C — False; D — True; E — False) G6PD-deficient individuals cannot manufacture NADPH, the major reducing compound of the red cell. These cells are therefore susceptible to oxidative stresses that result in the oxidation of ferrohemoglobin, glutathione, and the sulfhydryl groups of the globin chains of hemoglobin. The denatured hemoglobin forms precipitates (Heinz bodies) along the red cell membrane. The red cell becomes less deformable, leading to hemolysis and premature destruction. Sulfa drugs, antimalarials, and vitamin K are oxidant compounds capable of causing hemolysis. *(Cecil, pp. 64–65, 867)*

75. (All are True) Although all these observations have their correlates in the experimental laboratory or have been reported in hypertensive patients, none provides an unequivocal explanation for the pathophysiology of essential hypertension. *(Cecil, pp. 230–232)*

76. (All are True) About 2–5% of patients taking penicillin develop a hypersensitivity reaction that may be either immediate (e.g., anaphylaxis, urticaria) or delayed (e.g., serum sickness). The semisynthetic penicillins, in particular, have been associated with nephritis. *(Cecil, pp. 77–78)*

77. (A — True; B — True; C — True; D —False; E — True) With the exception of hydrops fetalis, all of these are common results of hypertension in pregnant patients. Adequate hypertensive control (mainly with methyldopa) can prevent most, if not all, of these complications. *(Cecil, pp. 227–228)*

78. (All are True) *(Cecil, pp. 227–228)*

79. (A — False; B — False; C — False; D — True; E — False) Of the listed choices, being male is the only proved risk factor for coronary artery disease. Although there is no question that exercise rehabilitation has a role in the treatment of patients with coronary artery disease and that being physically active is a reasonable recommendation for the public, proof that physical inactivity is a major risk factor for coronary disease is lacking. Similarly, there is little evidence that a high-cholesterol diet, per se, is a risk factor for coronary artery disease. Only a family history of premature coronary artery disease in *both* parents would be a risk factor. Hypertriglyceridemia, once diabetes, body weight, and cholesterol are controlled, is not an independent risk factor. *(Cecil, pp. 225, 241–242)*

80. (A — True; B — True; C — True; D — True; E — False) In western societies blood pressure rises with age. Heredity is also an important factor. There is no question that body weight correlates with blood pressure, but there is controversy as to whether weight loss itself or the concomitant reduction of salt intake that is part of a weight-loss diet contributes to the blood pressure lowering. Similarly, there is controversy over the role of salt intake in hypertension, but there is convincing epidemiologic evidence that salt does play a role and that salt restriction is a reasonable component of antihypertensive therapy. *(Cecil, pp. 224–225)*

81. (A — True; B — True; C — True; D — False; E — False) Peripheral edema could represent right-sided heart failure, a finding that is not specific for the etiology of the pulmonary hypertension. The high-frequency diastolic decrescendo murmur may represent pulmonary regurgitation, and again any cause of pulmonary hypertension could cause this lesion. The cephalization of pulmonary venous blood flow suggests left atrial hypertension and, when seen in concert with a diastolic rumble, suggests the presence of mitral stenosis. Cough and sputum production are typical of bronchitis and suggest that the pulmonary hypertension may be secondary to chronic pulmonary disease. *(Cecil, pp. 194, 215, 219–221)*

82. (A —True; B — True; C — True; D — True; E — False) Anything that decreases blood pressure can cause problems in these patients because of their inability to augment cardiac output owing to the obstruction of blood flow at the pulmonary vascular level. Lung biopsy would almost always induce pneumothorax, which can be disastrous in this entity. *(Cecil, pp. 215–216)*

83. (A — False; B — True; C — False; D — True; E — True) Arguments rage, but evidence that ACTH is superior to glucocorticosteroids in a number of diseases (including ulcerative colitis) is less than convincing. Dexamethasone is the most potent of the commonly used glucocorticosteroids (0.75 mg of dexamethasone equals 25 mg of cortisone). A patient with peptic ulcer disease should not receive glucocorticosteroids and, because of the salt and water retention associated with steroid use, hypertension is typically worsened. There is no convincing evidence that glucocorticosteroids are teratogenic. *(Cecil, pp. 86, 89)*

84. (A — True; B — False; C — True; D — True; E — True) With the exception of spontaneous remission, which is extremely rare (one reported case), all the other complications are common in patients with primary pulmonary hypertension. *(Cecil, pp. 216–217)*

85. (A — True; B — True; C — True; D — False; E — True) Cyanosis and clubbing usually are not part of the clinical presentation of primary pulmonary hypertension; their presence should suggest other etiologies such as primary lung disease or a shunt lesion. The diagnosis of multiple pulmonary emboli may be missed even with pulmonary angiography and found only on careful postmortem examination. Several recent reports have documented a significant drop in the pulmonary vascular resistance and increased cardiac output with vasodilators such as hydralazine. *(Cecil, pp. 213–216; Rubin and Peter)*

86. (A — False; B — True; C — True; D — False) The treatment of choice is oxygen while the affected individual is returned to sea level, where the pulmonary edema typically resolves in a very rapid fashion. Diuretics and digitalization have no role in treatment. *(Cecil, p. 213)*

87. (A — True; B — True; C — True; D — False; E — False) The role of the autonomic nervous system in controlling pulmonary vascular resistance has not been well documented, although it has been diligently sought. The effect of hypoxia on the pulmonary vascular resistance has been shown not to be mediated by histamine. *(Cecil, pp. 212–213)*

88. (A — True; B — True; C — False; D — False; E — False) Amyl nitrite drops peripheral vascular resistance (and blood pressure) without much effect on preload. The resultant tachycardia causes an increased cardiac output. The murmur of aortic regurgitation, and therefore the Austin Flint murmur, diminishes with amyl nitrite inhalation. The murmur of mitral stenosis increases because the tachycardia reduces the time available for left atrial emptying and because of the increase in cardiac output. All outflow murmurs increase with amyl nitrite, but the murmur of mitral regurgitation softens. The murmur of tricuspid regurgitation is quite variable, and therefore amyl nitrite may not help to differentiate tricuspid regurgitation from mitral regurgitation. The murmur of an AV fistula would soften, whereas right-sided outflow tract murmurs would increase. *(Cecil, pp. 200, 205; Dohan and Criscitiello)*

89 (A — False; B — True; C — False; D — False; E — True; F — False) Atrial fibrillation may occur with acute mitral regurgitation, but sinus rhythm is the rule. A fourth heart sound, particularly if loud and/or palpable, is distinctly unusual in chronic severe mitral regurgitation. A third heart sound and mid-diastolic murmur may occur with either. Pulmonary hypertension is expected in acute mitral regurgitation and is a relatively late finding in chronic regurgitation. Wide splitting of the second heart sound may occur with either. *(Cecil, pp. 198–200)*

90. (A — True; B — True; C — False; D — False; E — True; F — False) This patient has classic, stable angina pectoris and a history of treated hypertension. Most physicians would want to review an electrocardiogram and chest film in such a patient. The ECG provides a valuable baseline and may provide evidence of a previous unrecognized myocardial infarction or hypertensive cardiovascular disease. Screening chest films are no longer recommended, but in this patient roentgenography is indicated for baseline determination of heart size and to look for intracardiac calcifications, evidence of a previous myocardial infarction, the configuration of the aorta, and so forth. The indications for, and the timing of, the remaining tests are more controversial. The various types of exercise testing have three principal uses: (1) diagnosis; (2) prognosis; and (3) assessment prior to undertaking an exercise program. In this patient, exercise testing adds little to diagnosis because the pre-test likelihood of his having coronary artery disease is so great. The predictive accuracy of inexact tests (of which exercise testing is a classic example) is dependent on the population to which it is applied. When used in a population with a high prevalence of the condition being tested for, and given a reasonable sensitivity and specificity, the test will have a "good" performance characteristic (i.e., a high predictive accuracy). This performance characteristic of inexact tests and its obverse (i.e., in a population with a low prevalence of the condition being tested for, the test will have a lower predictive accuracy, even assuming reasonable sensitivity and specificity) is stated mathematically by Bayes' theorem, and limits the usefulness of such tests when used for diagnosis. The sensitivity, specificity, and predictive accuracy of radionuclide angiography pose the same problem but to a lesser degree (the sensitivity, specificity, and predictive accuracy are better). The other uses of exercise testing for prognosis and for prescribing exercise are more relevant to this patient. Radionuclide angiography provides a direct index of rest and exercise left ventricular performance (ejection fraction and wall motion) as compared with treadmill exercise testing, but whether this information significantly enhances the determination of prognosis and is worth the increased cost (double or triple depending on the type of RNA study) is a subject of current research. In this patient, exercise testing (and I have selected the cheaper treadmill method as the right answer) is indicated in order to help in his exercise prescription and to identify any potential hazards of exercise. The role of Holter monitoring at this point is a matter of clinical judgment. The patient has a stable 15-year history of palpitations, and the indications for treating arrhythmias discovered by Holter monitoring in this clinical setting are controversial. *(Cecil, pp. 245, 284–285; McNeer et al.; Rifkin and Hood)*

91. (A — False; B — False; C — True; D — True; E — False) There is "ischemic" S-T segment depression of 0.25 millivolts (note the double standard) in the lateral precordial leads in stage I of the Bruce protocol. This is an "early positive exercise test" and correlates with a 25–35% incidence of main left three-vessel coronary artery disease. In this patient, with a classic history of angina pectoris and the early and striking degree of changes, the test is extremely unlikely to be falsely positive but, as previously discussed, it adds little to the diagnosis. Although the absence of pain with exercise is of some theoretic concern in that the patient's "body alarm" system is not sounding, there are no studies documenting the validity of this concern. Although this early positive response demands attention, we should not lose sight of the fact that the clinical syndrome is stable and there is no need for emergency cardiac catheterization. Most cardiologists, however, would advise elective cardiac catheterization to define this patient's coronary anatomy followed by surgery if significant main left coronary artery disease or three-vessel coronary artery disease is detected *(McNeer et al.; Rifkin and Hood)*

92. (A — False; B — False; C — False; D — False; E — True) The rhythm strip shows multifocal premature ventricular contractions (PVCs). Since such arrhythmias are frequently absent in patients with coronary artery disease and may be present in those without coronary artery disease, they cannot be used as criteria for interpreting an exercise test. Whether or not this patient should receive antiarrhythmic therapy in addition to the propranolol is controversial. The patient is clinically stable with many years of palpitations. Antiarrhythmic therapy is expensive and associated with side effects, and the quinidine-like drugs (quinidine, procainamide, disopyramide), particularly in the setting of a long Q-T interval, have even been incriminated as a cause of sudden death. I would need more information before undertaking additional antiarrhythmic therapy. In patients with coronary artery disease, arrhythmias correlate most closely with the degree of left ventricular dysfunction, which in turn is a rough correlate of the extent of coronary artery disease. PVCs of this type in the setting of coronary artery disease and normal left ventricular function carry little additional prognostic significance. There is nothing about this exercise test result that contraindicates an exercise program, particularly in the setting of close monitoring, but most physicians would feel more comfortable deferring such a program until after the catheterization has excluded left main coronary artery disease. *(Cecil, pp. 246, 264, 284–285; Califf et al.)*

93. (All are True) Depending on maturity, atherosclerotic plaques may contain all of these elements as well as phospholipids, dead and dying cells, collagen, and various other other lipoproteins. *(Cecil, pp. 239–240)*

94. (A — False; B — False; C — False; D — True; E — True; F — True) The history is typical of Prinzmetal's variant angina with coronary artery spasm. The Holter monitor recording confirms the diagnosis, with dramatic S-T segment elevation indicating transmural ischemia with epicardial injury secondary to spasm of a proximal coronary artery. The ventricular arrhythmias (note the run of ventricular tachycardia at 3 AM) are also quite typical. Cardiac catheterization showed normal coronary arteries at rest, with inducible vasospasm of the left anterior descending coronary artery. Repeat exercise testing, with or without various types of radionuclide imaging, probably has little to offer in the management of this patient. In the United States 10–20% of patients with Prinzmetal's angina have no underlying occlusive coronary artery disease. With a clinical history such as this patient's, the incidence of normal coronary arteries is probably even higher. In Japan, it may approach 40–50%. A repeat Holter monitor may show similar S-T segment changes without any symptoms presumably related to vasospasm of differing severity. *(Cecil, pp. 244–245)*

95. (A — True; B — False; C — True; D — False; E — False) Various nitrate preparations continue to be effective in relieving vasospasm. Nifedipine, a calcium channel blocker, is probably the treatment of choice, particularly if the clinical syndrome is due entirely to vasospasm. Coronary artery surgery has not been particularly helpful in patients with isolated spasms, possibly because the spasm may involve the entire extent of the coronary artery. If, however, there is a combination of plaque and vasospasm, coronary artery surgery may be helpful. Similarly, the indications for or against angioplasty would depend on the underlying coronary artery anatomy. *(Cecil, pp. 245–247, 259)*

96. (A — False; B — True; C — True; D — True; E — False) Carotid sinus massage typically slows the ventricular rate by speeding the atrial rate (acetylcholine shortens the refractory period of atrial tissue) and through vagal effects on the AV node. Conversion to normal sinus rhythm, however, is unusual. Although it has been reported, atrial flutter as a toxic manifestation of digitalis is unlikely. Digitalis toxicity may occur during attempts to control the ventricular rate. This is particularly likely when the patient's atrial rate does not increase in response to digitalis. Relatively large doses of digitalis are then required to produce AV block, and the possibility of toxicity is enhanced. Low-energy direct current cardioversion and atrial pacing are both likely to restore sinus rhythm. Quinidine, by slowing the atrial rate and enhancing AV node conduction, may increase the ventricular response, sometimes with catastrophic consequences. *(Cecil, pp. 269–270, 284)*

97. (A — True; B — True; C — True; D — False; E — True) Myocardial fiber disarray has been reported in other cardiac diseases, mainly congenital heart disease with pressure overload of the right side of the heart. An echocardiographic study of relatives of patients with documented IHSS showed that it was familial with the genetic characteristics described. Preoperatively, systolic anterior motion of the mitral valve correlates very well with the presence of a gradient. Postoperatively, however, systolic anterior motion may persist in the absence of a gradient. The mitral regurgitation typically resolves after myectomy, even when the preoperative outflow gradient was relatively mild. The electrocardiogram in IHSS typically shows left ventricular hypertrophy with abnormal initial forces reflecting abnormal septal activation; it can simulate the electrocardiographic appearance of myocardial infarction. *(Cecil, pp. 291–292)*

98. (All are True) All these agents are potentially toxic to the heart. Intravenous alcohol causes a measurable deterioration in cardiac function even in normal volunteers. Cobalt added in minuscule amounts to beer as a stabilizing agent for the foam in 1965 caused a very distinctive acute cardiomyopathy associated with polycythemia and hypothyroidism. In a model of epidemiologic detective work, cobalt was determined to be the offending agent. Its removal was associated with the end of the cardiomyopathy epidemic. *(Cecil, pp. 290, 296–297, 297–300)*

99. (A — True; B — True; C — False; D — True; E — False) *(Cecil, pp. 307–308)*

100. (A — True; B — True; C — False; D — True; E — True) Passive rewarming subjects the damaged part to the least trauma. Vasoconstriction is an important contributing factor in both entities. Sympathectomy may be of some help acutely for frostbite (if the timing of the surgery is appropriate) and, with immersion foot, may help attenuate long-term sequelae. Since it may take a considerable time for healthy and damaged tissue to demarcate, a conservative operative approach is indicated. *(Cecil, pp. 325–327)*

101. (A — False; B — True; C — True; D — False; E — True) Thrombocytopenia with heparin therapy may be an immunologic phenomenon, but regardless of its mechanism the occurrence of thrombocytopenia is an indication to stop heparin therapy. *(Cecil, p. 330)*

102. (A — False; B — True; C — True; D — True; E — False) In the absence of sepsis, antibiotics have no role in superficial thrombophlebitis. *(Cecil, pp. 330–331)*

103. (All are True) There is controversy over the likelihood of continuing hypertension following repair, but it does appear to be more likely the older the patient is at the time of operation. An aneurysm may form at the suture line, and with the high incidence of concomitant bicuspid aortic valve, the subsequent occurrence of aortic stenosis and/or aortic regurgitation is not unusual. Paraplegia may result in patients who have a mild coarctation and inadequately developed collateral circulation. With cross-clamping of the aorta during operation, blood flow to the descending aorta may be severely limited. Normal longevity, of course, is also a likely possibility. *(Cecil, p. 308; Rudolph, pp. 358–359)*

104. (A — False; B — True; C — True; D — True; E — True) Dissections originating distal to the aortic arch are most likely to respond to medical therapy; operative repair can be done at a more remote, elective time. When the dissection is bleeding, causing congestive heart failure, causing continued pain, or occurring in the absence of hypertension, early operative intervention is probably indicated despite the attendant risks. *(Cecil, p. 314)*

105. (A — True; B — True; C — True; D — True; E — False; F — True) With the exception of vasodilator drugs, all these modalities have a role in the treatment of arteriosclerosis obliterans. There is little objective evidence that vasodilator drug therapy relieves intermittent claudication or favorably affects blood flow in the affected extremity. *(Cecil pp. 317–318)*

106. (A — True; B — False; C — True; D — True; E — True; F — True) *(Cecil, pp. 316–321, 322–324)*

107. (A — False; B — True; C — False; D — False; E — True) By convention, Raynaud's disease is a term reserved for paroxysmal ischemia of the digits induced by cold or emotional stimuli. The etiology is unknown. A history of exposure to polyvinyl chloride or signs and symptoms suggestive of collagen vascular disease removes it from the idiopathic category or "disease," and the vasospasm is termed Raynaud's phenomenon. Lumbar sympathetic ganglionectomy typically gives complete relief. The response to vasodilator therapy is usually less than dramatic. There is optimism that the newer calcium blocking drugs (e.g., nifedipine) may be effective, but results are still preliminary. *(Cecil, pp. 322–323)*

108. (A — True; B — False; C — False; D — False; E — False) Although pleural effusion may occur with either isolated right or left ventricular failure, it is much more common when high venous pressures in both the pulmonary and systemic circulations impair the removal of fluid from the pleural space. The occurrence of a pleural effusion with cor pulmonale should raise the suspicion of another cause for the effusion. Early left heart failure causes a rise in pulmonary venous pressure, but CVP may remain normal. Intravascular blood volume goes up in congestive heart failure, but to a modest extent (approximately 50% in severe heart failure). Fatigue and weakness, notoriously nonspecific symptoms, may occur with either isolated right or left ventricular failure, particularly when there is poor cardiac output. *(Cecil, pp. 133–135, 136–137, 139)*

109. (All are False) Most young athletes who die suddenly have hypertrophic cardiomyopathy. Aortic rupture, myocarditis, coronary artery anomalies, and, infrequently, coronary artery disease account for the remainder. Most survivors of near sudden death do not evolve a myocardial infarction and appear to be at higher risk for subsequent sudden death than those who do. Although sudden death and mitral valve prolapse have been reported, documented instances (particularly given the high prevalence of the condition in the United States population) are rare. Prevention of sudden death with antiarrhythmic therapy, although a laudable goal, is frequently elusive. Current research efforts center around the efficacy of electrophysiologic testing of high-risk patients in order to tailor their antiarrhythmic therapy and to obtain some estimate of the likelihood of success. *(Cecil, pp. 256–257)*

110. (A); 111. (D); 112. (E) *(Cecil, p. 224)*

113. (E); 114. (F); 115. (D); 116. (C); 117. (A) 113. The Rauwolfia alkaloids are associated with a small but definite incidence of significant depression, even when used in low doses. On the other hand, reserpine is cheap and is also one of the three antihypertensive agents used in the Veterans Administration trial, the study that provides the best evidence of the salutary effects of antihypertensive treatment. **114.** The main side effect of guanethidine is postural hypotension, but there is a definite incidence of the inhibition of ejaculation. **115.** Methyldopa is converted to methyl-norepinephrine before it exerts its centrally mediated antihypertensive effect via the stimulation of alpha-receptors in the brain stem. Unfortunately, this also causes slowing of the heart rate and sedation. In some patients, this side effect may decrease with time. **116.** Propranolol, a beta-blocker, is generally well tolerated but, by blocking beta-receptor–mediated smooth muscle relaxation, may cause bronchospasm. The combination of arterial vasoconstriction and a reduced cardiac output may contribute to the occasional worsening of claudication that has been reported. **117.** The thiazide diuretics invariably cause hyperuricemia via a reduction in the renal clearance of uric acid. The thiazides also reduce urinary calcium excretion and cause a small rise in serum calcium concentration. This usually is not clinically significant, and dramatic increases in the serum calcium level or failure of the calcium level to return to normal on the discontinuance of thiazide should raise the suspicion of another cause for the hypercalcemia. *(Cecil, pp. 151–152, 234–238, 1327)*

118. (C); 119. (A); 120. (C); 121. (E); 122. (E) 118. Hurler's syndrome is clinically associated with coronary artery disease, valvular heart disease, and endocardial fibroelastosis. Pathologically, the mitral valve is most likely to be involved. Mitral regurgitation is more likely than mitral stenosis, although the latter has been reported. Aortic regurgitation may also occur. **119.** Ankylosing spondylitis is a well-recognized cause of aortic regurgitation. Indeed, the presence or absence of this valvular lesion may be the prime determinant of longevity. **120.** An aneurysm involving either papillary muscle interfers with mitral valve coaptation and typically produces mitral regurgitation. **121.** Although drug addicts may have left-sided valvular endocarditis, the presence of right-sided endocarditis should inspire a diligent search for evidence of parenteral drug abuse. **122.** The carcinoid syndrome is classically associated with right-sided valvular lesions of which the most likely is tricuspid regurgitation. Pulmonic stenosis and tricuspid stenosis, however, are not unusual. *(Cecil, pp. 198, 206, 209–210, 1313; Krovetz et al.)*

123. (A); 124. (C); 125. (D); 126. (E); 127. (C) 123. Isolated aortic stenosis, tricuspid regurgitation, mitral regurgitation, and aortic regurgitation are unlikely to be due to previous rheumatic fever. Mitral stenosis with or without associated mitral regurgitation has a rheumatic etiology in 95% or more of cases. **125.** Mitral regurgitation is compatible with the longest latent period because of the very favorable hemodynamic situation created by the low-pressure atrial runoff. Aortic regurgitation is also compatible with a relatively long asymptomatic interval. **126.** Aortic regurgitation, because of the very large stroke volume following the compensatory pause of a premature ventricular contraction, is most likely to produce symptomatic palpitations in which the patient feels the augmented beat associated with this post-PVC contraction. **127.** Neck pulsations are most likely to be due to tricuspid regurgitation, although an occasional patient with aortic regurgitation may be aware of neck pulsations, and (very occasionally) patients with pulmonary hypertension and markedly accentuated A waves may become aware of venous pulsations in the neck. In men this is likely to be noted while shaving. *(Cecil, pp. 193–195, 199–200, 207–208, 210)*

128. (C); 129. (A); 130. (B); 131. (D) 128. Rubella in the first trimester is a known teratogen, with patent ductus arteriosus and peripheral pulmonic stenosis the most likely resulting heart diseases. **129.** A ventricular septal defect with associated aortic regurgitation mimics a continuous murmur by virtue of the holosystolic VSD murmur merging with the diastolic blowing murmur of aortic regurgitation. Typically, however, these murmurs are quite distinctive and the differentiation is not difficult. **130.** A coronary AV fistula may mimic, in virtually every way, patent ductus arteriosus. Hints that the continuous murmur is not due to PDA include an atypical location for the murmur, and peaking of the murmur in systole instead of around the time of S2. **131.** Anomalous origin of the left coronary artery from the pulmonary artery classically produces a lateral myocardial infarction pattern on electrocardiogram and, in infants, may cause congestive heart failure. An occasional patient, however, presents as an adult with ischemic chest pain. *(Cecil, pp. 182–185)*

132. (B); 133. (A); 134. (E); 135. (F); 136. (D); 137. (A) 132. Atrial septal defect classically produces 0.05- to 0.07-second splitting of the second heart sound. There may be some variation when documented by phonocardiography, but to the examining ear the second heart sound is split and fixed. **133.** A murmur at the upper left sternal edge should be judged by the company it keeps and, in particular, by the character of S2. Requirements for normality of S2 include normal inspiratory splitting of the second heart sound (defined by respiratory variation greater than 0.025 seconds), a pulmonary component that is softer than the aortic component at the upper left sternal edge (although, in children, P2 may be accentuated in the absence of pulmonary hypertension), and a sound that closes to within less than 0.04 seconds on expiration. In most patients the second heart sound becomes single on expiration, particularly if they are examined in the sitting position. **134.** In shunt patients with pulmonary vascular disease (Eisenmenger's syndrome), S2 becomes narrowly split with little or no respiratory variation and a markedly accentuated pulmonary component. **135.** The patient with mild valvular pulmonic stenosis may have an entirely normal second heart sound, but there may be exaggerated respiratory splitting of the second heart sound, particularly if there is poststenotic dilatation. **136.** Severe infundibular pulmonic stenosis, like severe valvular pulmonic stenosis, may produce very wide splitting of the second heart sound with a softened pulmonary component. Auscultation with the bell and light pressure over the upper left sternal edge is sometimes necessary to discern this soft pulmonary closure sound. **137.** Patients with mild-to-moderate supravalvular pulmonic stenosis may have an unremarkable second heart sound. *(Cecil, pp. 179–180; Perloff, pp. 9–10, 206–207, 297–300)*

138. (E); 139. (C); 140. (B); 141. (A); 142. (D) 138. In supravalvular aortic stenosis, the murmur is usually louder in the right neck, the opposite finding to that typical of valvular aortic stenosis. **139.** Discrete membranous subvalvular aortic stenosis carries a 10% incidence of associated aortic regurgitation. **140.** Valvular aortic stenosis, particularly in younger patients, is usually associated with a prominent aortic ejection sound. **141.** Muscular subvalvular aortic stenosis (IHSS or hypertrophic obstructive cardiomyopathy) invariably has a brisk carotid pulse that, on occasion, may be bifid. The normal pulse pressure helps to separate this entity from aortic regurgitation. **142.** If coarctation of the aorta involves the origin of the left subclavian artery, the left brachial pulse may be absent or diminished. *(Cecil, pp. 175–176, 182, 291; Perloff, pp. 81–113)*

143. (C); 144. (B); 145. (A); 146. (D); 147. (C) 143. Membranous subvalvular aortic stenosis is classically associated with a normal aortic root. In approximately 10% of cases, however, there is associated aortic regurgitation that may produce generalized dilatation of the entire thoracic aorta. **144.** Aortic regurgitation, particularly if severe, may also produce dilatation of the entire thoracic aorta. **145.** Valvular aortic stenosis is associated with localized poststenotic dilatation of the root alone. This is especially likely with congenital valvular aortic stenosis. **146.** With coarctation of the aorta, the dilated left subclavian artery, the coarctation itself, and localized poststenotic dilatation of thoracic aorta combine to form a "3" sign. With barium in the esophagus, the barium column is indented by these same structures, producing the "E" or reversed "3" sign of coarctation. **147.** Muscular subvalvular aortic stenosis (IHSS), like membranous subvalvular aortic stenosis, does not alter the aortic root. Associated hypertension is common, however, and can affect the radiographic appearance of the thoracic aorta. *(Cecil, pp. 175–176, 182, 204, 208, 291, 308)*

148. (B); 149. (C); 150. (D); 151. (A); 152. (E) 148. A bruit is present in a high percentage of patients with renal arterial stenosis, although its absence does not exclude the possibility of this diagnosis. **149.** Although not all patients with pheochromocytoma are thin, weight gain is distinctly unusual, and weight loss is the rule. **150.** Cushing's syndrome is commonly associated with diabetes and skin changes, including striae. **151.** Coarctation of the aorta is a clinical diagnosis with a continuous murmur that may originate either at the site of the coarctation or over the collateral intercostal arteries. **152.** Hyperaldosteronism is associated with hypokalemia and hypernatremia. *(Cecil, pp. 232–234)*

153. (B); 154. (C); 155. (E); 156. (D); 157. (A) 153. Chloramphenicol, by inhibiting hepatic enzymes that metabolize warfarin, can potentiate the anticoagulant effects of warfarin and cause bleeding. **154.** The combination of calcium chloride and sodium bicarbonate leads to the formation of calcium carbonate, an insoluble precipitate formed by chemical bonding. **155.** Phenylbutazone, by displacing warfarin from albumin, may markedly potentiate the anticoagulant effects of warfarin and cause clinically significant bleeding. **156.** Phenothiazines are bound by antacid preparations, which leads to decreased absorption. **157.** Phenobarbital induces hepatic enzymes that metabolize and diminish the effects of warfarin. Therefore, the addition of phenobarbital to the regimen of a patient already taking warfarin typically results in a larger requirement for warfarin in order to maintain a suitable state of anticoagulation. If the patient is already taking warfarin and phenobarbital, the discontinuance of the latter is typically associated with a diminished requirement for the former. Occasionally, the potentiation of the warfarin effects may be associated with significant bleeding. *(Cecil, pp. 58–59)*

158. (B); 159. (C); 160. (D); 161. (E) 158. The thiazide diuretics are associated with increased excretion of salt and water, with a secondary contraction of the extracellular and plasma fluid volume. This is associated initially with a reduction in cardiac output. Long-term treatment, however, is usually associated with a restoration of blood volume and cardiac output, but with a continuing antihypertensive effect. This fall in peripheral vascular resistance appears to be mediated by changes in the salt content of the arteriolar vessel wall, but the precise mechanism of action remains to be defined. **159.** Propranolol, a beta-blocker, reduces cardiac output, inhibits renin release, blocks central sympathetic receptors, and blocks the presynaptic receptors of adrenergic nerve endings. Although this is controversial, the predominant antihypertensive effect of beta-blockers is probably mediated by a reduction in cardiac output in concert with a blunting of the baroreceptor-mediated increase in peripheral vascular resistance. **160.** Methyldopa, by means of stimulation of central nervous system alpha-receptors, decreases CNS sympathetic activity. **161.** Hydralazine acts directly on the arteriolar wall to cause vasodilatation and a decrease in peripheral vascular resistance. *(Cecil, pp. 234–236)*

162. (F); 163. (D); 164. (C); 165. (C); 166. (E); 167. (E) 162. Propranolol, a beta-blocker, decreases contractility and may cause a small rise in preload with no significant change in afterload in the normotensive patient. **163.** Nitroprusside is primarily an arteriolar vasodilator and therefore has its effects primarily on afterload, with a secondary drop in preload particularly if preload was elevated to begin with. **164. and 165.** Digoxin and paroxysmal atrial tachycardia (the latter via the Bowditch effect of increased inotropy with increases in heart rate) increase the contractility of both normal and diseased hearts. **166. and 167.** The nitrates are primarily venous vasodilators and have their effects on preload. *(Cecil, pp. 135–137, 145–151)*

168. (D); 169. (A); 170. (E); 171. (B); 172. (B); 173. (C) Beta$_1$-adrenergic receptors mediate the cardiac responses to sympathetic stimulation; beta$_2$-adrenergic receptors mediate smooth muscle relaxation in the arteriolar and bronchial walls. Alpha$_1$-adrenergic receptors mediate arteriolar vasoconstriction; alpha$_2$-adrenergic receptors mediate platelet aggregation and inhibit norepinephrine release from presynaptic nerve terminal. Dopaminergic receptors mediate renal and mesenteric arteriolar vasodilatation. *(Cecil, pp. 66–67)*

174. (B); 175. (A); 176. (E); 177. (C) 174. Kerley's B lines, particularly if greater than 2 cm in length and extending to the lateral chest wall, are associated with chronic pulmonary venous hypertension that is typically greater than or equal to 20 mm Hg. **175.** Well-compensated severe chronic aortic regurgitation is typically associated with cardiomegaly (as defined by cardiothoracic ratio greater than 55%) with no radiographic findings suggestive of congestive heart failure. On the lateral view, this cardiomegaly can be shown to be due primarily to left ventricular dilatation. **176.** Cardiac calcifications (including valvular, myocardial, coronary, and pericardial) are best detected by cardiac fluoroscopy. **177.** In early left-sided congestive heart failure, cephalization of pulmonary blood flow occurs as a result of distention and recruitment of upper lobe vessels that is, in turn, due to diversion of blood flow from the constricted lower-lobe pulmonary vessels. *(Cecil, pp. 112, 195–196, 208)*

178. (E); 179. (F); 180. (D); 181. (G); 182. (B); 183. (I) Volume expansion (e.g., fluids) or depletion (e.g., diuretics, bleeding) moves patients up and down on the same ventricular function curve. Responses **E** and **F** identify such volume changes in patients with normal ventricular function. Response **D** identifies a patient with normal ventricular function whose peripheral vascular resistance (an index of afterload) has decreased. The generalized vasodilatation, in the absence of fluid replacement, shifts the patient to a new ventricular function curve, but because of the concomitant drop in preload the stroke volume and cardiac output may fall. Response **G** identifies a patient with abnormal resting ventricular function who is given volume expansion; stroke volume and cardiac output increase. Response **B** identifies the shift in ventricular function that occurs in a patient with abnormal resting ventricular function who is placed on a vasodilator. The decrease in afterload causes a rise in stroke volume, and secondarily a drop in preload. The opposite results (response **I**) occur when a patient with abnormal ventricular function is given a pure alpha-stimulator (phenylephrine). The afterload rises in association with a diminution in stroke volume, and secondarily a rise in filling pressure. *(Cecil, pp. 102–104, 149–151)*

184. (B); 185. (C); 186. (E); 187. (A); 188. (F); 189. (D) 184. In a patient with chest pain and an irregular rapid pulse, a 12-lead electrocardiogram accomplishes the dual goals of identifying abnormal initial forces and S-T segments and documenting rhythm status. **185.** In a patient with left bundle branch block and atypical chest pain, rest and exercise radionuclide angiography may help define the probability that coronary artery disease is or is not the cause. **186.** In a patient with changing murmurs, echocardiography can provide early identification of intracardiac mass lesions such as tumors or vegetations. **187.** Although the role of phonocardiography in the evaluation of suspected heart disease has come under some criticism, its ability to provide temporal resolution of events in the cardiac cycle is unrivaled. **188.** For patients with coronary artery disease and syncope, Holter monitoring should be undertaken to evaluate significant arrhythmias as a potential cause. **189.** Although controversy continues about exactly when to perform cardiac catheterization and whom to perform it on, most would agree that a relatively young man receiving beta-blockers and nitrates who still has class IV angina is a candidate for cardiac catheterization as a preliminary to consideration for coronary artery bypass surgery. *(Cecil, pp. 116–117, 123–126; Craige)*

190. (A); 191. (B); 192. (D); 193. (E); 194. (A) Propranolol and timolol are nonselective beta-blocking agents. When used to treat angina or hypertension, they may cause unwanted bronchospasm. Metoprolol is a relatively selective beta$_1$-blocker that, in low doses, is not associated with bronchospasm. Unfortunately, higher doses of the drug are frequently required, and significant beta$_2$-blockade then ensues. Phentolamine is a nonselective alpha-adrenergic blocker. Prazosin is a selective alpha$_1$-blocker that results in vasodilatation. *(Cecil, pp. 66–67)*

195. (A); 196. (C); 197. (B); 198. (D); 199. (A); 200. (A); 201. (F) 195. The powerful "loop" diuretics are by far the most likely to cause severe electrolyte imbalance. **196.** Agranulocytosis is most likely to result from the organomercurial diuretics, and very rarely results from the potassium-sparing diuretics. **197.** The thiazide diuretics cause hypercalcemia by diminishing urinary calcium excretion and possibly by other, as yet undefined, mechanisms. **198.** All the diuretics with the exception of the aldosterone antagonists cause hypokalemia, but triamterene may cause hyperkalemia, particularly in patients with underlying renal disease. **199.** Furosemide produces hypercalciuria and, in combination with isotonic sodium chloride infusion, is used to treat symptomatic hypercalcemia. **200.** The rapid intravenous administration of either ethacrynic acid or furosemide has been reported to cause deafness. **201.** The aldosterone antagonists (in particular, spironolactone) at high dosages produce reversible gynecomastia. *(Cecil, pp. 152 [Table 6], 234)*

202. (E); 203. (A); 204. (A); 205. (F); 206. (C); 207. (B) 202. In the Holt-Oram syndrome, the thumb is hypoplastic and often has an accessory phalanx (although occasionally the thumb may be completely absent), and there is hypoplasia of the radius. In this syndrome, ASD may be inherited in an autosomal dominant pattern. **203 and 204.** Prematurity is associated with both ventricular septal defect and patent ductus arteriosus. The latter probably results from decreased cholinergic innervation and reduced constrictor response to oxygen of the ductus arteriosus. A PDA may persist for as long as four to six months postpartum before closing spontaneously. The increased incidence of ventricular septal defect in premature infants is probably due to the fact that the normal terminal phase of the fusion of the endocardial cushion has not yet occurred. **205.** Aortic valve disease, although not exclusively a disease of men, has a well-known male predominance. **206.** Turner's syndrome is most likely to be associated with coarctation of the aorta, although valvular pulmonic stenosis has also been reported. **207.** Down's syndrome is particularly likely to be associated with a complete endocardial cushion defect, and more rarely with an isolated septal defect of the endocardial cushion type. *(Cecil, p. 169; Perloff, pp. 152, 352)*

208. (C); 209. (D); 210. (A); 211. (B) Congenitally corrected transposition of the great vessels is associated with an increased incidence of congenital AV block, which when present produces the typical findings of AV dissociation. More commonly, however, such patients may have incompetence of the systemic AV valve (morphologic tricuspid valve) because of associated Ebstein's anomaly of the tricuspid valve. The loud S_2 results from malposition of the aorta such that it is anterior and just underneath the chest wall. The reversal of the stomach bubble position identifies inversion of the abdominal viscera, a necessary component of situs inversus. Cor triatriatum may produce a picture clinically indistinguishable from mitral stenosis. This disorder is usually detected in childhood, but occasionally symptoms do not appear until adulthood. *(Cecil, pp. 172–174; Perloff, pp. 47–51, 66–68)*

212. (E) This electrocardiogram shows normal sinus rhythm with first-degree AV block and pathologic Q waves with S-T segment elevation and T-wave inversion in leads II, III, AVF, and V_6 characteristic of a diaphragmatic lateral myocardial infarction. The prominent wide R waves in V_1-V_2 and the S-T segment depression in V_1 reflect true posterior involvement (i.e., they are the reciprocal changes of the Q waves and S-T segment elevation that would be recorded over the posterior surface of the heart). The first-degree AV block, in the absence of QRS prolongation, reflects increased vagal tone and/or AV node ischemia. Ninety per cent of AV node arteries arise from the right coronary artery, suggesting that occlusion of this patient's dominant right coronary artery explains the location of the myocardial infarction and AV block. The symptoms, which suggest a gastrointestinal etiology, are particularly likely when infarction involves this region of the heart. *(Cecil, pp. 249–251)*

213. (A) The lack of salt restriction in combination with thiazide therapy is particularly likely to cause hypokalemia via enhanced sodium-potassium exchange in the distal tubule. This electrocardiogram shows sinus bradycardia, first-degree AV block, and a nonspecific intraventricular conduction disturbance. The prominent S-T segment sagging is probably due to digitalis, and the low T waves and prominent U waves are typical of hypokalemia. This patient's serum potassium was 2.2 mEq/L. *(Cecil, p. 152)*

214. (B) This electrocardiogram shows sinus bradycardia and symmetric T-wave inversion in I, II, AVL, and V_4-V_6. These T-wave changes resolved completely in a second ECG obtained ten minutes later; they therefore were due to reversible left ventricular ischemia and correlate well with this patient's transient bout of angina. *(Cecil, pp. 245, 249–250)*

215. (D) This electrocardiogram shows normal sinus rhythm with right bundle branch block and right axis deviation of the initial 0.08 seconds of the QRS, reflecting concomitant left posterior hemiblock. Such conduction disturbances are found with increasing frequency in older patients and may be due to any one of a number of degenerative conditions associated with aging such as coronary artery disease, idiopathic fibrosis of the conduction system (Lenegre's disease), calcification of the cardiac skeleton (Lev's disease), or calcification of adjacent valvular structures. The small Q waves in leads II, III, and AVF are due to the posterior hemiblock, and not to previous infarction. These conduction disturbances commonly appear in an asymptomatic patient. *(Cecil, p. 117; Rosenbaum et al. pp. 121–130, 138–155)*

216. (C) This electrocardiogram shows a P-R interval of from 0.12 seconds (lead I) to 0.16 seconds (lead II) and a delta wave (leads I and V_4-V_6) identifying an accessory conduction pathway (i.e., Wolff-Parkinson-White syndrome). The orientation of the delta wave superiorly, anteriorly, and to the left causes the "pseudo"-Q waves in leads II, III, and AVF that may be mistaken for a diaphragmatic myocardial infarction. In some leads (e.g., II) the P-R interval appears longer because of the increased duration of the P wave as a result of the patient's associated mitral regurgitation. The absence of a short P-R interval in this patient is therefore explained by the prolonged intra-atrial conduction time. Note, however, that the terminal portion of the P wave virtually merges with the delta wave (e.g., leads V_5-V_6) typical of the W.-P.-W. syndrome. This patient's symptoms suggest a re-entry arrhythmia that, in this electrocardiographic setting, is most likely AV junctional re-entry or reciprocation (so-called paroxysmal atrial tachycardia). The impulse utilizes the normal antegrade pathway but then conducts retrograde through the accessory pathway, re-enters the atrium, and initiates a reciprocating tachycardia utilizing the AV node, ventricular conduction system (antegrade), and accessory pathway (retrograde). Typically, the delta wave is lost during this arrhythmia because it is now activated late in the cardiac cycle in a retrograde fashion. *(Cecil, pp. 275–278)*

217. (B) This film (p. 39) is within normal limits. The most likely cause for this patient's collapse is heat syncope or heat dehydration with heat exhaustion. *(Cecil, p. 109, Figs. 1 and 2)*

218. (D) This patient's history is compatible with previous rheumatic fever. The chest film (p. 40) shows a calcified mitral valve (lateral view—open arrows) along with left atrial enlargement (the "double density" [open arrow] and the dilated left atrial appendage [closed arrow] on the PA film, and the enlarged atrium [closed arrows] on the lateral film). These findings are typical of rheumatic mitral stenosis with or without associated mitral regurgitation. *(Cecil, pp. 111 [Fig. 11], 112 [Fig. 12], 193, 195–196)*

219. (A) This film (p. 39) shows left ventricular enlargement with a calcified left ventricular aneurysm (note rim of calcification on the lateral view), which is compatible with this patient's history of a previous myocardial infarction. Congestive heart failure and ventricular arrhythmias are two common sequelae of such aneurysms. This patient also had a transvenous pacemaker placed for symptomatic sinus bradycardia. *(Cecil, pp. 112, 251)*

220. (C) This film (p. 40) shows evidence of a pericardial effusion with cardiomegaly on the PA view and inward displacement of the subepicardial fat line on the lateral view (arrows). The pericardial effusion is most likely a cardiovascular complication of mediastinal irradiation. Radiation-induced effusions may occur anytime from immediately to as late as several years after such treatment. Most appear within three to 12 months. *(Cecil, pp. 110 [Fig. 8], 112, 304)*

221. (E) This film (p. 41) shows generalized cardiomegaly typical of a cardiomyopathy. In addition, there is hilar vascular congestion and cephalization typical of congestive heart failure with early pulmonary edema, explaining the patient's recent deterioration. *(Cecil, pp. 289–290)*

222. (B) These clinical findings are typical of a pulmonary hypertension with right ventricular hypertrophy. The absence of a left ventricular impulse is highly significant and places possible etiologies proximal to the left ventricle.

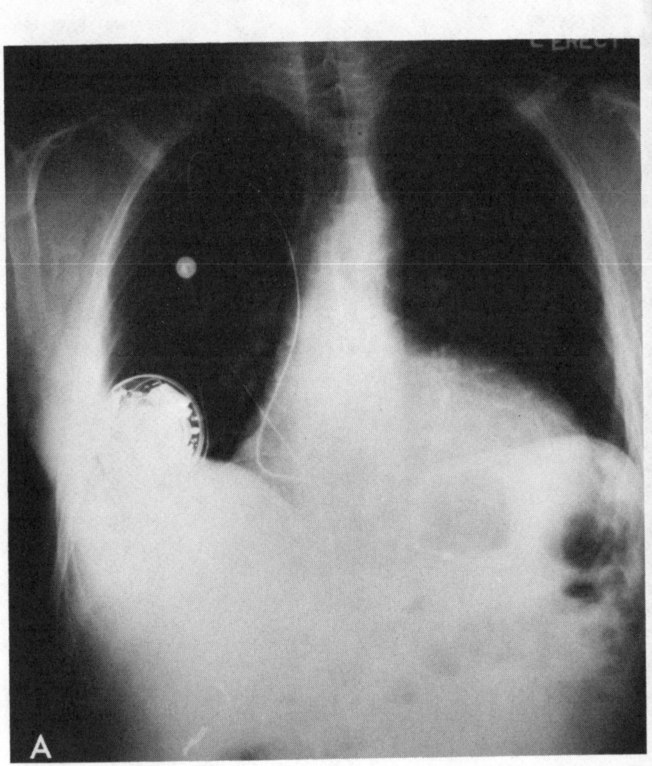

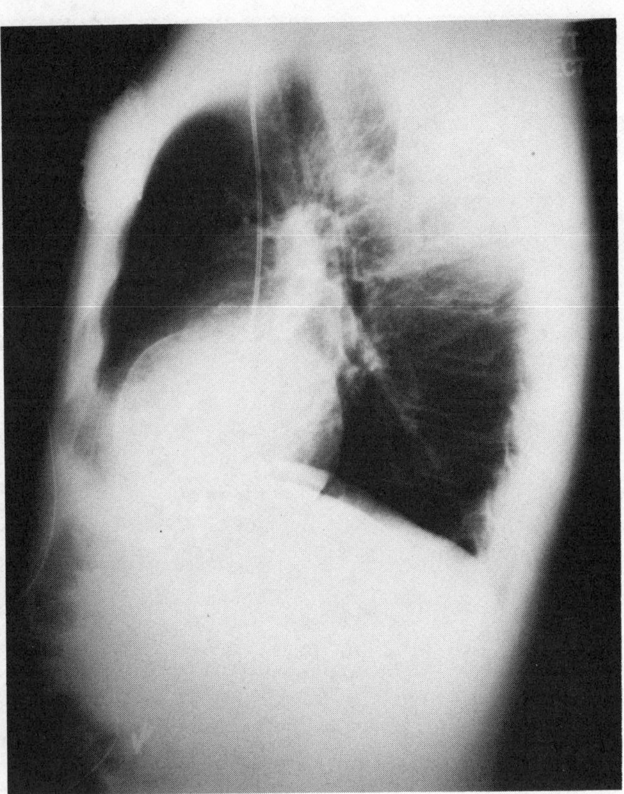

219.

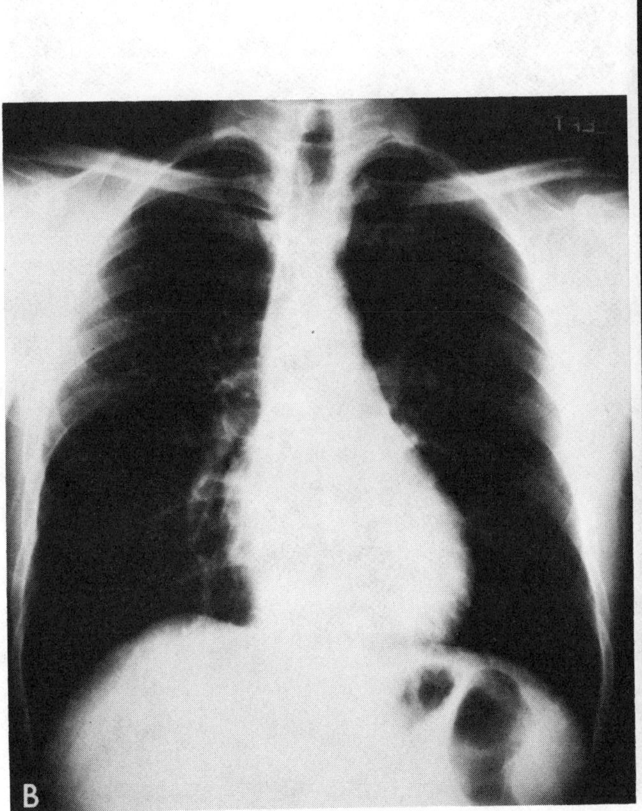

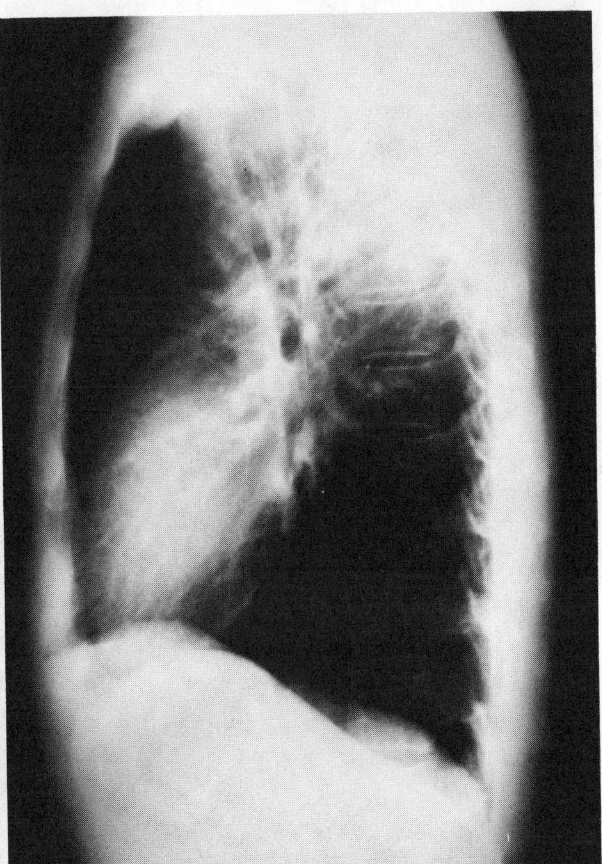

217.

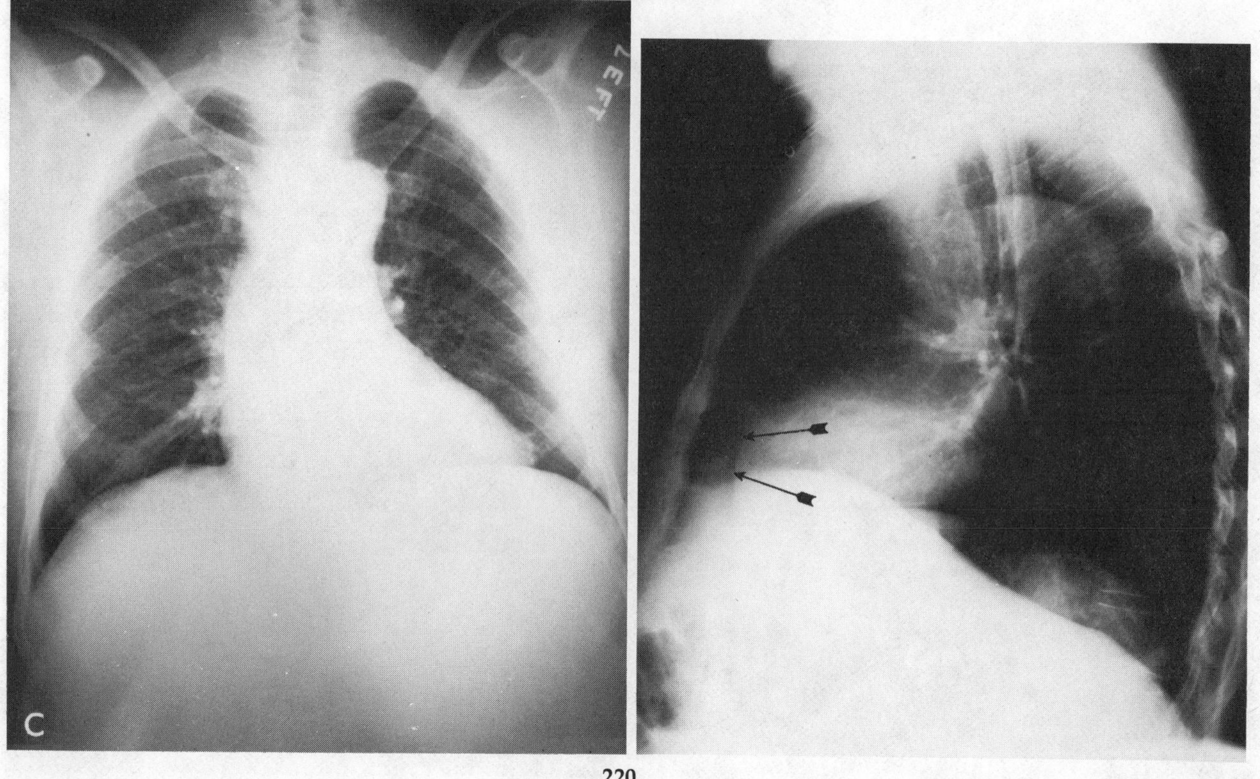

220.

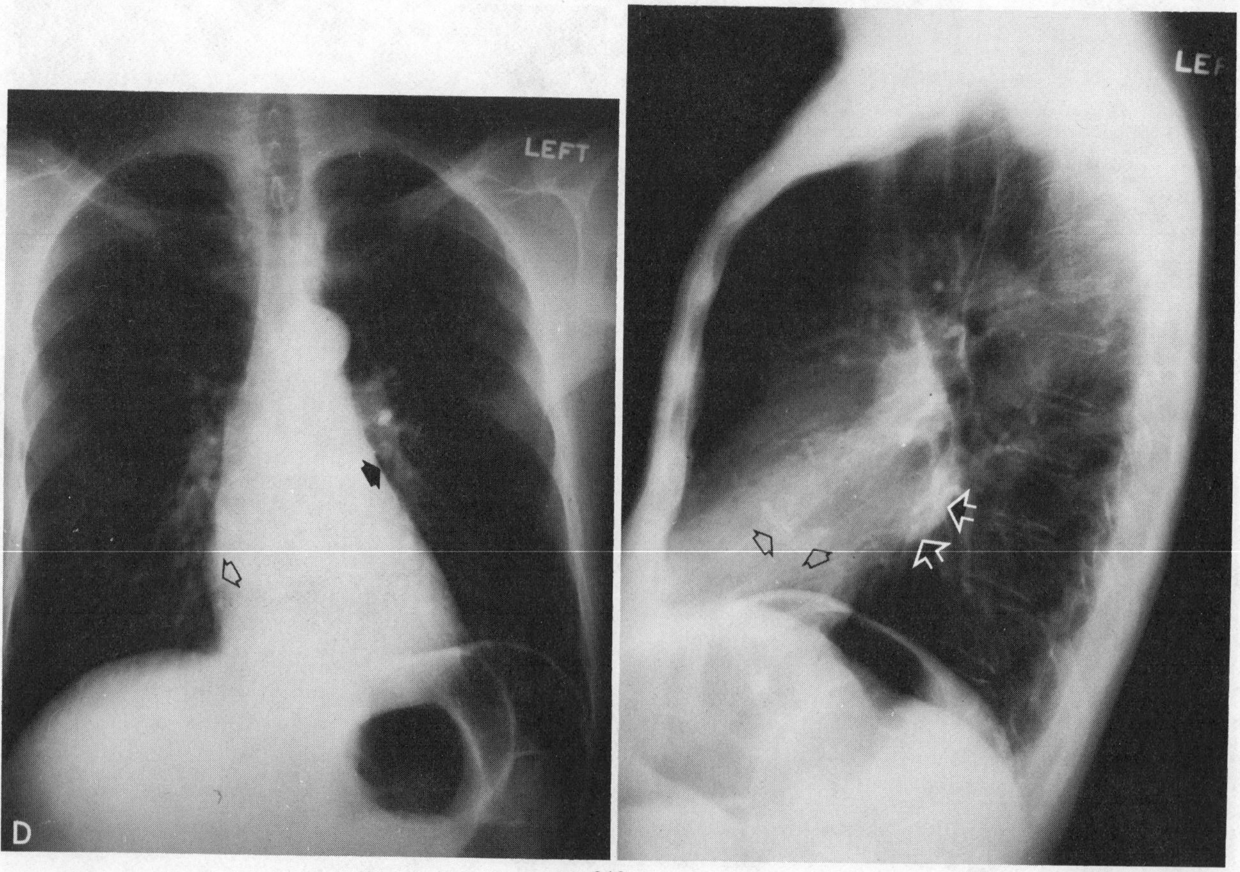

218.

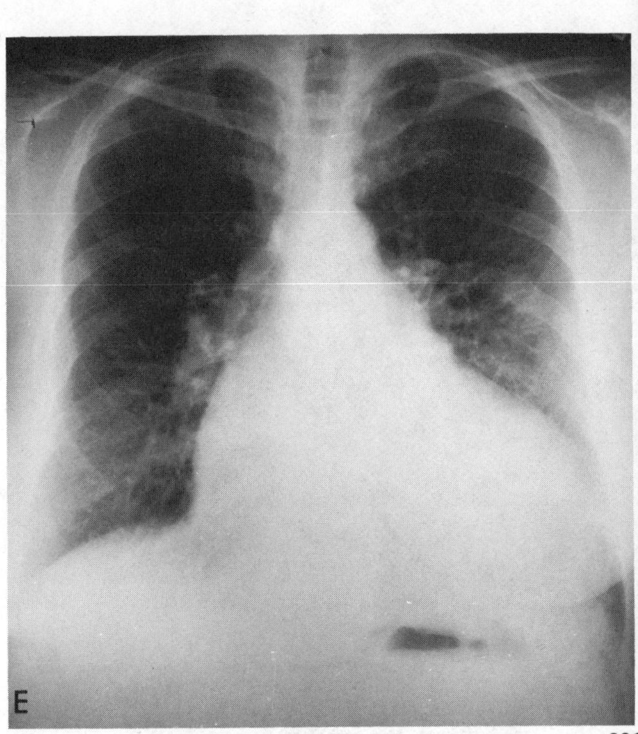

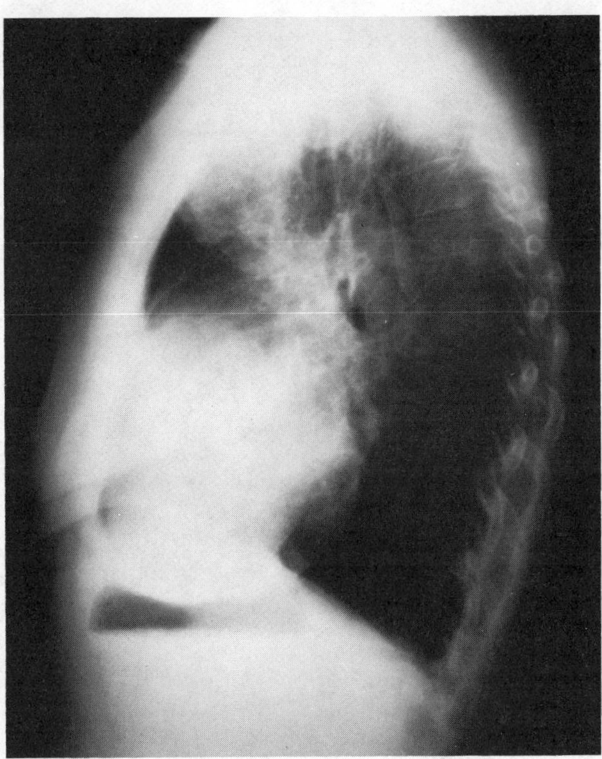

221.

Mitral stenosis is a likely culprit. This echocardiogram (p. 42) shows the four classic findings of rheumatic mitral valve disease: thickened leaflets, a slow-diastolic slope of the anterior mitral valve leaflet (AML), a diminutive A wave (arrowheads), and paradoxic motion of the posterior leaflet (PML). RV = right ventricle; IVS = interventricular septum; PLV = posterior left ventricle. *(Cecil, pp. 193–196)*

223. (A) These clinical findings are those of moderate-to-severe aortic regurgitation most likely secondary to congenital aortic valve disease (e.g., bicuspid leaflet). The echocardiogram (below) shows a dilated left ventricle (LV), diastolic flutter of the anterior mitral valve leaflet (arrows), and interventricular septum (IVS, asterisks) typical of aortic regurgitation. RV = right ventricle; PLV = posterior left ventricle. *(Cecil, pp. 206–208)*

224. (C) These clinical findings raise the possibility of infection. The soft first heart sound and the short diastolic murmur in the absence of a wide pulse pressure are compatible with acute severe aortic regurgitation with a high left ventricular end-diastolic pressure. This echocardiogram (p. 42) is a sweep from the aortic valve to the mi-

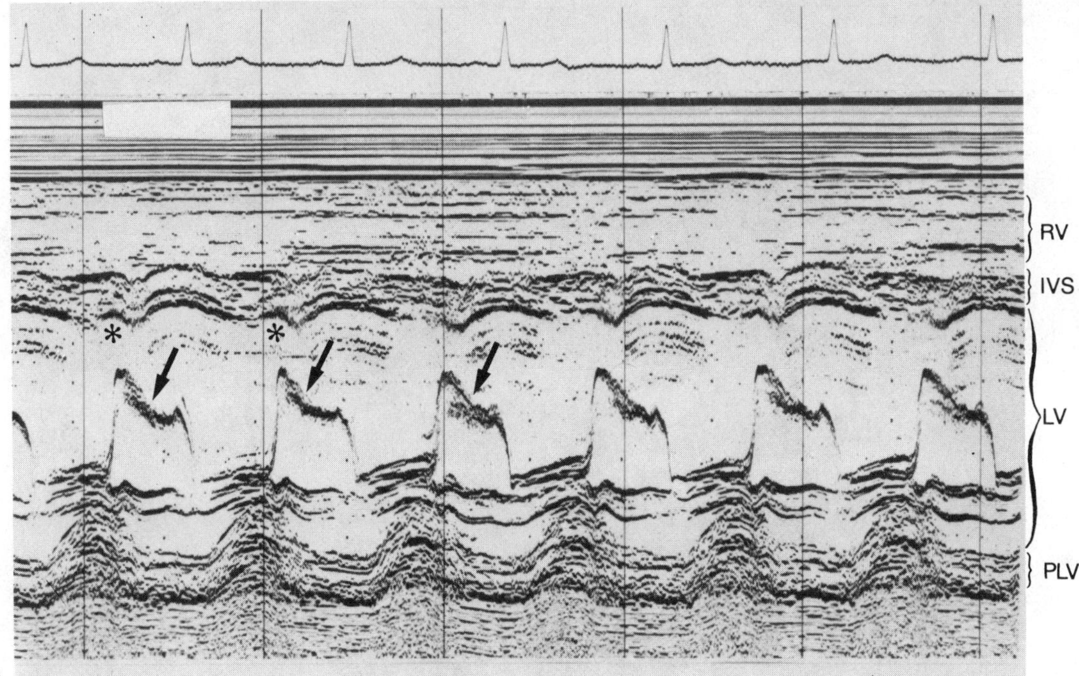

223.

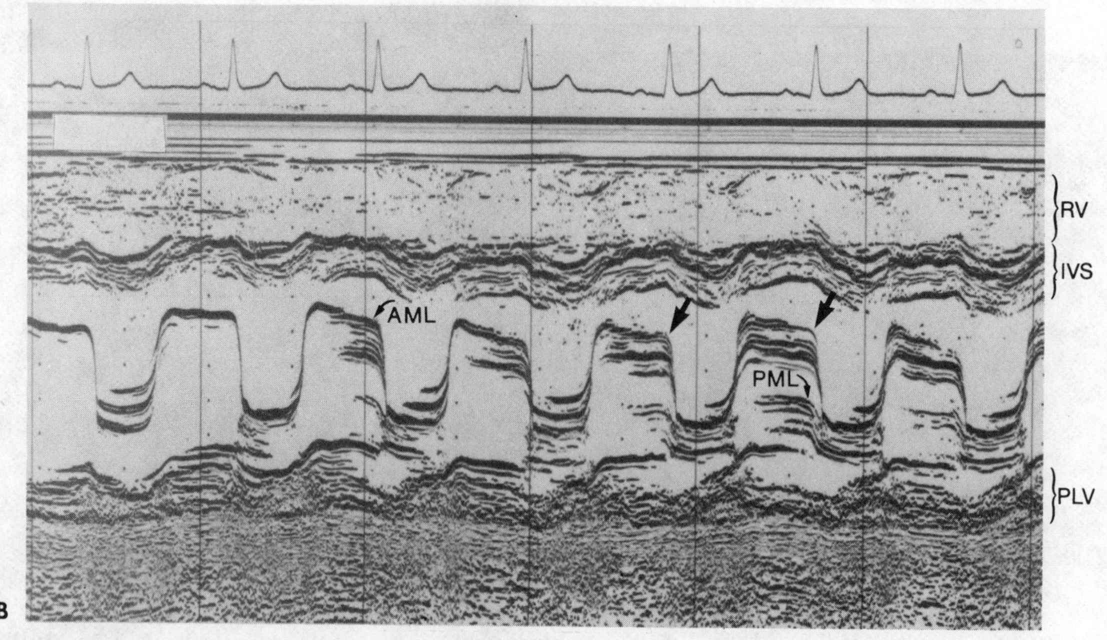

222.

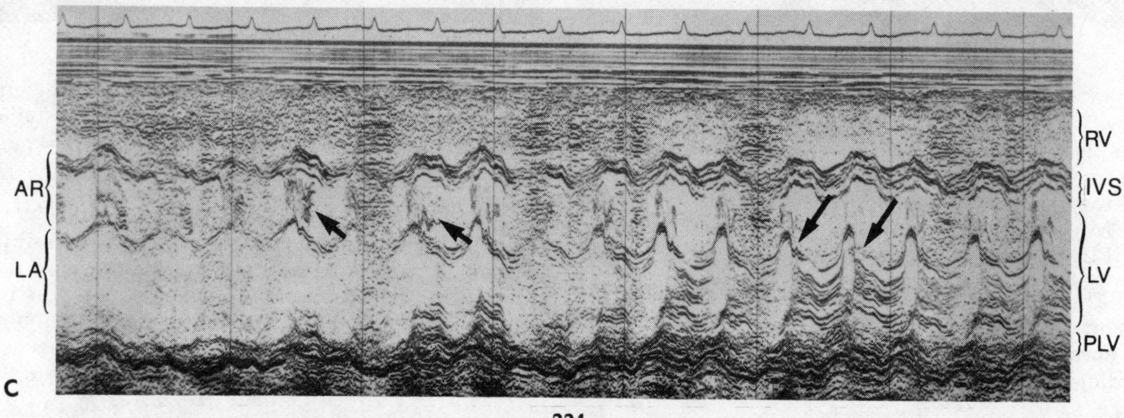

224.

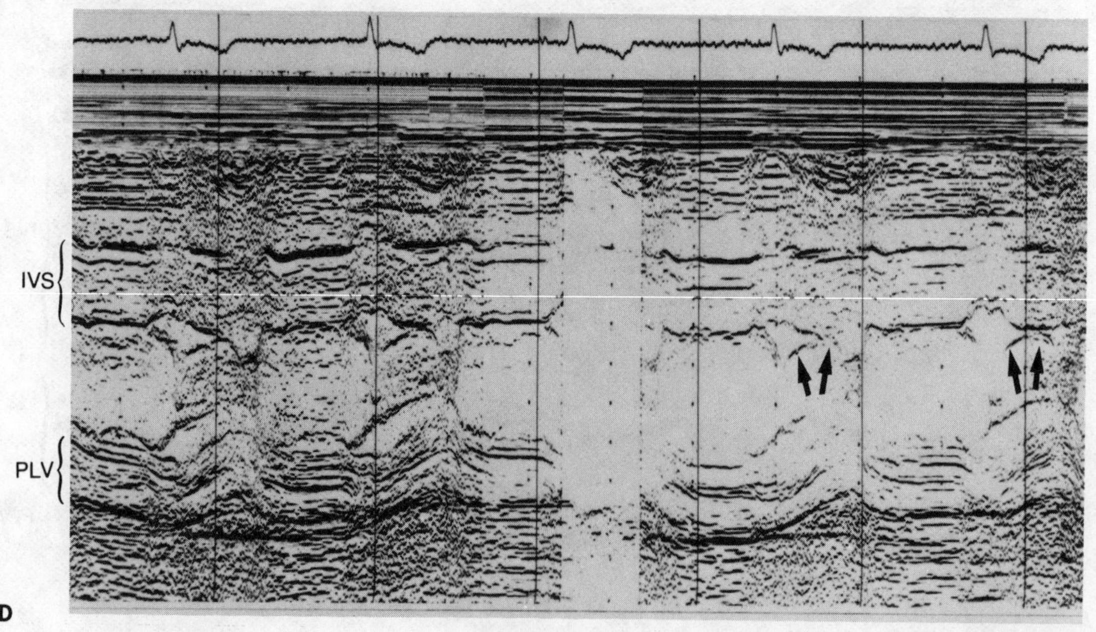

225.

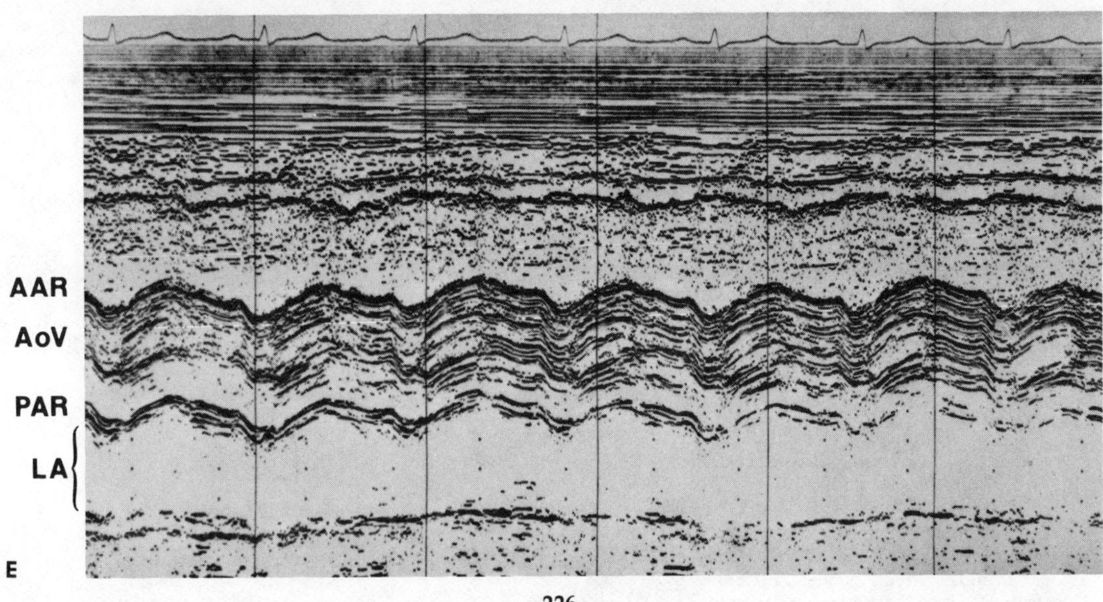

226.

tral valve. It shows abnormal echoes prolapsing into the left ventricular outflow tract in diastole (arrowheads) typical of a vegetation on the aortic valve with disruption of the aortic valve leaflets. There is also presystolic closure of the mitral valve (arrows) typical of severe acute aortic regurgitation with a high left ventricular end-diastolic pressure. This premature mitral valve closure explains the soft first heart sound. AR = aortic root; LA = left atrium; RV = right ventricle; IVS = interventricular septum; LV = left ventricle; PLV = posterior left ventricle. *(Cecil, pp. 208–209)*

225. (D) These clinical findings are typical of a hypertrophic cardiomyopathy with muscular subaortic obstruction. The echocardiogram (p. 42) shows the typical features of a hypertrophic obstructive cardiomyopathy (IHSS): a thickened interventricular septum (IVS) and anterior motion of the anterior mitral valve leaflet during systole (arrows). PLV = posterior left ventricle. *(Cecil, pp. 193, 290–292)*

226. (E) These clinical findings suggest obstruction to blood flow that is due to a pressure-loaded left ventricle. Aortic stenosis is a reasonable possibility and in this clinical setting could be due to calcification of either a bicuspid or tricuspid leaflet. This echo (above) is typical of calcific aortic valve disease with multiple linear echoes within the aortic root throughout systole and diastole. No discrete leaflet motion is identified. If a single aortic valve cusp with normal mobility had been seen, significant aortic stenosis would be very unlikely. AAR = anterior aortic root; PAR = posterior aortic root; LA = left atrium; AoV = aortic valve. *(Cecil, pp. 202–205)*

227. (A); 228. (A); 229. (D); 230. (D); 231. (A) Marfan's syndrome, osteogenesis imperfecta, and syphilis are particularly likely to involve the ascending thoracic aorta. The presence of calcification, particularly if it involves the sinuses of Valsalva, is a helpful differential point implicating underlying syphilitic aortic involvement. Pseudoxanthoma elasticum and arteriosclerosis are almost exclusively clinically significant diseases of the abdominal aorta. *(Cecil, pp. 309, 310, 312)*

BIBLIOGRAPHY

Califf, R., Burks, J., Behar, V. S., et al.: Relationships among ventricular arrhythmias, coronary artery disease and angiographic and electrocardiographic indicators of myocardial fibrosis. Circulation, *57*:725, 1977.

Craige, E.: Heart Sounds. *In* Braunwald, E. (ed.): Heart Disease: A Textbook of Cardiovascular Medicine. Philadelphia, W. B. Saunders Company, 1980, pp. 39–42.

Doering, W.: Quinidine-digoxin interaction: pharmacokinetics, underlying mechanisms and clinical implications. N. Engl. J. Med., *301*:400, 1979.

Dohan, M. C., and Criscitiello, M. G.: Physiological and pharmacological manipulations of heart sounds and murmurs. Mod. Concepts Cardiovasc. Dis., *39*:121, 1970.

Krovetz, L. J., Lorincz, A. E., and Schiebler, G. L.: Cardiovascular manifestations of the Hurler syndrome. Hemodynamic and angiocardiographic observations in 15 patients. Circulation, *31*:132, 1965.

McNeer, J. F., Margolis, J. R., Lee, K. L., et al.: The role of exercise testing in the evaluation of patients for ischemic heart disease. Circulation, *47*:64, 1978.

Perloff, J. K.: The Clinical Recognition of Congenital Heart Disease. 2nd ed. Philadelphia, W. B. Saunders Company, 1978.

Radtke, W. E., Tajik, A. J., Gau, G. T., et al.: Atrial septal defect: echocardiographic observations. Ann. Intern. Med., *84*:246, 1976.

Rifkin, R. D., and Hood, W. B.: Bayesian analysis of electrocardiographic exercise stress testing. N. Engl. J. Med., *297*:681, 1977.

Roberts, W. C.: The congenitally bicuspid aortic valve: a study of 85 autopsy cases. Am. J. Cardiol., *26*:72, 1970.

Rosenbaum, M. B., Elizari, M. V., and Lazzari, J. D.: The Hemiblocks. Oldsmar, FL, Tampa Tracings, 1970.

Rubin, L. J., and Peter, R. H.: Oral hydralazine therapy for primary pulmonary hypertension. N. Engl. J. Med., *302*:69, 1980.

Rudolph, A. M.: Congenital Diseases of the Heart. Chicago, Year Book Medical Publishers, 1974.

PART 2

RESPIRATORY DISEASE

Homer A. Boushey

DIRECTIONS: For questions 1 to 29, choose the ONE BEST answer to each question.

1. In a resting patient with severe diffuse interstitial fibrosis, hypoxemia is predominantly due to which one of the following?

A. Alveolar hypoventilation
B. Thickening of the air blood barrier (alveolar-capillary block syndrome)
C. Reduction in alveolar-capillary blood volume
D. Increased wasted ventilation
E. Ventilation-perfusion mismatching

2. Lung abscess is frequently caused by any of the following organisms EXCEPT

A. *Klebsiella pneumoniae*
B. *Staphylococcus aureus*
C. microaerophilic streptococci
D. *Hemophilus influenzae*
E. *Mycobacterium tuberculosis*

3. In a normal adult in the upright position, the air inspired with a tidal breath taken from functional residual capacity is distributed

A. predominantly to upper lung zones
B. predominantly to lower lung zones
C. predominantly to central, perihilar regions
D. uniformly throughout the lungs
E. to match precisely the distribution of pulmonary perfusion

4. A 52-year-old alcoholic man is admitted to the hospital with fever, cough productive of putrid sputum, and a chest radiographic finding of a thick-walled cavity in the superior segment of the right lower lobe. Ziehl-Nielsen stain of the sputum is negative for acid-fast organisms; Gram stain shows many neutrophils and pleomorphic gram-positive and gram-negative organisms. The patient has a history of severe wheezing with use of penicillin. Which of the following is the most appropriate initial antibiotic in this patient?

A. Gentamicin
B. Ampicillin
C. Trimethoprim-sulfamethoxazole
D. Vancomycin
E. Clindamycin

5. Hypersensitivity pneumonitis may be caused by exposure to all of the following EXCEPT

A. compost
B. talc
C. bird droppings
D. flour
E. redwood dust

6. A 28-year-old woman with chronic asthma comes to the emergency room because of increased dyspnea and cough following a recent viral upper respiratory infection. Oxygen is given by face mask and two doses of epinephrine are given subcutaneously. Thirty minutes later, arterial blood gases are Po_2 68 mm Hg, Pco_2 41 mm Hg, and pH 7.43. The patient appears anxious and fatigued. Which one of the following should you do next?

A. Increase the flow of supplemental oxygen
B. Give an additional dose of epinephrine
C. Administer a central nervous system stimulant such as methylphenidate (Ritalin)
D. Administer methylprednisolone and aminophylline intravenously and begin therapy with an aerosol of an adrenergic agent.
E. Administer a sedative such as diazepam (Valium) or phenobarbital

7. Bronchoscopy would be of value in all the following circumstances EXCEPT

A. hemoptysis (of undetermined cause) of more than 200 ml in 12 hours
B. aspiration of a peanut by a 13-year-old girl
C. hyponatremia and hyposthenuria in a 50-year-old smoker with a normal chest roentgenogram
D. fever, tachypnea, and leukocytosis in an alcoholic who has a left lower lobe infiltrate on chest film and who is unable to raise sputum
E. a 48-year-old woman with a 2.2-cm nodule of unknown age in the right midlung field on chest film, a positive tuberculin skin test (PPD), and recent travel to Bakersfield, California

8. A 23-year-old woman has a single breath diffusing capacity for carbon monoxide (DL_{CO}) that is 45% of predicted. This abnormality is consistent with all the following disease processes EXCEPT

A. scleroderma
B. recurrent pulmonary emboli
C. sarcoidosis
D. cystic fibrosis
E. systemic lupus erythematosus

9. A 23-year-old man complains of progressive dyspnea six weeks after discharge from the hospital, where he had been treated with prolonged intubation and mechanical ventilation for management of an overdose with glutethimide (Doriden). The pulmonary function test most likely to be *abnormal* is

A. maximal inspiratory force (MIF)
B. peak expiratory flow rate (PEFR)
C. flow-volume curve
D. arterial Po_2
E. diffusing capacity for carbon monoxide (DL_{CO})

10. The alveolar-arterial oxygen difference is LEAST increased in which one of the following conditions?

A. Lobar pneumonia
B. Pulmonary edema
C. Barbiturate overdose
D. Influenza pneumonia
E. Status asthmaticus

11. A 50-year-old miner with a 40 pack-year smoking history is found to have a well-differentiated epidermoid tumor occluding 95% of the lumen of the right bronchus intermedius. No hilar, mediastinal, or distant metastases can be detected. Pulmonary function tests reveal that vital capacity, forced expiratory volume in one second (FEV_1), and maximal voluntary ventilation are approximately 40% of predicted and do not improve with bronchodilator therapy. Which one of the following would you do now?

A. Recommend right pneumonectomy
B. Recommend radiotherapy
C. Offer no treatment at present, but treat metastatic lesions with radiotherapy as they appear
D. Recommend palliative resection of a portion of the tumor via the bronchoscope to restore ventilation to the right lower lobe
E. Initiate an exercise training program and repeat pulmonary function tests in six to ten weeks

12. The first test to become abnormal in the progression of chronic obstructive pulmonary disease is

A. arterial P_{CO_2}
B. roentgenogram of the chest
C. peak expiratory flow rate (PEFR)
D. forced expiratory volume in one second (FEV_1)
E. maximal expiratory flow at low lung volumes (MMF, $\dot{V}max_{75\%}$)

13. Analysis of pleural fluid obtained from a patient with severe, biventricular congestive heart failure is likely to reveal which one of the following?

A. Specific gravity greater than 1.015
B. A total protein of 3 gm/dl
C. A pH of 7.20
D. A lactic dehydrogenase level about 60% of the serum level
E. Protein content less than half of the serum protein content

14. Restrictive lung disease with diffuse alveolar fibrosis may result from chronic exposure to any of the following agents EXCEPT

A. silica
B. talc
C. cotton bract
D. beryllium
E. pigeon guano

15. A 21-year-old woman has a wedge-shaped density in the posterior basal segment of the left lower lobe, thought to represent an intralobar bronchopulmonary sequestration. Contrast material could best be introduced into this abnormal portion of the lung by

A. selective bronchial arteriography
B. bronchography
C. abdominal aortography
D. pulmonary arteriography
E. lymphangiography

16. A patient with the "blue-bloater" (type B) prototypic form of chronic obstructive pulmonary disease differs from the "pink-puffer" (type A) form in that he has

A. scant, mucoid sputum production
B. normal or low arterial P_{CO_2}
C. increased residual volume
D. increased inspiratory airway resistance
E. reduced maximal expiratory flow

17. A reduction in total lung capacity in a patient with diffuse systemic sclerosis is most likely caused by

A. sclerosis of the costovertebral joints
B. intimal thickening of small pulmonary arteries and arterioles
C. decreased elasticity of the skin overlying the chest
D. diffuse alveolar fibrosis
E. neuropathic degeneration of the phrenic nerves

18. Radiation therapy may control or improve all the following complications of bronchogenic carcinoma EXCEPT

A. superior vena caval obstruction
B. hypertrophic pulmonary osteoarthropathy
C. hemoptysis
D. pancytopenia
E. painful rib metastases

19. Heroin addiction is associated with all the following pulmonary complications EXCEPT

A. pulmonary hypertension
B. pulmonary veno-occlusive disease
C. septic emboli
D. pulmonary edema
E. aspiration pneumonia

20. Rheumatoid arthritis is associated with all the following changes in the respiratory system EXCEPT

A. lobar atelectasis
B. pleural effusion
C. fibrosing alveolitis
D. pulmonary hypertension
E. upper airway obstruction

21. The chest roentgenograms of a 54-year-old housewife show an irregular left upper lobe infiltrate that has increased in size over the past six months. The most recent films reveal possible areas of cavitation. Tuberculin skin test (PPD) produces 8 mm of induration at 48 hours. Sputum culture yields several colonies of "atypical mycobacteria, Group III, probable *M. intracellulare*." Which one of the following would you do now?

A. Begin a course of isoniazid and rifampin
B. Begin a clinical and roentgenographic survey for underlying malignancy
C. Refer the patient for left upper lobectomy
D. Begin chemotherapy with five or six antituberculous drugs while awaiting results of sensitivity testing
E. Begin chemotherapy and advise the patient to avoid contact with children or other potentially susceptible individuals until sputum cultures are negative

22. The chest roentgenogram (*A*) and tomogram (*B*) illustrated below are most likely from which one of the following patients?

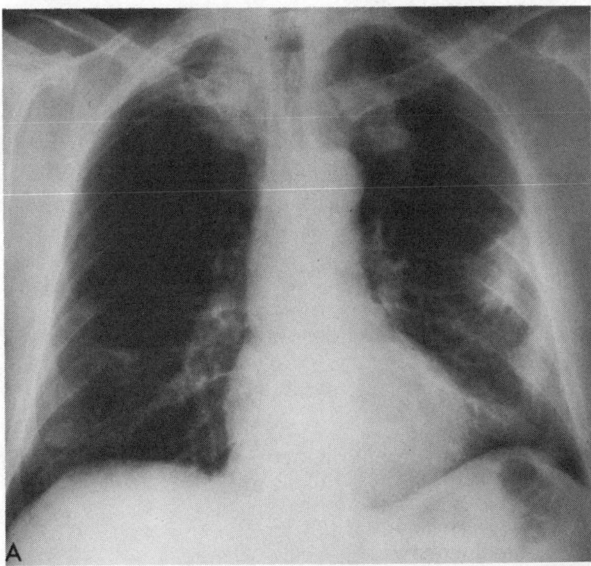

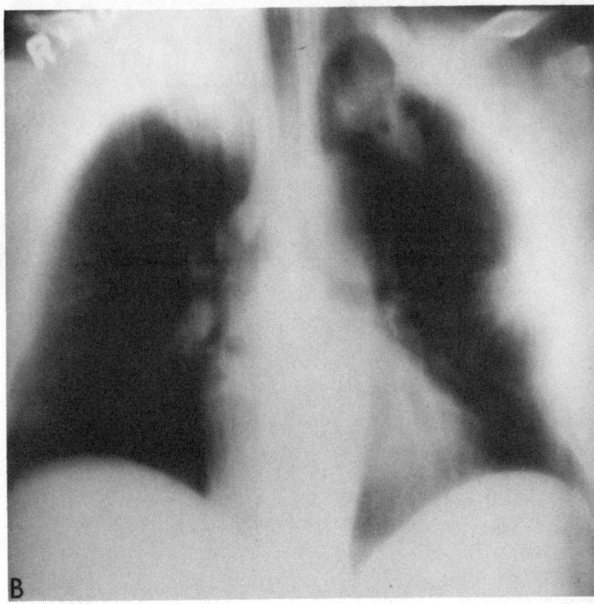

A. A 22-year-old black man with recent onset of night sweats, fever, and arthralgias; ophthalmologic examination shows uveitis
B. A 17-year-old student with fever, cough, and headache who is found to have circulating cold agglutinins
C. A 55-year-old man with pleuritic pain, shaking chills, fever, and cough that began suddenly two days ago
D. A 31-year-old man with fever, malaise, and nasal congestion who is found to have hematuria
E. A 34-year-old unconscious fireman who was rescued from a burning building 30 minutes ago; soot is noted in the nares; scattered rales and wheezes are heard over the chest

23. The chest roentgenogram illustrated at the top of the next column suggests that the patient may have been employed as which one of the following?

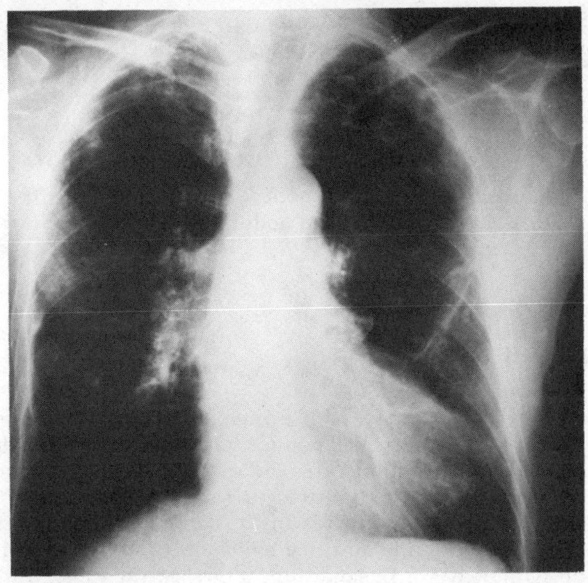

A. Chicken farmer
B. Shipyard plumber
C. Welder
D. Migrant farm worker in California
E. Sandblaster

24. A 39-year-old man with a three-week history of fever, weight loss, and left-sided chest pain has the chest roentgenogram illustrated below. All the following statements are true EXCEPT

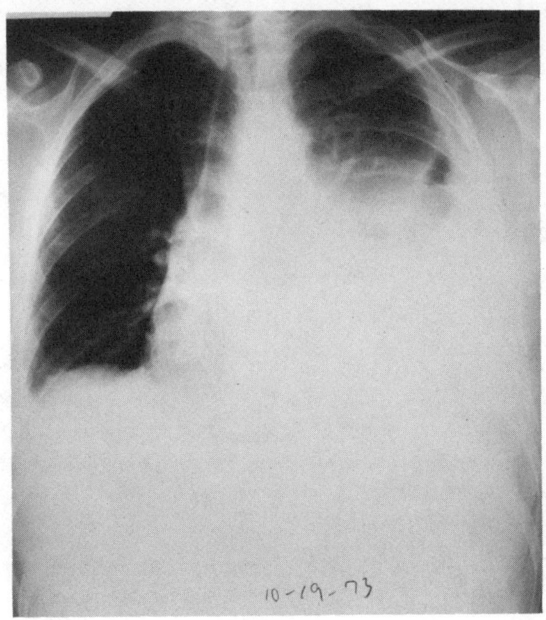

A. Aerobic cultures of fluid obtained at thoracentesis are likely to be negative
B. Pleural fluid pH is probably lower than 7.30
C. Surgical decortication may be necessary three to six months after initial therapy
D. Therapy should include instillation of tetracycline into the pleural space
E. Tube drainage or rib resection with open drainage will be required

25. In sarcoidosis, noncaseating granulomas are likely to be found in biopsies taken from all the following EXCEPT

A. lung
B. liver
C. lacrimal gland
D. mediastinal lymph nodes
E. painful, red, swollen nodules on the anterior tibial surface

QUESTIONS 26–28

A 34-year-old woman with a lifelong history of obesity who currently weighs 340 pounds has had exercise intolerance, daytime somnolence, and nocturnal sleepwalking and enuresis for the past two years. Her husband reports that she has become increasingly inattentive and forgetful during this time and that she snores loudly at night. The patient has a flushed appearance and a short, thick neck. Blood pressure (leg cuff) is 180/100 mm Hg, pulse rate is 85/minute, respirations are 18/minute. Examination of the chest is normal, although breath sounds are poorly heard; cardiac examination is normal. There is pitting edema of both ankles. Laboratory studies reveal:

Hemoglobin	17.8 gm/dl
Hematocrit	54%
White blood cell count	6700/cu mm
Arterial blood studies:	
Po_2	62 mm Hg
Pco_2	48 mm Hg
pH	7.37

The chest roentgenogram shows a poor inspiratory effect but is otherwise unremarkable.

26. The daytime somnolence is most likely caused by

A. carbon dioxide retention
B. hypoxemia
C. exhaustion secondary to the increased work of breathing
D. lack of restful sleep
E. acidosis secondary to increased fatty acid metabolism

27. Study of this patient during sleep will probably reveal

A. intermittent apnea due to upward displacement of the diaphragm by abdominal contents
B. severe insomnia
C. rapid progression to deep, REM sleep without passing through earlier phases
D. recurrent apnea despite vigorous respiratory efforts
E. decrease in Pco_2 secondary to a decrease in metabolic rate

28. Performance of a permanent tracheostomy will probably improve all the patient's symptoms EXCEPT

A. daytime somnolence
B. ankle edema
C. exercise intolerance
D. snoring
E. sleepwalking

---

29. Clinical syndromes that may result from sarcoidosis include all the following EXCEPT

A. unilateral facial paralysis
B. severe crampy flank pain with hematuria
C. painless ulceration of the skin overlying the lateral malleolus
D. polyuria and polydypsia
E. recurrent syncope and a slow, regular pulse

DIRECTIONS: For questions 30 to 80, you are to decide whether EACH choice is true or false. Any combination of answers, from all true to all false, may be present. Mark the answer sheet "T" or "F" in the space provided.

30. Which of the following statements regarding acute tuberculous pleurisy is/are true?

A. Tuberculin skin test is positive in almost every case
B. Acid-fast bacilli are usually found in the pleural fluid
C. The risk of subsequent clinically apparent tuberculosis is high
D. The pleural effusion is transudative
E. The causative organisms are usually resistant to isoniazid

31. Causes of chronic, nonproductive cough include

A. asthma
B. bronchogenic carcinoma
C. congestive heart failure
D. brachial neuropathy
E. diffuse interstitial fibrosis

32. A 42-year-old woman who has smoked a pack of cigarettes daily for 20 years has a cough productive of mucoid sputum on awakening each morning. When the patient has viral upper respiratory infections, the sputum increases in volume and appears purulent. Which of the following statements regarding this patient is/are true?

A. Daily use of a broad-spectrum antibiotic is likely to reduce the frequency of bouts of purulent sputum
B. Progressive respiratory insufficiency is likely to develop if she continues smoking
C. Culture of sputum obtained by transtracheal aspiration probably would *not* yield bacterial organisms on culture
D. Bronchography would probably reveal enlarged mucous gland ducts
E. Cough and sputum production will probably improve if she stops smoking

33. A reduction in expiratory flow when 50% of the vital capacity has been exhaled can be produced by which of the following?

A. Loss of lung recoil
B. Inadequate expiratory effort
C. Reduction in cross-sectional area of small airways
D. Tracheal stenosis
E. Breathing a helium-oxygen gas mixture

34. Static lung compliance is reduced in which of the following conditions?

A. Pulmonary edema
B. Obesity
C. Asthma
D. Bilateral pleural fibrosis
E. Diffuse interstitial fibrosis

35. A 28-year-old woman with a history of nasal polyps complains of episodes of dyspnea, chest tightness, and shortness of breath that have recently begun to occur whenever she takes aspirin. She should be advised to avoid the use of medications containing

A. codeine
B. indomethacin
C. sodium salicylate
D. acetaminophen
E. H_2-receptor blocking antihistamines (e.g., cimetidine)

36. Cystic fibrosis is

A. transmitted as an autosomal dominant trait
B. associated with abnormal levels of sodium and chloride in sweat, urine, feces, and transbronchial secretions
C. fatal in the first five years of life in about 75% of cases
D. properly treated with frequent use of positive pressure breathing (IPPB) to deliver aerosolized saline
E. associated with recurrent pneumonia caused by *Pseudomonas aeruginosa* and *Staphylococcus aureus*

37. Which of the following statements about involvement of the lung in systemic lupus erythematosus (SLE) is/are true?

A. Pulmonary and pleural involvement occurs in less than 20% of patients with SLE
B. Pleural effusions associated with SLE are exudative
C. A positive antinuclear antibody titer with interstitial pulmonary infiltrates establishes the diagnosis of lupus pulmonary disease
D. The low-pressure pulmonary circulation is spared in lupus vasculitis
E. The characteristic pulmonary function abnormalities are volume restriction, decreased diffusing capacity, and arterial hypoxemia

38. Necrotizing granulomatous vasculitis on open lung biopsy is characteristic of which of the following?

A. Goodpasture's syndrome
B. Wegener's granulomatosis
C. Caplan's syndrome
D. Löffler's syndrome
E. Lymphomatoid granulomatosis

39. Asbestos exposure is associated with an increased incidence of which of the following?

A. Hilar lymphadenopathy
B. Pleural effusions
C. Mesothelioma
D. Laryngeal cancer
E. Gastrointestinal cancer

40. Characteristics of allergic bronchopulmonary aspergillosis include which of the following?

A. Pulmonary infiltrates with eosinophilia
B. Parenchymal invasion with *Aspergillus* organisms
C. Expectoration of rubbery, brownish plugs of sputum
D. Proximal bronchiectasis
E. Type I, IgE-mediated reaction

41. Disorders that predispose to the development of bronchiectasis include

A. cystic fibrosis
B. immotile cilia syndrome

C. pulmonary tuberculosis
D. hypogammaglobulinemia
E. atopic asthma

42. Which of the following is/are associated with the protease inhibitor (Pi) phenotype of ZZ?

A. Hepatitis in infancy
B. Emphysema appearing by the age of 40 years
C. Centrilobular emphysema
D. Decrease in serum alpha$_1$ globulin
E. Predominantly basilar emphysema

43. Marked flattening of the diaphragms and increase in the retrosternal air space on roentgenogram of the chest are characteristic of which of the following disorders?

A. Pulmonary emphysema
B. Primary pulmonary hypertension
C. Bilateral diaphragmatic paralysis
D. Asthma
E. Chronic obstructive bronchitis

44. The *nonmetastatic* effects of bronchogenic carcinoma include which of the following?

A. Back pain, leg weakness, loss of bowel and bladder control
B. Unilateral ptosis and miosis
C. Arthralgias, limitation of movement, and tenderness of wrists and ankles
D. Truncal ataxia, poor coordination, and frequent falling
E. Numbness and tingling over the soles of both feet

45. In evaluating a solitary pulmonary nodule, which of the following findings strongly favor(s) its being benign?

A. The patient is less than 35 years old
B. Sputum cytology is reported as benign in three induced samples
C. A central nidus of calcification
D. Increase in diameter from 0.8 to 1.1 cm over six months
E. Positive skin test for coccidioidomycosis

46. A patient with tachypnea and diminished respiratory excursions has diffuse bilateral alveolar infiltrates on the chest radiograph. Arterial blood gases are Po_2 51 mm Hg, Pco_2 31 mm Hg, and pH 7.47. This patient's condition is compatible with which of the following events in the preceding 48 hours?

A. Fracture of the left femur and pelvis in a motorcycle accident
B. Acute, severe abdominal pain and vomiting following heavy alcohol intake
C. Resuscitation by mouth-to-mouth breathing after near-drowning in a fresh water pool
D. Profound hypotension after ingestion of 2.5 gm of secobarbital in a suicide attempt
E. Hypotension, tachycardia, and fever after urethral catheterization

47. Which of the following statements regarding hypoxemia in patients with large pulmonary emboli is/are true?

A. It invariably occurs in such patients
B. It is temporarily reversed if a breath as large as 80% of the predicted inspiratory capacity is taken
C. It usually resolves within 24 hours of beginning heparin therapy
D. The alveolar-arterial oxygen difference (on 100% oxygen) will usually be normal
E. Its presence is an indication of pre-existing cardiopulmonary disease

48. A patient has coughed up 100 ml of blood in the past eight hours. Initial management should include which of the following?

A. Placing the patient in the decubitus position with the site of bleeding lowermost
B. Sedation to suppress coughing
C. Deferral of bronchoscopy until the bleeding has ceased
D. Intubation of the right main-stem bronchus with inflation of the balloon cuff to confine the bleeding to one lung
E. Pulmonary angiography to identify the site of bleeding

49. Which of the following findings on roentgenogram of the chest would favor a diagnosis of Hodgkin's disease or non-Hodgkin's lymphoma over a diagnosis of sarcoidosis?

A. Bilateral hilar and right paratracheal adenopathy
B. Diffuse infiltration of both lung fields
C. Anterior mediastinal adenopathy
D. Diffuse interstitial fibrosis with apical bullae
E. Pleural effusion

50. Carbon monoxide poisoning results in hypoxic damage by

A. reducing the arterial Po_2
B. shifting the oxygen-hemoglobin dissociation curve to the left
C. decreasing alveolar ventilation
D. reducing the number of oxygen binding sites available on hemoglobin
E. "uncoupling" oxidative metabolism and ATP production

51. A 54-year-old man with a history of chronic productive morning cough and recurrent hemoptysis is found on chest roentgenography to have coarse lung markings and ring shadows in the right lower lobe. Conditions predisposing to this disorder include

A. tuberculosis
B. gingivitis and periodontitis
C. cystic fibrosis
D. intravenous drug abuse
E. agammaglobulinemia

52. A 55-year-old man with a two-week history of fever and cough productive of foul-smelling sputum has the chest roentgenogram shown at the top of p. 51. Conditions predisposing to this disorder include

A. alcoholism
B. hiatus hernia with esophagitis
C. periodontitis
D. mycoplasma pneumonia
E. seizure disorder

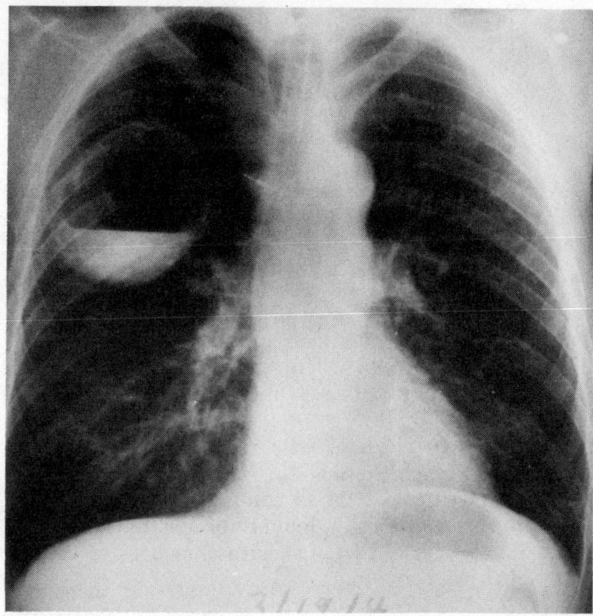

53. Hemosiderin-laden macrophages would be expected in bronchial washings from patients with

A. Wegener's granulomatosis
B. Goodpasture's syndrome
C. hemolytic anemia
D. primary pulmonary hypertension
E. mitral stenosis

54. A pleural fluid glucose concentration of less than 25 mg/dl is compatible with

A. pancreatitis
B. tuberculosis
C. hepatic cirrhosis and ascites
D. rheumatoid pleuritis
E. pulmonary infarction

55. Increasing the fraction of inspired air that is oxygen (FI_{O_2}) to 0.40 would be expected to correct the hypoxemia of which of the following conditions?

A. Far-advanced pulmonary emphysema
B. Acute respiratory failure occurring two days after severe trauma with multiple fractures
C. Large intrapulmonary arteriovenous malformation
D. Acute exacerbation of chronic bronchitis and cor pulmonale following a viral upper respiratory infection
E. Pulmonary hypertension in an adult with an uncorrected atrial septal defect

56. Elevation of the bases of the fingernails may be related to the primary disease in which of the following patients?

A. A 44-year-old woman with intense pruritus for three months and painless jaundice for the past month
B. A 52-year-old man with a heavy smoking history and recent onset of cough with trace hemoptysis
C. A 32-year-old woman with chronic cough productive of copious, sometimes foul-smelling sputum for several years
D. A 28-year-old woman with recurrent bouts of bronchospasm and persistent peripheral eosinophilia
E. A 22-year-old man with recurrent pneumonia, chronic productive cough, infertility, and intestinal malabsorption

57. The flow-volume curve pictured here would be expected in which of the following patients?

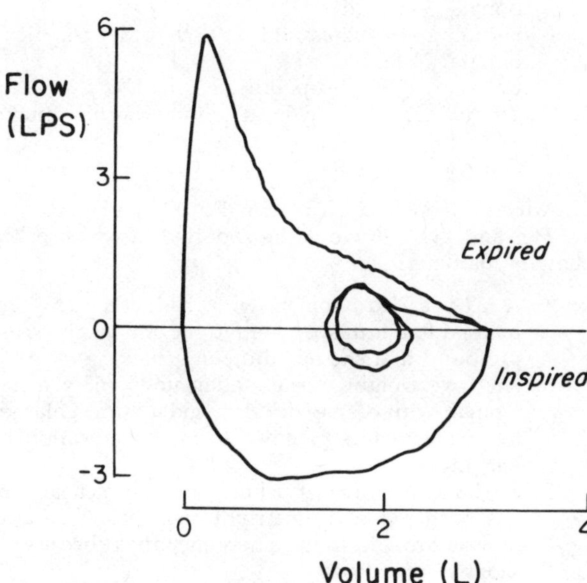

A. A 58-year-old foundry worker with a 50 pack-year smoking history who has dyspnea on exertion and a chronic productive cough
B. A 21-year-old woman with a three-month history of joint pains, hematuria, and recurrent pleuritic chest pain
C. A 36-year-old woman with loss of vascular markings over both bases on chest roentgenogram and a low $alpha_1$ globulin peak on serum protein electrophoresis
D. A 38-year-old laborer with episodic chest pain and recent onset of dyspnea two weeks after sustaining soft tissue injury of his right thigh
E. A 28-year-old man with episodic wheezing and dyspnea

58. When tested against appropriate antigens, precipitating antibodies would be found in the serum of which of the following patients?

A. A 19-year-old farm worker who recently arrived in central California and who has headache, fever, an erythematous rash, and a pulmonary infiltrate on chest film
B. A 38-year-old woman carder who complains of chest tightness, wheezing, and shortness of breath on entering the cotton mill, particularly on Monday mornings
C. A 19-year-old man with pulmonary fibrosis secondary to advanced sarcoidosis, hemoptysis, and a new, oval density within a left upper lobe bulla on chest film
D. A 41-year-old man admitted to the hospital with cyanosis, tachypnea, and diffuse pulmonary infiltrates on chest film four hours after entering a silo filled with corn silage
E. A 35-year-old man with a history of recurring episodes of bronchospasm, fever, eosinophilia, and transient infiltrates on chest film

59. A 63-year-old accountant who has smoked a pack of cigarettes a day for 50 years presents with hemoptysis of recent onset. Roentgenogram of the chest reveals a new right hilar mass. Which of the following serum values might be related to the primary disease process?

A. Sodium, 132; potassium, 2.8; chloride, 95; bicarbonate, 34 mEq/L
B. Sodium, 118; potassium, 3.9; chloride, 88; bicarbonate, 24 mEq/L
C. Calcium, 12.8; phosphorus, 2.1 mg/dl
D. Thyroxine, 14.1 μg/dl; triiodothyronine uptake, 39%
E. Glucose, 35 mg/dl

60. Arterial blood studies showing Po_2 40 mm Hg, Pco_2 75 mm Hg, and pH 7.19 would be expected in which of the following patients?

A. A 37-year-old woman who had recently complained to her husband of fatigue and weakness so profound that she had difficulty chewing meat
B. An overweight, pale, edematous 68-year-old woman with coarse, dry skin and a thick, enlarged tongue who was given a sleeping medication by her physician
C. A 24-year-old man in whom an endotracheal tube has been placed in the right main bronchus after he was brought to the emergency room because of sedative overdose
D. A 28-year-old man with hemoptysis who was thrown against the steering wheel of his sports car when he drove it into a telephone pole 45 minutes ago
E. A 6-year-old boy who ingested 40 aspirin tablets 45 minutes ago

61. Acute pulmonary embolism

A. is excluded if thoracentesis reveals nonbloody pleural effusion
B. is confirmed by demonstrating a perfusion defect on perfusion lung scan
C. causes hypoxemia by increasing the respiratory dead space
D. causes pulmonary infarction in less than 20% of cases
E. is unlikely if the patient's temperature exceeds 39° C

62. Which of the following statements regarding the treatment of sputum-positive active tuberculosis is/are true?

A. The patient should be kept in hospital isolation on chemotherapy until sputum smears become negative
B. Annual chest roentgenograms should be obtained for at least ten years after completion of chemotherapy
C. At least three effective antituberculous drugs should be used pending results of sensitivity studies
D. Treatment with isoniazid and ethambutol for nine months is appropriate
E. Household contacts should be treated with isoniazid only if their tuberculin skin tests are positive

63. Which of the following findings might be related to an occupational history of working in a shipyard for ten years, 20 years before presentation?

A. Diffuse interstitial fibrosis on chest roentgenography
B. Encasement of the left lung by pleural thickening
C. Perihilar mass; class V sputum cytology
D. Obstruction to airflow, increase in residual volume, reduction in diffusing capacity for carbon monoxide
E. Recurrent pleural effusion

64. Arterial blood studies showing Po_2 65 mm Hg, Pco_2 32 mm Hg, and pH 7.48 would be expected in which of the following patients?

A. A 45-year-old woman with chronic rheumatoid arthritis and diffuse increase in interstitial markings on chest roentgenogram
B. A 19-year-old student complaining of dyspnea, circumoral numbness, and paresthesias on the eve of a final exam
C. A 49-year-old man with recent myocardial infarction and basilar rales
D. A 22-year-old woman complaining of dyspnea 48 hours after normal delivery of healthy twins
E. An 18-year-old woman with an acute exacerbation of chronic asthma

65. *Pneumocystis carinii* pneumonia can usually be diagnosed by

A. methenamine silver staining of tissue obtained by open lung biopsy
B. staining of sediment of centrifuged sample of pleural fluid
C. staining of sample obtained by transbronchial biopsy
D. serologic studies
E. typical pattern of diffuse bilateral infiltrates on chest film

66. Complications of fiberoptic bronchoscopy and transbronchial biopsy include which of the following?

A. Pneumothorax
B. Hemorrhage
C. Laryngospasm
D. Fever
E. Hypoxemia

67. Definitive pulmonary angiographic findings of pulmonary embolism include

A. appearance and persistence of contrast material in an alveolar pattern in a localized portion of the lung
B. an intraluminal filling defect
C. delayed filling of a portion of the pulmonary arterial tree
D. a shift in flow of contrast material away from a region of the lung
E. cut-off of a large branch of the pulmonary artery

68. The respiratory effects of massive obesity include

A. increase in functional residual capacity
B. tracheal compression
C. decrease in residual volume
D. hypoxemia
E. decrease in chest wall compliance

QUESTIONS 69–72

A confused 55-year-old woman is brought by ambulance to the emergency room. Her husband tells you that she has a

50 pack-year smoking history, a chronic cough, and a four-year history of progressive dyspnea on exertion, especially after upper respiratory infections. She recently complained to her husband of a 10-pound weight gain over her usual weight of 150 pounds. She contracted a cold one week ago and has had progressive cough, dyspnea, and headache. When she entered the ambulance one hour ago, she was oriented and responsive.

The patient appears flushed. Blood pressure is 160/85 mm Hg; pulse rate is 106/minute and bounding; respirations are 14/minute. She is afebrile. Funduscopic examination reveals mild papilledema; chest expansion is poor, and there are scattered coarse rhonchi on inspiration with a prolonged expiratory phase. Neck veins are distended to the jaw; there is a left parasternal lift but no cardiac murmurs or gallops. The liver is enlarged, and there is pitting ankle edema. Laboratory data include:

Hemoglobin	16.0 gm/dl
Hematocrit	55%
White blood cell count	12,800/cu mm
Serum sodium	134 mEq/L
Serum chloride	81 mEq/L
Serum potassium	6.1 mEq/L
Serum bicarbonate	34 mEq/L
Arterial blood studies:	
Po_2	105 mm Hg
Pco_2	95 mm Hg
pH	7.25

Electrocardiogram shows an axis of 115° with a persistent S wave in V_5–V_6. The chest roentgenogram is shown. Gram stain of sputum shows numerous PMNs and mixed bacterial flora.

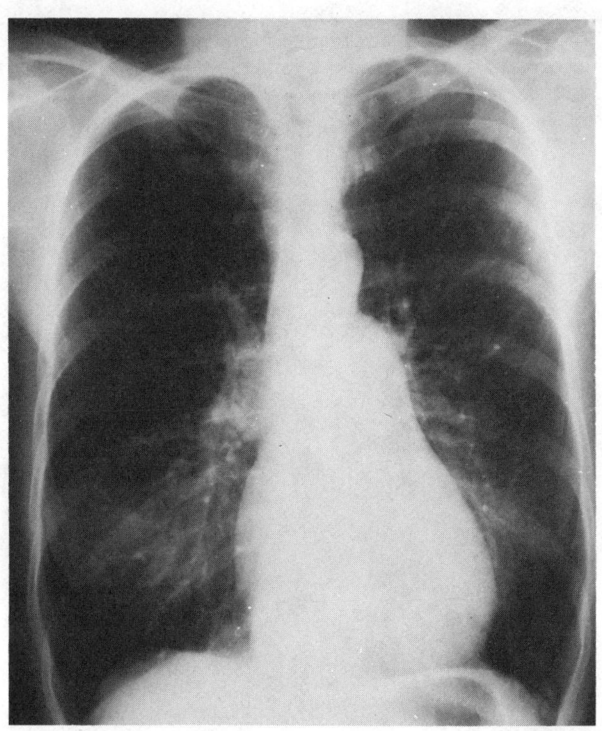

69. The arterial blood gases indicate

A. that the patient should be immediately switched to breathing room air, so that the hypoxic drive to breathing will be restored
B. that the patient was given supplemental oxygen in the ambulance
C. that carbonic anhydrase should be given to eliminate excess bicarbonate
D. alveolar hypoventilation of more than three to five days' duration
E. probable lactic acidosis

70. Initial therapy should include

A. a loading dose of 500 mg of aminophylline followed by a constant infusion of 70 mg/hour
B. digoxin, 0.5 mg intravenously
C. an oral cation exchange resin to correct hyperkalemia
D. administration of a nebulized bronchodilator aerosol (metaproterenol, terbutaline)
E. sedation and bed rest

71. The abnormal appearance of the pulmonary artery on the chest roentgenogram and the right axis deviation on the electrocardiogram should be treated with

A. heparin, until perfusion lung scan, angiogram, or both exclude acute pulmonary embolization
B. morphine sulfate to reduce cardiac preload
C. hydralazine or diazoxide to reduce pulmonary vascular resistance
D. phlebotomy of 2 units or more to reduce the hematocrit to less than 50%
E. measures to increase alveolar ventilation and to maintain arterial Po_2 over 55 mm Hg.

72. Despite appropriate management, the patient's condition deteriorates to the point at which mechanical ventilatory assistance is initiated. Ventilatory treatment should include

A. 10 to 15 cm of positive end-expiratory pressure (PEEP)
B. an FI_{O_2} adequate to maintain arterial oxygen saturation in the range of 90 to 95%
C. careful avoidance of endotracheal suctioning or tracheal manipulation to avoid precipitating reflex bronchospasm
D. adjusting tidal volume and rate to maintain arterial Pco_2 at approximately 50 to 55 mm Hg
E. water delivered by ultrasonic nebulization

QUESTIONS 73–76

A 32-year-old woman with mitral stenosis is late in her second trimester of pregnancy during an outbreak of type A influenza. She presents with fever, headache, myalgias, a nonproductive cough, dyspnea, and conjunctival burning and redness. She appears apprehensive, tachypneic, and cyanotic. Her chest expands poorly with inspiration; breath sounds are distant; a few inspiratory rales are noted. Her neck veins are flat with 30° elevation. The point of maximal cardiac impulse (PMI) is normally located. S_1 is prominent, and an opening snap and faint diastolic rumble can be heard. Laboratory data include:

Hemoglobin	11.2 gm/dl
Hematocrit	34%
White blood cell count	14,000/cu mm with 90% PMNs
Arterial blood studies:	
Po_2	38 mm Hg

Pco_2	44 mm Hg
pH	7.28

Roentgenogram of the chest is shown below. Sputum is scanty, and Gram stain shows scattered mixed flora.

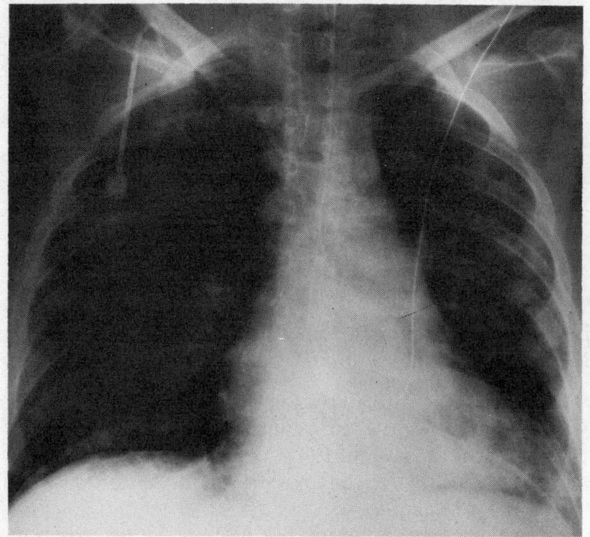

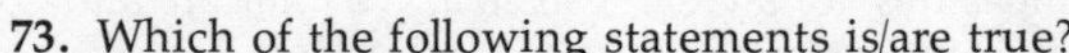

73. Which of the following statements is/are true?

A. End-expiratory lung volume is decreased
B. There is a greater-than-normal change in pleural pressure with inspiration of 500 ml of air
C. The hypoxia is largely caused by widespread narrowing of bronchi throughout the lungs
D. The acidosis will be corrected by normalizing alveolar ventilation
E. Excessive extravascular lung water will be cleared by normalizing left atrial pressure

The patient is intubated and placed on a volume-cycled ventilator. Tidal volume is set at 10 ml/kg, frequency at 16 breaths/minute and $F_{I_{O_2}}$ at 0.4 (40%). One-half hour later, arterial blood gases are Po_2, 49 mm Hg; Pco_2, 39 mm Hg; and pH, 7.35.

74. The patient's hypoxemia may be improved by

A. giving large amounts of intravenous fluid
B. increasing minute ventilation by increasing respiratory frequency
C. infusing a pulmonary arterial vasodilator
D. applying positive end-expiratory pressure (PEEP)
E. halving the tidal volume and doubling respiratory frequency

Eight hours later, the patient develops sudden hypotension, tachycardia, and cyanosis. Breath sounds are decreased over the left chest; the point of maximal cardiac impulse is no longer palpable.

75. At this point, appropriate therapy would include

A. administering a 500-ml saline load
B. inserting a chest tube
C. withdrawing the endotracheal tube 2 to 3 cm
D. inserting a catheter to measure pulmonary arterial and wedge pressure
E. performing pericardiocentesis

Five days after admission, hypoxemia has worsened and a roentgenogram of the chest now appears as shown below, despite appropriate therapy.

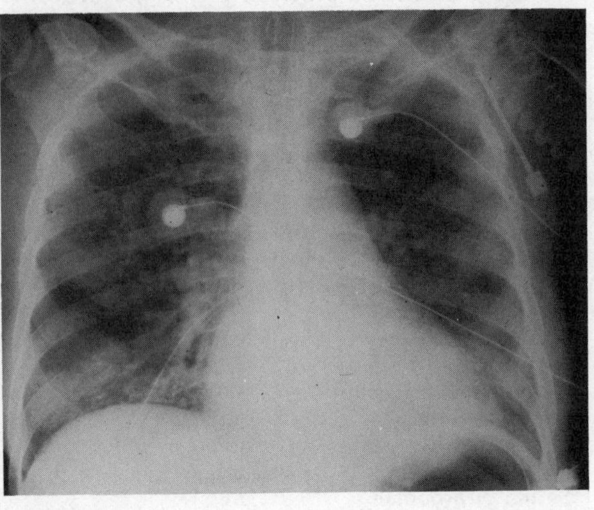

76. This picture is consistent with

A. multiple staphylococcal pneumatoceles
B. bacterial suprainfection
C. oxygen toxicity
D. progression of the primary disease
E. pulmonary congestion from high left atrial pressure

---

77. A 22-year-old black male schoolteacher complains of a nonproductive cough and dyspnea on jogging 2 miles, a distance he formerly covered with ease. Roentgenogram of the chest is shown below.

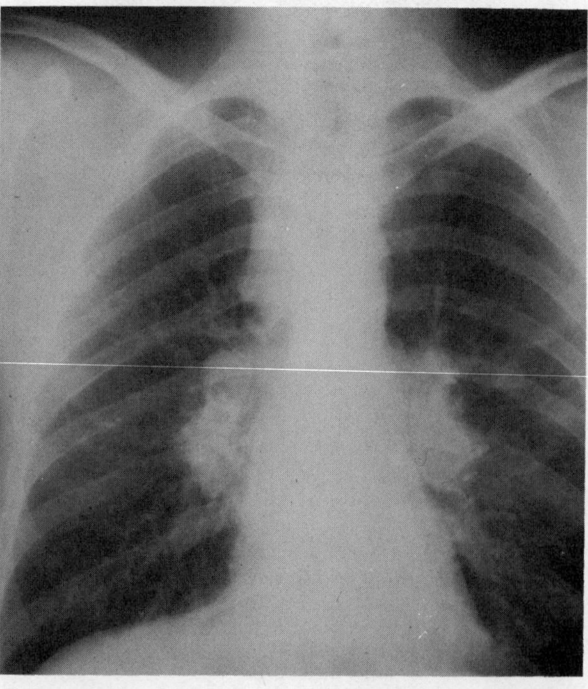

The roentgenographic abnormalities are consistent with

A. Hodgkin's disease
B. diffuse interstitial fibrosis
C. sarcoidosis
D. asbestosis
E. Wegener's granulomatosis

QUESTIONS 78–79

A 19-year-old student with a lifelong history of asthma developed increasing dyspnea, wheezing, and a cough productive of yellowish sputum ten days ago, shortly after contracting a "cold." Despite regular use of aminophylline tablets and increasingly frequent use of his isoproterenol cannister, the symptoms have worsened to the point at which he now has trouble finishing sentences without stopping to inhale. On examination the patient appears apprehensive, diaphoretic, and fatigued. Respirations are 28/minute, with prolonged expiration and audible wheezing. Blood pressure is 140–115/90 mm Hg, pulse rate is 135/minute. Examination of the chest reveals poor inspiratory expansion and diffuse, high-pitched wheezing. FEV_1/FVC is 500/1100 ml. Arterial blood studies show Po_2 58 mm Hg, Pco_2 42 mm Hg, and pH 7.38; the chest film shows overinflation with no lung infiltrate. Gram stain of sputum shows scattered flora.

78. Appropriate therapy includes which of the following?

A. Aminophylline, 500 mg infused intravenously over 30 minutes, followed by continuous infusion of 0.7 mg/kg/hr
B. Methylprednisolone, 50–100 mg intravenously
C. Diazepam, 5–10 mg orally
D. Aerosolized isoproterenol, terbutaline, or metaproterenol
E. Supplemental oxygen by face mask

Appropriate therapy is begun. After initial slight improvement the patient fails to improve further over the next 48 hours.

79. Probable reasons for the failure to improve include

A. inspissation of mucus in the airway lumen
B. abnormally prolonged theophylline half-life owing to undetected liver disease
C. edema and cellular infiltration of the bronchial mucosa.
D. the patient's airway obstruction being in part due to coexistent pulmonary emphysema
E. untreated bacterial bronchitis

---

80. A 23-year-old female schoolteacher with a history of mild perennial asthma comes to the emergency room at 2 o'clock on Sunday morning complaining of shortness of breath, right-sided inspiratory chest pain, and lightheadedness beginning suddenly two hours earlier. She has been using oral contraceptives for two years. On examination she appears anxious. Blood pressure is 105/70 mm Hg, pulse rate is 115/minute, respirations are 24/minute. There is a faint ventricular gallop (S_3) and poor inspiratory expansion of the right chest; wheezing is detected on forced exhalation. No other abnormalities are noted. Laboratory data include:

Hemoglobin	13.5 gm/dl
Hematocrit	40%
White blood cell count	11,200/cu mm
Arterial blood studies:	
Po_2	95 mm Hg
Pco_2	30 mm Hg
pH	7.53

Roentgenogram of the chest shows slight elevation of the right diaphragm; the electrocardiogram is unremarkable. A lung scan shows a segmental perfusion defect in the right midlung field. Which of the following would be appropriate?

A. Treat with bronchodilators for 24 hours and repeat the lung scan
B. Obtain pulmonary angiography
C. Measure pulmonary arterial and wedge pressure with a balloon-tipped catheter
D. Order I^{131} fibrinogen scanning of both lower extremities
E. Treat with anticoagulants for three to six months

DIRECTIONS: Questions 81 to 136 are matching questions. For each numbered item, choose the most likely associated lettered item from those provided. Each numbered item has ONLY ONE answer. Within each group, each lettered item may be the answer to one, more than one, or none of the numbered items, unless otherwise specified.

QUESTIONS 81–85

For the following chest radiographic findings, select the most likely primary malignancy. Use each lettered item only once.

A. Thyroid carcinoma
B. Breast carcinoma
C. Osteogenic sarcoma
D. Laryngeal carcinoma
E. Testicular carcinoma

81. Diffuse linear and reticulonodular markings throughout both lung fields

82. Isolated subpleural nodule in left lower lobe

83. Multiple small nodules throughout both lung fields

84. Several rapidly enlarging, irregular masses with calcification

85. Several irregular masses, some with central cavitation

QUESTIONS 86–90

For each description of clinical findings, select the most likely responsible condition.

A. Goodpasture's syndrome
B. Chronic eosinophilic pneumonia
C. Miliary tuberculosis
D. Eosinophilic granulomatosis
E. Idiopathic pulmonary hemosiderosis

86. Hemoptysis, bilateral pulmonary infiltrates, hematuria

87. Diffuse pulmonary infiltration, diabetes insipidus

88. Diffuse pulmonary fibrosis, microcytic hypochromic anemia

89. Fever, night sweats, diffuse micronodular infiltration

90. Fever, dyspnea, bilateral peripheral pulmonary infiltrates, eosinophilia

QUESTIONS 91–95

For each of the descriptions listed below, select the drug most likely to be responsible for the condition.

A. Busulfan
B. Methysergide
C. Hydralazine
D. Nitrofurantoin
E. Prednisone

91. Fever, pleuritic pain, pleural effusion

92. Fever, cough, pulmonary infiltrates, eosinophilia

93. Parenchymal and pleural fibrosis

94. Fever, dyspnea, diffuse pulmonary infiltrates, type II cell hyperplasia

95. Mediastinal widening

QUESTIONS 96–99

For the following chest radiographic findings, select the most likely associated disease.

A. Sarcoidosis
B. Pulmonary alveolar proteinosis
C. Silicosis
D. Asbestosis

96. Fine granular perihilar and lower lobe infiltrates

97. Calcified hilar nodes with interstitial upper lobe infiltrates

98. Bilateral hilar adenopathy with chiefly lower lobe interstitial infiltrates

99. Diffuse lower lobe interstitial infiltrates with pleural plaques

QUESTIONS 100–102

For each type of sputum that follows, select the lung disease with which it is most likely to be associated.

A. Amebic abscess of lung
B. Resolving pulmonary hemorrhage
C. Anaerobic abscess
D. Coal-worker's pneumoconiosis
E. Cavitating Wegener's granulomatosis

100. Melanoptysis

101. Chocolate- or anchovy sauce–like sputum

102. Putrid sputum

QUESTIONS 103–107

For the following patients, select the most likely set of pulmonary function test results. Use each lettered item only once.

A. Isolated reduction in diffusing capacity
B. Reduction in total lung capacity, residual volume, and diffusing capacity
C. Reduction in the percentage of the vital capacity exhaled in the first second (FEV_1), increase in residual volume, normal diffusing capacity
D. Reduction in total lung capacity, arterial hypoxemia, chronic respiratory acidosis
E. Increase in total lung capacity and residual volume, reduction in maximal expiratory flow, reduction in diffusing capacity

103. A 58-year-old heavy cigarette smoker with progressive dyspnea on exertion and loss of vascular markings on the chest radiograph

104. A 25-year-old woman with Raynaud's phenomenon, dysphagia, and thickening of the skin over the back of the hands

105. A 35-year-old woman with cough and exertional dyspnea following a viral upper respiratory infection

106. A 50-year-old male shipyard worker with progressive exertional dyspnea and cough

107. A 46-year-old man with massive obesity, daytime somnolence, and polycythemia

QUESTIONS 108–112

For each of the listed conditions, choose the most likely associated term. Use each lettered item only once.

A. Hyperpnea
B. Hypoventilation
C. Hyperventilation
D. Dyspnea
E. Orthopnea

108. Morphine overdose

109. Gradual ascent to high altitude

110. Exercise

111. Acute asthmatic attack

112. Bilateral diaphragmatic paralysis

QUESTIONS 113–116

For each of the following side effects, select the drug most likely to have caused it.

A. Isoproterenol
B. Terbutaline
C. Aminophylline
D. Beclomethasone
E. Cromolyn

113. Seizures

114. Hoarseness and sore throat

115. Tremor

116. Palpitations

QUESTIONS 117–121

For each of the following characteristics, select the most likely associated type of pulmonary tumor.

A. Oat cell carcinoma
B. Squamous cell carcinoma
C. Adenocarcinoma
D. Alveolar cell carcinoma
E. Bronchial carcinoid

117. Has multicentric origin

118. Metastasizes early to bone marrow

119. Produces episodic flushing and syncope

120. Most common in cigarette smokers

121. Secretes mucin

QUESTIONS 122–126

For each of the disorders described below, select the organism most likely to have caused it.

A. *Nocardia asteroides*
B. *Pneumocystis carinii*
C. *Pseudomonas aeruginosa*
D. *Aspergillus fumigatus*
E. *Streptococcus pneumoniae*

122. Diffuse, bilateral infiltrates in a kidney transplant recipient with low-grade fever and hypoxia

123. Acid-fast septa on sputum stain

124. Necrotizing pneumonia in a patient receiving immunosuppressive therapy for severe lupus erythematosus

125. Necrotizing pneumonia complicating adult respiratory distress syndrome

126. Dense lobar infiltrate in a patient with multiple myeloma

QUESTIONS 127–131

For each of the following characteristics, select the most likely associated pulmonary disorder.

A. Emphysema
B. Bronchitis
C. Asthma
D. Bilateral vocal cord paralysis
E. Diffuse interstitial fibrosis

127. Maximal inspiratory flow less than maximal expiratory flow

128. Abnormally large decrease in FEV_1 after inhalation of histamine aerosol

129. Greater-than-normal change in pleural pressure during slow inhalation of 500 ml of air

130. Goblet cell hyperplasia

131. Transpulmonary pressure of 7.5 cm H_2O at total lung capacity

QUESTIONS 132–136

For each of the following findings, select the most likely associated disorder.

A. Coccidioidomycosis
B. Histoplasmosis
C. Mucormycosis
D. Tuberculosis
E. Cryptococcosis

132. Cavitary pneumonia, sinusitis, brain abscess

133. Splenic calcification

134. Thin-walled cavity in left upper lobe

135. Pericarditis

136. Hodgkin's disease

PART 2

RESPIRATORY DISEASE

ANSWERS

1. (E) In patients with severe interstitial lung disease, widespread inequalities in matching of ventilation and perfusion have been shown to be responsible for resting hypoxemia. *(Cecil, p. 345)*

2. (D) Aspiration is by far the most common background cause of lung abscess. The infecting organisms are therefore most often the anaerobic bacteria found in the mouth. Aerobes that cause lung abscess are those that cause necrotizing pneumonia, especially *Staphylococcus aureus, Klebsiella pneumoniae,* and *Mycobacterium tuberculosis. Hemophilus influenzae* most often causes exacerbations of chronic bronchitis or bacterial pneumonia, but rarely causes lung abscess. *(Cecil, pp. 383–384)*

3. (B) Because of the vertical gradient of pleural pressure at normal resting lung volume, the alveoli in the lung bases have a smaller initial volume and are on a steeper portion of their pressure-volume curve than are the alveoli in upper lung zones. With inspiration, the volume of these basal alveoli changes more than the volume of apical alveoli. Perfusion does not precisely match this distribution of ventilation, so that mean alveolar oxygen tension is higher at the apex than at the base of the lungs. *(Cecil, pp. 342, 345; Murray, pp. 957–958)*

4. (E) The working diagnosis in this patient is anaerobic lung abscess. The anaerobes found in lung abscess or necrotizing pneumonia are generally susceptible to penicillin, ampicillin, and amoxicillin. Ampicillin would not be acceptable in this patient because of the history of penicillin allergy. Clindamycin, chloramphenicol, and second-generation cephalosporins are active against most anaerobes found in pulmonary infections. *(Cecil, p. 385)*

5. (B) Hypersensitivity pneumonitis is an inflammatory interstitial pneumonitis that results from an Arthus-type immunologic reaction in response to a variety of inhaled organic dusts, e.g., fungal spores or fungal particles from compost or redwood dust, insect particles from wheat weevils, and avian proteins from bird droppings. Inhalation of talc, an inorganic magnesium silicate, causes pulmonary fibrosis and pleural plaques, not hypersensitivity pneumonitis. *(Cecil, pp. 377, 402)*

6. (D) Asthma is associated with an increased drive to ventilation, so that the arterial P_{CO_2} is typically in the low to mid-30s during an acute attack. A normal or increased P_{CO_2} therefore indicates bronchospasm so severe that the patient is unable to match the ventilatory demand, and aggressive treatment is required. *(Cecil, pp. 361, 362–363)*

7. (D) Because the bronchoscope is contaminated by oral or nasopharyngeal flora on insertion, it is unsatisfactory for obtaining material for bacteriologic examination. Sputum samples should be obtained by transtracheal aspiration if the patient is unable to raise sputum on his own. In the other patients, bronchoscopy is indicated for evaluation of the site and cause of hemoptysis, removal of an aspirated foreign body, evaluation of suspected lung carcinoma, and biopsy (under fluoroscopic guidance) of a peripheral nodule. *(Cecil, p. 357)*

8. (D) The uptake of carbon monoxide is determined by the volume of capillary blood in contact with alveolar air (Vc) and the mean thickness of the alveolar-capillary membrane (Dm). Of the diseases listed, all but cystic fibrosis may reduce pulmonary capillary blood volume. Cystic fibrosis affects ciliary function and mucus secretion, and results in severe, progressive obstructive lung disease with recurrent infection and bronchiectasis, but spares pulmonary capillaries. *(Cecil, pp. 344–345)*

9. (C) The history of progressive dyspnea after prolonged intubation suggests that tracheal stenosis has developed in response to ischemic damage caused by excessive pressure in the cuff of the endotracheal tube. Upper airway obstruction causes characteristic changes on the flow-volume curve, depending on whether the lesion is intra- or extrathoracic. *(Cecil, p. 371)*

10. (C) Simple alveolar hypoventilation, as from barbiturate overdose, reduces mean alveolar oxygen tension with consequent arterial hypoxemia. Abnormal widening of the difference between mean alveolar and arterial oxygen tensions is caused by mismatching of ventilation and perfusion, as in status asthmaticus, a diffusion defect, or "shunting" of blood through nonventilated alveoli. Alveolar filling with inflammatory exudate or edema fluid causes a shuntlike effect in lobar or influenza pneumonia and in pulmonary edema. *(Cecil, p. 430)*

11. (A) In assessing the probable effects of pulmonary resection on pulmonary function, it is important to consider whether the tumor is significantly impairing function preoperatively. In this case, the nearly complete obstruction of the right bronchus intermedius prevents the participation of the right lower lobe in the FEV_1, vital capacity, and maximal voluntary ventilation. Removal of this nonfunctioning lung should not greatly impair postoperative pulmonary function. *(Cecil, p. 418)*

12. (E) Histologic studies of the lungs of cigarette smokers show that irreversible obstructive changes first occur in airways less than 2 mm in diameter. These airways contribute little to total airway resistance when the lungs are fully inflated, but contribute a greater proportion at lower lung volumes. A reduction in maximal expiratory flow when 75% of the vital capacity has been exhaled therefore precedes changes in flows at higher lung volumes, such as the peak expiratory flow rate or FEV_1. *(Cecil, p. 364; Murray, pp. 1022–1023)*

13. (E) Examination of pleural fluid from patients in whom a definitive diagnosis could be established has shown that transudates are distinguished by low concentrations of protein and LDH, both in absolute terms and as a proportion of serum values. *(Cecil, pp. 356–357)*

14. (C) Workers exposed to cotton bract develop asthma, probably from chronic irritation of the airways with resultant sensitization of irritant receptors, potentiating reflex cough and bronchoconstriction. Silica, talc, and beryllium cause collagenous pneumoconiosis. Pigeon guano produces diffuse alveolar fibrosis through type III and type IV immune responses. *(Cecil, pp. 399–404)*

15. (C) Bronchopulmonary sequestration is a congenital malformation arising from accessory budding of the tracheobronchial tree in fetal development. The sequestered segment does not communicate with the normal bronchial tree and receives its vascular supply from a branch of the aorta. *(Cecil, p. 373)*

16. (D) The fundamental abnormality in the type B or "bronchial" form of COPD is chronic inflammatory damage to the bronchial wall, with mucous gland hypertrophy, edema, cellular infiltration, and smooth muscle hyperplasia, so that the airway lumen is narrowed during both inspiration and expiration. In the type A (emphysematous) form, the airway lumen narrows during expiration because of the loss of support of the surrounding lung parenchyma. During inspiration, negative pleural pressures hold the airways open. *(Cecil, pp. 367–370; Murray, pp. 1023–1024)*

17. (D) Diffuse alveolar fibrosis is frequently found on lung biopsy or postmortem examination of patients with diffuse systemic sclerosis. Although intimal proliferation is frequently found in small pulmonary vessels in this disorder, pathologic changes in the lung vasculature do not directly affect lung volumes. *(Cecil, p. 380)*

18. (D) Radiation provides valuable palliative therapy for relief of symptoms due to localized metastases, whether to mediastinal nodes (superior vena caval obstruction) or to bone. Irradiation of the primary lesion often relieves local effects, such as obstruction or hemoptysis. Hypertrophic osteoarthropathy remits with surgical or irradiation-induced reduction in the tumor mass. Pancytopenia reflects extensive metastatic replacement of bone marrow and is not amenable to radiotherapy. *(Cecil, pp. 417–418)*

19. (B) Foreign materials such as talc crystals or cotton fibers may be injected with heroin into peripheral veins and are filtered from the circulation by precapillary pulmonary vessels. A fibrotic inflammatory response in vascular or perivascular tissues obliterates the vascular bed and causes eventual pulmonary hypertension. Septic emboli may result from direct injection of contaminated material or from embolization of valvular vegetations from right-sided endocarditis. Pulmonary edema often complicates heroin overdose and is presumed to be due to a transient change in permeability of the alveolar-capillary membrane. Aspiration may result from drug-induced impairment of consciousness or from misguided attempts to resuscitate an unconscious drug user by pouring milk or other material into the mouth and throat. Veno-occlusive disease is a disorder of unknown etiology, but develops in postcapillary vessels, which are protected from the effects of intravenous injection of foreign matter by the filtering action of pulmonary arteries, arterioles, and capillaries. *(Cecil, pp. 2008–2009)*

20. (A) Rheumatoid arthritis, in common with other collagen-vascular diseases, often causes pleural inflammation with local pain and effusion. It is also associated with diffuse fibrosis of the lung parenchyma ("rheumatoid lung"); pulmonary hypertension may be seen with far-advanced pulmonary fibrosis from any cause. Upper airway obstruction may be caused by rheumatoid involvement of the cricoarytenoid joints. Lobar atelectasis is most commonly caused by obstruction of a large bronchus by inspissation of a large mucus plug or by local tumor growth, and is not associated with rheumatoid arthritis. *(Cecil, pp. 379–380)*

21. (D) *M. intracellulare* is a Group III atypical mycobacterium that may cause primary pulmonary disease in an apparently normal host. It is resistant to standard antituberculous chemotherapy, and prolonged treatment with a multiple-drug regimen is required. If the infection progresses despite therapy, surgical resection may be required. The mode of spread of infection is unknown, but person-to-person communication does not occur. *(Cecil, p. 1555)*

22. (D) The chest roentgenogram and whole lung tomogram show multiple localized infiltrates with central cavitation. The symptoms of sinusitis and the finding of hematuria suggest a systemic disorder involving the upper respiratory tract and kidneys as well as the lungs. This triad is characteristic of Wegener's granulomatosis, a necrotizing granulomatous vasculitis of the upper and lower respiratory tract with focal glomerulitis or glomerulonephritis. The absence of hilar or mediastinal adenopathy and the presence of central cavitation distinguishes the roentgenographic appearance from sarcoidosis (patient A). Cavitation is very rarely seen with mycoplasma pneumonia (patient B). The patchy, localized infiltrates are inconsistent with typical lobar pneumonia (patient C) or pulmonary edema from smoke inhalation (patient E). *(Cecil, pp. 1869–1871)*

23. (E) Involvement of hilar and mediastinal nodes with eggshell calcification is almost pathognomonic of silicosis, but it has been reported in sarcoidosis. *(Cecil, pp. 399–400)*

24. (D) The clinical history of a subacute illness with fever and chest pain and the chest roentgenogram shown suggest an aerobic bacterial empyema. Advanced infections such as this one are often associated with low pleural fluid pH, perhaps reflecting the accumulation of metabolic products of leukocyte activity. Severe pleural inflammatory disease may lead to persistent fibrous entrapment of the underlying lung even after the infection has been controlled. Proper therapy includes parenteral antibiotics (usually with penicillin alone) and adequate drainage of the pleural space. Instillation of tetracycline into the pleural space would elicit further inflammatory reaction and would add little to systemic antibiotic therapy. *(Cecil, pp. 423–424)*

25. (E) Sarcoidosis is a systemic disorder with noncaseating granulomas found in lymphatic tissue, lungs, liver, spleen, skin, and other sites. Erythema nodosum is immunologically mediated, and biopsies reveal vasculitic changes rather than direct granulomatous involvement of the skin. *(Cecil, pp. 1891–1896, 2280)*

26. (D); 27. (D); 28. (C) Studies of obese patients with similar complaints have shown repeated interruption of sleep by apneic spells caused by recurrent obstruction of the upper airway by opposition of the tongue against the posterior pharyngeal wall. Despite vigorous respiratory efforts, no air movement occurs. The resulting hypoxia and hypercapnia stimulate pulmonary arterial vasoconstriction, overloading the right ventricle. Eventually, reflex responses to the worsening gas values rouse the patient, who typically resumes breathing with a sonorous snore, sometimes thrashing about or rising from bed. These episodes occur hundreds of times nightly, so that compensatory polycythemia and chronic right-sided heart failure may develop. Deprivation of normal restful sleep (stage IV or V) leads to daytime exhaustion. Tracheostomy bypasses the obstructed upper airway and relieves the consequences of recurrent nocturnal apnea. Because upper airway obstruction does not occur when the patient is awake, it is not responsible for the exercise intolerance associated with obesity. *(Cecil, pp. 432, 1934–1935; Walsh et al.; Murray, pp. 1042–1044)*

29. (C) Sarcoid granuloma may compress the seventh cranial nerve, damage the posterior pituitary, or interrupt the conduction system of the heart. Crampy flank pain and hematuria suggest renal calculi, possibly secondary to the increased gastrointestinal absorption of calcium seen in sarcoidosis. Painless ulceration of the skin over the ankles suggests a vasculitic process rather than sarcoidosis. *(Cecil, pp. 1891–1896)*

30. (A — False; B — False; C — True; D — False; E — False) Tuberculous pleurisy often occurs shortly after primary infection; pleural involvement results from extension of disease from the lung where the infection developed. The effusion in this setting results from hypersensitivity to tubercular protein in pleural tubercles. Acid-fast bacilli are rarely seen in the effusion itself. Skin-test conversion may not yet have occurred in some patients, but about two thirds of patients will go on to develop clinically apparent disease if left untreated. The infecting organisms are those that are responsible for new cases of pulmonary tuberculosis, so the incidence of isoniazid resistance does not differ from that ordinarily found. *(Cecil, p. 423)*

31. (A — True; B — True; C — True; D — False; E — True) Cough is a nonspecific symptom that may be produced by any condition that alters the distending pressure across airways (congestive heart failure, diffuse interstitial fibrosis), constriction of airway smooth muscle (asthma), or growth of tissue over the mucosal surface (bronchogenic carcinoma). Primary disorders of efferent nerves do not cause cough, but may cause hiccup. *(Cecil, p. 335)*

32. (A — False; B — False; C — False; D — True; E — True) Simple chronic bronchitis is diagnosed when productive cough is present on most days for at least three months of the year. Cough and mucous gland hypertrophy (detected as abnormally enlarged ducts on bronchography) develop in response to chronic irritation, usually by cigarette smoke, and improve when the irritant is removed. The effect of cigarette smoking on airway function seems to be independent of its effect on mucous secretion, as smokers with productive cough do not have a greater decline in lung function than asymptomatic smokers. Regular use of an antibiotic would reduce the duration and severity of exacerbations, which are due to overgrowth of bacteria that have colonized the respiratory tract, but would not reduce the frequency of exacerbations. *(Cecil, pp. 365–366)*

33. (A — True; B — True; C — True; D — True; E — False) Maximal expiratory flow is determined by the lung's tendency to recoil inward, the resistance of the airways to flow, and the generation of a critical positive pleural pressure. Only when this pressure has been achieved will further expiratory effort fail to further increase flow ("effort-independent flow"). Breathing a low-density gas mixture results in an increase in flow. *(Cecil, p. 342; Murray, pp. 953–956)*

34. (A — True; B — False; C — False; D — True; E — True) Compliance, the change in lung volume for a given change in pressure, is reduced by any process that reduces the number of patent air-filled alveoli communicating with the airways (pulmonary edema, interstitial fibrosis), that increases the stiffness of lung tissue (interstitial fibrosis), or that prevents the expansion of the alveoli when transalveolar pressure is increased (pleural fibrosis). Asthma is associated with a reversible increase in lung compliance. Obesity reduces the compliance of the chest wall, not of the lungs. *(Cecil, p. 340; Murray, pp. 947–951)*

35. (A — False; B — True; C — False; D — False; E — False) About 10% of asthmatic patients have a peculiar triad of bronchospasm, nasal polyps, and sensitivity to aspirin. The mechanism is unknown, but may have to do with drug-induced alteration in prostaglandin metabolism. Indomethacin, aminopyrine, and yellow food dyes (e.g., tartrazine yellow) may also trigger attacks of severe bronchospasm, urticaria, and even hypotension. These patients do not react to sodium salicylate, further suggesting that the condition is not immunologically mediated. *(Cecil, p. 361)*

36. (A — False; B — False; C — False; D — False; E — True) Cystic fibrosis is transmitted as an autosomal recessive disorder. The diagnosis is supported by finding elevated levels of chloride in eccrine sweat. Other biologic fluids have normal electrolyte concentrations. With improving medical therapy, approximately 50% of all patients now survive to age 18. Pneumothorax often complicates the illness, and IPPB should be avoided. *Pseudomonas* and staphylococcal infections so often cause exacerbation of pulmonary symptoms that empiric treatment with tobramycin and methicillin is often given. *(Cecil, pp. 387–388)*

37. (A — False; B — True; C — False; D — False; E — True) Pulmonary and pleural involvement in SLE is common, occurring in more than 50% of patients. This high frequency is largely due to the frequency of polyserositis with pleuritis. Pleural effusions are exudative and may have LE cells. Pulmonary infiltrates may be due to pulmonary vasculitis, infection, or interstitial pneumonitis. A positive antinuclear antibody associated with interstitial infiltrates is found in a number of interstitial lung diseases. *(Cecil, p. 399)*

38. (A — False; B — True; C — False; D — False; E — True) Pulmonary granulomatous vasculitis is characterized by granuloma formation in addition to vasculitis. Pulmonary diseases that show this pattern are Wegener's granulomatosis, allergic granulomatosis, and lymphomatoid granulomatosis. *(Cecil, pp. 378–379)*

39. (A — False; B — True; C — True; D — True; E — True) The inhalation of asbestos fibers can produce interstitial pulmonary fibrosis, pleural effusions and fibrosis, pleural plaques, mesotheliomas of the pleura and peritoneum, lung cancer, and cancer of the larynx and gastrointestinal tract. Unlike silica exposure, asbestos exposure does not cause lymphadenopathy. *(Cecil, pp. 400–402)*

40. (A — True; B — False; C — True; D — True; E — True) Allergic bronchopulmonary aspergillosis is one of the many causes of pulmonary infiltrates with eosinophilia and should be considered when these findings are associated with asthma. The disease is most commonly caused by an allergy to a *noninvasive colonization* of the bronchial airways by species of *Aspergillus*. Patients with this disorder frequently cough up brownish, rubbery bronchial casts, which on microscopic examination are found to be packed with the septate hyphae of the aspergilli. Bronchiectasis restricted to the proximal bronchi has often been said to be pathognomonic of this disorder. The allergic reaction is characterized by a Type I reaginic response

(IgE), which appears to pave the way for the Type III antigen-antibody–mediated reaction. The aspergillus skin test in affected individuals typically causes a dual response with an immediate wheal-and-flare reaction, followed in four to ten hours by an Arthus lesion at the test site. *(Cecil, p. 376)*

41. (All are True) The prevalence of bronchiectasis has decreased since antibiotics have come into common use. Distortion of the bronchial anatomy and airway obstruction by tuberculosis, other bacterial pneumonias, foreign bodies, tumors, and chronic asthma continue to predispose to the development of bronchiectasis. In a young person without an evident predisposing cause, one must consider cystic fibrosis, immotile cilia syndrome, and immunodeficiency syndrome. *(Cecil, pp. 386–387)*

42. (A — True; B — True; C — False; D — True; E — True) Severe deficiency of alpha$_1$ globulin, which contains most of the serum's antiproteolytic activity, occurs in patients homozygous for the Z phenotype for protease inhibitor (Pi phenotype). This genetic abnormality is associated with hepatitis in infancy and with the early onset of panacinar emphysema that is most apparent in the lung bases on the chest radiograph. *(Cecil, p. 367)*

43. (A — True; B — False; C — False; D — True; E — True) These radiographic findings (typical of overinflation) are found in patients with any of the obstructive airway diseases. Diseases primarily affecting the lung vasculature do not result in an increase in alveolar volume and may, by producing right ventricular hypertrophy, result in a decrease in retrosternal air space. With paralysis, the diaphragms are displaced upward into the thoracic cage by the abdominal contents. *(Cecil, p. 368)*

44. (A — False; B — False; C — True; D — True; E — True) Nonmetastatic effects of bronchogenic carcinoma include hypertrophic pulmonary osteoarthropathy (C), spinocerebellar degeneration (D), and peripheral neuropathy (E). These syndromes do not progress further, and may improve, with treatment of the primary malignancy. Spinal cord compression (A) requires prompt therapy directed toward the epi- or subdural metastasis, regardless of the state of the primary tumor. Horner's syndrome (B) is due to extension or metastasis of the malignancy to a cervical ganglion. *(Cecil, pp. 415–416)*

45. (A — True; B — False; C — True; D — False; E — False) Youth and central calcification provide strong evidence that a solitary pulmonary nodule is benign. Bronchogenic carcinoma is very rare in patients under 35 years old. A dense central nidus of calcification almost always indicates that a lesion is granulomatous. Sputum cytologic examination is generally negative even in patients with malignant peripheral nodules. A doubling time (remembering that volume is a function of the third power of the radius) of between five weeks and 18 months is compatible with malignancy. A positive coccidioidin skin test suggests another possible cause for the nodule, but positive skin tests are so common in endemic areas that the finding cannot be considered strong evidence against malignancy. *(Cecil, pp. 420–421)*

46. (All are True) Pulmonary edema resulting from increased alveolar capillary permeability is an important cause of acute respiratory failure, especially in patients hospitalized with serious medical and surgical illnesses that initially do not involve the lungs. The resulting clinical syndrome, known as the adult respiratory distress syndrome, has been reported as a complication of many apparently unrelated conditions, including fat embolism (A), pancreatitis (B), fresh water near-drowning (C), drug overdose (D), and gram-negative sepsis (E). *(Cecil, pp. 431–432)*

47. (A — False; B — True; C — False, D — False; E — False) Hypoxemia on room air in patients with angiographically proved pulmonary emboli can be accounted for by the amount of true shunting measured by the 100% oxygen technique. The temporary reversibility of hypoxemia with inhalation of breaths equal to 80% or more of the predicted inspiratory capacity suggests that hypoxemia is due to microatelectasis. Even with large pulmonary emboli, the Po_2 can be deceptively normal: capillary perfusion is best maintained in normally ventilated areas. Furthermore, an increase in alveolar ventilation may raise mean alveolar oxygen tension to levels where the arterial Po_2 is normal despite an abnormal widening of the alveolar-arterial oxygen difference [(A-a)dO_2]. The (A-a)dO_2 gradually returns to normal over about two months after the embolus. *(Cecil, pp. 389, 390–394)*

48. (A — True; B — False; C — False; D — False; E — False) Fortunately, intrapulmonary bleeding usually stops spontaneously. Until it does, the affected lung should be kept lowermost to keep the airways free of blood. Heavy sedation, which may suppress cough, should be avoided. Bronchoscopy should be performed in virtually every patient with significant hemoptysis to determine the site of bleeding and its cause, and the site is most easily found when bleeding is ongoing. Isolation of the healthy lung from the hemorrhagic lung by intubation of the right main-stem bronchus is reserved for massive, life-threatening hemoptysis. Hemoptysis is frequently due to bleeding from the bronchial circulation and will not be localized by pulmonary angiography. *(Cecil, pp. 336–337)*

49. (A — False; B — False; C — True; D — False; E — True) Lymphomatous malignancies may involve intrathoracic lymph nodes and may extend to the lung parenchyma or pleura via lymphatic vessels. The roentgenogram of the chest may therefore reveal hilar or mediastinal adenopathy, parenchymal infiltration, or pleural effusion. Anterior mediastinal adenopathy and pleural effusion are rare in sarcoidosis. Diffuse interstitial fibrosis complicates chronic sarcoidosis; bullae may result from retraction of lung tissue and distortion of airway architecture. *(Cecil, pp. 382, 419, 1891–1896)*

50. (A — False; B — True; C — False; D — True; E — False) The binding of carbon monoxide to hemoglobin not only reduces the number of sites available for oxygen transport but also increases the affinity of hemoglobin for oxygen, so that hemoglobin desaturation does not occur at normal tissue Po_2. Arterial oxygen tension is proportional to the quantity of oxygen dissolved in plasma and is not influenced by the replacement of oxygen by carbon monoxide in erythrocytic hemoglobin. The lack of oxygen reduces oxidative metabolism, but the link between metabolism of glucose and generation of ATP is unimpaired. *(Cecil, p. 409; Roughton)*

51. (A — True; B — False; C — True; D — False; E — True) The history and roentgenographic findings suggest bronchiectasis, which is usually caused by peripheral bronchial obstruction, stasis, and infection, with destruction of muscle and elastic tissue in the bronchial wall. Common predisposing conditions include severe bronchopneumonia or tuberculosis in childhood. In cystic fibrosis, thick secretions obstruct the bronchial lumen, and normal mucociliary clearance is impaired. Recurrent infections in individuals with agammaglobulinemia also lead to bronchiectasis. Gingivitis and periodontitis may predispose to anaerobic abscess or pneumonia, but not to recurrent airway obstruction and infection. *(Cecil, p. 386)*

52. (A — True; B — True; C — True; D — False; E — True) The fluid-filled cavity on the chest roentgenogram suggests lung abscess, and the most important background factor for lung abscess or necrotizing pneumonia is aspiration, usually related to altered consciousness. Common causes of altered consciousness in such patients are alcoholism, cerebral vascular accident, general anesthesia, drug overdose or addiction, seizure disorder, diabetic coma, shock, or other serious illness. Other factors in aspiration include dysphagia caused by esophageal disease or neurologic disease. Next to aspiration, the most important factor predisposing to lung abscess or necrotizing pneumonia is periodontal disease or gingivitis. Although abscess has been reported with primary infection with *Mycoplasma pneumoniae,* it is extremely uncommon. Mycoplasmal pneumonia does not predispose to secondary bacterial infection. *(Cecil, pp. 383–386, 1427–1429)*

53. (A — True; B — True; C — False; D — False; E — True) Hemosiderin-laden macrophages simply reflect the presence of intra-alveolar blood, and are a nonspecific finding. Intra-alveolar bleeding is a late and unusual event in primary pulmonary hypertension. As hemolytic anemia is associated with intravascular destruction of red cells, blood does not enter the alveolar space. *(Cecil, p. 356)*

54. (A — False; B — True; C — False; D — True; E — False) A low value for glucose in pleural fluid is virtually diagnostic of rheumatoid arthritis, but only if tuberculous and malignant effusion can be excluded. *(Cecil, pp. 356–357)*

55. (A — True; B — False; C — False; D — True; E — False) Increasing alveolar Po_2 will not correct hypoxia due to shunting of blood through an intracardiac defect (patient E), through fluid-filled alveoli (as in the post-traumatic adult respiratory distress syndrome—patient B), or through an arteriovenous malformation (patient C). Hypoxia due to mismatching of ventilation and perfusion (patients A and D) is distinguished by its correction on administration of supplemental oxygen. *(Cecil, pp. 346–348)*

56. (A — True; B — True; C — True; D — False; E — True) Clubbing is not specific for diseases of the respiratory system. It occurs in patients with ascending cholangitis (patient A) as well as in patients with bronchiectasis, lung cancer, or cystic fibrosis (patients C, B, and E). Clubbing is not associated with asthma. *(Cecil, pp. 387, 416)*

57. (A — True; B — False; C — True; D — False; E — True) The flow-volume curve is concave, suggesting a reduction in maximal expiratory flow at mid- and low lung volumes; this pattern results from loss of lung recoil, as in emphysema (patient C) or from an increase in airway resistance, as in chronic obstructive bronchitis or asthma (patients A and E). The interstitial diseases associated with collagen-vascular diseases increase lung recoil, causing abnormally high flow rates (patient B). Recurrent pulmonary emboli (patient D) obliterate pulmonary vessels, reducing diffusing capacity, but do not affect lung recoil or airway resistance. *(Cecil, pp. 339–345)*

58. (A — True; B — False; C — True; D — False; E — True) Precipitating antibodies are found in patients with primary infection from *Coccidioides immitis* (patient A); they precede the appearance of complement-fixing antibodies. Precipitating antibodies against *Aspergillus fumigatus* are typically found in the serum of patients with bronchopulmonary aspergillosis (patient E) or with mycetoma occurring in cysts or bullae from pre-existing lung disease (patient C). "Silo filler's diseae" (patient D) is an acute pulmonary edema caused by inhalation of toxic levels of nitrogen dioxide, and is not mediated immunologically. The pathogenesis of byssinosis (patient B) is unknown, but it appears that some fraction of the offending dust causes the nonantigenic release of histamine, thus triggering bronchoconstriction. *(Cecil, pp. 376, 403, 408, 1700–1701)*

59. (A — True; B — True: C — True; D — False; E — False) Adrenocorticotropin (ACTH), antidiuretic hormone (ADH), and parathyroid hormone (PTH) may be secreted by primary lung tumors, particularly of the small cell, anaplastic type. Secretion of thyroid-stimulating hormone (TSH) has been reported with choriocarcinoma metastatic to the lung, but neither TSH nor insulin secretion has been found with primary lung cancer. *(Cecil, pp. 415–416, 1022–1026)*

60. (A — True; B — True; C — False; D — False; E — False) The arterial blood gases suggest acute alveolar hypoventilation with a normal alveolar-arterial oxygen difference [(A-a)dO_2]. Such a pattern might be found in rapid failure of the respiratory musculature in myasthenia gravis (patient A) or from depression of the respiratory center, as in the patient with myxedema given a sedative (patient B). The lung contusion or bronchial laceration causing hemoptysis in patient D and the intubation of the right main bronchus in Patient C would interfere with the lung as an organ of gas exchange and widen the (A-a)dO_2. Aspirin ingestion in children (patient E) produces a mixed metabolic acidosis and respiratory alkalosis. *(Cecil, pp. 346–348)*

61. (A — False; B — False; C — False; D — True; E — False) Pulmonary embolism is most often associated with a clear, amber, nonhemorrhagic effusion. Although an embolus does increase the respiratory dead space by blocking perfusion of ventilated lung, such a disorder does not produce hypoxemia. The hypoxemia associated with pulmonary embolism is probably due to atelectasis in adjacent areas of the lung where perfusion is maintained. A perfusion defect on a lung scan simply demonstrates decreased perfusion of a portion of the pulmonary vascular bed and is compatible with localized pulmonary infiltration, localized airway constriction (with local reflex vasoconstriction), lung cysts or bullae, or other disorders. The diagnosis can be confirmed only by angiography. Fever of 39°C or higher may occur in the first 48 hours after an acute embolus. *(Cecil, pp. 389–394)*

62. (All are False) Effective antituberculous therapy reduces infectivity so rapidly that isolation (or even hospitalization) of patients with uncomplicated pulmonary tuberculosis is no longer considered necessary. After completion of a course of chemotherapy, the chances of reactivation are so remote as to make prolonged follow-up unnecessary. Primary isoniazid resistance is unusual in the United States, so that treatment with isoniazid and ethambutol is usually adequate and a third antituberculous drug is not needed to cover the remote possibility that a resistant strain is present, except in recent immigrants. A nine-month course of therapy is effective only if two bactericidal drugs (e.g., isoniazid and rifampin) are used. All household contacts of a new active case should be treated, regardless of their skin-test status. *(Cecil, pp. 1541–1542, 1544–1548)*

63. (A — True; B — True; C — True; D — False, E — True) Asbestos exposure has been causally related to diffuse alveolar fibrosis, bronchogenic carcinoma (especially in cigarette smokers), and mesothelioma. It has not been implicated in causing obstructive lung disease, suggested by the pattern of abnormal function in answer D. Recurrent pleural effusions may also result from asbestos exposure and do not necessarily indicate an underlying mesothelioma. *(Cecil, pp. 400–402)*

64. (A — False; B — False; C — True; D — True; E — True) The arterial blood gases show acute, uncompensated respiratory alkalosis with an abnormally great alveolar-arterial oxygen difference. Acute pulmonary embolism (patient D), asthma (patient E), and congestive heart failure (patient C) are associated with an abnormal drive to ventilation (causing the Pco_2 to fall) and with hypoxemia. Diffuse alveolar fibrosis (patient A) is associated with hyperventilation, but because the disorder is chronic, renal excretion of bicarbonate should have normalized the pH. In a patient with normal lungs (patient B), acute hyperventilation *increases* arterial Po_2. *(Cecil, pp. 346–348, 429–430)*

65. (A — True; B — False; C — True; D — False; E — False) The diagnosis of *Pneumocystis carinii* infection is made by demonstrating the organism histologically. The disease involves the peripheral, gas-exchanging portion of the lung, so tissue must ordinarily be obtained by bronchoscopy with transbronchial or brush biopsy or by open lung biopsy. Pleural effusions are not associated with the infection and no reliable serologic test is available. Many disorders cause diffuse bilateral infiltrates on the chest radiograph, and a specific diagnosis cannot be made on this basis. *(Cecil, pp. 1742–1744; Williams et al.)*

66. (All are True) Although flexible fiberoptic bronchoscopy is ordinarily safe and well tolerated, all the listed complications have occurred. Pneumothorax results from puncture of the visceral pleura, hemorrhage from laceration of a bronchial artery, and hypoxemia (10–15 mm fall in Po_2) from ventilation-perfusion mismatching. Laryngospasm is probably due to a reflex response to mechanical irritation of the larynx, and is made less likely by careful application of a topical anesthetic to the upper airway before insertion of the bronchoscope. Fever has been reported in 10% of patients who have undergone bronchoscopy, but it is rarely associated with sepsis or radiographic evidence of pneumonia. *(Cecil, p. 357)*

67. (A — False; B — True; C — False; D — False; E — True) Abrupt "cut-off" of a large vessel or an intraluminal filling defect confirms the diagnosis of pulmonary embolism. Delayed filling, "pruning" of arteries, and shifts in perfusion to other regions are helpful findings but are nonspecific. *(Cecil, pp. 392–393)*

68. (A — False; B — False; C — False; D — True; E — True) The reduction in chest wall compliance caused by obesity decreases functional residual capacity (the point at which the opposing tendencies of the chest wall to recoil outward and of the lung to recoil inward are equal and opposite), but does not alter residual volume (determined by airway closure). Air inspired at low lung volumes is distributed to mid- and upper lung regions, so that the well-perfused lung bases are poorly ventilated. This mismatching of ventilation and perfusion results in hypoxemia. *(Cecil, pp. 346–348)*

69. (A — False; B — True; C — False; D — True; E — False) Mean alveolar Po_2 can be estimated from the formula $PA_{O_2} = PI_{O_2} - 1.25 \times Paco_2$. Breathing room air at sea level, this patient's calculated PA_{O_2} would be 32 mm Hg. As it is impossible for arterial Po_2 to be *greater* than alveolar Po_2, the PI_{O_2} must have been greater than 150, implying that supplemental oxygen was given. Switching the patient to room air would mean that unless alveolar ventilation improved, alveolar Po_2 would be 32 mm Hg — a dangerously low value. One cannot count on the respiratory system responding rapidly enough to avoid a precipitous fall in Po_2. The increase in Pco_2 largely reflects alveolar hypoventilation. The high bicarbonate excludes superimposed metabolic acidosis and implies chronic respiratory insufficiency. With uncompensated respiratory acidosis of this severity, pH would be about 7.15. Carbonic anhydrase should not be used in an unstable patient already acidotic from respiratory failure. *(Cecil, pp. 433–435)*

70. (A — True; B — False; C — False; D — True; E — False) The hyperkalemia reflects acute acidosis and will improve as alveolar ventilation is increased. No additional therapy is required. The right-sided heart failure evident on physical examination will improve as gas exchange is improved and pulmonary vascular resistance decreases. Digoxin is unnecessary and carries the risk of toxicity with the shifts in potassium ion that will follow correction of the respiratory acidosis. A normal loading dose of aminophylline should be given if the patient has been taking no theophylline-containing medications. Because the drug is metabolized in the liver, half of the usual maintenance dose should be used in the presence of right-sided heart failure with hepatic congestion. Aerosolized bronchodilators are safe and effective in reducing bronchospasm and in increasing mucociliary clearance. Sedation is contraindicated in a patient already on the verge of CO_2 narcosis. *(Cecil, pp. 362–363)*

71. (A — False; B — False; C — False; D — False; E — True) Pulmonary embolism need not be invoked to account for pulmonary hypertension and right ventricular strain in a hypoxic, hypercapnic patient with chronic obstructive lung disease. Hypoxia and hypercapnic acidosis are responsible for contraction of vascular smooth muscle; pulmonary hypertension will resolve as gas exchange is improved. Phlebotomy is not necessary for polycythemia with a hematocrit of less than 60%. At higher levels, an increase in blood viscosity significantly impedes blood flow in small vessels. Morphine sulfate would further depress the respiratory center and is contraindicated. Intravenous aminophylline and methylprednisolone, aerosolized adrenergic agents, verbal stimulation, and judicious use of supplemental oxygen are all appropriate. *(Cecil, pp. 435–437)*

72. (A — False; B — True; C — False; D — True; E — False) PEEP is indicated for increasing lung volume and for stabilizing alveolar units in conditions in which intra-alveolar exudation of fluid and loss of surfactant reduce lung compliance and lead to closure of peripheral airways. In chronic bronchitis, lung compliance is normal or increased. Tracheal suction should be performed frequently, as inspissation of abnormally thick mucus contributes to airway obstruction. Because the serum bicarbonate level is elevated, reducing Pco_2 to the normal range of 40 ± 1.5 mm Hg would produce severe alkalosis. A Pco_2 of 50 to 55 mm Hg would be an appropriate first goal for this patient. Adequate saturation of hemoglobin is achieved at a Po_2 of 60 mm Hg. The FI_{O_2} should be kept no higher than necessary to avoid oxygen toxicity. With oxygen saturation less than 90%, there is potential danger of ischemic damage to tissues supplied by partially obstructed vessels. Water droplets may actually cause reflex bronchoconstriction, worsening airway obstruction. Even with ultrasonic nebulization, only very small amounts are delivered beyond the ductal airways. Increasing the water content of mucus is best attempted with parenteral or oral hydration. *(Cecil, pp. 433–435)*

73. (A — True; B — True; C — False; D — False; E — False) With influenza pneumonia, increased permeability of the alveolar-capillary membrane leads to transudation of abnormal quantities of fluid and large molecular weight proteins into the alveolar space, decreasing lung volumes, reducing lung compliance, and interfering with normal oxygenation of blood. Because the fundamental abnormality is in the permeability of the membrane, fluid is not removed by simply normalizing left atrial pressure. Arterial pH is disproportionately low for the modest degree of hypercapnia indicating a combined metabolic and respiratory acidosis. *(Cecil, pp. 2187–2198)*

74. (A — False; B — False; C — False; D — True; E — False) Because the hypoxemia is largely due to "shunting" of blood through nonventilated or fluid-filled alveoli, infusion of an arterial vasodilator would worsen the hypoxemia. Maintaining airway patency and stabilizing lung units with positive end-expiratory pressure (PEEP) will reduce the severity of shunting and improve arterial Po_2. Decreasing the volume and increasing the frequency of ventilation would result in an increase in wasted ventilation, reducing alveolar ventilation and worsening hypoxemia. *(Cecil, pp. 2187–2198)*

75. (A — False; B — True; C — False; D — False; E — False) Tension pneumothorax must be considered in the presence of an asymmetric decrease in breath sounds and the sudden appearance of hypotension in a patient on a mechanical ventilator. Prompt insertion of a chest tube to decompress the pleural space is imperative. *(Cecil, pp. 2187–2198)*

76. (A — False; B — True; C — True; D — True; E — True) The radiographic and physiologic data suggest progressive filling of alveoli by fluid or inflammatory cells. Pneumatoceles are rounded, subpleural cysts surrounded by densely infiltrated tissue; none can be seen on this roentgenogram. *(Cecil, pp. 2187–2198)*

77. (A — True; B — False; C — True; D — False; E — False) Diffuse interstitial fibrosis and asbestosis spare hilar nodes. The roentgenographic picture is typical of sarcoidosis, but Hodgkin's disease may rarely present with bilateral hilar adenopathy and parenchymal infiltration. Wegener's granulomatosis presents roentgenographically as nodules of varying size that frequently cavitate. Hilar and mediastinal adenopathy rarely occur. *(Cecil, pp. 382, 955–956)*

78. (A — False; B — True; C — False; D — True; E — True) A loading dose of aminophylline should not be given in a patient who has been using it chronically. Maintenance intravenous therapy, methylprednisolone, and inhaled adrenergic aerosols are appropriate for initial therapy for a patient who has worsened despite outpatient use of full doses of bronchodilators. Sedation should be avoided in an already fatigued asthmatic patient as it may reduce respiratory drive. Unlike some patients with chronic obstructive bronchitis, asthmatics do not depend on the hypoxic drive to breathing, and oxygen should be given if the Po_2 is less than 60 mm Hg. *(Cecil, pp. 362–363)*

79. (A—True; B—False; C—True; D—False; E—True) Bronchial obstruction is due not only to constriction of smooth muscle, but also to inspissation of mucus and to edema and cellular infiltration of the mucosa, which may by worsened by coexistent bronchitis. *(Cecil, pp. 359–363)*

80. (A — False; B — True; C — False; D — False; E — False) A defect on lung scan indicates only that perfusion of a portion of the lung is diminished. Such defects may be caused by bullae, by pulmonary infiltrates, or by local vasoconstriction in response to regional hypoventilation. The last mechanism is probably responsible for the segmental and subsegmental perfusion defects noted in patients with asthma. Since this patient has asthma, the defect on the lung scan does not prove the diagnosis of pulmonary embolism, and definitive pulmonary angiography should be obtained. The angiogram is the "gold standard" for the diagnosis of pulmonary embolism. It is conceivable that it may miss very small emboli, but the correlation of findings at postmortem examinations done in close proximity to the radiographic study suggests that pulmonary angiography has a high level of sensitivity. The high mortality rate of untreated pulmonary embolism does not permit delay in obtaining definitive diagnostic information and beginning therapy. *(Cecil, pp. 362, 390–393; Moser; Robin)*

81. (B); 82. (E); 83. (A); 84. (C); 85. (D) The chest radiograph may provide clues as to the source of primary lesions that have metastasized to the lungs. Solitary metastatic lesions commonly originate from carcinomas of the colon, rectum, breast, kidney, testis, and cervix. Diffuse hematogenous metastasis, as from thyroid, renal, or trophoblastic tumors, may present as multiple micronodular shadows. Cavitation in metastatic lesions suggests an epidermoid carcinoma from the head and neck region, female reproductive organs, or colon. Calcification suggests an osteogenic sarcoma or a chondrosarcoma as the primary source. Diffuse lymphatic metastasis is often caused by carcinoma of the breast, stomach, pancreas, thyroid, and lung. *(Cecil, p. 420)*

86. (A); 87. (D); 88. (E); 89. (C); 90. (B) The number of conditions causing pulmonary infiltration is great, but diagnostic clues with important clinical implications may be provided in reviewing the function of other organ systems. The association of episodic hemoptysis, dyspnea, and evidence of glomerulonephritis suggests Goodpasture's syndrome. The symptoms of anemia may predominate in patients with chronic, recurrent extravasation of blood into lung parenchyma (idiopathic pulmonary hemosiderosis). Findings of adrenal insufficiency, hypothyroidism, or diabetes insipidus suggest that the nonspecific finding of diffuse interstitial fibrosis may be due to eosinophilic granulomatosis. Miliary tuberculosis must be considered in patients with a diffuse micronodular infiltrate, as it responds to effective chemotherapy. Similarly, chronic eosinophilic pneumonia should be considered in patients with bilateral peripheral infiltrates and eosinophilia, as the response to corticosteroids is often dramatic. *(Cecil, pp. 373–383)*

91. (C); 92. (D); 93. (B); 94. (A); 95. (E) A vast number of drugs are associated with pulmonary toxicity. Hydralazine may produce a lupus-like condition with acute pleurisy. Nitrofurantoin may cause slowly progressive diffuse infiltrative disease if taken chronically for suppression of bacterial urinary tract infections; it may also produce an acute syndrome with fever, cough, pulmonary infiltrates, and eosinophilia. Methysergide may provoke fibrosis of the lung parenchyma and pleura. Diffuse pulmonary infiltration, cough, fever, and dyspnea may appear long after the initiation of treatment with busulfan. The changes in Type II alveolar cells may be mistaken for malignancy. Corticosteroids can lead to an increase in mediastinal fat, causing mediastinal widening on the chest radiograph. *(Cecil, pp. 380–381)*

96. (B); 97. (C); 98. (A); 99. (D) Although infiltrative lung diseases cause a spectrum of radiographic findings, certain patterns are suggestive of specific diagnoses. The association of bilateral hilar adenopathy with bilateral lower lobe infiltrates is common with sarcoidosis. Few other diseases that cause interstitial infiltrates also cause symmetric enlargement of hilar nodes. Egg-shell calcification of lymph nodes suggests silicosis, which, in its early stage, also usually causes upper lobe infiltrates. Pleural plaque associated with interstitial infiltrates suggests asbestos exposure. The infiltrates of pulmonary alveolar proteinosis tend to be finely granular, may have associated air bronchograms, and often are perihilar and in the lower lobes. *(Cecil, pp. 382, 399–402)*

100. (D); 101. (A); 102. (C) Melanoptysis is the coughing up of jet-black fluid that occasionally occurs in coal-worker's pneumoconiosis. Amebic abscess of the lung is associated with a peculiar chocolate- or anchovy sauce–like sputum. Putrid sputum is frequently present with anaerobic lung abscess, and much less frequently with anaerobic pneumonitis prior to abscess formation. *(Cecil, pp. 383–384, 398–399)*

103. (E); 104. (A); 105. (C); 106. (B); 107. (D) Knowledge of the structural determinants of pulmonary function allows one to predict the pattern of abnormality that results from different diseases of the respiratory system. Thus, the enlargement of air-containing spaces and loss of lung tissue in emphysema (103.) results in an increase in lung volumes, a reduction in maximal expiratory flow, and a loss of diffusing capacity. Scleroderma (104.) may affect the small vessels of the lungs, reducing the diffusing capacity, without altering the alveolar volume or airway patency. Cough and exertional dyspnea (105.) may be the presenting symptoms of asthma, associated with obstruction of large and small airways throughout the lung. The diffuse parenchymal fibrosis of asbestosis (106.) reduces lung volumes and obliterates alveolar vessels. The reduction in total lung capacity in massive obesity (107.) reflects the decrease in chest wall compliance. Arterial blood gases may reflect the alveolar hypoventilation sometimes associated with this condition. *(Cecil, pp. 340–348)*

108. (B); 109. (C); 110. (A); 111. (D); 112. (E) Dyspnea refers to an awareness of a disproportionate degree of shortness of breath for a given level of activity, and thus describes the breathlessness experienced by a patient with acute asthma but not the increase in minute ventilation (hyperpnea) associated with exercise. Hyper- and hypoventilation refer to a disturbance in the relationship between alveolar ventilation and CO_2 production, as may be caused by the increased hypoxic drive to breathing at high altitude or by drug-induced depression of the respiratory center. Orthopnea, the worsening of dyspnea on recumbency, is caused by the upward displacement of the diaphragm by the abdominal contents in patients with diaphragmatic paralysis. *(Cecil, p. 339)*

113. (C); 114. (D); 115. (B); 116. (A) Seizures may occur as a complication of aminophylline therapy, but are usually associated with plasma theophylline levels so far above the therapeutic range that the risk of their occurrence should be minimal unless an error in dosage is made or the patient metabolizes theophylline abnormally. Laryngeal candidiasis may complicate treatment with beclomethasone aerosol, presumably because of local suppression of immune mechanisms. The infection usually resolves with simple discontinuation of the steroid aerosol. Terbutaline is a selective beta$_2$-agonist and therefore stimulates skeletal muscle tremor. Isoproterenol stimulates both beta$_1$- and beta$_2$-adrenergic receptors, and therefore increases the rate and force of cardiac contraction if the drug is absorbed into the circulation. *(Cecil, p. 362)*

117. (D); 118. (A); 119. (E); 120. (B); 121. (C) Although the point is not proved, the nearly simultaneous appearance of malignant infiltrates due to alveolar cell carcinoma in several widely separate parts of the lung suggests a possible multicentric origin of the tumor. Oat cell or small cell carcinoma has so often metastasized widely by the time the chest roentgenogram has become abnormal that surgical treatment is not attempted for this form of lung cancer. Bone marrow biopsy reveals metastatic malignant cells in a high proportion of cases. Bronchial carcinoid tumors may produce the "carcinoid syndrome" of flushing, diarrhea, bronchoconstriction, and cardiovascular lesions. Squamous or epidermoid cancers constitute approximately 40% of all primary lung malignancies, oat cell carcinomas about 25%, and adenocarcinomas (including bronchoalveolar tumors) 20 to 25%. Large cell carcinomas and other tumors make up the remainder. Secretion of mucin in the glandular-like tissue of adenocarcinoma is a typical histologic finding. *(Cecil, pp. 414–419)*

122. (B); 123. (A); 124. (D); 125. (C); 126. (E) *Pneumocystis* infection is common in immunosuppressed patients and classically presents with diffuse, bilateral, alveolar infiltrates on chest roentgenography. *Nocardia* septa are acid-fast. *Aspergillus* pneumonia is an invasive, necrotizing pneumonia that occurs almost exclusively in immunologically compromised hosts. *Pseudomonas* pneumonia is a common and lethal complication of the prolonged intubation and ventilatory support required for treatment of respiratory failure. Multiple myeloma is associated with impairment of humoral immunity, and patients with myeloma are more prone to common bacterial infections. *(Cecil, pp. 969–970, 1433–1435, 1533–1534, 1708–1710, 1742–1744; Williams et al.)*

127. (D); 128. (C); 129. (E); 130. (B); 131. (A) On inspiration, the subatmospheric pressure in the trachea and upper airway tends to pull the cords together, worsening the obstruction caused by vocal cord paralysis. Asthma is characterized by exaggerated bronchial reactivity to nonspecific irritants, such as histamine and methacholine. Lung compliance is decreased with diffuse fibrosis, so that greater changes in transpulmonary (alveolar-pleural) pressure are required for lung expansion. Bronchitis is defined by chronic overproduction of mucus, and is associated with enlargement of the submucosal mucous glands and with hyperplasia of goblet cells in the respiratory epithelium. Normal transpulmonary pressure at total lung capacity is 25 to 35 cm H_2O. The abnormally compliant lungs of an emphysematous patient are fully inflated at low distending pressures. *(Cecil, pp. 341–342, 371)*

132. (C); 133. (B); 134. (A); 135. (D); 136. (E) Mucormycosis may present with primary involvement of the nose and paranasal sinuses or as a rapidly progressive, dense bronchopneumonia. Hematogenous dissemination from the lung may involve the sinuses, brain, and gastrointestinal tract. A roentgenographic finding of multiple punctate calcifications of the spleen permits the diagnosis of previous infection with histoplasmosis. A thin-walled cavity is normally an innocuous complication of coccidioidomycosis infection, unless accompanied by hemoptysis or complicated by rupture into the pleural space. Tuberculous pericarditis requires early recognition and prompt, effective therapy to minimize the chance of progression to chronic, constrictive pericarditis. Pericarditis occurs rarely with the other listed organisms. Cryptococci have been found so often in patients with Hodgkin's disease that they were once suspected of causing the malignancy. *(Cecil, pp. 958, 1551, 1697–1713)*

BIBLIOGRAPHY

Moser, K.M.: Pulmonary embolism. Am. Rev. Respir. Dis., *115*:829, 1977.

Murray, J.F.: Respiration. *In* Smith, L.H., Jr., and Thier, S.O. (eds.): Pathophysiology: The Biological Principles of Disease. Philadelphia, W.B. Saunders Company, 1981.

Robin, E.D.: Overdiagnosis and overtreatment of pulmonary embolism: the emperor may have no clothes. Ann. Intern. Med., *87*:775, 1977.

Roughton, F.J.W.: Transport of oxygen and carbon dioxide. *In* Fenn, W.O., and Rahn, H. (eds.): Handbook of Physiology. Vol. 1. New York, Williams & Wilkins Company, 1964, pp. 767–825.

Walsh, R.E., Michaelson, E.D., Harkleroad, L.E., et al.: Upper airway obstruction in obese patients with sleep disturbance and somnolence. Ann. Intern. Med., *76*:185, 1972.

Williams, D.W., Krick, J.A., and Remington, J.S.: Pulmonary infection in the compromised host. Am. Rev. Respir. Dis., *114*:359, 593, 1976.

PART 3
RENAL DISEASE

David G. Warnock

DIRECTIONS: For questions 1 to 11, choose the ONE BEST answer to each question.

1. A 35-year-old woman with the nephrotic syndrome is being treated with sodium restriction and diuretics pending admission to the hospital for further studies. She comes to the emergency room with acute shortness of breath and right-sided pleuritic chest pain. Roentgenogram of the chest shows a right lower lobe infiltrate and a small pleural effusion. Electrocardiogram shows sinus tachycardia. Arterial blood gases include Po_2 70 mm Hg and Pco_2 30 mm Hg. Urinalysis reveals 4+ protein and 2–6 RBCs/hpf. Blood urea nitrogen is 15 mg/dl, and serum creatinine is 0.8 mg/dl. Which one of the following studies is the most appropriate at this time?

A. Selective renal venography
B. Fluorescent test for antinuclear antibodies
C. Intravenous urogram
D. Renal arteriogram
E. Renal biopsy

2. The diuretic phase of acute renal failure may result from each of the following EXCEPT

A. increases in glomerular filtration rate
B. impaired tubular reabsorption of fluid
C. expansion of extracellular volume during the oliguric phase
D. hypocalcemia
E. solute diuresis

3. An asymptomatic 26-year-old woman is found to have a blood pressure of 160/100 mm Hg on a routine physical examination. Urinalysis shows 2+ protein, a few granular casts, and rare WBCs/hpf. Which of the following conditions is most likely?

A. Renovascular hypertension
B. Essential hypertension
C. Orthostatic proteinuria
D. Urinary tract infection
E. Renal parenchymal disease

4. Optimal treatment of severe acute renal failure includes all the following EXCEPT

A. restriction of dietary protein
B. restriction of sodium and water intake
C. restriction of potassium intake
D. early and frequent dialysis
E. continuous administration of high-dose diuretics

5. Acquired nephrogenic diabetes insipidus may be caused by all the following EXCEPT

A. hypokalemia
B. hypercalcemia
C. chronic interstitial renal disease
D. methoxyflurane anesthesia
E. chlorpropamide therapy

6. Which of the following is LEAST likely to be useful in evaluating patients with calcium-containing renal stones?

A. Dietary history
B. Serum electrolytes
C. Serum uric acid level
D. 24-hour urinary excretion of calcium
E. 24-hour urinary excretion of uric acid

7. The 20-year-old daughter of a man with polycystic kidney disease is engaged to be married and consults you for an examination. She has no symptoms, and results of a physical examination are normal. Urinalysis reveals 3–5 WBCs and 0–1 RBCs/hpf; qualitative test for protein is negative. Intravenous urogram reveals no abnormalities. Which one of the following is true?

A. She does not have polycystic kidney disease
B. Her chance of having polycystic kidney disease is about 1 out of 2
C. Her chance of having polycystic kidney disease is less than 1 out of 4
D. Her brother is more likely than she to develop polycystic kidney disease
E. She cannot transmit polycystic kidney disease to her children

8. Pending results of culture and sensitivity, which of the following is the best initial treatment for a urinary tract infection in patients with moderately advanced chronic renal insufficiency?

A. Tetracycline
B. Gentamicin
C. Ampicillin
D. Nitrofurantoin
E. Trimethoprim-sulfamethoxazole

9. Electrocardiographic signs of hyperkalemia include all the following EXCEPT

A. absent P waves
B. peaked T waves
C. prominent U waves
D. prolonged P-R interval
E. widened QRS complex

10. A 34-year-old man with a long history of indigestion that is relieved by Tums is brought to the emergency room after 24 hours of repeated vomiting of coffee-ground material. He is drowsy but cooperative. Skin turgor is poor; blood pressure is 100/70 mm Hg; pulse rate is 125 per minute. Epigastric tenderness is noted.

Serum sodium concentration is 125 mEq/L. He weighs 55 kg, whereas his usual weight is 60 kg. Which one of the following would be required to restore body fluids to normal?

A. A positive balance of 420 mEq of cations
B. A positive balance of 1,000 mEq of cations
C. A shift of 420 mEq of sodium from the intracellular into the extracellular volume
D. A urine sodium concentration of under 1 mEq/L
E. Administration of 5 liters of 5% dextrose solution to increase total body water

11. Three years ago an apparently healthy 70-kg man had a serum creatinine concentration of 0.8 mg/dl and a creatinine clearance of 100 ml/minute. Sodium excretion rate was 100 mEq/24 hr. At this time he is still without symptoms, he has not changed his diet, and he still weighs 70 kg. Creatinine clearance, however, is now 25 ml/minute. Routine blood chemistries are normal except for a blood urea nitrogen of 40 mg/dl and a serum creatinine of 3.5 mg/dl. Which of the following statements regarding this patient's present renal function, compared with that of three years ago, is true?

A. The creatinine excretion rate is now about one fourth as much
B. The fractional excretion of filtered sodium is higher
C. The fractional excretion of phosphate is unchanged
D. The renal phosphate excretion rate is higher
E. The urinary volume has increased

DIRECTIONS: For questions 12 to 51, you are to decide whether EACH choice is true or false. Any combination of answers, from all true to all false, may be present. Mark the answer sheet "T" or "F" in the space provided.

12. A 69-year-old man undergoes repair of an abdominal aneurysm. He is hypotensive during surgery; urinary output during the first 24 hours after the operation is 300 ml. Which of the following statements regarding this patient is/are true?

A. A urine/plasma creatinine ratio of 40 would indicate acute parenchymal renal failure
B. A urinary sodium concentration greater than 25 mEq/L would indicate acute parenchymal renal failure.
C. The blood urea nitrogen will probably be elevated because of increased protein catabolism
D. Administration of fluids should be minimized in this patient
E. The severity of renal functional impairment is related to the duration of ischemia

13. Which of the following statements regarding the adult form of minimal change disease (lipoid nephrosis) is/are true?

A. Hypertension is common
B. It affects women more often than men
C. Hematuria is frequently observed
D. It occurs in association with Hodgkin's disease
E. It preferentially affects juxtamedullary glomeruli

QUESTIONS 14–16

A 55-year-old man is admitted to the hospital in a confused, disoriented state. He is a known alcoholic and has been drinking heavily and eating little for the last three weeks. He has vomited intermittently during the past week. Physical examination reveals an unkempt, wasted man with poor skin turgor. Blood pressure is 100/60 mm Hg; pulse rate is 100 per minute. Admission laboratory studies are as follows:

Blood urea nitrogen	60 mg/dl
Serum electrolytes:	
Sodium	110 mEq/L
Potassium	2.3 mEq/L
Chloride	62 mEq/L
Bicarbonate	42 mEq/L
Serum osmolality	220 mOsm/kg H_2O
Arterial blood pH	7.52
Urinary electrolytes:	
Sodium	60 mEq/L
Potassium	72 mEq/L
Chloride	5 mEq/L
Urinary osmolality	410 mOsm/kg H_2O
Urinary pH	7.5

14. Which of the following factors probably contributed to the hypokalemia in this patient?

A. Starvation
B. Vomiting
C. Renal potassium wasting
D. Alkalemia
E. Bicarbonaturia

15. Which of the following factors probably contributed to the high urinary potassium concentration in this patient?

A. Extracellular volume depletion
B. Bicarbonate diuresis
C. Secondary hyperaldosteronism
D. Underlying chronic renal disease
E. Acute tubular necrosis

16. Which of the following factors probably contributed to the generation and maintenance of the metabolic alkalosis in this patient?

A. Potassium deficiency
B. Vomiting
C. Extracellular volume contraction
D. Hyperventilation
E. Bicarbonate diuresis

---

17. Which of the following is/are true of peritoneal dialysis?

A. Clearance rates for urea and creatinine are lower with peritoneal dialysis than with extracorporeal hemodialysis.
B. It is useful in patients in whom heparin must be avoided
C. It is more efficient than extracorporeal hemodialysis in correcting the platelet disorder of chronic renal failure
D. It increases the tendency of hospitalized patients to develop atelectasis
E. It is contraindicated following recent abdominal vascular surgery

18. Which of the following statements regarding renal involvement in multiple myeloma is/are true?

A. Light-chain proteinuria may be the first manifestation of multiple myeloma
B. Non–light-chain proteinuria suggests deposition of amyloid in the glomeruli
C. Acute renal failure is a frequent occurrence
D. Bence-Jones proteinuria causes progressive renal failure
E. Significant hypercalcemia is common

19. A 65-year-old man with longstanding congestive heart failure and marked peripheral edema has been treated with furosemide. When treatment was started, he lost 2 to 3 kg/day, but after three days the weight loss ceased. The following values were obtained prior to (day 0) and on the fifth day of diuretic therapy.

	Plasma		Urine	
	Day 0	*Day 5*	*Day 0*	*Day 5*
Creatinine	1.2 mg/dl	2.6 mg/dl	–	–
Sodium	1.40 mEq/L	128 mEq/L	1 mEq/L	15 mEq/L
Potassium	4.0 mEq/L	3.1 mEq/L	42 mEq/L	75 mEq/L
Volume	–	–	800 ml/24 hr	1300 ml/24 hr

Which of the following statements is/are true?

A. The patient is continuing to show a tubular response to furosemide on day 5

B. Diuresis should improve by switching to ethacrynic acid
C. One would expect a natriuretic response to spironolactone on day 5
D. More vigorous diuresis should improve cardiac function and thereby improve renal function

20. A 62-year-old woman who has adult-onset diabetes is brought to the emergency room in coma. Her husband tells you that she had complained of increased thirst and polyuria during the last few days. The patient's therapy had been switched from insulin to an oral hypoglycemic agent one year ago. On physical examination she is comatose, responding only to deep pain; there are no localizing neurologic signs. Skin turgor is slightly decreased, and mucous membranes appear dry. Blood pressure is 120/60 mm Hg; pulse rate is 122 per minute and regular. Laboratory studies show:

Serum electrolytes:	
Sodium	149 mEq/L
Potassium	4.8 mEq/L
Chloride	109 mEq/L
Bicarbonate	15 mEq/L
Serum glucose	1200 mg/dl
Serum ketones	Negative on 1:2 dilution

Which of the following statements regarding this patient is/are true?

A. She has severe diabetic ketoacidosis
B. The coma is probably due to severe intracellular dehydration
C. The ketone measurement is probably an error
D. Hypotonic saline and insulin should be started immediately

21. Which of the following is/are true concerning preeclampsia?

A. Normal blood pressure during the first trimester differentiates preeclampsia from essential hypertension
B. It occurs primarily during first pregnancies
C. Women who have preeclampsia during their first pregnancy have an increased incidence of hypertension in later life
D. Patients with preeclampsia have diminished sensitivity to the pressor effects of infused angiotensin II
E. The magnitude of proteinuria correlates with the severity of renal involvement

22. Which of the following causes of metabolic alkalosis would be expected to result in a very low (<10 mEq/L) urinary chloride concentration?

A. Protracted vomiting
B. Diuretic therapy
C. Primary hyperaldosteronism
D. Cushing's syndrome
E. Bartter's syndrome

23. Which of the following statements concerning renal cell carcinoma is/are true?

A. Radiologic or clinical evidence of metastases is fairly common (25%) at the time of initial presentation
B. It often presents as a palpable abdominal mass
C. Hepatomegaly and hepatic dysfunction usually indicate metastases to the liver
D. Tumor calcification on roentgenogram is associated with a relatively poor five-year survival rate (less than 20%).
E. Renal vein and vena caval involvement is associated with a significantly worse prognosis than if the tumor were confined to the kidney

24. Which of the following is/are true concerning simple renal cysts?

A. Ultrasound scanning is helpful for determining whether a mass is solid or fluid-filled
B. Coexistence of renal cyst and tumor is common enough to warrant routine arteriography
C. Needle aspiration of a cyst has supplanted arteriography for the evaluation of simple cysts in elderly patients
D. The late nephrographic phase is the most useful aspect of a nephrotomogram for diagnosing simple renal cysts
E. Large, benign, simple cysts cause hypertension with elevated renin secretion from that kidney

25. Which of the following statements regarding polycystic kidney disease is/are true?

A. Approximately one third of adult patients also have hepatic cysts
B. Urinary tract obstruction in this disorder can be caused by blood clots
C. It predisposes to transitional cell carcinoma
D. Renal calculi are found in less than 5% of these patients
E. The adult form is inherited as an autosomal dominant condition

26. Which of the following is/are more consistent with chronic, rather than acute, renal failure?

A. Hypertension
B. Bilaterally small kidneys
C. Anemia
D. Oliguria
E. Hyperphosphatemia

27. Which of the following is/are true concerning the metabolic complications of chronic renal failure?

A. Hyperphosphatemia may necessitate use of phosphate-binding antacids
B. Hypocalcemia is usually associated with hyperphosphatemia
C. Vitamin D will correct hypercalcemia
D. Hypermagnesemia occurs when the glomerular filtration rate is less than 20 ml/minute
E. Hypercalcemia results from excess secretion of parathyroid hormone

28. Ureteral calculi can cause acute obstruction at the ureterovesicular junction. Which of the following is/are true?

A. Intravenous urogram will show ipsilateral renal enlargement with delayed calyceal visualization
B. Surgical removal of the stone is indicated if it does not pass within 24 hours
C. Postobstructive diuresis is common following relief of unilateral obstruction
D. Postobstructive diuresis is caused by renal salt wasting
E. Partial ureteral obstruction causes vasopressin resistance

29. Which of the following statements regarding the treatment of nephrolithiasis is/are true?

A. Loop diuretics are useful for decreasing urinary calcium excretion
B. Increased dietary salt intake will overcome the hypocalciuric effects of thiazide diuretics
C. If stones recur, it usually happens within five to ten years of the initial episode
D. Acidification of the urine is beneficial in the treatment of uric acid nephrolithiasis

30. Which of the following statements regarding diuretics is/are true?

A. Loop diuretics inhibit maximal concentration of the urine
B. Loop diuretics inhibit maximal dilution of the urine
C. Thiazide diuretics inhibit maximal concentration of the urine
D. Thiazide diuretics inhibit maximal dilution of the urine

31. Renal papillary necrosis is frequently associated with which of the following?

A. Diabetic nephropathy
B. Sickle cell disease
C. Analgesic-induced nephropathy
D. Gentamicin nephrotoxicity

32. Which of the following is/are true of sarcoidosis?

A. The nephrotic syndrome is a manifestation of glomerular involvement in patients with sarcoidosis
B. Disordered calcium metabolism is the most common cause of renal dysfunction in sarcoidosis
C. Granulomatous interstitial nephritis rarely causes renal failure in sarcoidosis
D. Hypercalcemia is usually associated with elevated levels of serum parathyroid hormone in sarcoidosis

33. Which of the following is/are true of the nephrotic syndrome?

A. It consists of heavy proteinuria, hypoalbuminemia, and edema
B. It occurs with proliferative forms of glomerulonephritis
C. It occurs with diffuse but not with focal glomerular disease
D. It results only from glomerular diseases
E. Most patients with the nephrotic syndrome also have hypertension

34. Which of the following is/are true of poststreptococcal glomerulonephritis?

A. It is an immunologically mediated disorder
B. It occurs in all age-groups
C. It is frequently associated with hypocomplementemia
D. It follows streptococcal skin infections as well as pharyngitis.

35. Which of the following is/are true of anti-glomerular basement membrane (anti-GBM) antibody disease in adults?

A. It is a common cause of the nephrotic syndrome
B. Linear deposits of antibody can be demonstrated in the glomerular capillary wall
C. It is a hypocomplementemic form of glomerulonephritis
D. It frequently results in rapidly progressive renal failure

36. Glomerular diseases associated with persistent activation of complement

A. are typically characterized morphologically as membranoproliferative glomerulonephritis
B. involve the alternate pathway
C. tend to recur in transplanted kidneys
D. respond to immunosuppressive therapy

37. Which of the following statements is/are true concerning renal osteodystrophy in adults?

A. Myopathy is likely to be present
B. Osteomalacia is more common than osteitis fibrosa
C. A bone biopsy would probably reveal increased osteoclastic activity
D. It is prevented by the low-grade metabolic acidosis that develops in chronic renal failure

38. Which of the following is/are true of Alport's hereditary nephritis?

A. It is inherited as an autosomal dominant trait
B. It is phenotypically more severe in men than in women
C. It is characterized by the presence of fat-laden foam cells in the renal interstitium
D. It is associated with deafness for high-frequency sounds

39. A 48-year-old man is admitted to the hospital for evaluation of a chronic cough and a 15-pound weight loss over the past six weeks. The patient has smoked a pack of cigarettes daily for 30 years. Physical examination is unremarkable. Roentgenogram of the chest shows a large mass in the right perihilar region. Scalene node biopsy shows oat cell carcinoma. Laboratory studies are as follows:

Serum electrolytes:	
Sodium	110 mEq/L
Potassium	3.8 mEq/L
Chloride	80 mEq/L
Bicarbonate	22 mEq/L
Serum alkaline phosphatase	Two times normal
Serum bilirubin	3.0 mg/dl (total)
Serum creatinine	0.8 mg/dl
Blood urea nitrogen (BUN)	8.0 mg/dl
24-hour urinary volume	530 ml
Urinary sodium	85 mEq/L

Which of the following statements regarding this patient is/are correct?

A. The low BUN is probably related to liver metastases
B. The low BUN is probably related to an excess of total body water
C. "Salt-losing nephritis" is probably a cause of the hyponatremia
D. The aldosterone excretion rate is likely to be markedly elevated
E. The clinical picture is more compatible with the syndrome of inappropriate secretion of antidiuretic hormone than with adrenal insufficiency

40. Which of the following is/are true of bacteriuria?

A. The prevalence of bacteriuria in school-age girls is about 1%
B. Bacteriuria is more common in diabetic than in nondiabetic school-age girls
C. The prevalence of bacteriuria in school-age girls is considerably greater than in boys of similar age
D. For a relatively healthy patient, the risk of developing persistent bacteriuria after a single bladder catheterization is greater than 10%

41. Which of the following is/are true concerning the effects of lithium on the kidney?

A. Thirst and urinary frequency are common in patients taking lithium
B. Impaired concentrating ability can persist for months following cessation of therapy
C. Focal tubular atrophy with interstitial fibrosis occurs in patients who have taken lithium for a long time
D. The impaired diluting ability can be overcome by administration of vasopressin

42. Which of the following statements is/are true regarding drug-induced tubulointerstitial disease?

A. It does not produce severe proteinuria (>3.5 gm/day)
B. Fever, rash, and eosinophils in the blood and urine are diagnostic clues
C. Aminoglycoside antibiotics characteristically cause acute tubulointerstitial nephritis
D. Antibody to tubular basement membrane is seen in methicillin-induced nephritis

43. Which of the following is/are true of acquired distal (type I) renal tubular acidosis?

A. It is frequently associated with autoimmune diseases
B. Urinary pH is always greater than 5.5
C. It is characterized by a renal leak of bicarbonate, often exceeding 10% of the filtered load
D. It is associated with severe hypokalemia and muscular weakness

44. Which of the following is/are true of renal transplantation?

A. The use of azathioprine for immunosuppression has been associated with anemia, leukopenia, and jaundice
B. Antibody-mediated rejection (hyperacute as well as chronic, indolent humoral rejection) responds to aggressive steroid therapy
C. Hypophosphatemia following successful transplantation necessitates parathyroidectomy
D. Renal allograft recipients have a strikingly increased incidence of lymphoproliferative disorders

45. Which of the following statements is/are true of primary hyperparathyroidism?

A. Hypercalciuria and hypercalcemia are frequently observed
B. Hypercalcemia produces a concentrating defect with resulting polyuria
C. Calcium phosphate nephrolithiasis is associated with primary hyperparathyroidism
D. Pruritus observed in chronic renal failure correlates better with serum calcium levels than with dermal calcium content

46. Which of the following is/are true of type IV renal tubular acidosis (hyporeninemic hypoaldosteronism)?

A. It develops when the glomerular filtration rate is less than 25 ml/minute
B. Anion-gap acidosis is usually present
C. Hyperkalemia is an important feature of the syndrome
D. Treatment increases the delivery of sodium to distal nephron sites

47. Which of the following is/are associated with furosemide therapy?

A. Hyperchloremic metabolic acidosis
B. Hypokalemic metabolic alkalosis
C. Magnesium wasting
D. Hypercalcemia
E. Hyperkalemia

48. Which of the following is/are associated with acetazolamide therapy?

A. Hyperchloremic metabolic acidosis
B. Hypokalemic metabolic alkalosis
C. Magnesium wasting
D. Hypercalcemia
E. Hyperkalemia

49. Which of the following is/are associated with triamterene therapy?

A. Hyperchloremic metabolic acidosis
B. Hypokalemic metabolic alkalosis
C. Magnesium wasting
D. Hypercalcemia
E. Hyperkalemia

50. Which of the following is/are associated with hydrochlorothiazide therapy?

A. Hyperchloremic metabolic acidosis
B. Hypokalemic metabolic alkalosis
C. Magnesium wasting
D. Hypercalcemia
E. Hyperkalemia

51. Which of the following is/are associated with indomethacin therapy?

A. Hyperchloremic metabolic acidosis
B. Hypokalemic metabolic alkalosis
C. Magnesium wasting
D. Hypercalcemia
E. Hyperkalemia

DIRECTIONS: Questions 52 to 89 are matching questions. For each numbered item, choose the most likely associated lettered item from those provided. Each numbered item has ONLY ONE answer. Within each group, each lettered item may be the answer to one, more than one, or none of the numbered items.

QUESTIONS 52–54

For each of the following patients, select the most likely associated radiocontrast study (*A–D* below).

52. A 54-year-old woman with chronic headaches, pyuria, and mild azotemia

53. A 24-year-old woman with 1+ proteinuria, headaches, and hypertension (blood pressure 160/105 mm Hg)

54. A 46-year-old man who had hepatitis nine months ago who now has hematuria, proteinuria, and severe hypertension (blood pressure 205/115 mm Hg)

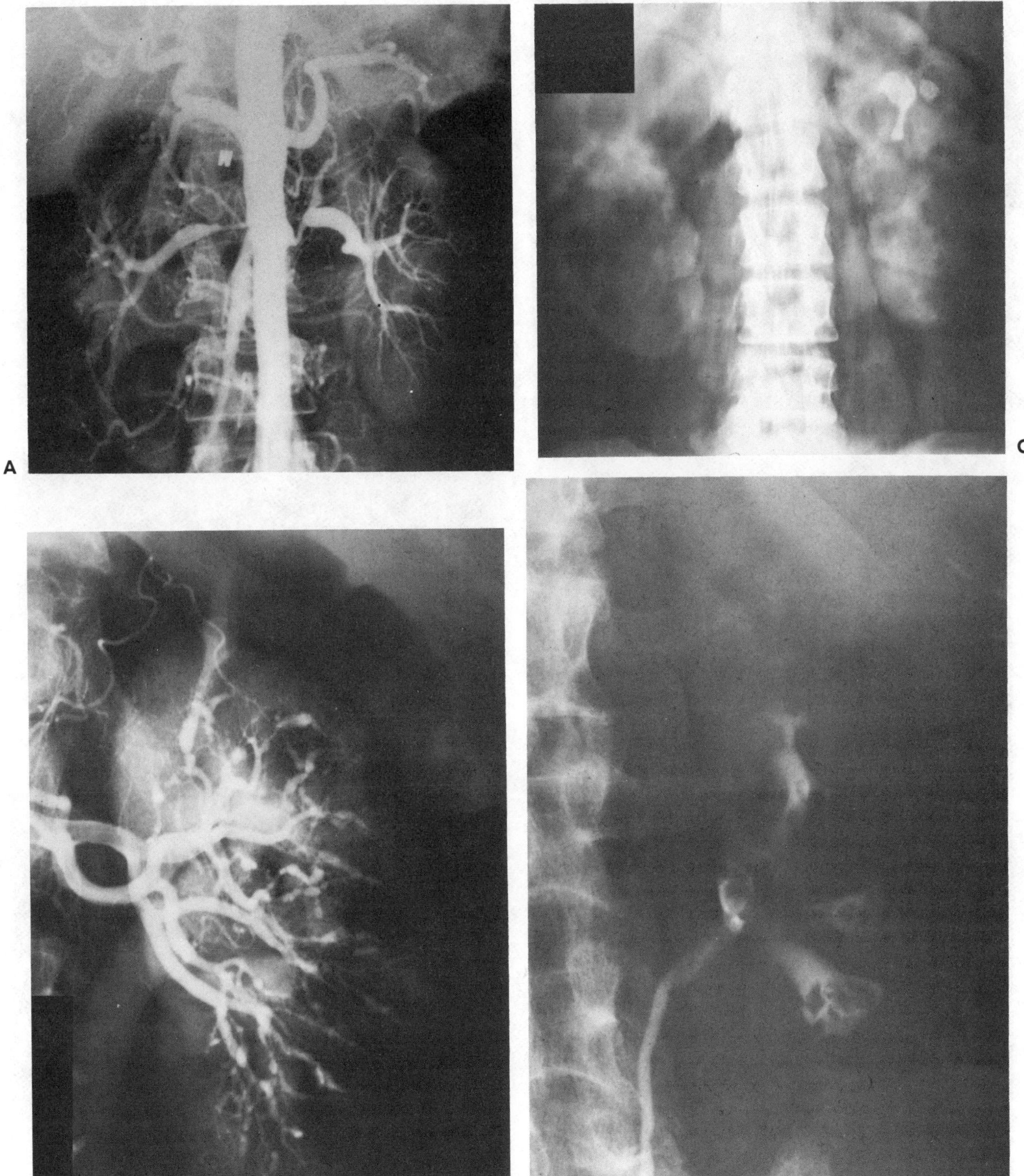

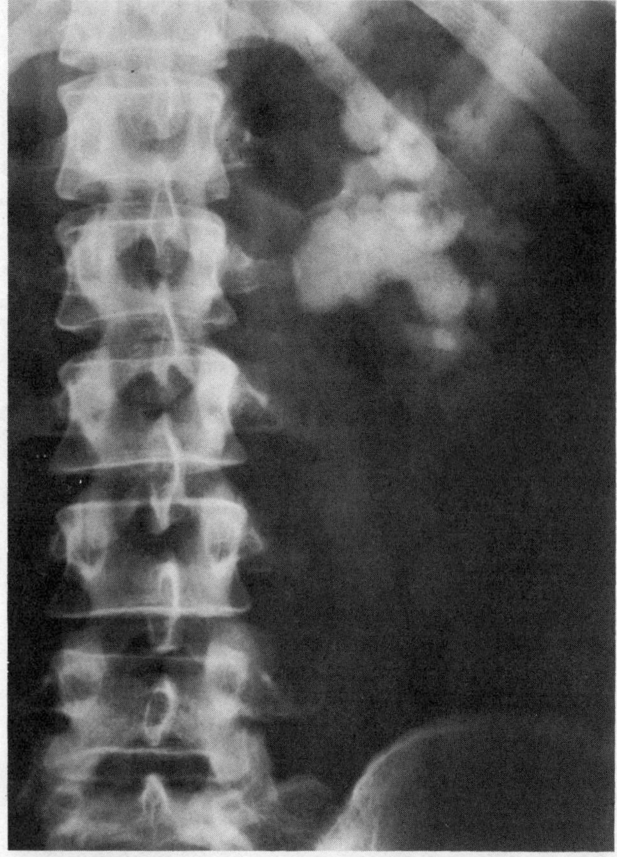

A

QUESTIONS 55–57

For each of the following patients, select the most likely associated radiocontrast study (*A–D*).

55. A 60-year-old man with fever, weight loss, and polycythemia

56. A 23-year-old woman with hypokalemia and hyperchloremic metabolic acidosis; urinary pH is 6.0

57. A 26-year-old man with a 14-year history of hematuria and multiple renal stones who now complains of dysuria and flank pain

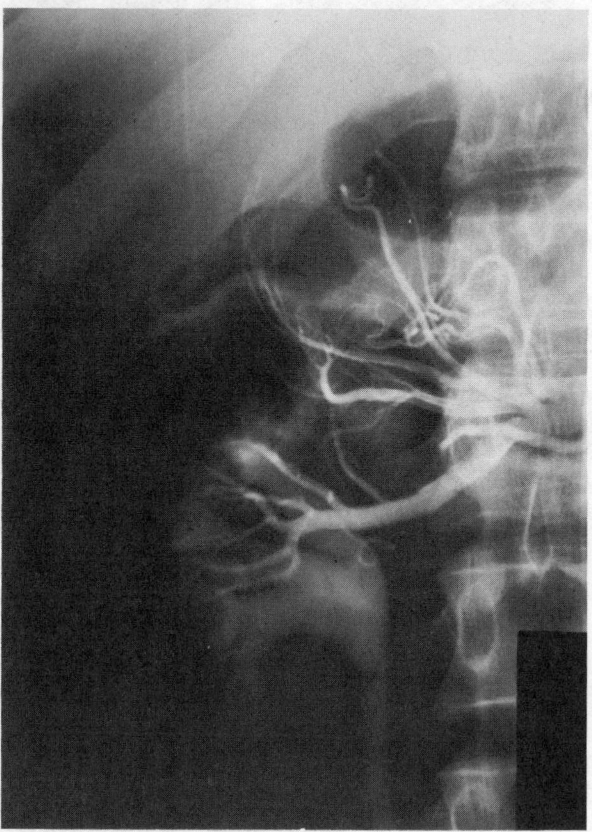

C

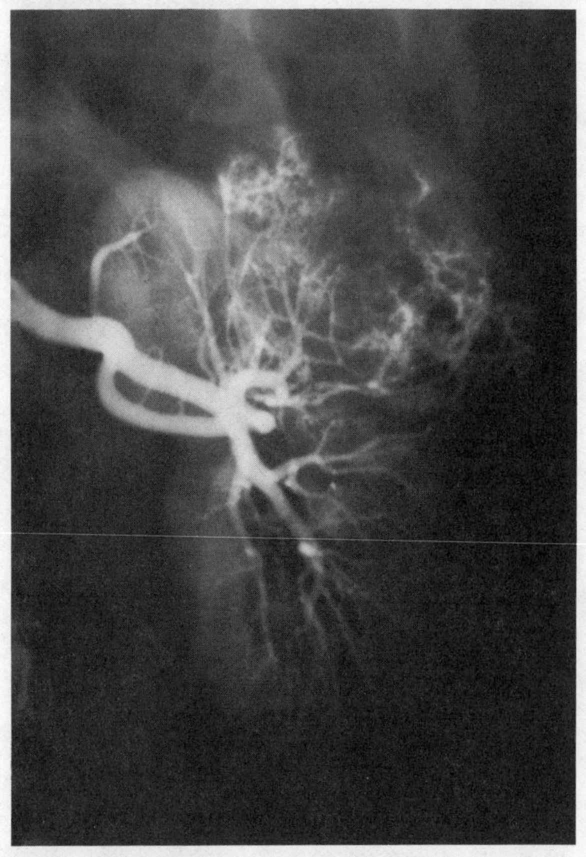

B

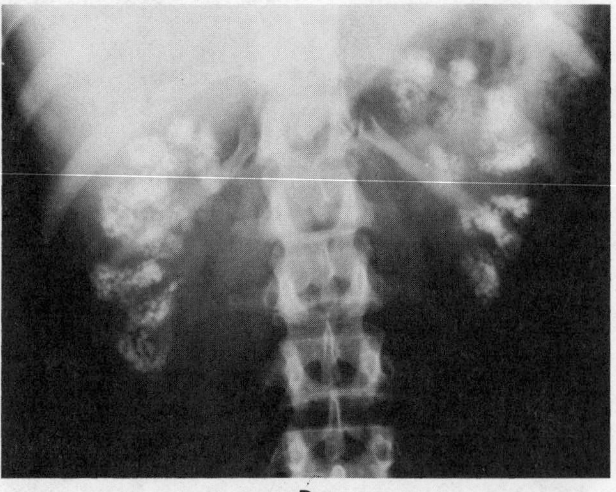

D

QUESTIONS 58–63

For each of the diseases listed below, select the most likely suggested mechanism of renal injury.

A. Anti-glomerular basement membrane antibodies
B. Immune complex–mediated disease
C. Activation of complement by the alternate pathway
D. Inflammatory or obliterative disease of renal blood vessels

58. Progressive systemic sclerosis (scleroderma)

59. Lupus nephritis

60. Acute poststreptococcal glomerulonephritis

61. Type 2 membranoproliferative glomerulonephritis ("dense-deposit" disease)

62. Wegener's granulomatosis

63. Glomerulonephritis in acute bacterial endocarditis

QUESTIONS 64–67

For each of the patients listed below, select the most likely associated renal complications.

A. Acute renal failure
B. Proteinuria
C. Nephrogenic diabetes insipidus
D. Renal calculi

64. A patient receiving demeclocycline

65. A 58-year-old neuropathic, insulin-dependent diabetic man who recently had intravenous urography because of moderate azotemia

66. A massively obese woman who had a jejunoileal bypass procedure three months ago

67. A 45-year-old woman receiving gold therapy for rheumatoid arthritis

QUESTIONS 68–72

Each of the following patients is being seen because of hyponatremia. For each patient, select the most appropriate set of data from the table below.

	Blood Pressure Standing		Serum		Urine	
	(mm Hg)	Peripheral Edema	*Na (mEq/L)*	*Osmolality ($mOsm/kg\ H_2O$)*	*Na (mEq/L)*	*Osmolality ($mOsm/kg\ H_2O$)*
A.	90/50	0	125	260	50	400
B.	90/50	0	125	260	5	800
C.	120/80	0	125	260	5	50
D.	150/100	2+	130	270	5	600
E.	110/80	0	125	280	15	300

68. A patient with hyperkalemia, increased blood urea nitrogen, and decreased serum cortisol

69. A patient who has received an excessive intravenous infusion of 5% glucose in water

70. A patient with severe hyperglycemia

71. A patient with severe diarrhea

72. A patient with untreated congestive heart failure

QUESTIONS 73–75

The following sets of data relate to patients being evaluated for polyuria. Select the most appropriate set of data for the clinical conditions described below.

	Serum Osmolality	Urinary Osmolality After Dehydration	Urinary Osmolality After Antidiuretic Hormone (ADH)
	($mOsm/kg\ H_2O$)	*($mOsm/kg\ H_2O$)*	*($mOsm/kg\ H_2O$)*
A.	260	700	700
B.	290	400	400
C.	290	1000	1000
D.	300	200	600

73. Psychogenic polydipsia

74. Chronic renal failure

75. Diabetes insipidus

QUESTIONS 76–83

A 55-year-old woman has longstanding chronic renal failure with a serum creatinine of 9.9 mg/dl and a creatinine clearance of 10 ml/minute. She is not receiving dialysis. You are considering the use of the following medications. Select from the lettered list below the statement that applies most appropriately to each of the numbered medications.

A. Should not be used in this patient
B. May be used for specific indication without dosage adjustment
C. May be used in DECREASED dosages
D. May need INCREASED dosages

76. Flurazepam

77. Allopurinol

78. Milk of magnesia

79. Hydrochlorothiazide

80. Spironolactone

81. Phenytoin sodium

82. Trimethoprim-sulfamethoxazole

83. Propranolol

QUESTIONS 84–89

For each of the following disorders, select the most likely site of electron-dense immune-complex deposition.

A. Mesangial
B. Mesangial and subepithelial
C. Subepithelial
D. Subendothelial
E. Mesangial and subendothelial

84. Idiopathic membranous nephropathy

85. IgG-IgA nephropathy

86. Poststreptococcal glomerulonephritis

87. Henoch-Schönlein syndrome

88. Membranoproliferative glomerulonephritis (type I)

89. Membranous lupus nephritis

PART 3

RENAL DISEASE

ANSWERS

1. (A) Pleuritic chest pain, mild hypoxemia, and hypocapnea occurring in a patient with the nephrotic syndrome suggest renal vein thrombosis and pulmonary embolism. Renal vein thrombosis most commonly occurs in the membranous form of the nephrotic syndrome. *(Cecil, p. 582)*

2. (D) Hypocalcemia is usually seen during the acute phase of oliguric renal failure. Hypercalcemia has been reported during the diuretic phase, especially in patients with extensive muscle injury. *(Cecil, pp. 497–498; Brenner and Rector, pp. 1187–1191)*

3. (E) Proteinuria is a very sensitive indicator of renal disease and is uncommon in essential hypertension or in urinary tract infections. The combination of hypertension, proteinuria, and granular casts increases the likelihood of parenchymal renal disease. *(Cecil, p. 439)*

4. (E) The evidence that the duration of azotemia may be shortened or that the dialysis requirement may be reduced is not convincing enough to justify continuous high-dose diuretic therapy in acute renal failure. *(Cecil, pp. 499–500; Brenner and Rector, p. 1194)*

5. (E) Chlorpropamide enhances the renal response to antidiuretic hormone and thus has an effect opposite to that expected in nephrogenic diabetes insipidus. The other conditions result in decreased renal concentrating capacity by various mechanisms. *(Cecil, pp. 573, 1195–1198)*

6. (C) Hyperuricemia is not necessarily associated with hyperuricosuria. Elevated uric acid excretion plays an important pathogenetic role in the formation of calcium oxalate stones as well as uric acid stones. *(Cecil, pp. 585–587)*

7. (B) Polycystic kidney disease is transmitted as a mendelian dominant trait with a very high degree of penetrance. Clinical evidence of disease may not be apparent until after the fourth or fifth decade. There is no sex predilection, and affected persons may transmit the gene. In the present case, no evidence of disease is present, but the patient is young and cysts may be developing. *(Cecil, pp. 590–591)*

8. (C) Dosage levels must be adjusted for the degree of renal failure if the antibiotic is excreted by the kidney. Tetracyclines and gentamicin may be used only with a major reduction of dosage; nitrofurantoin should be avoided. Trimethoprim-sulfamethoxazole may be used with only moderate reduction in dosage. Ampicillin is the treatment of choice, unless contraindicated by a history of allergic reaction. *(Cecil, p. 509)*

9. (C) Prominent U waves are an electrocardiographic sign of hypokalemia. *(Cecil, p. 485)*

10. (B) The acute weight loss indicates that at least 5 liters of fluids are needed to restore total body water to normal. The patient's cation deficit includes those 5 liters as well as the amount needed to raise the cation content of total body water from 125 to 140 mEq/L. Normal saline would be an appropriate replacement fluid for this patient, at least until whole blood becomes available. Infusion of 5% dextrose solution without replacing cation deficits would precipitate severe hyponatremia. *(Cecil, pp. 473–474, 479)*

11. (B) As renal excretory units are reduced in number, external balance is maintained by excretion of more filtered solute per nephron (fractional excretion). In this case, since neither diet nor weight has changed, sodium balance is being maintained by greater excretion of sodium per nephron. Similarly, fractional excretion of phosphate is increased. Urinary volume reflects mainly water intake. Creatinine excretion rate has not changed; the fall in GFR is matched by a rise in serum creatinine level. *(Cecil, pp. 502, 506)*

12. (A — False; B — True; C — True; D — True; E — True) A high U/P creatinine ratio indicates excellent tubular function, not the usual finding in acute parenchymal renal failure. Azotemia progresses at a rate determined by tissue catabolism. Enhanced urea reabsorption may also elevate BUN at low urinary flow rates. Salt and water overload may cause peripheral edema, pulmonary vascular congestion, cerebral edema, and hyponatremia. Judicious fluid administration may be necessary to treat any "prerenal" component of acute renal failure. The duration of ischemia and the presence of renal impairment before surgery are both related to the severity of renal impairment following surgery. *(Cecil, pp. 498–499)*

13. (A — False; B — False; C — False; D — True; E — False) The sex ratio is approximately equal in the adult form of minimal change disease. Microscopic hematuria is found in only about 15% of cases; macroscopic hematuria is extremely rare. Focal glomerulosclerosis in its early stages affects juxtamedullary glomeruli. Minimal change disease affects both juxtamedullary and cortical glomeruli. *(Cecil, p. 532; Brenner and Rector, pp. 1419–1421)*

14. (All are True) All these factors probably contributed to the hypokalemia. Vomiting and renal potassium wasting are probably most important in this patient. *(Cecil, p. 483; Brenner and Rector, pp. 887–889)*

15. (A — True; B — True; C — True; D — False; E — False) Vomiting with bicarbonate diuresis **(B)** is the primary event in this patient. Extracellular volume depletion and secondary hyperaldosteronism also contribute and result from the vomiting. *(Cecil, p. 483; Brenner and Rector, pp. 887–889)*

16. (A — False; B — True; C — True; D — False; E — False) Extracellular volume contraction related, in this case, to vomiting has a primary role in maintaining metabolic alkalosis. An important feature of this effect is the reduction of glomerular filtration rate that accompanies the volume contracted state. The alkalosis cannot be corrected until the volume deficits are restored. Alkalemia is usually corrected by saline administration, even though potassium deficits are not restored. Hyperventilation reduces P_{CO_2} and does not serve to maintain a chronic metabolic alkalosis. Potassium deficiency probably is not a primary factor in maintaining metabolic alkalosis, although there are a few reported cases of "saline-resistant" alkalosis that were corrected following potassium chloride administration. More commonly, "saline-resistant" alkalosis occurs in states of primary mineralocorticoid excess associated with hypokalemia. Bicarbonate diuresis represents incomplete reabsorption of the filtered level of bicarbonate. This effect may potentiate renal potassium wasting, but its primary effect is to lessen the severity of the metabolic alkalosis. *(Cecil, pp. 492, 562; Brenner and Rector, pp. 856–858)*

17. (All are True) *(Cecil, pp. 511–512; Brenner and Rector, pp. 2518–2519)*

18. (A — True; B — True; C — False; D — True; E — True) Progressive renal insufficiency is much more common than acute renal failure in patients with multiple myeloma, and it is strongly associated with Bence-Jones proteinuria (myeloma kidney). Hypercalcemia is found in up to 30% of patients with multiple myeloma. *(Cecil, pp. 571–572; Brenner and Rector, pp. 1654–1657)*

19. (A — True; B — False; C — True; D — False) The increased urinary volume, sodium, and potassium on day 5 are consistent with tubular effects of furosemide. Prerenal azotemia is indicated by the rise in serum creatinine to 2.6 mg/dl on day 5. Ethacrynic acid acts at the same tubular site (thick ascending limb) as furosemide; diuresis would not be improved and probably has been too vigorous already. The elevated urine potassium is consistent with secondary hyperaldosteronism due to volume depletion. Adding spironolactone would probably cause natriuresis, but this is not appropriate at this time. *(Cecil, pp. 234–235, 474–475)*

20. (A—False; B—True; C—False; D—True) This patient has hyperglycemic hyperosmolar coma owing to profound osmotic diuresis and severe intracellular dehydration. There is a large anion gap, but lactic acidosis is more likely than diabetic ketoacidosis because of the low serum ketone measurement. The patient's insulin requirement will be modest. "Hypotonic" saline could effectively be normal saline. The serum sodium concentration is approximately 165 mEq/L when corrected for the osmotic effect of hyperglycemia. The patient needs salt as well as water replacement. *(Cecil, pp. 472–474, 490, 1067)*

21. (A — False; B — True; C — False; D — True; E — True) Patients with essential hypertension may have normal blood pressure early in pregnancy. Preeclampsia is most common in first pregnancies; however, it also occurs in older, multiparous women, and these are the ones who develop hypertension in later life. *(Cecil, pp. 583–584)*

22. (A — True; B — False; C — False; D — False; E — False) Once established, metabolic alkalosis is sustained most commonly by mineralocorticoid activity, which promotes distal sodium reabsorption and hydrogen ion secretion. Mineralocorticoid hypersecretion may be a physiologic response to volume and chloride depletion caused by protracted vomiting or chloride-rich diarrhea, in which chloride depletion will result in a very low urinary chloride concentration. Pathologic hypersecretion of mineralocorticoids may occur in a variety of adrenocortical endocrine disorders and result in metabolic alkalosis, but without chloride depletion. Urinary chloride concentration in these situations will be greater than 10 mEq/L. Measurement of urinary chloride concentrations has little usefulness apart from evaluating possible causes of metabolic alkalosis. With regard to **B**, urinary electrolytes are difficult to interpret in the presence of diuretic therapy. *(Cecil, p. 493; Brenner and Rector, pp. 887–889)*

23. (A — True; B — True; C — False; D — False; E — False) Although only 10% of patients present with symptoms of metastases, as many as 25% have radiologic or clinical evidence of metastases when first seen for therapy. *(Cecil, p. 595)*

24. (A —True; B — False; C — True; D — True; E — True) Ultrasound is a simple, inexpensive test that can distinguish between solid masses and fluid-filled cysts. Computerized tomography may offer certain advantages over ultrasound but is more expensive at present. Coexisting renal tumors and cysts are uncommon. Regarding **C**, arteriography may be deferred if percutaneous aspiration, ultrasound, and nephrotomograms are consistent with a benign, simple renal cyst. **D** is true. The early arterial phase of a nephrotomogram is more useful for diagnosing renal cell carcinoma. **E** is also true, although this complication is fairly unusual. *(Cecil, pp. 464–467, 588–589, 595)*

25. (A — True; B — True; C — False; D — False; E — True) Ultrasonography demonstrates hepatic cysts in approximately 30% of adults with polycystic kidney disease. Obstruction may cause sudden deterioration of renal function in these patients. Stones are the usual cause (nephrolithiasis occurs in 10–20% of cases), but clots can also obstruct the collecting system, ureter, or both. *(Cecil, pp. 590–591; Brenner and Rector, pp. 1881–1883)*

26. (A — False; B — True; C — True; D — False; E — True) Bilaterally small kidneys, anemia, and hyperphosphatemia are typical findings in chronic renal failure. *(Cecil, p. 507)*

27. (A — True; B — True; C — False; D — True; E — True) The renal excretion of phosphate falls when the GFR is less than 20 ml/minute, and intestinal calcium absorption decreases. Calcium malabsorption may be corrected with vitamin D analogues. At this level of GFR, urinary excretion of magnesium is diminished while intestinal magnesium absorption continues normally. It is prudent to discontinue magnesium-containing antacids at this point. A subgroup of patients with chronic renal failure develop hypercalcemia after several months of dialysis. Most often the hypercalcemia is due to persistent secretion of PTH from glands that have previously undergone hyperplasia. Parathyroidectomy may be indicated if other causes of hypercalcemia (e.g., vitamin D intoxication) can be ruled out. *(Cecil, p. 503)*

28. (A — True; B — False; C — False; D — False; E — True) The key to diagnosis of urinary tract obstruction is the demonstration of a dilated urinary collecting system. The nephrogram will be delayed but quite dense in acute obstruction. Acute ureteral obstruction with calculi will usually correct spontaneously. If the ureter is not completely obstructed, one can delay for two to four weeks to see if spontaneous passage will occur. Postobstructive diuresis is associated with bilateral, but not with unilateral, obstruction. In most cases the diuresis is due to the excretion of salt, water, urea, and other solutes that were retained during the period of obstruction, rather than to true salt wasting. There may also be a vasopressin-resistant component to the diuresis, possibly caused by high levels of renal prostaglandins. *(Cecil, pp. 545–548)*

29. (A — False; B — True; C — True; D — False) Hypercalciuria may result from the use of loop diuretics. Two thirds of recurrences happen within seven years. Uric acid is much *less* soluble at an acid pH. *(Cecil, pp. 587–588; Brenner and Rector, pp. 1950–2007)*

30. (A — True; B — True; C — False; D — True) The "cortical" diluting segment is the site of action of thiazide diuretics, whereas loop agents affect the "medullary" diluting segment. As a consequence, loop agents (e.g., furosemide) may inhibit both urinary concentration and dilution, whereas thiazides primarily affect urinary dilution. *(Cecil, p. 472; Brenner and Rector, pp. 1097–1134)*

31. (A — True; B — True; C — True; D — False) Ischemic necrosis of the papilla and medulla is associated with severe pyelonephritis, especially in diabetics and in patients who ingest large amounts of analgesics. Infection and obstruction are the two major predisposing factors. Abnormalities of the medullary blood supply (e.g., sickle cell disease) constitute another factor to be considered. Aminoglycoside antibotics cause a reduction in GFR rather than papillary necrosis. *(Cecil, pp. 458–459, 567, 570)*

32. (A — True; B — True; C — True; D — False) Glomerular involvement is rare in sarcoidosis, but when it does occur the nephrotic syndrome is a common manifestation. Renal failure is more commonly related to hypercalciuria and hypercalcemia than to direct glomerular involvement. *(Cecil, pp. 538, 570; Brenner and Rector, pp. 1523, 1659)*

33. (A — True; B — True; C — False; D — True; E — False) Nephrotic syndrome can appear in any glomerular disease in which there is sufficient transglomerular passage of plasma proteins to cause proteinuria, with resultant hypoproteinemia and edema. Hypertension occurs in some patients and is determined by the type of underlying glomerular involvement. Hypertension is not usually observed unless there is an accompanying fall in GFR. *(Cecil, pp. 538–541)*

34. (All are True) Acute proliferative glomerulonephritis (following streptococcal or other infections) is believed to be immunologically mediated because of (1) the latent period between onset of infection and renal involvement, (2) decreased complement levels during the acute phase, and (3) morphologic similarities to experimental immune complex nephritis. Children and young adults are most frequently affected, but elderly patients have also been described. *(Cecil, pp. 521–523)*

35. (A — False; B — True; C — False; D — True) The diagnosis of anti-GBM antibody disease rests on two findings: linear immunofluorescent deposits of anti-GBM antibody in the glomerular (and occasionally tubular) capillary walls, and the presence of circulating anti-GBM antibodies. Rapidly progressive (crescentic) glomerulonephritis, with or without pulmonary hemorrhage, is the usual finding, but anti-GBM disease cannot always be equated with a rapidly progressive form of glomerulonephritis. Milder degrees of renal impairment are being recognized. Serum complement levels are usually normal. *(Cecil, pp. 454–458)*

36. (A — True; B — True; C — True; D — False) Membranoproliferative glomerulonephritis is typically associated with complement activation. There can be prominent glomerular deposition of complement, abnormalities in the circulating levels of complement, or both. Isolated glomerular deposition of C3 is seen without immunoglobulins or early-acting components (e.g., C1q, C4, C2), suggesting activation of the alternate pathway. These forms of primary glomerular disease are noted for recurring in transplant recipients. Therapy with steroids and cytotoxic agents has generally been unsuccessful in altering the progressive renal insufficiency. *(Cecil, pp. 457, 519, 528)*

37. (A — True; B — False; C — True; D — False) Myopathy of undetermined origin frequently accompanies the secondary hyperparathyroidism of chronic renal failure, and may contribute significantly to the musculoskeletal debility. Osteitis fibrosa is almost universal in terminal renal failure. Osteomalacia is less common, and only a minority of patients complain of bone pain. Bone biopsy material from patients with renal osteodystrophy shows variable degrees of increased osteoblastic and osteoclastic activity, as well as widened osteoid seams. With prolonged acidosis there is progressive bone resorption with resultant osteoporosis. Thus, metabolic acidosis, decreased levels of $1,25(OH)_2D_3$, and hyperparathyroidism all contribute to renal osteodystrophy. *(Cecil, p. 505)*

38. (All are True) Hereditary forms of nephritis are not uncommon, and detection rests on adequate inquiries into family history. *(Cecil, pp. 568–569)*

39. (A — False; B — True; C — False; D — False; E — True) This patient has the syndrome of inappropriate secretion of antidiuretic hormone (SIADH). Reduced blood urea nitrogen results from the volume expansion that occurs in this setting. Volume contraction and physiologically stimulated secretion of ADH are associated with prerenal azotemia. There is a period of negative salt balance during the initial phase of volume expansion in SIADH. Thereafter, normal salt balance is usually maintained in spite of the hyponatremia. Aldosterone secretion rates are normal, even though plasma renin levels are suppressed. The fact that the patient is not orthostatic and does not have prerenal azotemia is more consistent with SIADH than with Addison's disease. *(Cecil, pp. 477–479)*

40. (A — True; B — False; C — True; D — False) The prevalence of bacteriuria among school-age girls is 1.2%; it is only 0.03% in boys of the same age. The incidence in girls is 0.4% per year. Bacteriuria is not increased in diabetic girls. The risk of developing persistent bacteriuria following a single catheterization in relatively healthy individuals is 1 to 2%; the risk is much higher in debilitated patients and in men with prostatic obstruction. *(Cecil, p. 566)*

41. (A — True; B — True; C — True; D — False) C is true, although the causative role of lithium in the development of chronic renal insufficiency in psychiatric patients has not been established. Focal tubular atrophy and interstitial fibrosis have also been described in psychiatric patients who have never taken lithium. Regarding **D**, lithium causes a vasopressin-resistant nephrogenic diabetes insipidus. *(Cecil, p. 557; Brenner and Rector, pp. 2087–2089)*

42. (A — True; B — True; C — False; D — True) Heavy proteinuria is not a characteristic feature of acute interstitial nephritis; however, this has been described for the nonsteroidal anti-inflammatory agents. The findings of fever, rash, and eosinophilia, although classic, are not invariably present. Acute interstitial nephritis is not the usual finding in aminoglycoside-induced nephrotoxicity. Acute allergic interstitial nephritis has been observed as a drug allergy with anti-tubular basement membrane antibodies. *(Cecil, pp. 543, 553)*

43. (A — True; B — True; C — False; D — True) Acquired distal RTA is frequently observed among patients with diseases such as chronic hepatitis and Sjögren's disease. Occasionally the potassium losses and decreased bicarbonate reserves resulting from the renal defect contribute to the morbidity of these diseases. Although proximal acidification defects may be present despite urinary pH less than 5.5, distal defects always result in urinary pH greater than 5.5. The renal "leak" of bicarbonate is relatively mild compared with proximal forms of RTA, in which 15% of the filtered load of bicarbonate may be excreted in the urine if the serum bicarbonate is maintained at normal levels by replacement therapy. An understanding of how these differences may occur is fundamental to a grasp of the distinction between proximal and distal defects. *(Cecil, pp. 574–575)*

44. (A — True; B — False; C — False; D — True) Bone marrow suppression and hepatitis can occur during treatment with azathioprine. Responses to steroids may be only short-term, and the patients can encounter significant morbidity (infection and marrow depression) from the immunosuppressant therapy. Cell-mediated rejection responds more readily to immunosuppressants than antibody-mediated rejection. Other long-term complications of immunosuppression include a striking incidence of reticulum cell carcinoma with CNS involvement, aseptic necrosis, and other features of hypercortisolism. Hypophosphatemia can be seen after normal function is regained owing to persisting secondary hyperparathyroidism. This hyperplasia usually resolves spontaneously during the six months following transplantation. *(Cecil, pp. 518–519)*

45. (A — True; B — True; C — True; D — False) Ten to 40% of patients with primary hyperparathyroidism present with renal stones resulting from excessive bone resorption ("resorptive hypercalciuria"). Polydipsia and polyuria may be the presenting complaints in patients with hypercalcemic nephropathy. Pruritus seems more closely related to the dermal content of calcium. *(Cecil, pp. 506, 562–563, 585)*

46. (A — False; B — False; C — True; D — True) Hyperchloremic metabolic acidosis is the usual finding in this syndrome, and hyperkalemia can be life-threatening. Effective forms of therapy (furosemide, thiazides, volume expansion with mineralocorticoids, high-salt diet) all increase the delivery of sodium to the final segments of the nephron. Hyporeninemic hypoaldosteronism develops despite relatively well-preserved renal function (GFR greater than 25 ml/minute). *(Cecil, pp. 575–576)*

47. (B and C are True) Hypokalemic metabolic alkalosis results from the extracellular volume contraction, mineralocorticoid excess, and renal potassium wasting that accompany the use of loop diuretics such as furosemide. Loop diuretics cause proportionately greater increases in magnesium excretion than in sodium excretion and can cause clinically severe magnesium wasting. Calcium excretion is enhanced as long as severe volume contraction does not supervene. *(Cecil, pp. 454, 492–493; Brenner and Rector, pp. 567–570, 602–603, 1122–1123)*

48. (A is True) Acetazolamide inhibits renal carbonic anhydrase activity and causes increased urinary bicarbonate excretion. Chronic administration will cause bicarbonate wasting and a resultant hyperchloremic metabolic acidosis. Renal potassium wasting does occur, but chronic use of acetazolamide causes a metabolic acidosis. Carbonic anhydrase inhibitors have minimal effects on magnesium excretion. During acetazolamide administration, more calcium is delivered to and reabsorbed at distal nephron sites; however, hypercalcemia does not develop. *(Cecil, p. 453; Brenner and Rector; pp. 567–570, 602–603; 1122–1123)*

49. (A and E are True) Proton and potassium secretion by the distal tubule are limited by aldosterone antagonists such as triamterene; hyperkalemia and hyperchloremic metabolic acidosis may result. Magnesium excretion may actually be decreased. Triamterene is a potassium-sparing diuretic, and these can be associated with clinically significant hyperkalemia. *(Cecil, pp. 485, 490; Brenner and Rector, pp. 567–570, 602–603, 927, 1122–1123)*

50. (B and D are True) Hypokalemic metabolic alkalosis results from the extracellular volume contraction, mineralocorticoid excess, and renal potassium wasting that accompany the use of thiazide diuretics. Thiazides do have a mild magnesuric effect, but do not cause severe magnesium wasting like the loop diuretics. Thiazides enhance calcium absorption at distal sites and cause hypocalciuria. Hypercalcemia can be seen in severely volume-contracted patients or in those with primary hyperparathyroidism or vitamin D intoxication. Renal potassium wasting is more likely than hyperkalemia. *(Cecil, pp. 453, 472, 587; Brenner and Rector, pp. 567–570, 602–603, 1122–1123)*

51. (A and E are True) Renin is suppressed by the nonsteroidal anti-inflammatory agents. Hyperchloremic metabolic acidosis with hyperkalemia can occur, especially in patients with diminished renal function. A syndrome resembling hyporeninemic hypoaldosteronism has been reported. *(Brenner and Rector, p. 671)*

52. (D) The kidney has a distorted calyceal system and an irregular cortical surface. The radiocontrast material forms a ring sign in the lower calyx. These findings are most consistent with a chronic interstitial nephritis and papillary necrosis, as might occur with excessive intake of analgesics. *(Cecil, p. 550; Brenner and Rector, pp. 1640–1646)*

53. (A) This is a midstream aortogram showing bilateral proximal renal artery stenosis due to intimal hyperplasia. This condition is one of the forms of fibromuscular dysplasia, an important cause of hypertension in young women. *(Cecil, p. 233; Brenner and Rector; pp. 1725–1727)*

54. (B) Microaneurysms are seen throughout the renal vasculature and were also demonstrated in the superior mesenteric arterial branches. Their presence indicates vasculitis, as occurs in polyarteritis nodosa. Microaneurysms may also occur as a hypersensitivity reaction to sulfonamides or to intravenously administered amphetamines. *(Cecil, pp. 535–536; Brenner and Rector, p. 1519)*

55. (B) There is a large spherical mass that originates in the renal parenchyma and has a tumor blush consisting of complex vascular networks. This is renal cell carcinoma. *(Cecil, p. 595; Brenner and Rector, pp. 2111–2117)*

56. (D) This patient has distal renal tubular acidosis and nephrocalcinosis. Hypercalciuria with or without hypocalcemia, nephrocalcinosis, and osteomalacia with bone pain and pathologic fractures are common in distal RTA. *(Cecil, pp. 574–575, 585; Brenner and Rector, pp. 1853–1855)*

57. (A) This patient has a staghorn calculus. He has cystinuria and has passed numerous stones. The possibility of infection and obstruction must be considered. *(Cecil, p. 586; Brenner and Rector, pp. 1831–1836)*

58. (D) In the kidney, progressive systemic sclerosis is primarily a disease of blood vessels. There may be severe intimal thickening of the interlobular arteries with secondary severe interstitial fibrosis, tubular atrophy, and patchy glomerulosclerosis. Segmental fibrinoid necrosis may be present in the afferent arterioles and glomerular tufts. *(Cecil, pp. 537–538)*

59. (B) The pathogenesis of renal injury in lupus nephritis involves events triggered by the deposition of circulating immune complexes within the glomeruli. Proliferation and necrotizing lesions may be seen, but they are always associated with immune deposits. *(Cecil, pp. 456, 535)*

60. (B) The most significant ultrastructural finding in acute proliferative glomerulonephritis is subepithelial electron-dense deposits, scattered irregularly along the epithelial side of the glomerular capillary membrane. These are thought to be immune complexes that have deposited "humps" at these sites. *(Cecil, pp. 456, 521)*

61. (C) There is little evidence for an immune complex pathogenesis in type 2 membranoproliferative glomerulonephritis. Glomerular C3 localization without immunoglobulins is a constant finding. Intense glomerular localization of properdin is common, denoting activation of complement by the alternate pathway. *(Cecil, pp. 457, 526)*

62. (D) The renal lesion in Wegener's granulomatosis is a necrotizing, proliferative glomerulonephritis associated with an angiitis resembling the microscopic form of polyarteritis nodosa. *(Cecil, p. 536)*

63. (B) Acute proliferative glomerulonephritis with immune complex deposition ("humps") has been described in cases of acute bacterial endocarditis due to coagulase-positive staphylococci. *(Cecil, p. 521)*

64. (C) Demeclocycline interferes at a "post-cyclic AMP" site in the action of ADH, ultimately leading to reduced water permeability of the luminal membrane of the collecting duct. *(Cecil, p. 573)*

65. (A) The renal vascular bed tends to constrict when exposed to high concentrations of contrast media, leading to varying degrees of acute renal failure. The risk of nephrotoxicity is related to the state of hydration, the presence of pre-existent renal disease, and the dose of contrast media. *(Cecil, p. 560)*

66. (D) Alteration of intestinal lipid absorption by surgical or inflammatory alteration of the intestinal tract results in increased calcium binding in the gut, increased oxalate absorption, and hyperoxaluria. This may result in increased urolithiasis. *(Cecil, p. 585)*

67. (B) Renal damage during gold therapy is usually first manifested as microscopic hematuria or proteinuria. Acute tubular necrosis with anuria is rarely seen. More commonly, there may be an immune complex glomerulonephritis with proteinuria, and even the nephrotic syndrome. *(Cecil, p. 557)*

68. (A) The situation described is adrenocortical insufficiency. There is an inappropriately high urinary sodium concentration, and urinary osmolality is low, considering the low blood pressure and low serum osmolality. Thus, renal conservation of sodium is impaired, as might occur with adrenocortical insufficiency or potent diuretics. In this case, serum potassium is high, rather than low as might be expected with diuretics; plasma cortisol is decreased, confirming the diagnosis. *(Cecil, p. 450, 476–480; Brenner and Rector, pp. 815–816)*

69. (C) If excessive free water is administered either by mouth (polydipsia) or intravenously, at a rate that exceeds the maximal diluting ability of the kidney, serum sodium concentration and plasma osmolality will decrease despite maximally dilute urine. In this case the maximal diluting ability of the kidney seems normal, but in other instances, diluting capacity might be impaired by diuretics, glucosuria, reductions in glomerular filtration rate, or potent stimuli to ADH secretion, such as pain. *(Cecil, pp. 573–574; Brenner and Rector, pp. 812–819)*

70. (E) The key here is that the serum osmolality is high relative to the serum sodium concentration. This indicates the presence of significantly elevated concentrations of plasma solutes that do not normally contribute much to plasma osmolality. Glucose is the most common culprit. *(Cecil, pp. 573–574; Brenner and Rector, pp. 812–819)*

71. (B) There is evidence of volume contraction without renal losses of sodium. The urine is reasonably concentrated, indicating adequate ADH activity, which is appropriate given the degree of volume contraction. *(Cecil, pp. 449–450; Brenner and Rector, pp. 812–819)*

72. (D) Avid sodium conservation and free water conservation are present, leading to edema with a relative excess of free water over sodium. Clinical situations in which hyponatremia may be present with excess total body sodium include congestive heart failure, hepatic cirrhosis, the nephrotic syndrome, pregnancy, and acute and chronic renal failure. The mechanisms are obscure, but they seem to involve excess ADH activity, even though serum levels of ADH may be normal. *(Cecil, pp. 478–479; Brenner and Rector, pp. 812–815)*

73. (A) The serum osmolality is low originally, and maximal ADH effect is achieved after dehydration, since administering exogenous ADH does not increase the concentration of the urine. Maximal urinary osmolality is decreased, however, indicating impairment at the renal level, as might occur with "wash-out" of renal medullary hypertonicity from protracted water diuresis. *(Cecil, pp. 573–574; Brenner and Rector, p. 812)*

74. (B) Plasma osmolality is normal and urinary osmolality is slightly concentrated, but fixed after dehydration. This is the concentration defect observed in advanced renal failure. *(Cecil, pp. 501–502; Brenner and Rector, p. 814)*

75. (D) Plasma osmolality is slightly high originally; urinary osmolality is low, but responds to exogenous ADH. *(Cecil, pp. 573–574; Brenner and Rector, pp. 797–806)*

76. (B) Flurazepam is extensively metabolized by the liver. Two active metabolites are formed, but very little is excreted in the urine. *(Cecil, p. 509; Brenner and Rector, p. 2682)*

77. (C) Allopurinol and its active metabolite (oxypurinol) are excreted by the kidney. Oxypurinol accumulates in the total body water if GFR is less than 40 ml/minute. *(Cecil, p. 559; Brenner and Rector, p. 2680)*

78. (A) Intestinal absorption of magnesium is normal or near-normal in patients with chronic renal disease. In the face of impaired renal excretion, the tendency for hypermagnesemia to develop in uremic patients is not surprising. *(Cecil, p. 503; Brenner and Rector, p. 2257)*

79. (A) Thiazides are mostly (75%) excreted by the kidney and are generally thought to be ineffective if the GFR is less than 25 ml/minute. *(Brenner and Rector, p. 2694)*

80. (A) Spironolactone is extensively metabolized by the liver. Both the active form and inactive metabolites are excreted by the kidney. This drug is generally ineffective in chronic renal failure, and may cause severe, life-threatening hyperkalemia. *(Brenner and Rector, p. 2694)*

81. (B) Phenytoin is mostly metabolized by the liver, with very little renal excretion of the unchanged drug. Dosage does not necessarily have to be changed, but the therapeutic and toxic levels are lower in uremic patients owing to decreased plasma protein binding. *(Brenner and Rector, p. 2689)*

82. (C) Trimethoprim is largely (60–80%) excreted unchanged in the urine. Sulfamethoxazole is metabolized by the liver, and very little is excreted unchanged in the urine. The usual doses are needed to ensure adequate urinary concentrations if the GFR is less than 15 ml/minute. Nevertheless, the interval between doses should be extended in patients with reduced GFR. *(Cecil, p. 509; Brenner and Rector, p. 2672)*

83. (C) Propranolol is extensively metabolized by the liver. Both active and inactive metabolites are excreted by the kidney. Start therapy with *low* doses. *(Brenner and Rector, p. 2698)*

84. (C) The subepithelial localization of immune complexes is well accepted in membranous nephropathy. The nature of these complexes and the dynamics of their formation are controversial. *(Cecil, pp. 529–530; Brenner and Rector, pp. 1438–1441)*

85. (A) IgA, and to a lesser extent IgG, deposits in a granular pattern mainly involve the mesangium. *(Cecil, p. 456; Brenner and Rector, p. 1400)*

86. (C) The most characteristic electron-microscopic finding in acute poststreptococcal glomerulonephritis is the presence of discrete, electron-dense, dome-shaped deposits projecting outward from the epithelial side of the basement membrane. Although many morphologic, clinical, and serologic features suggest that this is an immune-complex disease, the precise nature of the antigen-antibody system operating in this disease remains undefined. *(Cecil, p. 522; Brenner and Rector, pp. 1379–1381)*

87. (A) By electron microscopy, the principal abnormalities of Henoch-Schönlein syndrome are found in the mesangium. Focal cellular proliferation, increase in mesangial matrix, and electron-dense deposits are seen. *(Cecil, p. 536; Brenner and Rector, p. 1572)*

88. (E) The hallmarks of this group of glomerular lesions are pronounced abnormalities of mesangial areas and peripheral capillary walls. The major feature on electron microscopy is extension and interposition of mesangial cells and matrix into subendothelial areas. Electron-dense deposits are very commonly seen in subendothelial locations or within the glomerular basement membrane. *(Cecil, p. 527; Brenner and Rector, pp. 1443–1451)*

89. (E) The pattern of complement and immunoglobulin deposition in membranous lupus nephritis resembles that of idiopathic membranous nephropathy except for the addition of subendothelial, intramembranous, and mesangial deposits. *(Cecil, p. 535)*

BIBLIOGRAPHY

Brenner, B. M., and Rector, F. C., Jr.: The Kidney, 2nd ed. Philadelphia, W. B. Saunders Company, 1981.

ACKNOWLEDGMENTS

The radiographs on page 73 (Figures C and D) were kindly provided by Dr. Robert A. Older, Department of Radiology, Duke University Medical Center. Figures A and B on page 73 and the figures on page 74 are courtesy of Drs. Anthony Sebastian, Stanley M. Linderfeld, and Morris Schambelan, Department of Medicine, University of California, San Francisco.

PART 4
GASTROINTESTINAL DISEASE

John P. Cello, James H. Grendell, Bruce F. Scharschmidt, and Rebecca W. Van Dyke

DIRECTIONS: For questions 1 to 68, choose the ONE BEST answer to each question.

QUESTIONS 1–2

1. A 44-year-old man who has drunk 6 ounces of whiskey daily for many years is evaluated for intermittent episodes of epigastric pain relieved by antacids. During an attack, moderate epigastric tenderness is present. Laboratory tests show:

Hematocrit	46%
White blood cell count	10,000/cu mm
Serum creatinine	1.2 mg/dl
Serum amylase	500 IU/L (N<110)
Urinary creatinine	120 mg/dl
Urinary amylase	50 IU/L

Examination of the stool for occult blood is positive (2+). Upper gastrointestinal series shows duodenal bulb deformity. The amylase:creatinine clearance ratio in this patient is

A. 0.001%
B. 0.1%
C. 1%
D. 10%

2. The most likely diagnosis is

A. acute pancreatitis with secondary spasm of duodenal bulb
B. coexistent acute pancreatitis and peptic ulcer disease
C. peptic ulcer disease and macroamylasemia
D. peptic ulcer disease with posterior penetration into the pancreas

QUESTIONS 3–6

A 35-year-old black male stockbroker has a three-month history of nocturnal epigastric burning pains relieved promptly by foods and sodium bicarbonate. For the past two days he has passed large amounts of liquid, black, tarlike stools. He denies using alcohol or salicylates. He smokes two packs of cigarettes and drinks 15 cups of coffee daily.

On physical examination the patient appears anxious. Pulse rate is 85/minute (supine) and 90/minute (sitting). Blood pressure is 120/70 mm Hg (supine) and 110/70 mm Hg (sitting). There is midepigastric tenderness on palpation of the abdomen. The stool is dark black in color and strongly positive (4+) for occult blood. Hemoglobin is 10 gm/dl; hematocrit is 32%. An upper gastrointestinal series is shown below.

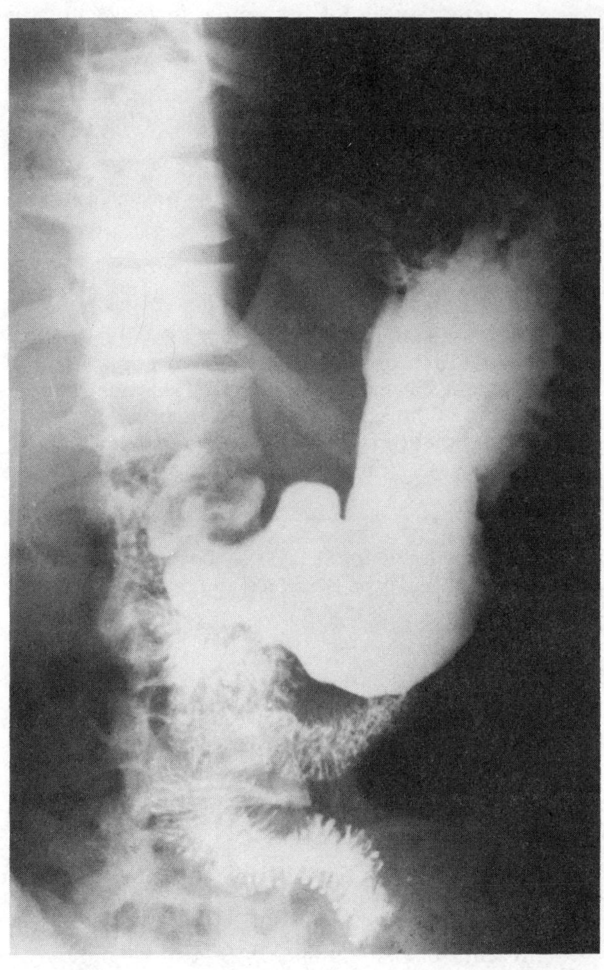

3. Further essential diagnostic work-up would include which one of the following?

A. Gastric acid secretory testing with pentagastrin, 6 μg/kg subcutaneously
B. Nasogastric lavage for cytology
C. Upper gastrointestinal endoscopy
D. Celiac angiography
E. None of the above

4. Which of the following is the most appropriate initial medical management for this patient?

A. Hourly administration of milk and cream (50 ml of each)

B. Propantheline (Pro-Banthine), 15 mg four times daily and diazepam (Valium), 10 mg four times daily
C. Liquid antacids, 80 to 140 mEq acid neutralizing capacity, one and three hours after meals and at bedtime
D. Cimetidine, 600 mg after meals and at bedtime
E. Antacid tablets (10 mEq/tablet) every two hours with two tablets at bedtime

5. Which of the following statements is correct regarding this patient's condition?

A. Salicylates and other nonsteroidal anti-inflammatory agents have *not* been shown to damage the mucosa in this portion of the gastrointestinal tract
B. Lesions similar to this are the most commonly encountered causes of gastrointestinal bleeding in stressed patients, such as those in burn and intensive care units
C. Compared with normal subjects, gastric acid secretion is likely to be increased only during the first 30 minutes following pentagastrin injection
D. This lesion on the anterior wall is more likely to bleed than a similar lesion on the posterior wall
E. None of the above

6. Which one of the following dietary programs would be most appropriate for this patient?

A. Low-roughage bland diet with six small feedings
B. Low-fat diet; broiled meats without pepper
C. Milk and cream every hour while awake, supplemented with clear liquids as tolerated
D. Regular diet (three meals) without bedtime snack
E. Regular diet (three meals) with a large bedtime snack

---

7. Which of the following is NOT seen in association with the presence of hepatitis B surface antigen (HB_sAg) in the serum?

A. Urticaria
B. Polyarteritis nodosa
C. Cryoglobulinemia
D. Primary biliary cirrhosis
E. Hepatocellular carcinoma

8. Which of the following statements regarding alpha$_1$-antitrypsin deficiency is INCORRECT?

A. It frequently is seen in the neonatal period as cholestatic jaundice
B. The most characteristic liver biopsy finding is the presence of eosinophilic, PAS-positive granules in periportal hepatocytes
C. Severe deficiency (Pi^{zz}) is almost always associated with clinically apparent liver disease
D. Liver disease and lung disease associated with alpha$_1$-antitrypsin deficiency frequently do not occur together in the same patient
E. Cirrhosis due to alpha$_1$-antitrypsin deficiency is a predisposing factor to the development of hepatocellular carcinoma

9. Which of the following statements about gastroesophageal reflux disease is true?

A. The occurrence of reflux in the upright position is the feature that distinguishes symptomatic individuals from the normal population
B. Diagnostic certainty requires direct manometric measurement of lower esophageal sphincter pressure
C. When it occurs during pregnancy, it usually resolves completely after completion of pregnancy
D. The presence of a Schatzki's ring on an esophagogram is an important clue to its presence
E. A bedtime snack, by buffering gastric acid, will reduce nocturnal symptoms in most patients

10. A 26-year-old woman is referred to you because of a recent episode of small bowel obstruction that resolved spontaneously. Physical examination is normal aside from melanin deposits on the buccal mucosa and palms. Stools are positive for occult blood. Family history reveals similar pigmentary changes in her mother and a maternal uncle, both of whom suffered recurrent attacks of abdominal pain and distention. Her uncle died at age 65 of an intestinal adenocarcinoma. Her mother is alive and well at the age of 68. Laboratory studies reveal a hematocrit of 34%, hemoglobin of 11.5 gm/dl, white blood cell count of 8000/cu mm, normal electrolytes, and normal urinalysis.

Which of the following is true of this woman's disorder?

A. She has a high risk of intestinal adenocarcinoma
B. The melanin spots were not present at birth
C. Consanguinity would be expected in her family
D. Histologic examination of the intestinal lesions would reveal hamartomas
E. Colectomy would be curative

11. A 49-year-old white woman with several radiolucent stones in the gallbladder has had repeated attacks of right upper quadrant discomfort after meals and was recently hospitalized for acute cholangitis due to choledocholithiasis. She is otherwise healthy. Which of the following is the most appropriate therapy for this patient?

A. Observation and a low-cholesterol diet
B. Chenodeoxycholic acid, orally
C. Ursodeoxycholic acid, orally
D. Endoscopic sphincterotomy
E. Cholecystectomy with common duct exploration

12. A 68-year-old woman with longstanding hypertension and atherosclerotic disease, who has recently undergone a long surgical procedure for placement of an aortofemoral bypass graft, is noted to be jaundiced on the fifth postoperative day. Serum bilirubin concentration is 16 mg/dl; prothrombin time is 12 seconds (control: 11); serum alkaline phosphatase is twice normal.

What is the most appropriate procedure for visualizing the biliary tree in this patient?

A. Ultrasonography
B. Percutaneous transhepatic cholangiography
C. Endoscopic retrograde cholangiography
D. Oral cholecystography
E. Computerized tomography

13. A 7-year-old girl has had postprandial irritability, headaches, and somnolence since early infancy. Physical examination and liver function tests are entirely within normal limits, but the blood ammonia is elevated. One male sibling died shortly after birth; another male sibling is normal. The most likely diagnosis is

A. type II glycogen storage disease
B. Wilson's disease (hepatolenticular degeneration)
C. alpha$_1$-antitrypsin deficiency
D. ornithine transcarbamylase deficiency
E. Reye's syndrome

14. Use of which one of the following drugs has been convincingly associated with the development of pancreatitis?

A. Digoxin
B. Heparin
C. Methotrexate
D. Penicillin
E. Azathioprine

15. Extraintestinal complications of Crohn's disease include all the following EXCEPT

A. cholelithiasis
B. amyloidosis
C. erythroderma
D. renal stones
E. conjunctivitis

16. A 42-year-old man consults you because of severe pain that occurs with defecation and resolves after a few minutes. Which of the following is the most likely diagnosis?

A. Thrombosed external hemorrhoids
B. Prolapsed thrombosed internal hemorrhoids
C. Anorectal abscess
D. Anal fissure
E. Anorectal fistula

QUESTIONS 17–18

A 68-year-old black male attorney is admitted to the hospital because of epigastric pain. He was well until two days ago when, following lunch, he noted severe sharp, steady, midepigastric pains that radiated to the back and right upper quadrant. He vomited food and "coffee-ground" material on three occasions. He slept poorly that night and awakened with severe right upper quadrant pains, chills, and a temperature of 102°F. This morning he noted abdominal distention and right lower quadrant pains. The abdominal distention was relieved somewhat by vomiting.

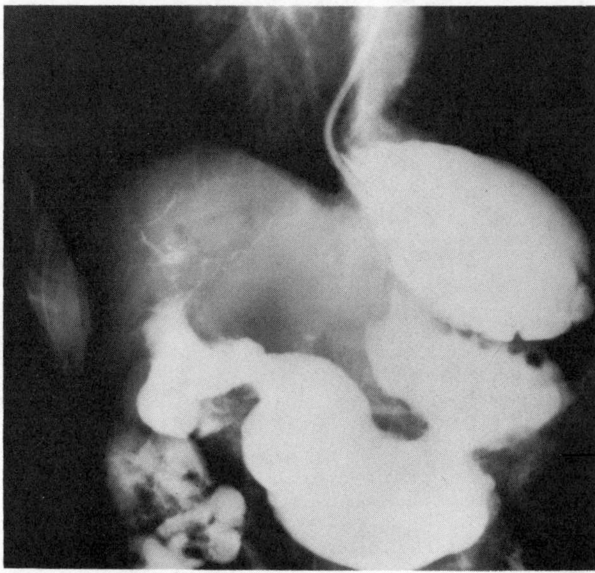

Physical examination reveals an acutely ill, febrile (temperature 101°F) man with anicteric sclerae and dry mucous membranes. The abdomen is distended and tympanitic with hyperactive bowel sounds, and there is tenderness on palpation in the epigastrium and right upper and lower quadrants. Hematocrit is 36%, white blood cell count is 6500/cu mm; serum amylase is 150 IU/L (N<110). Urinalysis is normal except for 1+ bilirubin. Upper gastrointestinal series is shown in the left column below.

17. These radiographic findings are seen in each of the following conditions EXCEPT

A. surgical choledochoduodenostomy
B. penetrating duodenal bulbar ulcer
C. perforating duodenal bulbar ulcer
D. choledocholithiasis
E. cholecystolithiasis

18. Which of the following is the most likely explanation for this patient's severe abdominal pains and abdominal distention on the day of admission?

A. Peritonitis
B. Pancreatitis
C. Peptic ulcer disease
D. Gallstone ileus
E. Cholangitis

---

19. Which one of the following would NOT be seen in a patient with steatorrhea due to pancreatic insufficiency?

A. Subacute combined degeneration of the spinal cord
B. Nyctalopia and keratomalacia
C. Osteomalacia
D. Calcium oxalate renal stones
E. Hypoprothrombinemia

20. A 75-year-old man is admitted to the hospital with severe periumbilical pains and abdominal distention. Tenderness is noted in the midepigastrium. Laboratory tests include the following (p. 88):

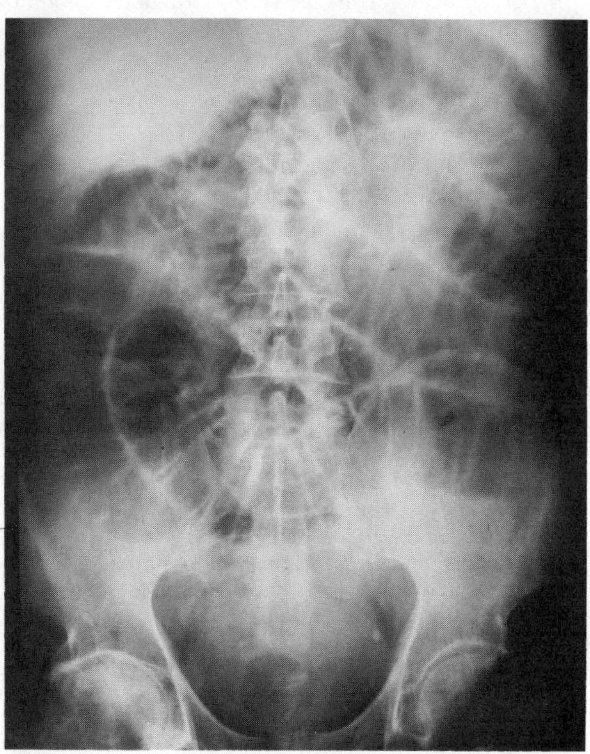

Hematocrit	40%
White blood cell count	15,000/cu mm
Serum amylase	300 IU/L (N<110)
Serum creatinine	1.0 mg/dl
Urinary amylase	1200 IU/L
Urinary creatinine	200 mg/dl

Examination of the stool for occult blood is positive (2+). Ultrasonography demonstrates a normal pancreas. A roentgenogram of the abdomen is done (see p. 87, right column). The most likely diagnosis is

A. bowel infarction
B. acute cholecystitis
C. ruptured abdominal aortic aneurysm
D. penetrating duodenal ulcer
E. pancreatic adenocarcinoma

21. A 27-year-old homosexual man is referred to the clinic because of mucoid diarrhea of 72 hours' duration. He has had three similar episodes over the past two years. He denies fever, chills, hematochezia, and weight loss. Stools are negative for ova and parasites, and routine bacterial cultures are negative. Sigmoidoscopy shows hyperemia, some friability of the mucosa, and thick mucus. Your next step would be

A. duodenal drainage for *Giardia lamblia*
B. phage typing of *Escherichia coli* isolated to look for enterotoxigenic organisms
C. hemagglutination test for ameba
D. rectal steroids (e.g., hydrocortisone, 100 mg) and suppositories
E. stool cultures for *Neisseria gonorrhoeae*

22. Which of the following statements regarding colonic diverticula is correct?

A. Diverticular disease mainly affects patients who are obese and of lower socioeconomic status
B. Diverticulitis is the result of a local perforation of a single diverticulum
C. Colonic diverticula are associated epidemiologically with a high-roughage, high-grain diet
D. Individuals over the age of 60 are rarely afflicted
E. Colonic diverticula usually develop in the right colon and cecum

23. An 18-year-old woman complains of excessive flatus without any other symptoms. Her weight and physical examination are normal. Which of the following statements is correct?

A. An increase in hydrogen on flatus analysis would suggest that excessive flatus is due to psychogenic air swallowing
B. A hydrogen breath test after oral administration of lactose would be the best laboratory study for evaluating the possibility of lactase deficiency
C. Adding vegetables high in indigestible carbohydrates (e.g., legumes) to the diet will usually reduce flatulence by increasing stool bulk
D. The absence of gas pains in this patient's history makes it unlikely that she actually passes more than normal quantities of flatus
E. An absence of methane on flatus analysis would suggest either significant malabsorption or the presence of abnormal colonic flora

24. Which of the following patients is most likely to have cholesterol cholelithiasis?

A. A 50-year-old oriental man with chronic *Clonorchis sinensis* infection
B. A 52-year-old white man who had a left hemicolectomy for colon cancer 10 years ago
C. A 52-year-old obese white woman who had an ileal resection ten years ago
D. A 52-year-old white woman with familial hypercholesterolemia
E. A 52-year-old white man with congenital spherocytosis who has never undergone splenectomy

25. Which of the following has NOT been found to be elevated in the blood or cerebrospinal fluid of patients with cirrhosis of the liver and hepatic encephalopathy?

A. Ammonia
B. False neurotransmitters such as octopamine
C. Short-chain fatty acids
D. Mercaptans
E. Branched-chain amino acids

26. A 31-year-old man has had blood-streaked stools and a muco-sanguineous rectal discharge for several months. Proctosigmoidoscopy reveals diffusely friable mucosa in the distal rectum that bleeds with swabbing. The more proximal rectum and distal sigmoid colon appear normal. Which one of the following would NOT cause these symptoms?

A. Lymphogranuloma venereum
B. Trauma
C. Nonspecific ulcerative proctitis
D. Granuloma inguinale
E. Radiation

QUESTIONS 27–28

A 55-year-old machinist is referred for evaluation of acute severe abdominal pains of five hours' duration. Since awakening this morning he has had nausea and right shoulder pains. He vomited forcefully on six separate occasions, producing only yellow-green fluid without

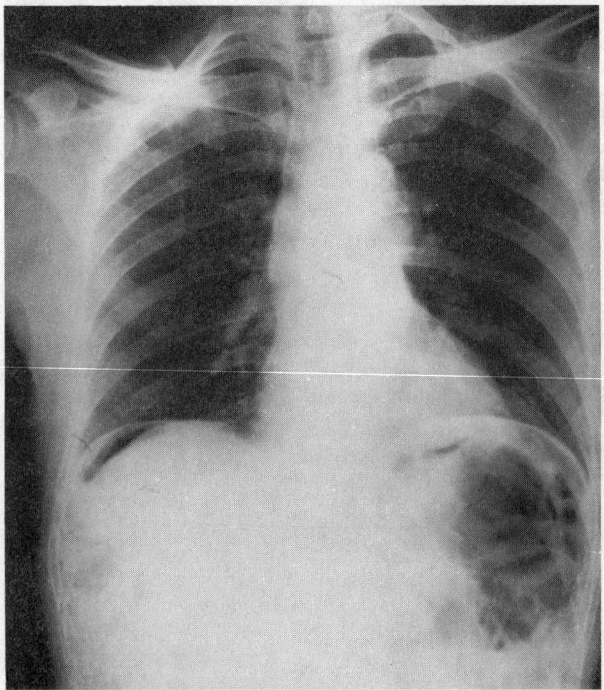

blood or coffee-ground material. On physical examination he appears acutely ill and icteric. The abdomen is distended; bowel sounds are hypoactive, and hepatomegaly is noted. Stool is negative for occult blood. Hematocrit is 40%, white blood cell count is 15,000/cu mm; serum amylase is 325 IU/L (N<110). Urinalysis is normal except for 2 + bilirubin. Roentgenogram of the chest is shown on p. 88.

27. Which one of the following conditions could account for the radiographic findings in this patient?

A. Hepatic abscess
B. Hemorrhagic pancreatitis
C. Acute cholecystitis
D. Posterior duodenal bulbar ulcer
E. Anterior gastric antral ulcer

28. Which one of the following therapeutic and diagnostic procedures should be performed?

A. Abdominal ultrasonography of liver, gallbladder, and pancreas
B. Nasogastric tube decompression
C. Abdominal paracentesis
D. Barium upper gastrointestinal series
E. Emergency endoscopy

---

29. A 59-year-old multiparous white woman consults you because of steady, severe right upper quadrant pain that began one day ago. Temperature is 99.5°F. There is tenderness in the right upper quadrant of the abdomen. The gallbladder is palpable. Serum bilirubin is 1.6 mg/dl. Serum transaminase (SGOT) and alkaline phosphatase are minimally elevated. White blood cell count is 11,000/cu mm. Which of the following statements regarding this patient is correct?

A. Computed tomography of the abdomen would be a useful diagnostic procedure in this patient
B. Ultrasonography is likely to demonstrate the cause of this patient's disorder
C. This patient's gallbladder is likely to visualize on oral cholecystography
D. This patient's gallbladder is likely to visualize on ^{99m}Tc-HIDA scan
E. This patient's gallbladder is likely to visualize on intravenous cholangiography

30. A 65-year-old woman with hypertensive cardiovascular disease (stable on antihypertensive agents and digoxin) is admitted for her second episode of painless hematochezia. Previous work-up included a negative single-contrast barium enema, sigmoidoscopy, and upper gastrointestinal series with small bowel follow-through. This time she passed three large (200-gm) bloody stools over the night, but she has not passed any blood for the past five hours. Sigmoidoscopy demonstrates normal mucosa to 25 cm, but dark bloody material mixed with stool is coming down from above. Your next diagnostic step would be

A. immediate angiography upon stabilization of the patient
B. emergency colonoscopy today
C. barium enemas after tap water enemas today
D. upper gastrointestinal series using air contrast technique today
E. double-contrast enema tomorrow; immediate angiography if brisk bleeding returns

31. A 48-year-old alcoholic man with a five-year history of chronic relapsing pancreatitis develops painless jaundice. Endoscopic retrograde cholangiopancreatography is performed (see illustration).

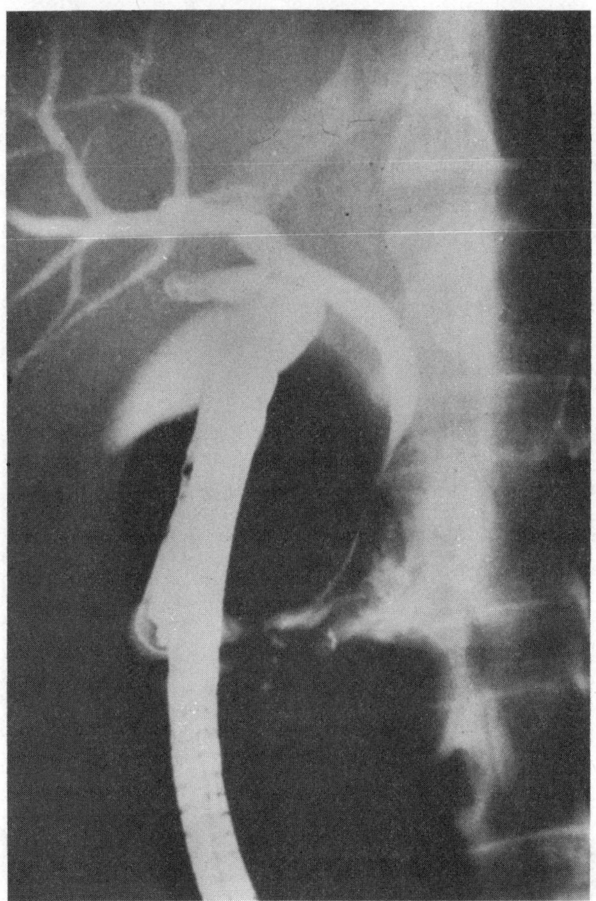

The most likely diagnosis is

A. periductal fibrosis of the common bile duct from chronic pancreatitis
B. common bile duct compression from pancreatic pseudocyst formation
C. carcinoma of the pancreas enveloping the common bile duct
D. carcinoma of the common bile duct
E. ductal stricture related to previous common duct stones

32. A 56-year-old woman is referred for evaluation of possible cancer of the pancreas, suspected on the basis of epigastric pain radiating to the back associated with an eight-pound weight loss. Physical examination and routine blood tests, including serum amylase, are normal. The next appropriate diagnostic test to detect pancreatic cancer is

A. urine amylase
B. upper gastrointestinal series
C. ultrasonography or computerized tomography of the pancreas
D. radioisotopic pancreatic scan with ^{75}Se-selenomethionine
E. visceral angiography

QUESTIONS 33–34

A 65-year-old man who had an abdominal aneurysmectomy three months ago consults you because of left lower quadrant cramping abdominal pains, constipation, and fever of two weeks' duration. For the past week he has noted intermittent passage of air on urination. Physical examination reveals an elderly man who appears ill. Temperature is 39°C. There is a tender mass in the left lower quadrant of the abdomen. Examination of stools for occult blood is positive. Hematocrit is 36%, and white blood cell count is 15,000/cu mm with 10% band forms. Barium enema is shown below.

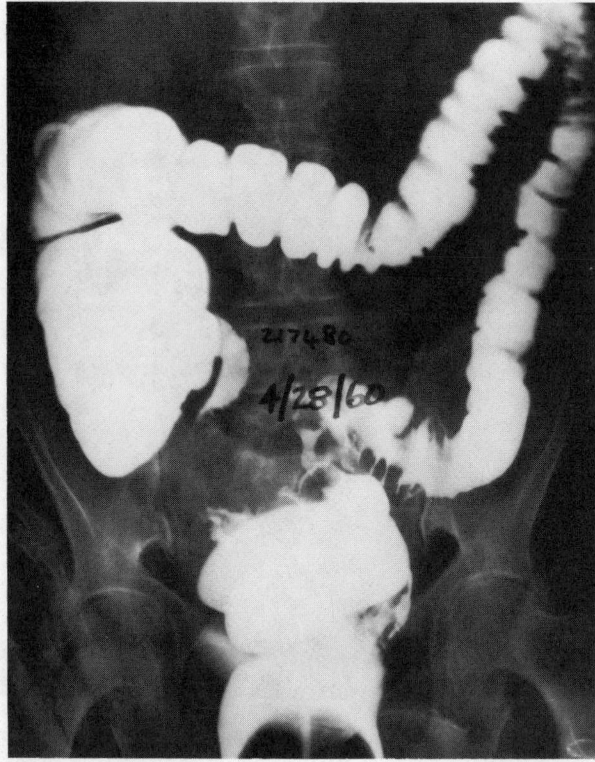

33. Which one of the following diseases can best explain the clinical presentation and barium radiography?

A. Colonic ischemia (ischemic colitis) following surgical repair of an aortic aneurysm
B. Crohn's disease of the sigmoid colon
C. Diverticulosis
D. Diverticulitis
E. Perforating sigmoid carcinoma

34. Further evaluation and treatment should include all the following EXCEPT

A. parenteral hyperalimentation or elemental, low-residue diet
B. broad-spectrum antibiotics, including clindamycin for anaerobic organisms
C. nonabsorbable oral antibiotics such as bacitracin, neomycin, or kanamycin to deliver high-dose antibiotics to the lower bowel lumen
D. consideration of a diverting colostomy to prevent continued local sepsis
E. intravenous pyelography to exclude obstruction of the ureters

---

35. A 60-year-old man with longstanding peptic ulcer disease is admitted with epigastric pain and vomiting. He has had morning vomiting of material ingested at suppertime over the past week. Physical examination demonstrates a fullness in the epigastrium and left upper quadrant, with tenderness to palpation in the right epigastric area. Stool is trace-positive for occult blood. Which one of the following would you order next?

A. Emergency endoscopy
B. Bed rest, light sedation, and antacids hourly
C. Nasogastric tube lavage to look for signs of recent bleeding
D. Nasogastric tube lavage followed by saline load (750 ml saline by nasogastric tube, aspiration back in 30 minutes)
E. Nothing by mouth, and cimetidine, 300 mg intravenously every six hours

36. A 52-year-old businesswoman is admitted because of recurrent epigastric burning pains two years after an antrectomy and vagotomy with Billroth II anastomosis (gastrojejunostomy). The pain is relieved by antacids and meals. One episode of hematemesis (mostly dark, coffee-ground material) occurred just before hospitalization. She denies alcohol or salicylate ingestion, and she does not smoke cigarettes. Physical examination reveals a thin woman (she has lost 15 pounds since surgery). Examination of the stool for occult blood is positive (1+). Upper endoscopy demonstrates a stomal ulceration. Gastric secretory testing shows a basal acid output of 4.0 mEq/hr and a peak acid output (after pentagastrin) of 8.2 mEq/hr; basal serum gastrin is 400 pg/ml ($N<150$ pg/ml). Following the intravenous injection of secretin (1 unit/kg), highest serum gastrin level is 375 pg/ml. This clinical picture is most compatible with which one of the following?

A. Zollinger-Ellison syndrome
B. Vasoactive intestinal polypeptide (VIP) tumor of the pancreas
C. Incomplete vagotomy
D. Retained antrum on duodenal stump
E. Incomplete gastric resection

37. A 27-year-old woman is admitted because of six hours of cramping right lower quadrant and suprapubic pains and gross hematochezia. She denies previous personal or

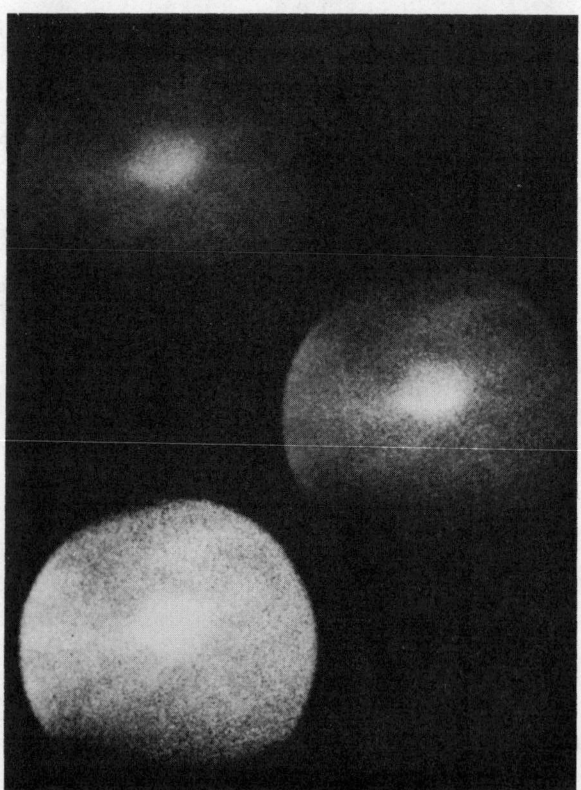

family history of bowel disease. She admits to consuming 2 quarts of Scotch over the past two days with a boyfriend, and she thinks she vomited bloody fluid one day before admission. Physical examination reveals a benign abdomen. Postural vital sign changes are noted. Sigmoidoscopy demonstrates normal mucosa to 25 cm with dark red blood clots coming down from above. Nasogastric aspiration reveals yellow fluid but no blood. A technetium scan of the abdomen is done (see illustration, p. 90, right column). Which of the following is the most likely diagnosis?

A. Carcinoid tumor
B. Crohn's disease with extensive ileal involvement
C. Lymphoma involving Peyer's patches
D. Meckel's diverticulum
E. Endometriosis of the bowel

38. Which of the following statements regarding pancreatic carcinoma is true?

A. Pancreatoduodenectomy (Whipple's procedure) is a good palliative measure when resection for cure is impossible
B. Direct surgical pancreatic biopsy is the only completely accurate means of making the diagnosis
C. Selenomethionine pancreatic scanning with ^{75}Se is a useful initial screening test
D. Most pancreatic carcinomas arise in the head of the gland and originate from ductular tissue
E. Pancreatic carcinoma, like gastric carcinoma, is decreasing in incidence in the United States

39. A 32-year-old American engineer who has just returned from a three-year visit to Central America is admitted because of nonbloody diarrhea and weakness. He has lost 20 pounds over the past eight months. There is no past history of bowel disorders. Stools are large, greasy, and foul-smelling. His appetite is good. Physical examination reveals a thin, obviously pale man. The liver is palpable 2 cm below the right costal margin; the spleen tip is also palpable. Loud borborygmi are audible. Laboratory values are as follows:

Hematocrit	22%
Mean corpuscular volume	110 cu microns
Mean corpuscular hemoglobin concentration	30%
White blood cell count	8000/cu mm
Serum vitamin B_{12}	200 pg/ml
Fecal fat	40 gm/24 hr (on 100 gm/day fat diet)
HB_sAg	Positive
Serum alkaline phosphatase	Normal
Serum transaminase (SGOT)	50 IU/L

Examination of stools for ova and parasites and stool cultures are negative. Correct evaluation and therapy would include all the following EXCEPT

A. serum folate
B. trial of gluten-free diet
C. upper gastrointestinal series
D. trial of tetracycline, 250 mg four times daily
E. small bowel biopsy

40. A 62-year-old housewife is admitted with midepigastric postprandial pains occurring 30 minutes after meals. She has lost 20 pounds over the past six months. She says she has a good appetite, but is afraid to eat because of the predictability of the pain. Physical examination is normal except for obvious signs of weight loss. An upper gastrointestinal series, endoscopy, oral cholecystogram, sigmoidoscopy, and barium enema are normal. Laboratory values are as follows:

Hematocrit	38%
White blood cell count	8100/cu mm
Serum albumin	4.0 gm/dl
Serum alkaline phosphatase	Normal
Serum bilirubin	Normal
Serum transaminase (SGOT)	Normal
Serum lactic dehydrogenase	Normal
Serum amylase	Normal

Stools are negative for occult blood on six successive days. Which one of the following tests would most likely give the correct diagnosis?

A. Exploratory laparotomy
B. Psychiatric evaluation
C. Computerized tomography of the abdomen
D. Laparoscopy
E. Mesenteric angiography

41. Which one of the following would reliably differentiate Crohn's disease from ulcerative colitis?

A. Deep mucosal ulcerations
B. Barium enema showing rectal sparing
C. Crypt abscesses
D. Perianal abscesses
E. "Skip" areas of normal colonic mucosa

42. A 27-year-old black man with sickle cell disease presents with chills, fever to 103°F, jaundice, and right upper quadrant pain. The patient has previously received a total of 67 units of blood, and five weeks ago he underwent a partial exchange transfusion prior to minor surgery. Physical examination reveals an enlarged liver and tenderness in the right upper quadrant of the abdomen. Laboratory studies show:

Serum bilirubin	27 mg/dl
Serum transaminases:	
SGOT	5 times normal
SGPT	2 times normal
Serum alkaline phosphatase	13 times normal
Prothrombin time	12 seconds (control:11)

Which of the following is the most likely cause of this patient's current illness?

A. Uncomplicated acute cholecystitis
B. Hemochromatosis
C. Hepatic infarction owing to sludging of sickled cells in the sinusoids
D. Choledocholithiasis with cholangitis
E. Viral hepatitis

43. The most common cause of traveler's diarrhea is

A. *Giardia lamblia*
B. *Shigella*
C. *Entamoeba histolytica* (amebic disease)
D. *Escherichia coli*
E. *Vibrio cholerae*

44. Characteristics of Crohn's disease include all the following EXCEPT

A. aphthous ulcers
B. arthralgias
C. "skip areas" of normal colonic mucosa
D. normal mesenteric lymph nodes
E. perianal fistulas

45. A 26-year-old man is noted to have a serum transaminase (SGOT) of five times normal, an elevated serum globulin, and a slightly decreased serum albumin on routine examination prior to discharge from the Armed Services. He feels well. Physical examination reveals hepatomegaly and cutaneous vascular spiders, and a liver biopsy shows findings compatible with chronic active hepatitis. Which of the following items in this patient's rather remarkable medical history is most likely to have led to his current liver disease?

A. An episode of jaundice caused by the use of chlorpromazine that cleared with discontinuation of the drug
B. An episode of hepatitis A that resulted from eating a salad prepared by an infected recruit
C. An episode of anicteric post-transfusion hepatitis
D. An episode of fulminant hepatic failure following exposure to carbon tetrachloride
E. A case of amebiasis contracted while serving overseas

QUESTIONS 46–47

A 75-year-old black man is brought to the emergency room with a one-day history of rectal bleeding. On the day before admission he passed four large stools containing large amounts of bright red blood within one hour. Bleeding stopped until this morning, when he passed large amounts of red blood and clots three times within two hours. Five hours later he passed bright red blood twice, and because of severe weakness and dizziness he came to the emergency room. The patient has severe hypertension being treated with propranolol, hydralazine, and furosemide. Five years ago he underwent resection of an abdominal aortic aneurysm with placement of a Dacron graft. Ten years ago he had an anterior myocardial infarction, and he has had occasional exertional angina pectoris since then. He has had five episodes of angina at rest today, each relieved by nitroglycerin.
Laboratory studies show:

Hematocrit	18%
White blood cell count	9500/cu mm
Platelet count	250,000/cu mm
Prothrombin time	11 seconds (control:11)
Serum electrolytes:	
Sodium	145 mEq/L
Potassium	3.5 mEq/L
Chloride	100 mEq/L
Bicarbonate	19 mEq/L
Liver function studies	All within normal range

Electrocardiogram is normal except for evidence of an old anterior myocardial infarction and hypertension. Sigmoidoscopy reveals normal mucosa with blood in the lumen. Nasogastric tube aspiration shows no blood and no bile.

46. After initial stabilization and blood replacement, which one of the following would be the most reasonable initial diagnostic test?

A. Colonoscopy
B. Selective inferior mesenteric artery arteriogram
C. Upper gastrointestinal panendoscopy
D. Barium enema
E. Computerized tomography of the abdomen

47. Which of the following lesions is LEAST likely to be the cause of the patient's hematochezia?

A. Duodenal ulcer
B. Aortoduodenal fistula
C. Angiodysplasia of the colon
D. Villous adenoma of the rectum
E. Bleeding diverticula

---

48. A 23-year-old man with a history of psychiatric hospitalizations and previous suicide attempts comes to the emergency room stating that he consumed about one half of a glass (4 oz) of a liquid lye preparation used to unclog drains. The patient's vital signs are normal except for a pulse rate of 110 per minute. Careful examination of the oropharynx reveals no lesions. The chest, abdomen, and roentgenogram of the chest are normal. Which of the following is the most appropriate next step?

A. Endoscopy with a pediatric endoscope to determine whether there is tissue damage in the esophagus
B. Esophagogram with a water-soluble contrast agent, followed by endoscopy if the esophagogram is abnormal
C. Placement of a nasogastric tube to preserve the esophageal lumen, and close observation for evidence of dysphagia or mediastinitis
D. Instillation of dilute hydrochloric acid into the esophagus to neutralize residual alkaline material
E. Psychiatric consultation with no further medical evaluation because the absence of pharyngeal lesions rules out significant lye injury to the esophagus

49. A 21-year-old man has had recurrent upper abdominal pain and intermittent jaundice for one month. The patient was in a motorcycle accident six months ago. Eight weeks ago he was stabbed in the upper abdomen. Exploratory laparotomy at that time revealed lacerations of the liver and colon, which were repaired without incident. Physical examination now reveals no abnormalities except for the laparotomy scar. The patient's stool is repeatedly positive for occult blood. Laboratory studies include a serum bilirubin of 2 mg/dl, a serum transaminase (SGOT) that is twice normal, and a serum 5'-nucleotidase that is three times normal. Proctosigmoidoscopy, barium enema, and upper gastrointestinal films are all normal. Which of the following tests is most likely to provide a definitive diagnosis?

A. Ultrasonography
B. Intravenous cholangiography
C. Arteriography
D. Laparoscopy
E. Liver biopsy

50. The presenting features of Wilson's disease (hepatolenticular degeneration) may include all the following EXCEPT

A. schizophrenia
B. chronic active hepatitis
C. fulminant hepatic failure
D. slowly progressive renal failure
E. hemolysis

51. Which one of the following stimuli of gastric acid secretion CANNOT be blocked by cimetidine?

A. Pentagastrin
B. Food
C. Vagally mediated gastric secretion
D. Histalog (betazole)
E. None of the above

52. A 25-year-old woman complains of three months of postprandial abdominal distention, bloating, and nausea that is partially relieved by vomiting of ingested food. Although symptoms were intermittent at first, they now appear about 15 minutes after each meal and last one to two hours. Symptoms are diminished by eating very small meals. The patient has lost 50 pounds in the past six months; however, she was on a weight-loss diet for the past seven months and at least 40 of the pounds were lost prior to the onset of symptoms. Recently she has noted partial relief of symptoms if she assumes a "hands-and-knees" position after eating. Physical examination reveals a thin woman with evidence of recent weight loss. No other abnormalities are noted. Which of the following diagnoses is most compatible with this patient's history?

A. Chronic cholecystitis
B. Pyloric channel ulcer with partial obstruction
C. Annular pancreas
D. Superior mesenteric artery syndrome
E. Intestinal pseudo-obstruction

53. A 32-year-old white man is referred to you for evaluation. The patient was healthy until nine weeks ago when he developed signs, symptoms, and laboratory studies suggestive of an acute hepatitis. (Liver function tests drawn five months ago as part of a pre-employment examination had been normal.) The patient has not recovered from the acute hepatitis. He is still jaundiced and, although somewhat fatigued, has recently returned to his job as a postal clerk. Laboratory studies show:

Serum transaminase (SGOT)	10 times normal
Serum alkaline phosphatase	2 times normal
Serum bilirubin	9 mg/dl
Hepatitis B surface antigen	Negative
Hepatitis B core antibody	Negative
Prothrombin time	14 seconds (control: 12)

Which one of the following would you recommend?

A. Liver biopsy for evaluation of possible chronic active hepatitis
B. An empiric six-month trial of corticosteroids
C. Continued observation
D. Staying off his job until liver function tests are normal
E. Gamma globulin injections for his fellow-workers

54. A 33-year-old woman who has spent the past three years living in Asia, Africa, and Scandinavia consults you because of jaundice of one week's duration. Serum bilirubin is 8.5 mg/dl, serum alkaline phosphatase is 450 IU/L (N<71); serum transaminase (SGOT) is 45 IU/L (N<37). Which of the following parasites is most likely to be responsible for the symptoms?

A. *Ancylostoma duodenale*
B. *Ascaris lumbricoides*
C. *Trypanosoma cruzi*
D. *Diphyllobothrium latum*
E. *Strongyloides stercoralis*

55. A 65-year-old man who has smoked two packs of cigarettes daily for 40 years is admitted to the hospital because of heartburn, regurgitation, and progressive dysphagia. An upper gastrointestinal series demonstrates a smooth tapered stricture of the distal esophagus. Laboratory studies reveal hematocrit, 49%; white blood cell count, 8600/cu mm; carcinoembryonic antigen (CEA), 2 ng/ml (N <2.5 ng/ml). Which one of the following should be ordered next?

A. Cine-esophagogram
B. Esophagoscopy and multiple lower esophageal biopsies
C. Antacids, cimetidine, elevate head of bed, restrict cigarettes
D. Dilatation (bougienage) of the strictured area
E. Bethanechol and antacids

56. A 43-year-old white woman consults a dermatologist with a complaint that her skin blisters and is "fragile," i.e., even minor trauma causes severe abrasions that are slow to heal. The patient admits to drinking several martinis daily for the past 20 years. She is taking no medications except oral contraceptives. Her health has been excellent. No other family members are similarly affected. Physical examination reveals intact and ruptured blisters, hypertrichosis, and hyperpigmentation in sun-exposed areas. Liver span is 15 cm in the midclavicular line. Serum transaminase (SGOT) is elevated to twice normal, but all other liver function tests are normal. The patient's hands are illustrated. Which of the following statements regarding this patient is INCORRECT?

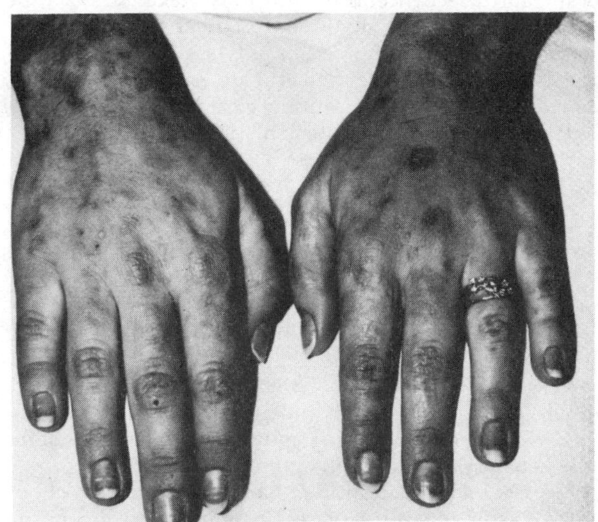

A. Urinary uroporphyrin is probably elevated
B. Urinary porphobilinogen is probably elevated
C. The oral contraceptives should be discontinued
D. The skin lesions will probably improve with phlebotomy
E. Her illness requires both an inherited enzyme deficiency and environmental factors for its full expression

57. A 50-year-old housewife complains of weight gain, intolerance to fatty foods, and increasing flatus. Physical examination reveals no abnormalities. Examination of stools for occult blood is consistently negative. A barium enema shows a 3-cm polyp on a stalk in the mid-descending colon, and a $1\frac{1}{2}$-cm polyp in the splenic flexure. Which of the following would be most appropriate?

A. Repeat barium enema examinations yearly to watch for increases in polyp size before considering surgery
B. Colonoscopic biopsy of both polyps
C. Laparotomy and colotomy with removal of known polyps, while looking for other polyps
D. Colonoscopic polypectomy of most distal larger (i.e., 3-cm) polyp and colonoscopy to splenic flexure
E. Pancolonoscopy (to cecum) and removal of both polyps

58. Which of the following has been shown to improve survival in patients with fulminant hepatic failure?

A. Cimetidine
B. Corticosteroids
C. Exchange transfusion
D. Artificial liver support systems
E. None of the above

59. All the small bowel parasites listed below can cause anemia in the host. Which one specifically results in vitamin B_{12} deficiency?

A. *Entamoeba histolytica*
B. *Schistosoma mansoni*
C. *Ancylostoma duodenale*
D. *Trichuris trichiura*
E. *Diphyllobothrium latum*

60. A 54-year-old man in an alcohol rehabilitation program is found on a routine set of blood tests to have a serum amylase concentration that is elevated 1½ times normal. He is asymptomatic, and all other serum chemistry values are normal. The serum amylase determination is repeated six months later and is again elevated to about the same degree. Amylase-creatinine clearance ratio is normal. Which of the following statements is correct?

A. The elevated serum amylase probably reflects an increase in the salivary amylase isoenzyme component of the total serum amylase
B. The elevated serum amylase reflects subclinical kidney disease with inadequate excretion of amylase
C. The patient should undergo oral cholecystography because of the likelihood that gallstones are present
D. The patient should undergo endoscopic retrograde cholangiopancreatography to evaluate whether pancreatic disease is present
E. Oral administration of pancreatic enzymes should result in return of serum amylase to the normal range

QUESTIONS 61–62

A 65-year-old male engineer who has been taking ampicillin for the past five days begins to have loose, watery, nonbloody diarrhea and passes ten stools during the day and night. On the sixth day of ampicillin therapy he develops abdominal cramps, nausea, and a fever to 39°C. On the seventh day he consults a physician. The patient has a history of intermittent episodes of diarrhea over the past ten years, but he denies hematochezia or nocturnal diarrhea. On sigmoidoscopy the rectal mucosa is hyperemic and friable with a thick mucous plaque adherent. A rectal biopsy and a barium enema are performed (see illustrations).

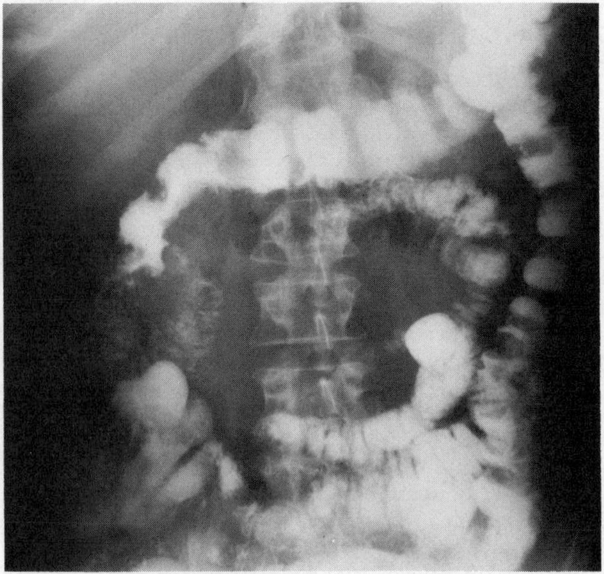

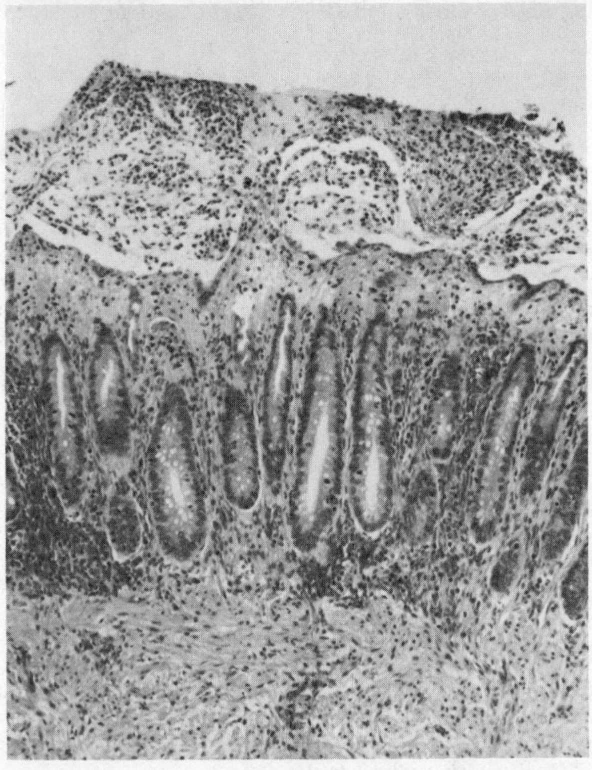

61. Which of the following diagnoses best explains these findings?

A. Pancolonic ulcerative colitis
B. Acute amebic colitis exacerbated by ampicillin
C. Pseudomembranous enterocolitis
D. Ischemic colitis
E. Acute Crohn's disease of the colon with rectal involvement

62. Which one of the following mechanisms can best explain the alteration in colonic structure and function in this patient?

A. Invasion of the mucosa by enteric pathogens
B. An immune-related phenomenon with "K" lymphocytes lysing mucosal cells
C. Altered mucosal blood flow

D. An enterotoxin-related destruction of mucosa
E. Cytotoxic effect of antibodies on colonic epithelial cells

---

QUESTIONS 63–64

A 62-year-old man underwent resection of an abdominal aortic aneurysm under halothane anesthesia four days ago. The operation lasted eight hours, the patient received 12 units of blood, and he was hypotensive on several occasions during the procedure. The postoperative course has been complicated by renal failure and gram-negative sepsis. The patient has become progressively jaundiced since the operation. Liver function tests show:

Serum transaminase (SGOT)	72 IU/L
Serum alkaline phosphatase	2 times normal
Prothrombin time	12 seconds (control:11)
Serum bilirubin:	
Total	22 mg/dl
Direct	15 mg/dl

63. Which of the following is LEAST likely to be contributing to the patient's jaundice?

A. Increased bilirubin production
B. Sepsis
C. Halothane-induced liver injury
D. Renal failure
E. Intraoperative hypotension

64. Which diagnostic procedure would be most appropriate for this patient?

A. Ultrasonography
B. Liver biopsy
C. Endoscopic retrograde cholangiography
D. Percutaneous transhepatic cholangiography
E. Intravenous cholangiography

QUESTIONS 65–66

A 62-year-old Mexican-American farm worker has noted weight loss for a two-month period. His appetite has decreased substantially, and he has had dull right upper quadrant abdominal pains. He has also had a low-grade fever (temperature 38.6°C). He denies diarrhea, hematochezia, jaundice, or use of alcohol. He has never returned to Mexico since he emigrated to the United States 25 years ago. Physical examination demonstrates signs of recent weight loss and scleral icterus. Liver span is 18 cm in the midclavicular line; the hepatic edge is mildly tender to palpation. An ultrasonographic study is performed, and the transverse scan through the abdomen is illustrated. The bottom scale is in centimeters.

65. Which one of the following diagnostic procedures would you recommend as the next step in the patient's evaluation?

A. Percutaneous biopsy of the liver
B. Upper gastrointestinal series and barium enema examination to look for malignancy
C. A liver-spleen radioisotope scan
D. Alpha-fetoprotein determination followed by a liver biopsy
E. Serologic test for ameba *(Entamoeba histolytica)*

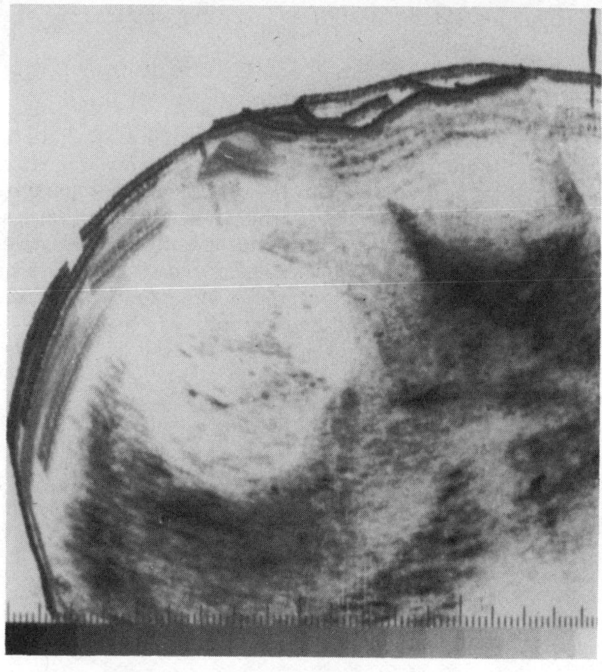

66. Treatment for this patient should include which one of the following?

A. Metronidazole (Flagyl), 750 mg three times daily for ten days
B. Laparotomy and drainage of the liver
C. Hemihepatectomy if angiography confirms no disease in the left lobe of the liver
D. Chemotherapy with hepatic artery infusion of 5-fluorouracil
E. Clindamycin, 600 mg intravenously every six hours for two weeks, and gentamicin, 5 mg/kg intravenously in three divided doses daily for two weeks

---

67. A 56-year-old white man is admitted to the hospital because of abdominal pain and vomiting. Physical examination reveals a temperature of 38°C, jaundice, vascular spiders, palmar erythema, and tender hepatomegaly. Laboratory studies reveal:

White blood cell count	20,000/cu mm
Serum transaminase (SGOT)	200 IU/L
Serum alkaline phosphatase	600 IU/L (N<71)
Prothrombin time	14 seconds (control: 11)
Total serum bilirubin	10 mg/dl

A liver biopsy shows diffuse large droplets of fat, hepatocellular disarray with areas of focal necrosis and infiltration by polymorphonuclear leukocytes, and eosinophilic cytoplasmic inclusions (Mallory bodies) in pericentral hepatocytes. Which of the following statements regarding this hepatic disorder is INCORRECT?

A. It may progress to cirrhosis even if the patient stops drinking alcohol
B. It may be accompanied by a leukemoid reaction
C. It may be accompanied by marked elevations of alkaline phosphatase and bilirubin, suggesting extrahepatic obstruction
D. The presence of eosinophilic cytoplasmic inclu-

sions (Mallory bodies) is pathognomonic of this disorder

E. Alcohol alone has produced this disorder in primates ingesting a balanced diet

68. A 52-year-old white man with longstanding diabetes mellitus and the recent onset of arthropathy and congestive heart failure is noted by an astute medical student to have a "grayish hue" to his skin. The patient denies excess alcohol intake or use of vitamin preparations, and states that both his parents and his 37-year-old sister are living and healthy. A liver biopsy reveals markedly increased iron in both parenchymal and reticuloendothelial cells by special staining, and a quantitative analysis for iron also reveals abnormally high values. Which statement regarding this patient is correct?

A. His parents probably have normal liver iron concentrations
B. His asymptomatic sister cannot have the same disease as he
C. Because of the patient's age and advanced disease, phlebotomy is *not* advisable
D. This patient's disorder is transmitted by a chromosomal locus closely linked to the HLA locus
E. Serum iron, transferrin saturation, and ferritin values for this patient's father are no different from those for age- and sex-matched controls

DIRECTIONS: For questions 69 to 119, you are to decide whether EACH choice is true or false. Any combination of answers, from all true to all false, may be present. Mark the answer sheet "T" or "F" in the space provided.

69. Which of the following statements about infection of the esophagus is/are true?

A. Infection is a frequent complication of gastroesophageal reflux disease because gastric juice disrupts the esophageal mucosal barrier
B. Infection should be suspected in any immunocompromised individual complaining of odynophagia or dysphagia
C. Identification of the etiologic agent is *not* essential because the treatment is the same for all
D. A barium study of the esophagus is usually sufficient to enable diagnosis to be made
E. The contiguous spread of streptococcal pharyngitis is a frequent source of esophageal infection

70. Which of the following statements regarding isoniazid-associated hepatitis is/are true?

A. Isoniazid-associated hepatitis occurs most frequently in middle-aged and elderly individuals, in whom the incidence of severe liver disease may exceed 2% of those receiving the drug
B. Isoniazid produces a characteristic injury that is usually distinguishable from acute viral hepatitis and chronic active hepatitis on liver biopsy
C. In many patients, hepatotoxicity will not become evident until many months after beginning isoniazid therapy
D. Isoniazid-induced liver injury is typically accompanied by a skin rash or eosinophilia
E. Many patients will develop mild elevations of serum transaminases after beginning isoniazid therapy, but most of these do not develop severe liver disease

71. Which of the following statements about pancreatic insufficiency is/are correct?

A. Significant protein and fat absorption continues even when postcibal secretion of enzymes by the pancreas is 1% of normal
B. Clinical symptoms of malabsorption begin to appear when about half of the exocrine secretory capacity of the pancreas is lost
C. Megaloblastic anemia commonly occurs unless vitamin B_{12} is replaced
D. Symptoms of malabsorption often improve after a course of cholecystokinin and secretin
E. The presence of large amounts of undigested food in the intestinal tract predisposes patients with pancreatic insufficiency to acquire intestinal parasites

72. Which of the following statements concerning Mallory-Weiss tears of the gastroesophageal junction is/are true?

A. They are associated with mediastinitis
B. Alcohol abuse is common in patients with these lesions
C. Multiple episodes of forceful retching and vomiting are usually seen in patients with these lesions
D. They occur in the absence of a hiatus hernia
E. Bleeding is from submucosal arterioles

73. A 27-year-old woman was struck across the upper abdomen by a steering wheel during an auto accident one month ago. She was admitted to the hospital for observation because of abdominal pain and tenderness. Abdominal roentgenograms were normal, and peritoneal lavage was negative for blood. She felt better the next day and was discharged. She comes to see you now because of increasing abdominal girth. Which of the following statements regarding the evaluation and management of this patient is/are correct?

A. If the patient has pancreatic ascites with a high fluid amylase concentration, initial therapy should include vigorous diuresis and anticholinergic agents to suppress pancreatic secretion
B. Ultrasonography would be less reliable for diagnosing pancreatic pseudocyst in this patient than in the setting of alcoholic pancreatitis
C. If surgery becomes necessary, endoscopic retrograde cholangiopancreatography should be performed prior to the operation
D. If a pseudocyst is present in an accessible location, percutaneous aspiration under ultrasonographic guidance is the initial treatment of choice
E. Significant pancreatic injury is unlikely in this patient because it rarely occurs in the absence of clinically apparent damage to the spleen and liver

74. A 35-year-old white man who has had insulin-dependent diabetes mellitus for 20 years now complains of an 18-month history of loose, frequent stools up to 10 to 12 times per day with frequent occurrence at night and occasional incontinence. Which of the following is/are likely in this patient?

A. Improved control of serum glucose levels will alleviate the diarrhea
B. Diabetic nephropathy is present
C. Peripheral neuropathy is present
D. Small bowel radiographs will show prolonged transit times and dilated bowel loops
E. Diarrhea will respond to treatment with tetracycline

75. Which of the following statements about pancreatic carcinoma is/are correct?

A. It occurs less frequently than stomach cancer in the United States
B. It is often associated with symptoms of mental disorders such as depression or anxiety
C. Advances in diagnostic methods have significantly improved survival
D. Hypoglycemia is an important complication
E. It is seen less frequently than benign tumors of the exocrine pancreas

76. Which of the following statements regarding gastrin, cholecystokinin, secretin, gastrin inhibitory peptide, and vasoactive inhibitory peptide is/are true?

A. They show remarkable amino acid similarity in their carboxy-terminal regions
B. They show remarkable amino acid similarity in their amino-terminal regions
C. They are all produced by cells of the proximal small intestine
D. They all have physiologically important effects on gastric acid secretion

E. Hypersecretion of each has been shown to cause a human disease

77. Which of the following statements regarding gastrin is/are correct?

A. Markedly elevated serum gastrin levels differentiate patients with acid hypersecretion from patients with achlorhydria
B. A marked rise in serum gastrin levels after secretin injection differentiates patients with the Zollinger-Ellison syndrome from patients with other acid hypersecretory states
C. It circulates in serum in several different forms
D. Digested proteins and amino acids are the most powerful natural "releasers" of gastrin in humans
E. Vagotomy reduces the acid secretory response to gastrin

78. Which of the following pulmonary abnormalities is/are associated with acute pancreatitis?

A. Basal atelectasis
B. "Shock lung"
C. Pleural effusion
D. Tension pneumothorax
E. Elevation of the diaphragms

79. Gastroesophageal reflux may be induced by which of the following?

A. Gastrin
B. Metoclopramide
C. Bethanechol
D. Smoking
E. Anticholinergic drugs

80. Which of the following diseases is/are associated with ileocecal involvement?

A. Tuberculosis
B. Salmonellosis
C. Amebiasis
D. *Yersinia enterocolitica* infection
E. South American blastomycosis

81. Which of the following is/are pathogenetically linked to hepatocellular carcinoma?

A. Hepatitis A virus infection
B. Hepatitis B virus infection
C. Wilson's disease
D. Androgen administration
E. Aflatoxin ingestion

82. Which of the following statements about motor disorders of the esophagus is/are true?

A. Carcinoma of the gastric cardia can exactly mimic achalasia both clinically and radiographically
B. Endoscopy has little usefulness in the evaluation of most motor disorders
C. Gastroesophageal reflux accounts for most of the esophageal symptoms of scleroderma
D. Pneumatic bag dilatation, because of its high risk, generally has been superseded by surgery in the treatment of achalasia
E. A trial of sublingual nitroglycerin is a useful way to distinguish between the pain of diffuse esophageal spasm and that of angina pectoris

83. Which of the following conditions is/are associated with the weight loss experienced by patients following a subtotal gastrectomy with a Billroth II anastomosis?

A. Decreased dietary intake
B. Poor mixing of chyme and pancreaticobiliary secretions
C. Rapid gastric emptying of solids and liquids
D. Hypochlorhydria and bacterial overgrowth
E. Loss of antral gastrin secretion

84. A 16-year-old boy is referred to you because of postprandial abdominal pain, nausea, vomiting, and a 20-pound weight loss. Stools are large, bulky, and foul-smelling but without occult blood. White blood cell count is 7500/cu mm with 25% eosinophils. Which of the following would explain his problem?

A. *Giardia lamblia* infestation
B. Ascariasis
C. Eosinophilic granuloma
D. Eosinophilic gastroenteritis
E. Pancreatic insufficiency

85. Which of the following factors is/are associated with esophageal cancer?

A. Cigarette usage
B. Achalasia
C. Strictures of the esophagus following lye ingestion
D. Barrett's esophagus
E. Previous squamous carcinoma of the head and neck

86. Which of the following grains may be given to patients with celiac (nontropical) sprue?

A. Barley
B. Corn
C. Oats
D. Rice
E. Buckwheat

87. Which of the following statements concerning irritable bowel disease ("mucous colitis" or "spastic colitis") is/are correct?

A. Distinctive changes are seen on barium enema
B. Rectal biopsy is often abnormal
C. Exacerbations are often associated with periods of stress
D. Onset of disease is usually before the age of 40
E. The disease often responds to bulk laxatives and bran

88. Whipple's disease of the bowel is associated with

A. peripheral neuropathy
B. palpable, tender, enlarged lymph nodes
C. heart murmurs
D. distinctive PAS-positive macrophages in the lamina propria
E. intermittent migratory arthritis

89. Carcinoma of the colon may be associated with ulcerative colitis. Which of the following statements is/are correct?

A. Diagnosis can best be made by following serial carcinoembryonic antigen (CEA) levels
B. The incidence of malignancy correlates with activity and duration of illness
C. Annual barium enema examination can be relied on to exclude malignancy
D. Colonic malignancy is rarely associated with ulcerative proctitis

E. Malignant lesions tend to be flat and infiltrative rather than polypoid

90. Diseases caused by which of the following parasites may involve the biliary tract?

A. *Clonorchis sinensis*
B. *Giardia lamblia*
C. *Ascaris lumbricoides*
D. *Schistosoma mansoni*
E. *Trichuris trichiura*

91. A 35-year-old black woman who weighs 475 pounds undergoes a jejunoileal bypass procedure for weight loss. Recognized complications of this operation include which of the following?

A. Glomerulonephritis
B. Fatty liver
C. Pancreatitis
D. Renal stones
E. Hepatic failure

92. Which of the following statements regarding the serologic markers of hepatitis B virus is/are correct?

A. Hepatitis B surface antigen (HB_sAg) is typically the first marker to appear and generally precedes clinically evident hepatitis
B. Hepatitis B core antibody (HB_cAb) typically appears at the onset of clinical hepatitis and may be the only serologic marker of acute type B hepatitis present in some patients
C. Hepatitis B surface antibody (HB_sAb) appears late in the convalescent phase and is generally protective of a future hepatitis B infection
D. Hepatitis B core antibody (HB_cAb) is not protective and is found in nearly all chronic HB_sAg carriers
E. Hepatitis B core antibody (HB_cAb) is a marker of viral replication

93. Which of the following statements regarding hepatitis transmission is/are correct?

A. Hepatitis A virus is transmitted primarily by the fecal-oral route during the preicteric phase of the illness
B. Most post-transfusion hepatitis in the United States results from infectious agents other than those causing type A or type B hepatitis
C. Nonparenteral transmission of hepatitis B is now well documented and occurs via many body secretions, including saliva and semen
D. Most individuals who are stuck by a needle previously used in a patient with HB_sAg-positive serum will develop hepatitis B
E. Co-workers of patients found to have hepatitis B should receive injections of hepatitis B–immune globulin

94. A 65-year-old woman who underwent subtotal gastrectomy and Billroth II gastrojejunostomy two years ago is evaluated for a 30-pound weight loss and diarrhea. She passes four or five loose watery stools after each meal; there has been no nocturnal diarrhea. Proctoscopy is normal. Examination of the stool shows many muscle fibers and fat globules. Barium enema is illustrated. Which of the following statements is/are correct?

A. The patient was given a larger-than-normal volume of barium contrast material, which has refluxed to the proximal gastrointestinal tract

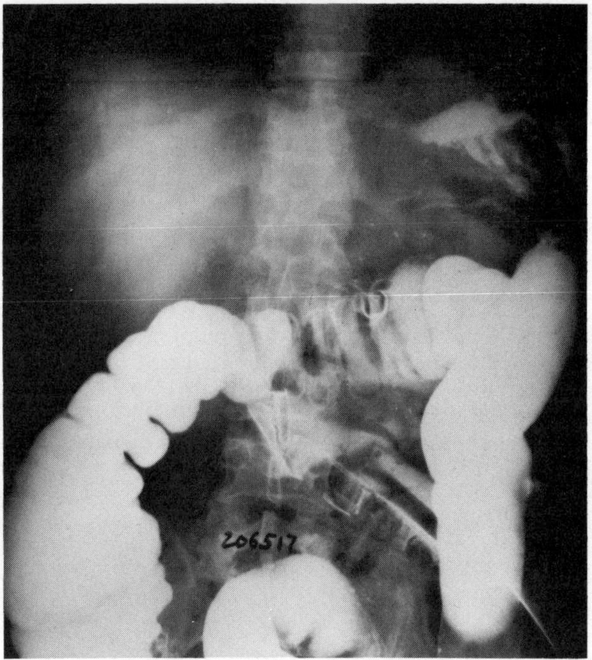

B. A subphrenic collection of barium suggestive of an abscess has developed from a perforating colonic carcinoma
C. The differential diagnosis includes Crohn's disease, carcinoma, and abdominal trauma
D. The diarrhea is due to fecal contamination and overgrowth of colonic flora in the upper gastrointestinal tract
E. An upper gastrointestinal series will reliably demonstrate the same findings

95. A 22-year-old white woman has been referred to you for evaluation of fatigue and jaundice of several months' duration. Liver function tests include a serum transaminase (SGOT) that is several times normal, a serum bilirubin concentration of 3 mg/dl, an albumin:globulin ratio of less than 1, and a prothrombin time that is 3 seconds prolonged compared with a control. A liver biopsy is interpreted as showing chronic active hepatitis. Which of the following might be causing this patient's illness?

A. Isoniazid therapy for tuberculosis
B. Methyldopa therapy for hypertension
C. Chronic hepatitis B virus infection
D. Liver disease associated with ulcerative colitis
E. Hepatic copper accumulation due to Wilson's disease

96. A 48-year-old man who does not drink alcohol is admitted to the hospital because of severe periumbilical pain radiating to the back. Three weeks ago he had an episode of similar but much less severe pain, and an oral cholecystogram at that time was normal. On physical examination the patient is acutely ill with shock, respiratory distress, and diffuse abdominal tenderness with rebound. Laboratory studies show:

Hematocrit	54%
White blood cell count	22,000/cu mm
Serum amylase	1800 IU/L
Serum albumin	4.5 gm/dl
Serum calcium	10.2 mg/dl

Serum glucose	360 mg/dl
Serum cholesterol	300 mg/dl
Serum triglycerides	2350 mg/dl

Which of the following might have caused this episode of severe pancreatitis?

A. Diabetic ketoacidosis
B. Hyperparathyroidism
C. Thiazide diuretics
D. Acute leukemia
E. Hyperlipoproteinemia

97. A 52-year-old man with longstanding alcoholism is seen for gradually increasing abdominal girth, weight loss, and intermittent vague abdominal pain. On physical examination the patient appears chronically ill with muscle wasting and massive ascites. Which of the following might be causing the ascites?

A. Cirrhosis with portal hypertension
B. Pancreatic pseudocyst
C. Methyl alcohol abuse
D. Splenic vein thrombosis
E. Hypothyroidism

98. Intestinal ischemia

A. frequently results in ischemic damage to the rectum with ulceration and submucosal hemorrhage
B. requires either complete venous or arterial occlusion
C. results in gangrenous bowel whenever any one of the three main mesenteric vessels is occluded (i.e., celiac axis, superior mesenteric artery, inferior mesenteric artery)
D. commonly involves the small bowel, splenic flexure, and descending colon
E. will be improved by the use of vasoconstrictors such as alpha-adrenergic agonists to combat shock

99. A 42-year-old white man is undergoing evaluation for recurrent hemorrhage from esophageal varices. Wedged hepatic vein pressure is found to be 3 mm Hg above that in the inferior vena cava (N<5). Which of the following causes of portal hypertension typically produce(s) the hemodynamic changes found in this patient?

A. Congenital hepatic fibrosis
B. Alcoholic cirrhosis
C. Portal vein thrombosis
D. Liver disease due to *Schistosoma mansoni* infection
E. Primary biliary cirrhosis

100. Which of the following statements about pancreatic pseudocysts is/are true?

A. Asymptomatic pseudocysts arising in patients with acute pancreatitis should be followed by sequential ultrasonography; if they are decreasing in size, no surgery is indicated.
B. Patients with pseudocysts should receive broad-spectrum antibiotics to reduce the risk of infection of the cyst contents
C. Internal drainage of a pseudocyst is acceptable if surgery is indicated
D. Endoscopic retrograde cholangiopancreatography (ERCP) is required in the initial evaluation of most pseudocysts to determine if cyst contents are leaking into the abdominal cavity
E. Spontaneous erosion of a pseudocyst into the stomach or colon is almost always a catastrophic event requiring emergency surgical intervention

QUESTIONS 101–102

101. A 39-year-old white woman initially sought medical attention because of pruritus. Physical examination revealed only excoriations, and routine laboratory studies included a serum alkaline phosphatase 4 times the upper limit of normal. No specific diagnosis was made. One year later she returns with jaundice and worsening of the pruritus. Physical examination reveals hepatomegaly and palmar xanthomas. Laboratory studies reveal:

Serum alkaline phosphatase	9 times normal
Total serum bilirubin	4 mg/dl
Total serum globulin	4.2 gm/dl
Serum albumin	3.7 gm/dl
Serum cholesterol	700 mg/dl
Serum calcium	7.8 mg/dl
Prothrombin time	15 seconds (control: 11)

Past medical history is noncontributory except that the patient had a cholecystectomy for gallstones three years ago. The differential diagnosis in this patient includes which of the following?

A. Neoplasm located near the junction of the right and left hepatic ducts
B. Surgical injury to the extrahepatic biliary tree
C. Chronic active hepatitis
D. Choledocholithiasis
E. Primary biliary cirrhosis

102. A liver biopsy shows many lymphocytes and some plasma cells in the portal tracts surrounding interlobular bile ducts, with some degeneration of the ductal epithelium. Bile plugs are present in some canaliculi, but there are no bile plugs in the interlobular ducts and no bile lakes. Serum antimitochondrial antibody is positive, and an intravenous cholangiogram fails to visualize the bile ducts. Which of the following statements regarding this patient is/are correct?

A. Serum immunoglobulin M is probably elevated
B. Visualization of the biliary tree by transhepatic or retrograde cholangiography is indicated
C. She is more likely than the general population to have Raynaud's phenomenon
D. She is more likely than the general population to be anergic to skin tests
E. Therapy will probably include supplementation with the fat-soluble vitamins A, D, and K

QUESTIONS 103–105

A 33-year-old homosexual man comes to the emergency room because of severe abdominal pain and distention, fever, and bloody diarrhea of two days' duration. For the past two years he has had frequent episodes of mucous and bloody diarrhea, tenesmus, and cramps lasting up to three weeks. Admission laboratory tests include: hematocrit 35%, white blood cell count 13,500/cu mm, serum sodium 142 mEq/L, serum potassium 3.2 mEq/L. A plain film of the abdomen is shown on p. 101.

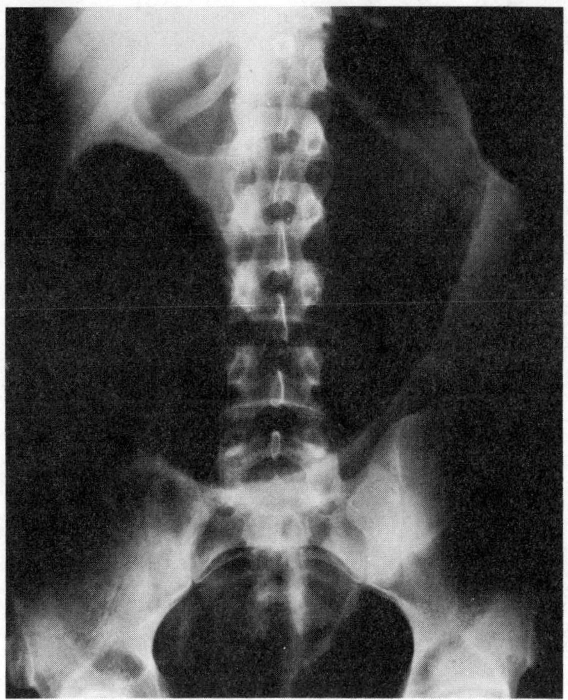

103. Which of the following would explain the patient's illness?

A. Shigellosis
B. Ulcerative colitis
C. Giardiasis
D. Crohn's colitis
E. Amebiasis

104. Stool cultures are negative, and no ova or parasites are visible on three successive stool examinations. Proctosigmoidoscopy reveals a diffusely granular friable mucosa to 15 cm. Which of the following diagnostic tests is/are indicated in this patient?

A. Barium enema
B. Serology for *Entamoeba histolytica*
C. Colonoscopy to the midtransverse colon
D. Blood cultures
E. Repeat plain film of abdomen within 24 hours

105. During the first 24 hours in the hospital the patient continues to complain of cramping pains and profuse bloody diarrhea. The abdomen increases in size, and bowel sounds become hypoactive. Which of the following is/are now indicated?

A. Oral hyperalimentation with elemental diet
B. Diphenoxylate and atropine (Lomotil)
C. Repeat serum electrolytes
D. Hydrocortisone, 100 mg intravenously every eight hours
E. Immediate emergency laparotomy and colectomy

---

106. A 57-year-old alcoholic black man with biopsy-proved cirrhosis of the liver is admitted to the hospital following a recent episode of heavy drinking. Physical examination reveals jaundice, hepatosplenomegaly, and petechiae on the lower extremities. Platelet count is 43,000/cu mm. Which of the following might be a cause of this patient's thrombocytopenia?

A. Toxic effect of alcohol on the bone marrow
B. Folic acid deficiency
C. Hypersplenism
D. Vitamin B_{12} deficiency
E. Disseminated intravascular coagulation

107. A 57-year-old reformed alcoholic with a well-documented history of chronic pancreatitis is referred to you because of severe, chronic epigastric pain only incompletely controlled by high doses of narcotic analgesics. Which of the following statements is/are true concerning this patient?

A. Endoscopic retrograde cholangiopancreatography (ERCP) should be performed before any surgical procedure
B. Pancreatoduodenectomy (Whipple's procedure) is the procedure of choice if pancreatic surgery is required
C. Celiac ganglionectomy (splanchnicectomy) provides the best chance for long-term relief of pain
D. About 20% of patients with this problem will continue to have pain even after appropriate surgical treatment
E. Longitudinal pancreaticojejunostomy (Puestow's procedure) successfully relieves pain in many patients with this disorder

108. Which of the following statements regarding the arthropathy of ulcerative colitis is/are true?

A. It always improves when the bowel disease is treated
B. It is much more common than the arthropathy of Crohn's colitis
C. It deforms and destroys the proximal interphalangeal joints
D. Involvement of the thoracolumbar spine is associated with the presence of HLA-B27 antigen
E. It most frequently affects large, weight-bearing joints

109. An elevated breath hydrogen level after oral administration of 50 gm of lactose is found in which of the following?

A. Cholestyramine administration
B. Bacterial overgrowth
C. Pancreatic insufficiency
D. Lactase deficiency
E. Adult celiac disease

110. A 52-year-old man is admitted to the hospital because of early satiety and epigastric pain. He has lost 20 pounds over the last three months. Stool is negative for occult blood. Upper gastrointestinal series is shown on p. 102. Which of the following statements is/are correct?

A. The presence of autoimmune atrophic gastritis in this patient would be strong evidence that the lesion is malignant
B. Nonsteroidal, anti-inflammatory drugs will not exacerbate this patient's disease
C. The presence of radiating gastric folds from the lesion reliably excludes malignancy
D. This is the most common site of gastric carcinoma
E. If the lesion is benign, the patient's peak acid output is likely to be higher than 40 mEq/hr

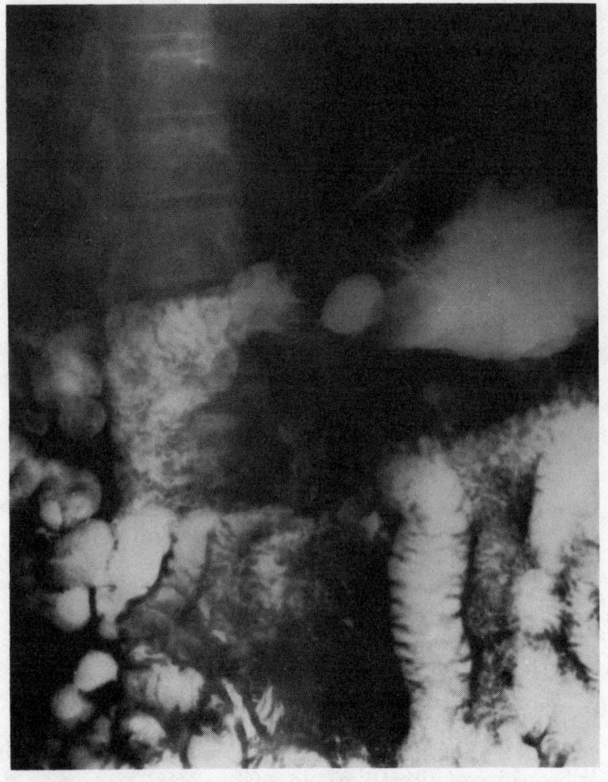

111. Which of the following statements concerning ulcerative proctitis is/are true?

A. It can cause substantial rectal bleeding
B. Rectal biopsy can distinguish this disease from ulcerative colitis
C. A normal barium enema excludes this diagnosis
D. In contrast to ulcerative colitis, complications in ulcerative proctitis are usually absent
E. The age of onset and sex distribution are different from those of ulcerative colitis

112. Measurement of serum lipase concentration may be helpful in making the diagnosis of acute pancreatitis for which of the following reasons?

A. It is specific for pancreatic inflammation
B. It is predictive of severe pulmonary complications
C. It provides information about the etiology of acute pancreatitis
D. It is not elevated in disorders of the salivary glands
E. It can suggest the appropriate approach to therapy

113. Which of the following statements regarding sexually transmitted diseases of the anus and rectum is/are true?

A. Primary and secondary syphilis involve the anus more often than the rectum
B. Gonococcal proctitis is most often asymptomatic or associated with only mild symptoms
C. Gonococcal septicemia seldom results from asymptomatic gonococcal proctitis
D. Condyloma acuminatum is caused by a papilloma virus
E. Lymphogranuloma venereum can cause rectal strictures

114. A 52-year-old man who has consumed at least 1 pint of whiskey each day for 20 years comes to you because of weight loss (despite a good appetite) and bulky, foul-smelling stools. After he has been on a 100-gm fat diet for three days, fecal fat excretion over 72 hours on the same fat intake averages 27 gm/24 hr. A widely used pancreatic enzyme replacement is prescribed, six tablets to be taken during each meal. The patient returns one month later because the symptoms have not improved. Which of the following possibilities could explain the failure of this therapy?

A. The patient is taking all six tablets before each meal
B. The patient has atrophic gastritis and hypochlorhydria
C. The dosage of the enzyme preparation is insufficient
D. The patient has primary small intestinal disease rather than chronic pancreatitis
E. Food particles are not sufficiently solubilized to allow absorption because of a decreased volume of pancreatic juice

115. Which of the following is/are associated with *Giardia lamblia* infections of the small bowel?

A. IgA deficiency
B. Hematochezia
C. Hypocalcemia
D. Absence of ova and parasites in the stool
E. Nodular lymphoid hyperplasia of the intestine

116. A 52-year-old woman has a five-year history of hemorrhoidal disease. The principal symptom has been bleeding, but within the past few months she has noted prolapse of hemorrhoids through the anus upon defecation. Examination discloses large, prolapsed internal hemorrhoids with overlying superficial ulceration. Which of the following would be likely to resolve this patient's problem?

A. Sitz baths, stool softeners, and suppositories
B. Submucosal injection of a sclerosing agent
C. Incision of the hemorrhoid with expression of clot
D. Rubber band ligation
E. Anal dilatation

117. A 38-year-old executive has just undergone an unusually thorough medical evaluation, including a physical examination, laboratory tests, glucose tolerance test, and roentgenograms of the chest and gastrointestinal tract. The only abnormality was an oral cholecystogram showing radiolucent gallstones, for which the patient is now referred to you. A careful history reveals no abdominal symptoms. Which of the following statements regarding this patient is/are correct?

A. There is a 75% or better chance that symptoms due to gallstones will develop in the future
B. Cancer is found more often in gallbladders with stones than in gallbladders without stones
C. There is about a 50% chance that a life-threatening complication of cholelithiasis will develop in the future
D. From a statistical standpoint, elective cholecystectomy performed now would increase this patient's lifespan
E. Percutaneous transhepatic cholangiography should be done to exclude choledocholithiasis

118. Which of the following patients is/are likely to have iron deficiency anemia?

A. A 12-year-old white girl with severe cystic fibrosis and pancreatic insufficiency
B. A 70-year-old white man with pernicious anemia and achlorhydria; he is a vegetarian
C. A 48-year-old woman with dysphagia, angular stomatitis, and an esophageal web
D. A 45-year-old man who had a Billroth II anastomosis for duodenal ulcer disease ten years ago; he has no recurrent ulcers
E. A 52-year-old reformed alcoholic man with a seizure disorder for which he is taking phenytoin

119. A 40-year-old woman is evaluated for diarrhea. A bile acid breath test (^{14}C-glycocholic acid) is performed, and 12% of the ingested dose is excreted as $^{14}CO_2$ in six hours (N<3%). Which of the following is/are consistent with this clinical picture?

A. A history of surgery six months ago to remove 90 cm of ileum because of intestinal ischemia
B. Peripheral arthritis and granulomas on small bowel biopsy
C. A five-year history of jaundice and pruritus, a positive antimitochondrial antibody test, and portal hypertension
D. A long history of alcohol abuse, midabdominal calcifications on an abdominal roentgenogram, and steatorrhea
E. Severe heartburn, tight shiny skin, and pulmonary fibrosis

DIRECTIONS: Questions 120 to 210 are matching questions. For each numbered item, choose the most likely associated lettered item from those provided. Each numbered item has ONLY ONE answer. Within each group, each lettered item may be the answer to one, more than one, or none of the numbered items, unless otherwise specified.

QUESTIONS 120–124

Match the clinical information with the gastric acid secretory test results. (*Note:* Each test result should be used only once.)

	Basal Acid Output (mEq/hr)	Peak Acid Output (After Pentagastrin, 6 μg/kg Subcutaneously) (mEq/hr)
A.	4	30
B.	0.1	0.2
C.	8	45
D.	12	15
E.	3	10

120. A 50-year-old executive admitted to the hospital with recurrent ulcer two years after a subtotal gastrectomy and incomplete vagotomy

121. A 20-year-old college senior with chronic dyspepsia and diarrhea; upper gastrointestinal series and endoscopy are negative

122. A 45-year-old housewife with two jejunal peptic ulcers one year after subtotal gastrectomy and vagotomy; exploratory laparotomy reveals a 2-cm mass in the tail of the pancreas

123. A 50-year-old man with a large fungating mass in the cardia of the stomach

124. A 37-year-old woman executive with two previous episodes of upper gastrointestinal bleeding; endoscopy discloses a 2-cm duodenal bulbar ulcer

QUESTIONS 125–129

For each of the following patients, select the most likely associated barium enema radiograph (*A–E*) below and on p. 105.

125. A 27-year-old woman with a six-year history of cramping abdominal pain, fever, and diarrhea with mucus and blood

126. A 30-year-old man referred for evaluation of intermittent hematochezia; several of his close relatives have developed colonic cancer before the age of 40

127. A 25-year-old man who has had periumbilical abdominal pains, constipation, fevers, and chills for the past 24 hours; white blood cell count is 17,500/cu mm

128. A 45-year-old Vietnamese refugee with postprandial cramping abdominal pains, constipation, and fever; roentgenogram of the chest shows apical pleural scarring

129. A 60-year-old woman with severe suprapubic cramping abdominal pains, fever, chills, and constipation

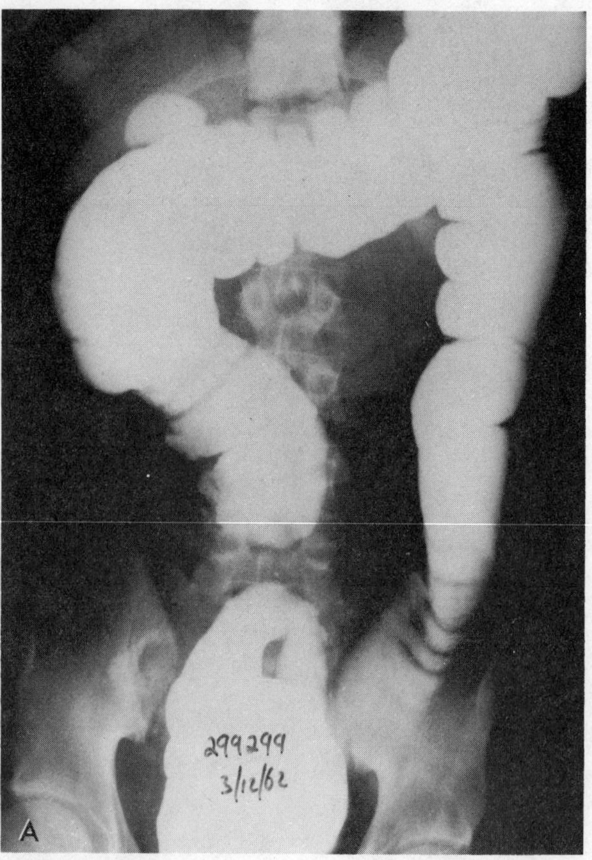

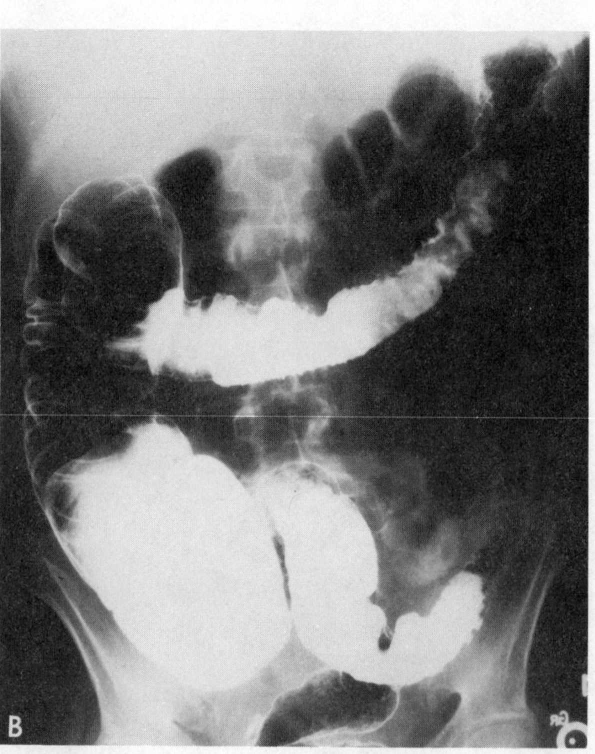

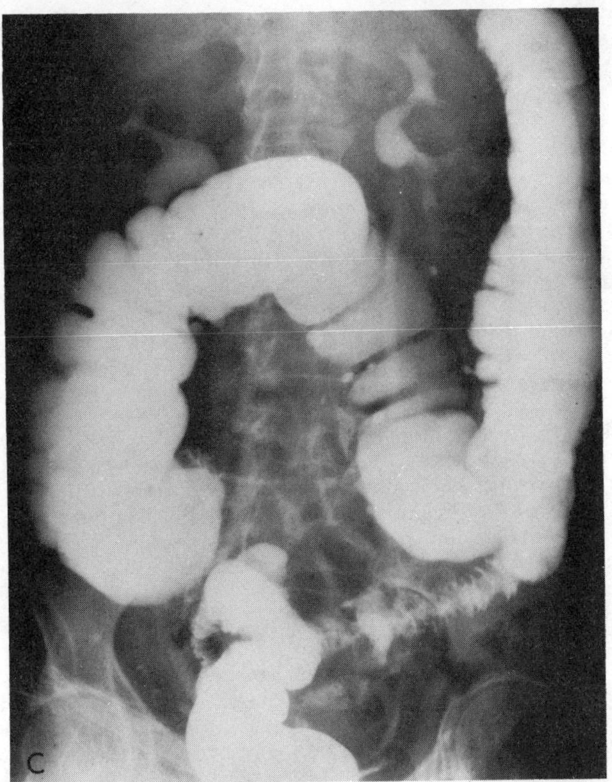

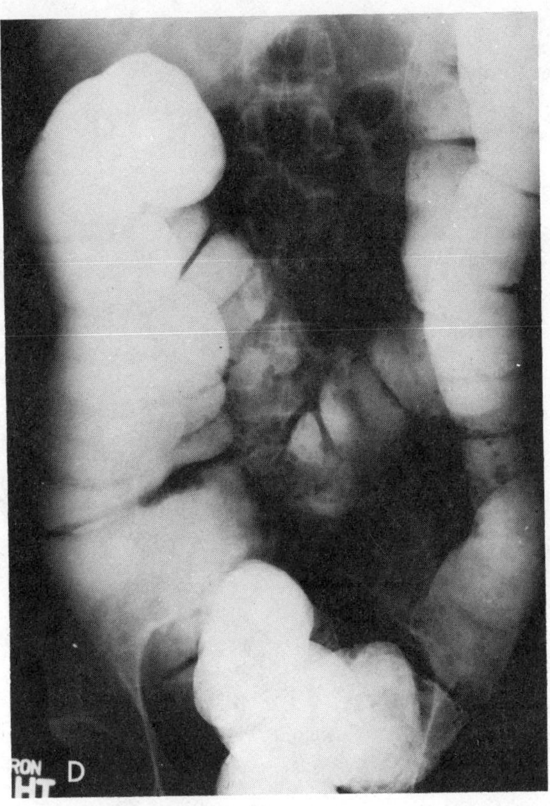

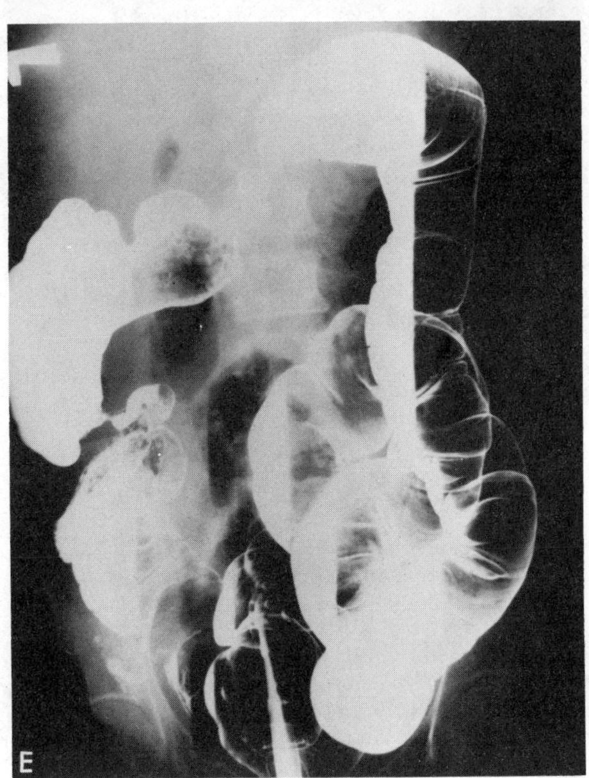

QUESTIONS 130–134

For each of the following descriptions, select the most likely associated substance.

A. Gastrin
B. Vasoactive intestinal polypeptide
C. Cholecystokinin
D. Secretin
E. None of the above

130. Trophic hormone for the gastric fundic gland mucosa and small bowel

131. Inhibits gastric acid secretion and stimulates pancreatic bicarbonate secretion; gastric pepsinogen secretion is stimulated

132. Associated with tumors of the pancreas producing hypokalemia and watery diarrhea

133. Stimulates pancreatic enzyme output with minor stimulation of bicarbonate

134. Release blocked by cimetidine, especially after a high-protein meal

QUESTIONS 135–137

The two photomicrographs (p. 106) show the jejunal histology of a patient before (*A*) and after (*B*) specific medical therapy for the bowel lesion. Each of the following patients could have had similar before-and-after small bowel histology. For each case history, select the treatment the patient is most likely to have received.

A. Quinacrine hydrochloride, 100 mg three times daily for seven days
B. Pancrease, two capsules with each meal or snack
C. Tetracycline, 250 mg four times daily and folic acid, 5 mg daily
D. Gluten-free diet
E. High-protein diet

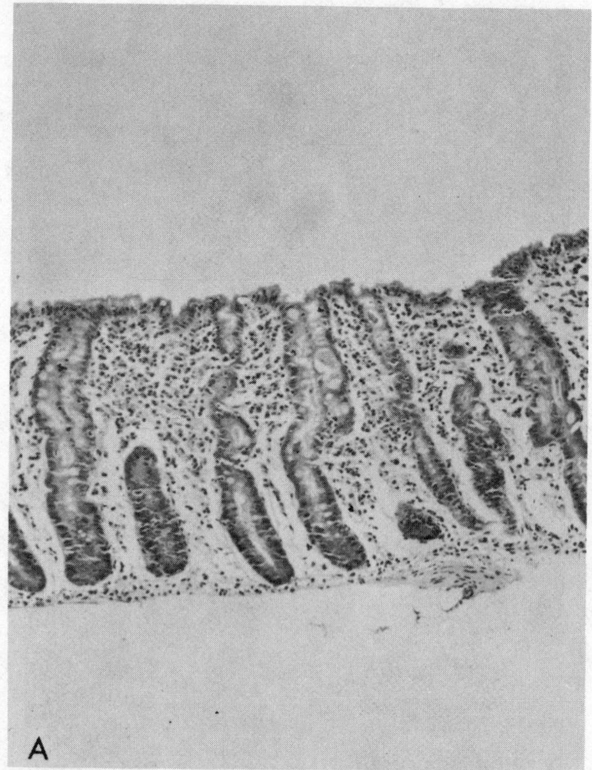

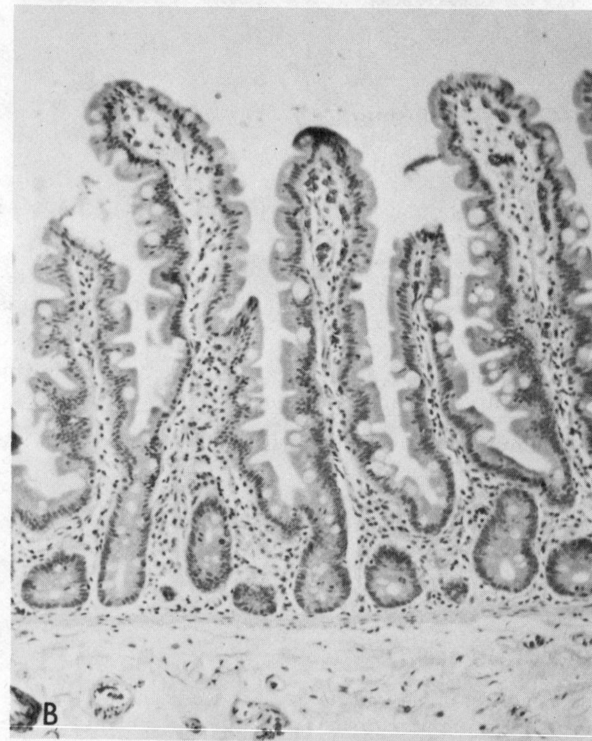

135. A 25-year-old white man returns to the United States from a six-week trip to Nepal. He consults you because of a two-week history of anorexia, watery diarrhea, flatulence, and weight loss (5 pounds). He has abdominal cramps prior to most episodes of diarrhea, which occur between three and six times per day. There has been no fever. Laboratory data and physical examination are unremarkable except for a 24-hour fecal fat excretion of 13 gm (N <5).

136. A 45-year-old retired British Army officer who operates a bar in Singapore has had progressive weight loss (50 pounds) and fatigue over the past 18 months. He notes bulky, frequent (two to four per day) stools, but states he has had frequent stools with rare episodes of diarrhea since he moved to Singapore six years ago. He has a sore tongue, dry skin, muscle weakness, and fatigue. There has been no abdominal pain. Physical examination reveals an emaciated man with glossitis. Abdominal examination is normal except for mild abdominal distention, and the stool is negative for occult blood and ova and parasites. Hematocrit is 29%, with a mean corpuscular volume of 110 cu microns; electrolytes and liver function tests are normal. Serum calcium is 7.5 mg/dl; serum albumin is 3.0 gm/dl. 24-hour fecal fat excretion is 30 gm.

137. A 45-year-old reformed alcoholic man with documented cirrhosis of the liver has lost 40 pounds over the past two years. He denies any alcohol intake in the past three years and claims to eat a normal diet. He notes mild abdominal distention, excessive flatus, and one to two soft stools per day. He denies abdominal pain. Two months ago he fell down three steps and suffered a crush fracture of the second lumbar vertebra. Physical examination reveals evidence of weight loss, mild abdominal distention, an enlarged hard liver palpable 4 cm below the right costal margin, and a normal rectum. Hematocrit is 29% with a mean corpuscular volume of 78 cu microns. Electrolytes are normal. Serum calcium is 7.5 mg/dl, serum phosphorus is 1.0 mg/dl; serum alkaline phosphatase is 320 IU/L (N<71). Serum transaminase (SGOT) is 45 IU/L (N<37), and serum bilirubin is 1.1 mg/dl. Prothrombin time is 14 seconds (control:11). 24-hour fecal fat excretion is 55 gm. A D-xylose test shows a five-hour urinary excretion of 1.5 gm (N>4).

QUESTIONS 138–142

Each of the following patients has an hepatic abnormality related to use of a drug. For each patient, choose the drug most likely to have caused the illness. (*Note:* Use each answer only once or not at all.)

A. Vincristine
B. Tetracycline
C. Methyldopa
D. Oral contraceptives
E. Ampicillin
F. Diazepam
G. Acetaminophen
H. Pentobarbital
I. Androgenic-anabolic steroids
J. Chlorpromazine

138. A 22-year-old white woman is brought to the emergency room after ingesting at least 30 tablets of an unknown medication. She is jaundiced and exhibits manic disorientation. Serum transaminase (SGOT) is elevated 40-fold. Prothrombin time is 35 seconds (control:11). She becomes comatose shortly after admission.

139. A 19-year-old man is evaluated for hepatomegaly and deteriorating liver function tests. Serum alpha-fetoprotein level is 50 times normal.

140. A 34-year-old previously healthy white woman is rushed to the emergency room in shock. Physical examination reveals a distended abdomen; paracentesis yields gross blood.

141. A 49-year-old black man is evaluated for chronically abnormal liver function tests. Liver biopsy demonstrates inflammatory cells in portal tracts that have "invaded" the surrounding parenchyma, evidence of hepatocyte necrosis, and fibrosis.

142. A 29-year-old white woman who is pregnant with her first child rapidly develops abnormal liver function and encephalopathy. Liver biopsy reveals diffuse microvesicular fatty changes in hepatocytes.

QUESTIONS 143–148

For each of the following patients, select the most likely colonic biopsy photomicrograph (*A–F*) below and on p. 108. (*Note:* Each figure should be used only once.)

143. A 32-year-old woman with multiple episodes of cramping right lower quadrant abdominal pains, nonbloody diarrhea, and a large, draining perianal fistula

144. A 50-year-old Egyptian man with splenomegaly and recurrent variceal hemorrhages

145. A 45-year-old woman with episodes of bloody diarrhea, cramping abdominal pains, and low-grade fever; the episodes occur two or three times a year each and last about two weeks

146. A 62-year-old woman treated for two weeks with clindamycin for a perforated appendix

147. A 22-year-old man with cramping abdominal pains, mucous and bloody diarrhea, and tenesmus after returning

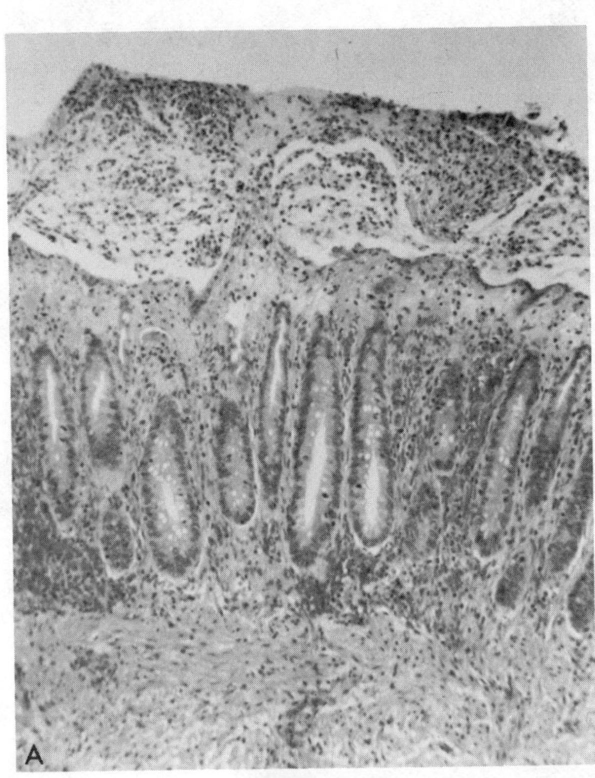
A

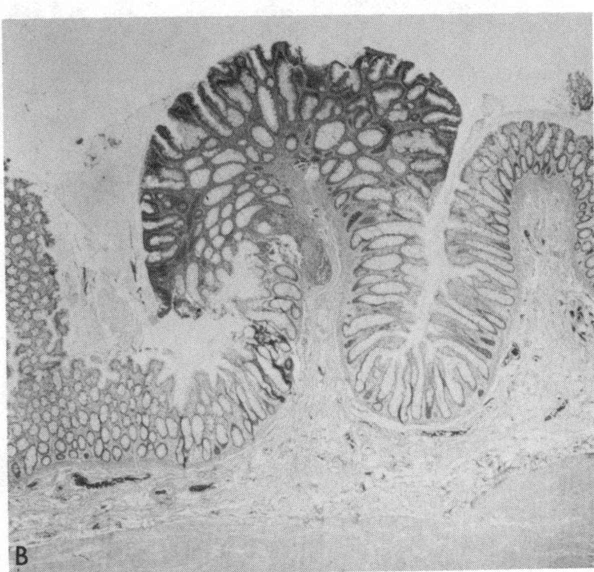
B

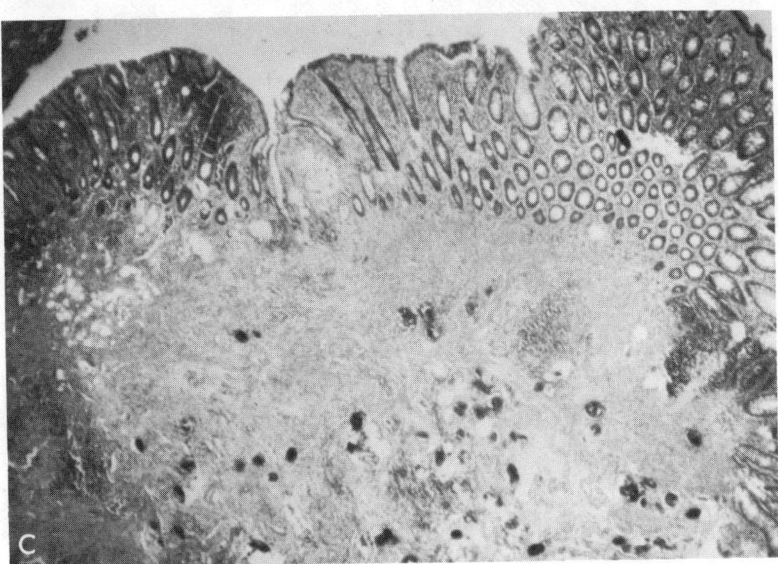
C

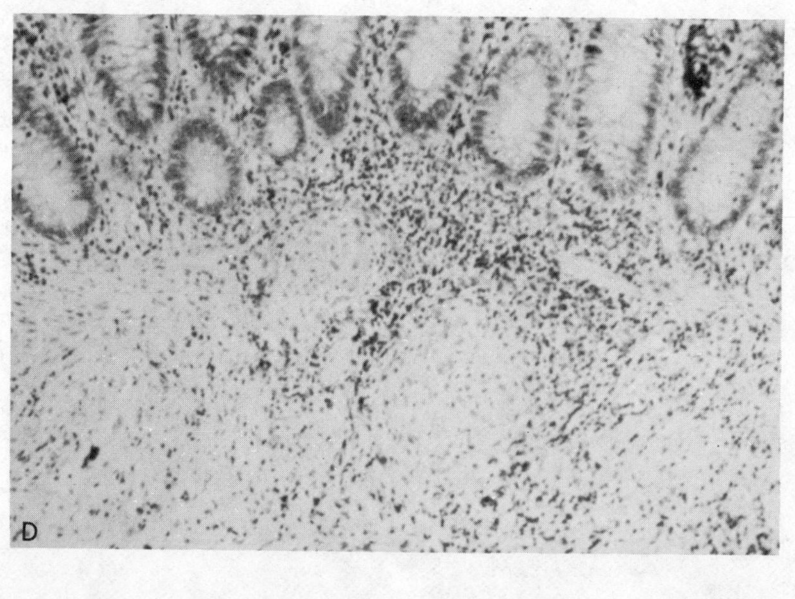
D

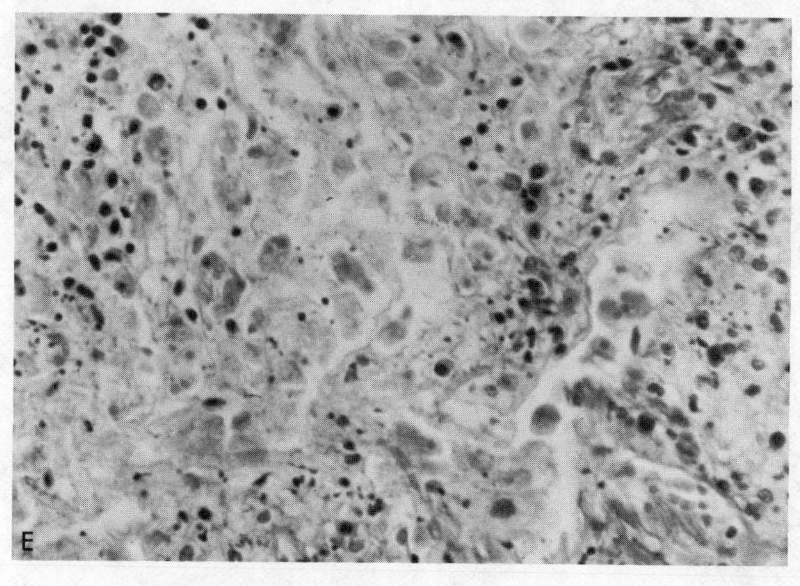
E

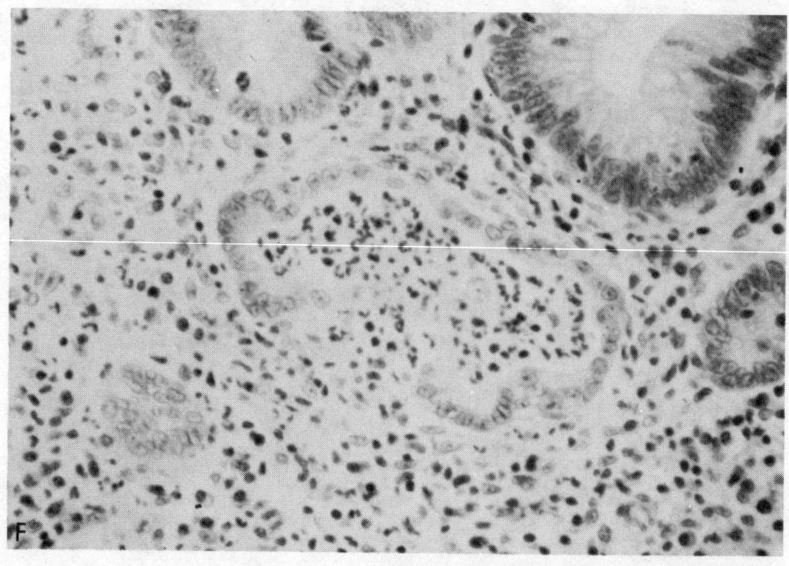
F

from a one-month scientific expedition to Central America

148. A 65-year-old man with iron deficiency anemia and weakness, but no altered bowel habits

QUESTIONS 149–152

For each statement below, select the disorder that best applies.

A. Chronic alcoholism
B. Gallstone disease
C. Protein-calorie malnutrition
D. Cystic fibrosis
E. Hyperparathyroidism

149. A potentially curable cause of pancreatic insufficiency seen mainly in children

150. A common cause of acute pancreatitis in the United States that rarely results in chronic pancreatitis

151. The most common cause of pancreatic insufficiency in the United States

152. Tests for trypsin activity in stools are helpful in making the diagnosis

QUESTIONS 153–156

For each of the following terms or descriptions, select the lettered answer that best applies.

A. Gastroesophageal reflux disease
B. Carcinoma of the esophagus
C. Both
D. Neither

153. Associated with columnar (Barrett's) epithelium

154. Associated with untreated or inadequately treated achalasia

155. The associated strictures can be successfully treated with esophageal dilatation

156. Cimetidine is useful for producing symptomatic relief

QUESTIONS 157–160

For each of the following case histories, select the most likely diagnosis.

A. Gilbert's syndrome
B. Benign recurrent cholestasis
C. Rotor's syndrome
D. Dubin-Johnson syndrome
E. Crigler-Najjar syndrome (congenital nonhemolytic jaundice), type I
F. Crigler-Najjar syndrome (congenital nonhemolytic jaundice), type II

157. An 18-year-old asymptomatic man is referred to you for evaluation of jaundice. Serum bilirubin is 8 mg/dl, essentially all indirect reacting. Liver function tests, complete blood count, and oral cholecystogram are all normal.

158. An 18-year-old asymptomatic man is referred to you for evaluation of jaundice. Total serum bilirubin is 8 mg/dl with 6 mg/dl direct reacting. Other liver function tests are normal except for a plasma sulfobromophthalein (BSP) disappearance curve that shows a secondary rise between 90 and 120 minutes. Urinary excretion of type I coproporphyrin isomer is increased, but total urinary coproporphyrin excretion is normal. An oral cholecystogram fails to visualize the gallbladder.

159. An 18-year-old man is referred to you for evaluation of jaundice with pruritus. Total serum bilirubin concentration is 8 mg/dl, with 6 mg/dl direct reacting. Serum alkaline phosphatase is also elevated. The patient felt well until two weeks ago. Both he and one of his siblings have had multiple self-limited attacks of jaundice with pruritus since early childhood.

160. An 18-year-old asymptomatic man is referred to you for evaluation of hyperbilirubinemia. Serum bilirubin is 2.2 mg/dl, with 0.2 mg/dl direct reacting. Other liver function tests and an oral cholecystogram are normal.

QUESTIONS 161–166

For each of the following diseases, select the appropriate set of laboratory data from the table below. (*Note:* Each set of data should be used only once.)

161. Chronic pancreatitis

162. Nontropical sprue in relapse

163. Scleroderma

164. Crohn's disease in a patient who has had a 100-cm ileal resection

165. Nontropical sprue in remission

166. Intestinal lymphangiectasia

	Schilling Test* (N > 7)	D-Xylose Test† (N ≥ 5)	Serum Albumin (gm/dl)	24-hr Fecal Fat (100-gm intake) (N ≤ 6)	Unconjugated Bile Salts in Duodenum
A.	9%	4.9 gm	4.0	4 gm	−
B.	9%	5.2 gm	3.6	60 gm	−
C.	4%	3.0 gm	3.2	15 gm	+
D.	8%	1.0 gm	2.8	30 gm	−
E.	2%	5.3 gm	3.9	12 gm	−
F.	8%	5.2 gm	2.1	6 gm	−

*% of ^{60}Co-labeled vitamin B_{12} excreted in urine/24 hr
†Urine excretion in 5-hr period after oral administration of 25 gm

QUESTIONS 167–170

A 35-year-old reformed alcoholic man with biopsy-proved cirrhosis was recently hospitalized for upper gastrointestinal hemorrhage shown by endoscopy to be due to bleeding varices. The bleeding was stopped by balloon tamponade; the course was complicated by stage III hepatic encephalopathy. The patient is currently feeling well and has returned to his usual job as a freight packer. He has no ascites and is not jaundiced. He is considering undergoing surgery, and two surgical procedures are being described to him. Which of the following choices best applies to each statement?

A. Standard portacaval shunt (end-to-side or side-to-side)
B. Distal splenorenal shunt (Warren shunt)
C. Both
D. Neither

167. Will decrease the likelihood of future variceal hemorrhage

168. Has/have clearly been shown to prolong useful life in patients such as this

169. The chance of this patient suffering intractable and disabling encephalopathy after surgery is greater than 50%

170. There is a substantial risk for further impairment of liver function postoperatively

QUESTIONS 171–173

For each of the following statements, select the lettered answer that applies.

A. Ulcerative colitis
B. Crohn's disease
C. Both
D. Neither

171. Proved to be caused by a microbial agent

172. Associated with ankylosing spondylitis that does not improve after total colectomy

173. Frequently accompanied by troublesome perianal fistulas and abscesses

QUESTIONS 174–175

For each of the following patients undergoing evaluation for possible biliary disease, select the most appropriate procedure for visualizing the biliary tree.

A. Percutaneous transhepatic cholangiography
B. Endoscopic retrograde cholangiography
C. Intravenous cholangiography
D. Cholescintigraphy with ^{99m}Tc-HIDA
E. Oral cholecystography
F. Computerized tomography

174. A 52-year-old accountant who has previously undergone vagotomy, antrectomy, and Billroth II anastomosis for peptic ulcer disease presents with pruritus, a markedly elevated serum alkaline phosphatase, and a serum bilirubin concentration of 2 mg/dl. Prothrombin time is 14 seconds (control:11). Sonographic examination shows dilated intrahepatic bile ducts.

175. A 49-year-old reformed alcoholic man with documented cirrhosis is admitted for evaluation of progressive pruritus, jaundice, and right upper quadrant pain. Serum bilirubin concentration is 11 mg/dl, prothrombin time is 17 seconds (control:11) and does not change after parenteral vitamin K. Serum alkaline phosphatase is elevated 15-fold. Ultrasonographic study does not show dilatation of the intrahepatic biliary tree and fails to visualize the extrahepatic bile ducts.

QUESTIONS 176–180

Match each of the following clinical histories with the appropriate motility/manometry tracing (*A–E*) below and on p. 111. (*Note:* Each tracing should be used only once.)

176. A 27-year-old woman with the sensation of a choking mass in the neck blocking the passage of solids; she has noted no weight loss, and a barium swallow was normal

177. A 62-year-old man with severe reflux esophagitis and regurgitation of sour material into the mouth

178. A 40-year-old man with sclerodactyly and Raynaud's phenomenon

179. A 53-year-old woman with sharp, stabbing retrosternal pains exacerbated by ice-cold drinks — some relief is obtained with nitroglycerin; a coronary angiogram shows normal vessels

180. A 30-year-old man with intermittent episodes of increasing dysphagia for both solid food and liquids after meals; vomiting of undigested material has been noted several hours after meals

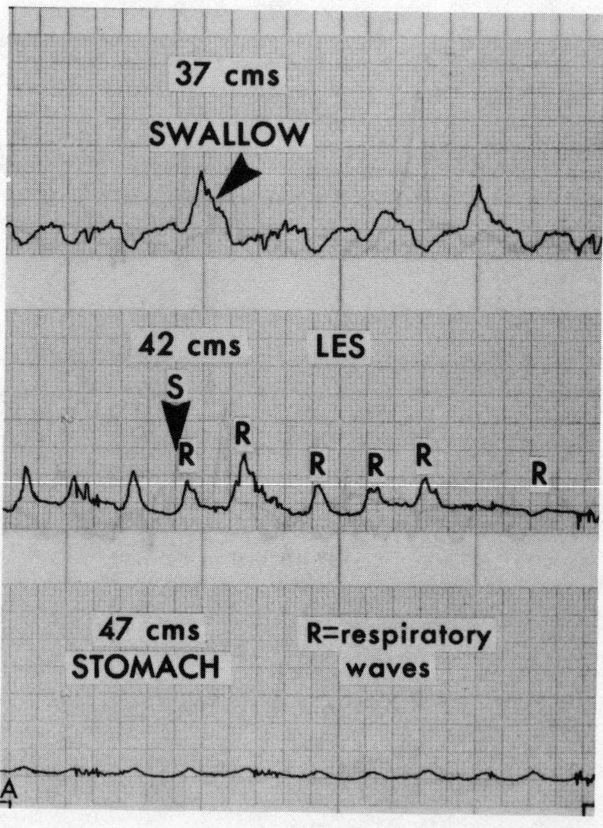

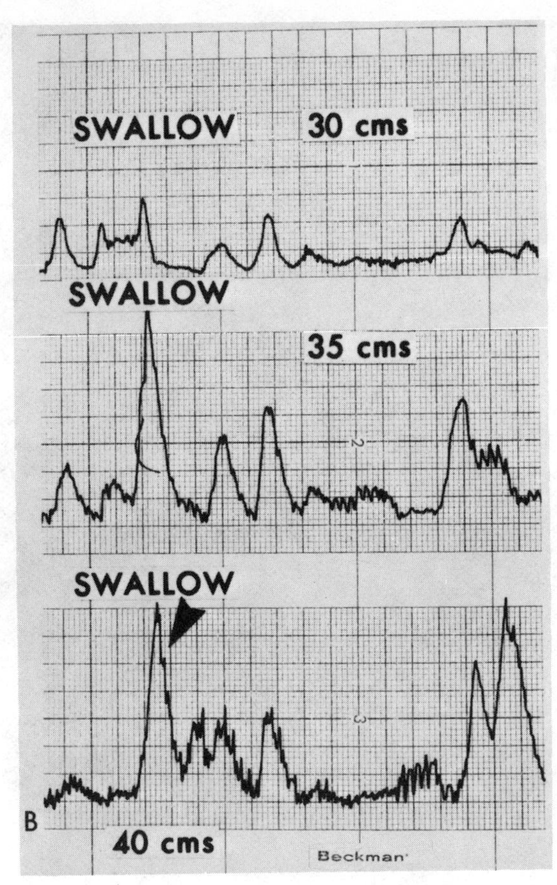
SWALLOW
30 cms
SWALLOW
35 cms
SWALLOW
40 cms
Beckman
B

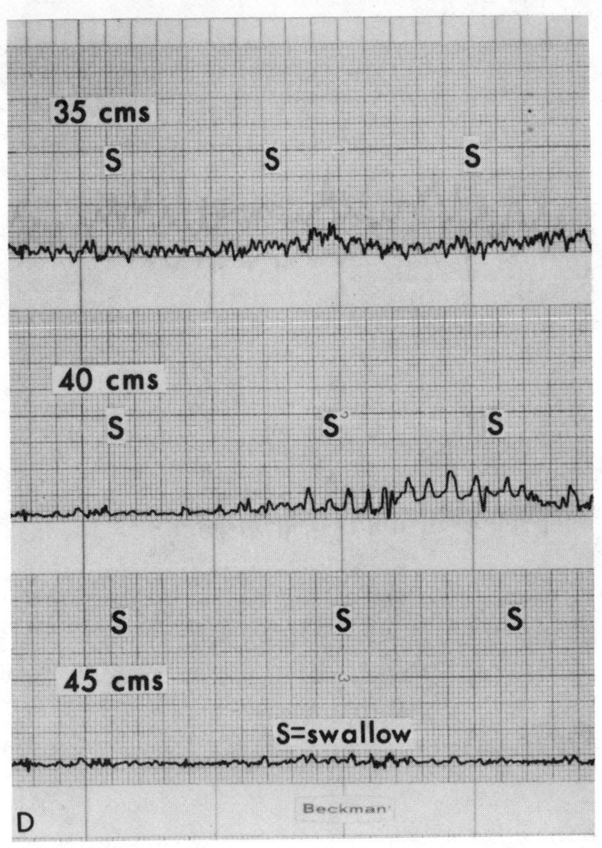
35 cms
S S S
40 cms
S S S
S S S
45 cms
S=swallow
Beckman
D

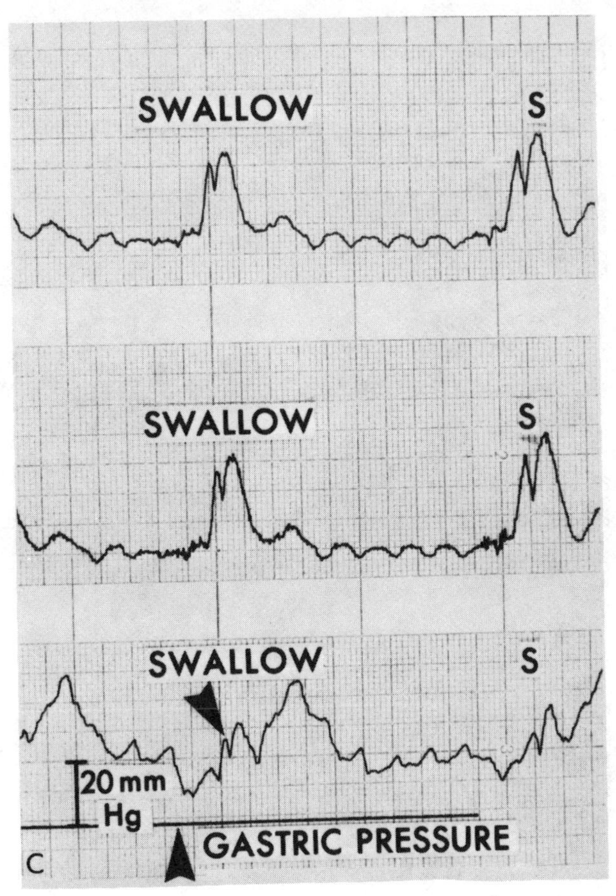
SWALLOW
S
SWALLOW
S
SWALLOW
S
20 mm
Hg
GASTRIC PRESSURE
C

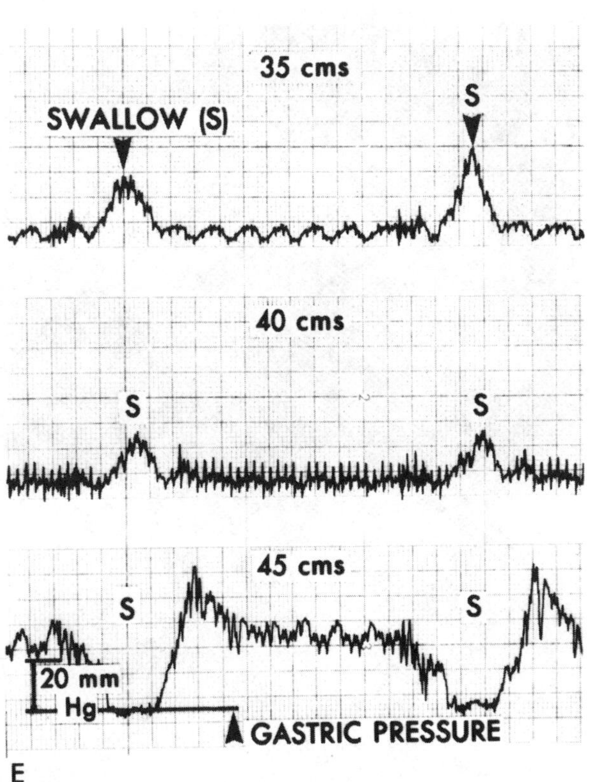
35 cms
SWALLOW (S)
S
40 cms
S
S
45 cms
S
S
20 mm
Hg
GASTRIC PRESSURE
E

QUESTIONS 181–185

For each of the following patients, select the most likely associated small bowel roentgenogram (*A–E*) below and on p. 113.

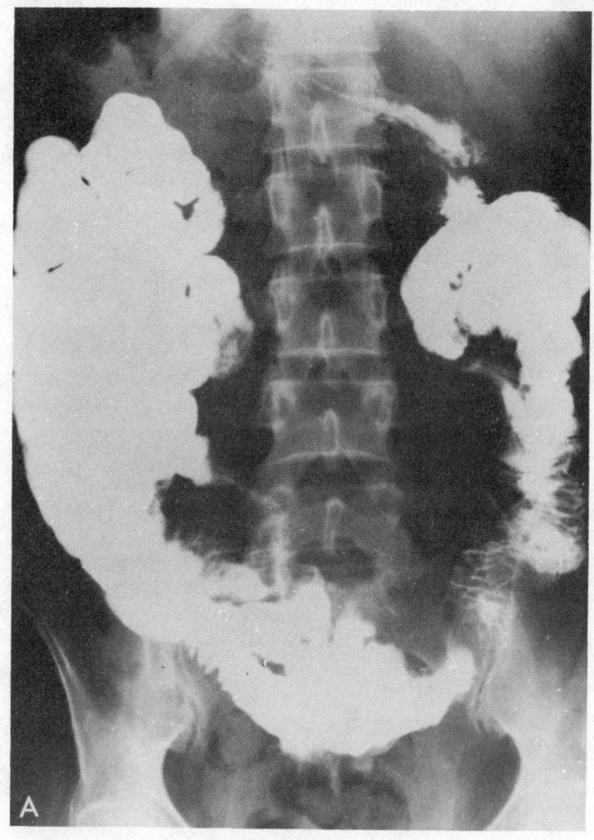

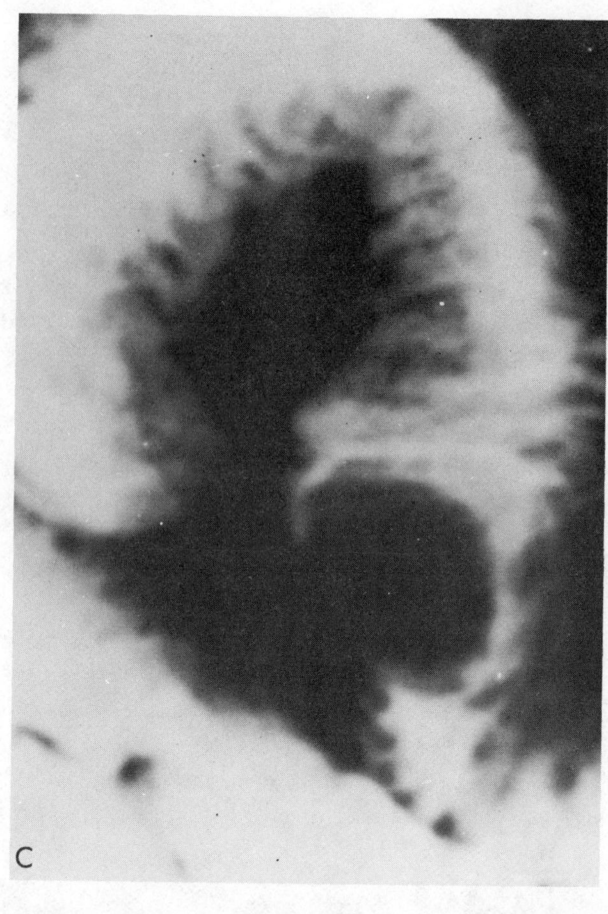

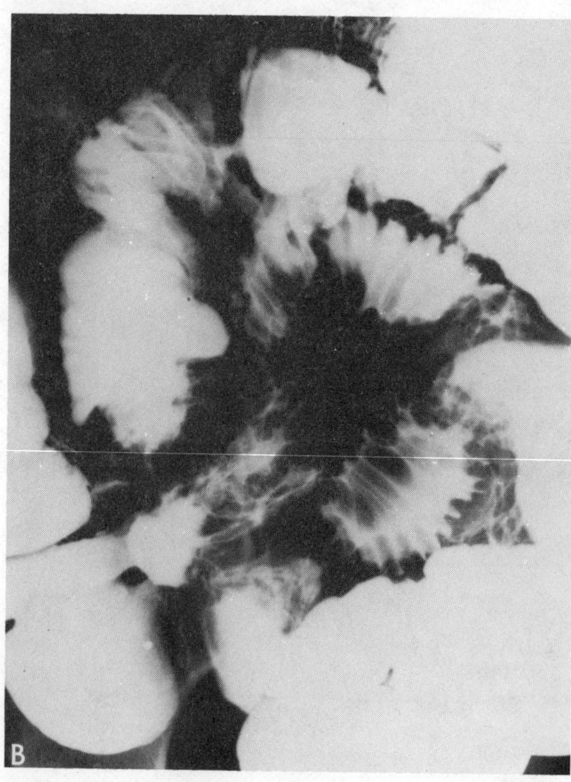

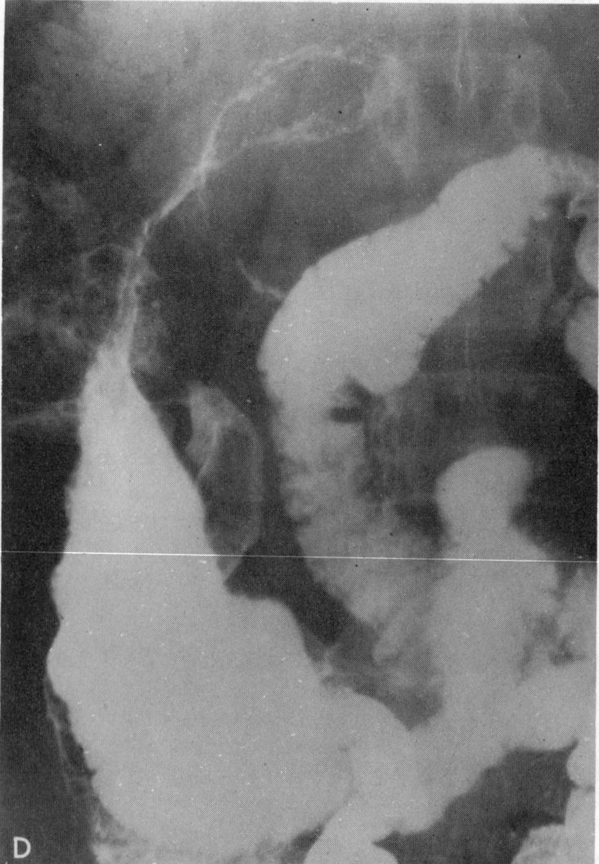

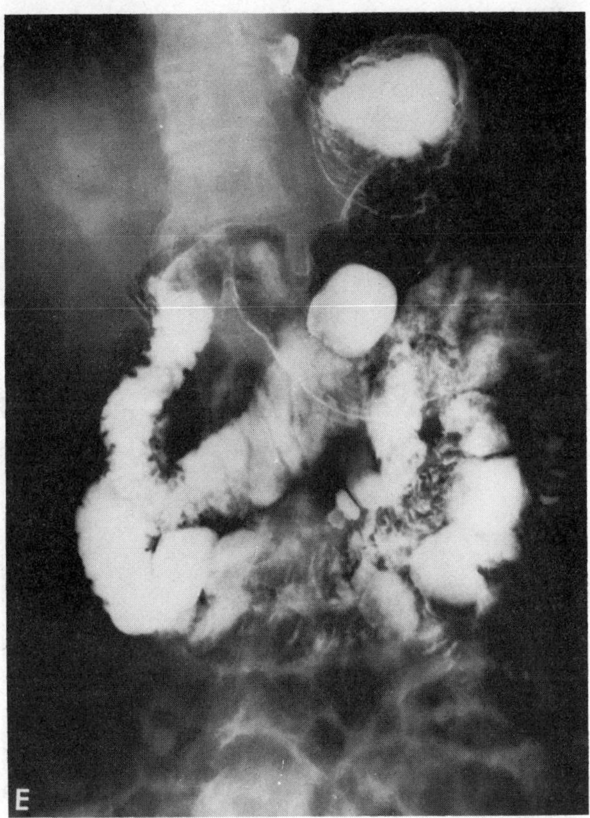

181. A 27-year-old white man has a six-year history of diarrhea. Stools are loose and occur four to six times per day; they do not contain visible blood. In the past six months the patient has noted intermittent episodes of crampy abdominal pain, nausea, and vomiting lasting six to 12 hours. Two years ago he experienced arthralgias in the hands and feet that persisted for five months. Physical examination reveals a thin man in no acute distress. The abdomen is scaphoid; bowel sounds are active, and there is a tender mass in the periumbilical-right lower quadrant region. Stools are positive for occult blood. Hematocrit is 32%; white blood cell count is 8500/cu mm with a normal differential; erythrocyte sedimentation rate is 45 mm/hr; electrolytes are normal.

182. A 59-year-old white man has had recurrent episodes of watery diarrhea for the past year. Each episode lasts 12 hours to two days and is accompanied by fatigue and malaise without nausea, vomiting, or fever. He has also noted episodes of flushing over the face and neck accompanied by a feeling of faintness during the diarrheal episodes. In the past six months he has lost 25 pounds, and over the past three months has had aching pain in the right shoulder and in the right upper quadrant of the abdomen. Physical examination reveals a thin, chronically ill–appearing man with a moderately distended abdomen and active bowel sounds. The liver is firm, nodular, and tender; liver span is 18 cm.

183. A 35-year-old Israeli man has had fatigue, anorexia, and occasional crampy abdominal pain for four months. He has lost 30 pounds over the same period. He has felt "feverish" but has never taken his temperature; there have been occasional night sweats. His stools have become soft, bulky, and foul-smelling in the past two months. On physical examination he appears chronically ill with evidence of weight loss. The liver is of normal size and the abdomen is nontender, obese, and moderately distended; bowel sounds are normal. The stool is negative for occult blood. Hematocrit is 35%; white blood cell count is 9500/cu mm; and electrolytes are normal. 24-hour fecal fat is 20 gm.

184. A 45-year-old black woman has a ten-month history of soft bulky stools and a 25-pound weight loss. She feels well and has no other medical problems. On physical examination the abdomen is obese with normal bowel sounds. No masses can be palpated, and the liver is of normal size. Stool is negative for occult blood; however, fat globules are readily apparent after Sudan staining. Cultures of aspirated jejunal fluid reveal 10^6 aerobic organisms and 10^7 anaerobic organisms per milliliter of fluid ($N<10^4$ aerobes and no anaerobes per ml).

185. A 15-year-old black boy has had five episodes of melena over the past year, each of which resolved spontaneously in one to two days. He now complains of fatigue. Physical examination is normal. Rectal examination reveals brown stool that is positive for occult blood. Hematocrit is 28%; white blood cell count is 7000/cu mm; platelet count is 350,000/cu mm. Electrolytes and liver function tests are normal.

QUESTIONS 186–189

Match each of the following clinical histories with the most likely set of ascitic fluid findings from the table below. (*Note:* Each fluid description should be used only once.)

186. A 43-year-old white man with decompensated alcoholic liver disease who is admitted for ascites and fever; physical examination reveals moderate generalized tenderness to abdominal palpation

187. A 43-year-old white man with the nephrotic syndrome

188. A 43-year-old white man who suffered a penetrating abdominal injury six months ago

189. A 43-year-old white man with established hemochromatosis who has recently lost 25 pounds; marked hepatomegaly and an hepatic friction rub have developed within the past two months

	Appearance	WBCs/cu mm	RBCs/cu mm	Protein (gm/dl)	Triglycerides (mg/dl)
A.	Milky	800	100	3.2	700
B.	Clear, straw-colored	50	50	0.9	Not performed
C.	Cloudy, straw-colored	1200	100	2.5	Not performed
D.	Serosanguineous	500	24,000	2.8	Not performed

QUESTIONS 190–194

For each of the following statements, select the lettered answer that best applies.

A. Gastric ulcer
B. Duodenal ulcer
C. Both
D. Neither

190. Male-to-female ratio is greater than one

191. Associated with elevated levels of both fasting and postprandial serum gastrin

192. Found most commonly at the junction of two dissimilar mucosal cell types

193. Associated with deficient duodenal secretin release and deficient pancreatic bicarbonate output

194. Associated with familial increased serum group I pepsinogen concentration

QUESTIONS 195–199

Match each of the following clinical histories with the appropriate radiograph (*A–E*) on this page and the left column of p. 115. (*Note:* Each figure should be used only once.)

195. A 62-year-old woman with epigastric pain; basal acid output is 1 mEq/hr, and peak acid output is 3 mEq/hr

196. A 42-year-old man with epigastric pain, melena, and a large liver

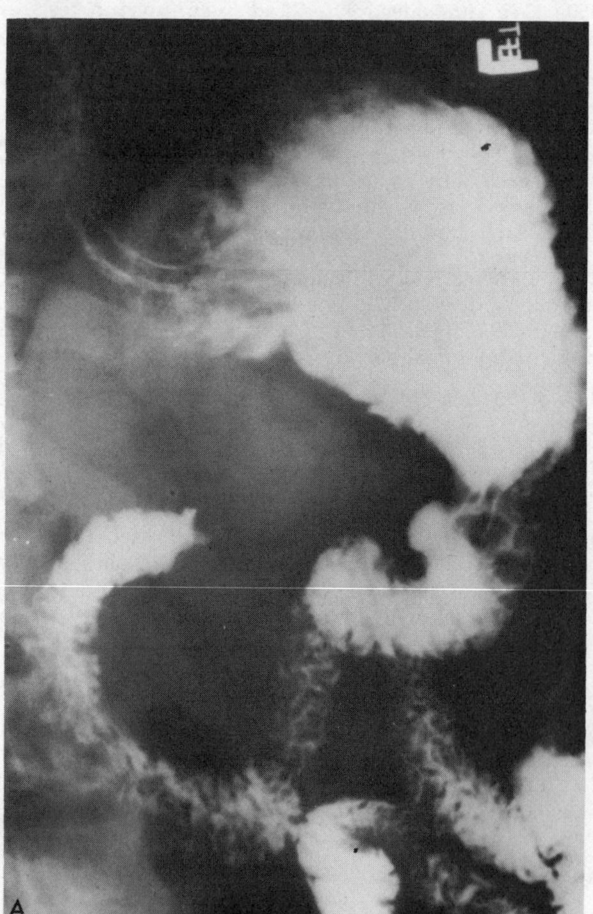

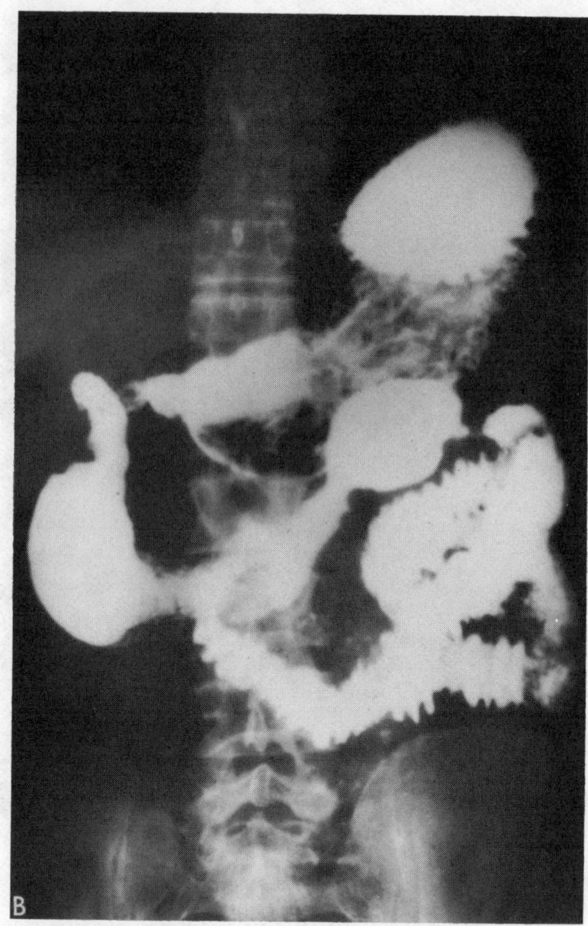

197. A 65-year-old woman with pernicious anemia

198. A 40-year-old woman who is a chronic aspirin abuser; she has dyspepsia, hematemesis, and melena

199. A 50-year-old man who has had previous gastric surgery for ulcer disease and who is admitted with hematemesis and a hematocrit of 20%

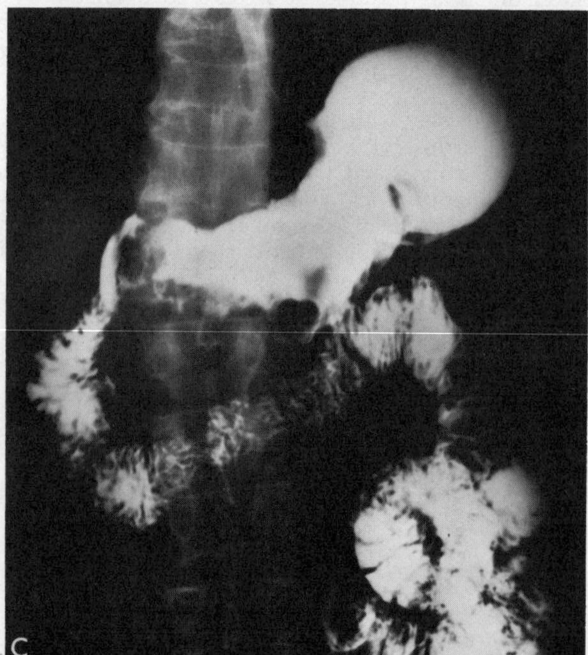

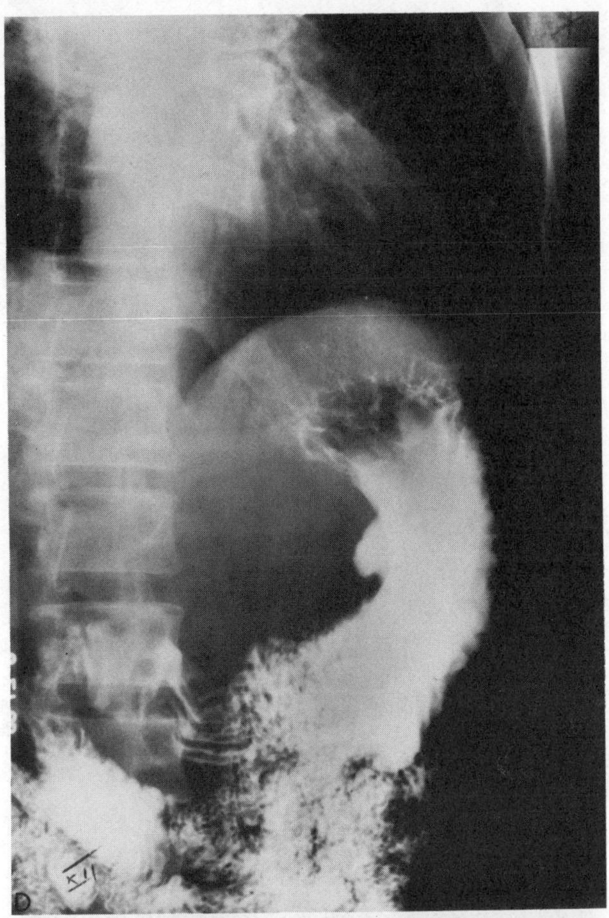
D

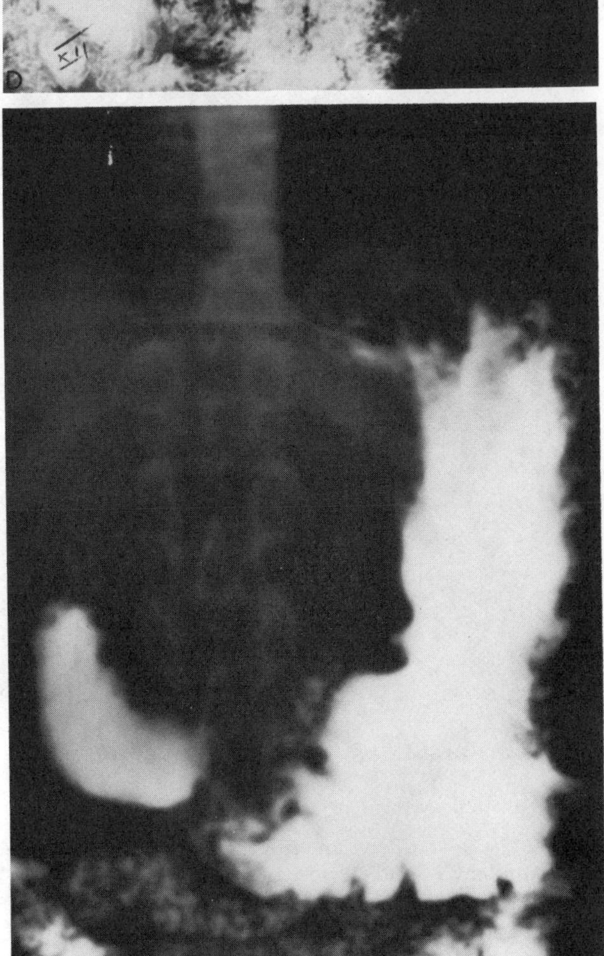
E

QUESTIONS 200–205

Match each of the following clinical histories with the most appropriate liver biopsy. (*A–F*) below and on p. 116. (*Note:* Each figure should be used only once.)

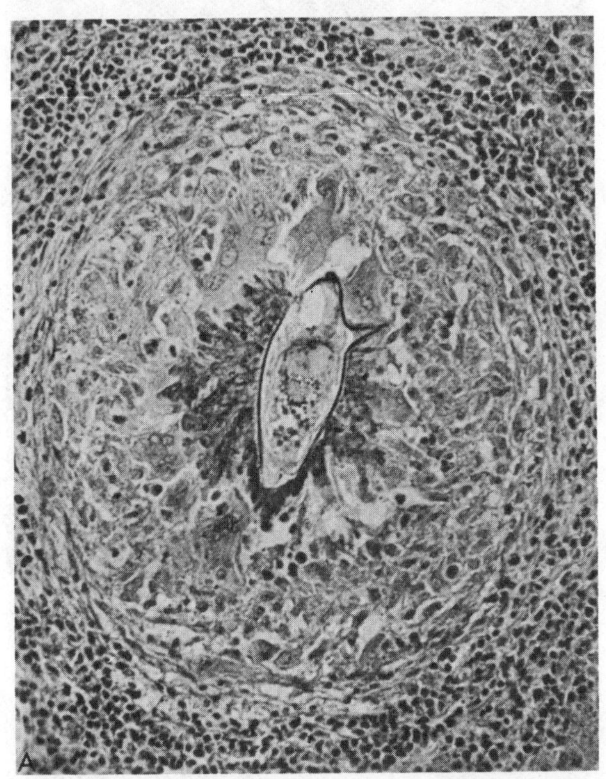
A

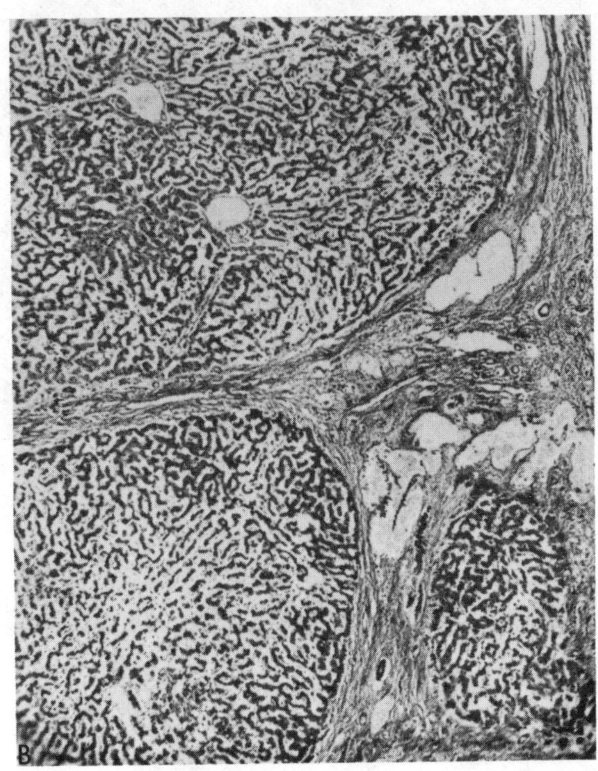
B

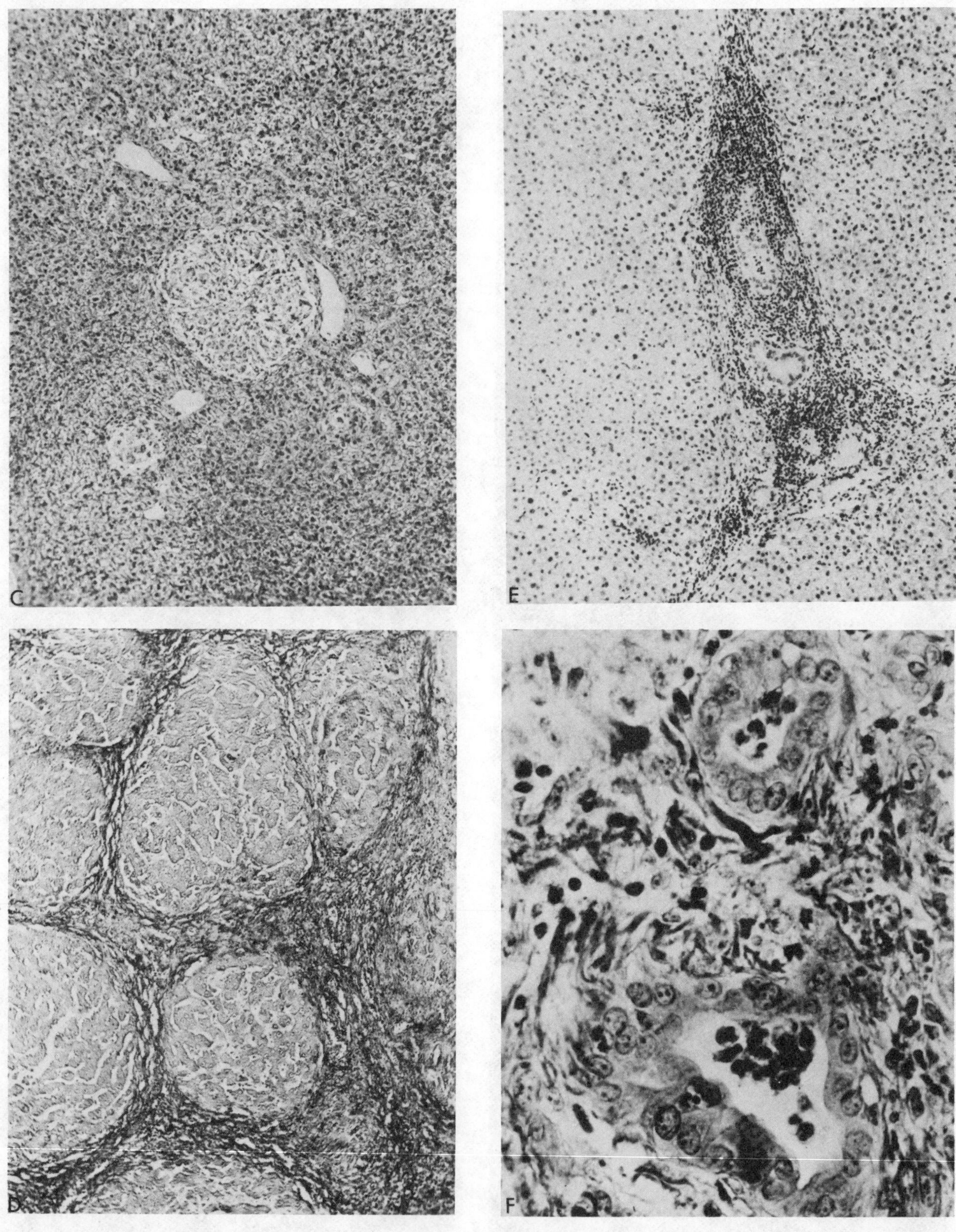

200. A 53-year-old alcoholic man with ascites, hepatosplenomegaly, and esophageal varices

201. A 46-year-old white man with chronic hepatitis B surface antigenemia, esophageal varices, and hepatosplenomegaly

202. A 42-year-old woman with pruritus, jaundice, hypercholesterolemia, and a positive antimitochondrial antibody test

203. A 36-year-old woman with documented cholelithiasis who now has fever, chills, right upper quadrant pain, and jaundice

204. A 43-year-old native Egyptian man who is undergoing evaluation for esophageal varices

205. A 39-year-old black woman with asymptomatic hilar adenopathy

QUESTIONS 206–210

Match each of the following infectious agents to the case history it most closely describes. Use each answer only once.

A. *Yersinia enterocolitica*
B. *Campylobacter fetus*
C. *Giardia lamblia*
D. *Salmonella typhimurium*
E. *Vibrio cholerae*

206. A 45-year-old woman who attended a neighborhood picnic two days ago consults you because of nausea, colicky abdominal pain, liquid diarrhea with mucus but without blood, and fever to 38°C. Hematocrit and white blood cell count are normal.

207. A 24-year-old male Peace Corps volunteer who returned home from India two days ago now experiences the abrupt onset of massive, painless, watery diarrhea. He is afebrile. Hematocrit is 55%; serum sodium is 152 mEq/L, and serum potassium is 2.8 mEq/L; pH is 7.21.

208. A 10-year-old boy with a three-day history of fever, right lower quadrant pain, diarrhea, and nausea is found to have right lower quadrant rebound tenderness. Hematocrit is 42%; white blood cell count is 13,500/cu mm; electrolytes and liver function tests are normal. The stool is positive for occult blood. At laparotomy for presumed appendicitis, mesenteric adenitis and terminal ileitis are seen; a normal appendix is removed.

209. A 27-year-old female graduate student consults you because of epigastric bloating, loose watery diarrhea, and anorexia of three weeks' duration. She has lost 10 pounds during this time. She returned from a backpacking trip in the Canadian Rocky Mountains 3½ weeks ago; there is no other travel history or medical problem. Physical examination, hematocrit, white blood cell count, and electrolytes are normal. The stool is negative for occult blood, ova, and parasites. Fat globules are seen after Sudan staining.

210. A 20-year-old male feed-lot worker with a three-day history of malaise, myalgias, and headache develops crampy lower abdominal pain, fever, and bloody diarrhea. Physical examination reveals an acutely ill–appearing man with a slightly distended, nontender abdomen and normal bowel sounds. Hematocrit is 40%; white blood cell count 14,000/cu mm; electrolytes and liver function tests are normal. Stool is bloody and contains numerous polymorphonuclear leukocytes. On sigmoidoscopy the rectum is inflamed and friable, and a biopsy shows acute and chronic inflammation and crypt abscesses.

PART 4

GASTROINTESTINAL DISEASE

ANSWERS

1. (B); 2. (C) The amylase:creatinine clearance ratio is derived from the general clearance formula U × V/P × T, and results in the following formula:

$$C_{am}/C_{cr}\% = \frac{\text{urine amylase}}{\text{serum amylase}} \times \frac{\text{serum creatinine}}{\text{urine creatinine}} \times 100$$

The normal range is 1 to 4%. From the data given in question 1, the C_{am}/C_{cr} ratio is 0.1%. This value is 10 times below the lower range of normal and typical of macroamylasemia, a benign chemical derangement associated with no specific disease state. In this entity, the serum amylase forms a macromolecular complex with a globulin whose size thus prevents urinary excretion. Peptic ulcer disease is a reasonable explanation for this patient's epigastric pain and deformed duodenal bulb. *(Cecil, p. 735; Salt and Schenker)*

3. (E) The upper gastrointestinal series demonstrates a duodenal bulbar ulcer. No essential diagnostic information will be gained by any of the diagnostic tests listed. The gastric acid secretory test may confirm gastric acid hypersecretion (peak acid output greater than 40 mEq/hr) seen in many patients with duodenal ulceration, but this information is not essential for management. Because there is no significant risk of malignancy in a duodenal ulcer, lavage cytology is not necessary. Endoscopy will invariably confirm the presence of a duodenal ulcer. It would have been the initial diagnostic procedure of choice had this patient presented with a hemodynamically significant hemorrhage (associated with shock or dramatic postural vital sign changes). In this patient, however, it is unlikely that any additional essential information would be gained by endoscopy. The celiac angiogram can assist in the location of occult bleeding in patients who continue to bleed briskly (greater than 0.5 ml/min), but there is little to justify its use here. *(Cecil, pp. 642–646; Sleisenger and Fordtran, pp. 226–233)*

4. (C) This dosage of liquid antacids is significantly better than placebo in healing endoscopically documented duodenal ulcers. The dosage is given in terms of acid neutralizing capacity rather than volume of antacids, since there is a wide range in the neutralizing capacities of commercially available antacids. The antacids are given one hour after meals, at a time when the gastric pH begins to fall. The bedtime antacid is essential to neutralize nocturnal acid production. Milk and cream are substantial stimulants of gastric acid secretion. The neutralizing capacity of milk is relatively weak compared with its ability to stimulate acid secretion. Anticholinergics and mild tranquilizers may have an adjunctive role in patients with acid peptic ulcer disease, but they are not drugs of choice for initial management. Cimetidine is an effective blocker of gastric acid secretion; however, it should be given *before* meals and at bedtime at a dose of 300 mg. Antacid tablets have only a limited place in the therapy of acid peptic ulcer disease. Their potency is relatively weak compared with standard liquid antacid preparations, and the compounding in tablet form results in an unpredictable availability of neutralizing base. *(Cecil, pp. 646–650; Sleisenger and Fordtran, p. 896)*

5. (D) Recent evidence gives substantial documentation that salicylates and other nonsteroidal anti-inflammatory agents are toxic to the mucosa in the stomach *and* duodenum. Prostaglandins E_2 and I_2, whose synthesis is blocked by salicylates, are probably essential for mucosal cytoprotection in the upper gastrointestinal tract. In patients with stress-related upper gastrointestinal tract bleeding, the most common lesions encountered (documented endoscopically or by postmortem studies) are multiple proximal gastric mucosal ulcerations. On occasion, stress-related duodenal ulcers are found, but these are far less common than superficial gastric mucosal ulcerations. Changes in proximal gastric mucosa blood flow, altered cytoprotection, and increased gastric acid secretion have all been postulated as being responsible for the rapid appearance of diffuse mucosal ulcerations in stressed patients.

Patients with duodenal ulcer disease may have a broad range of peak acid output in response to pentagastrin. In general, however, the peak acid output in these patients is significantly higher than that in patients with gastric ulcers or in normal individuals. This gastric acid hypersecretion is characteristically a delayed and prolonged hypersecretion in response to a variety of secretagogues. Duodenal ulcers throughout the duodenal bulb are associated with significant upper gastrointestinal tract hemorrhage. Because of the anatomic location of the posterior duodenal bulb juxtaposed to the gastroduodenal artery, an ulcer at this site is far more likely to be associated with substantial upper gastrointestinal tract hemorrhage. *(Cecil, pp. 637–640, 650; Sleisenger and Fordtran, pp. 816, 821; Silvoso et al.)*

6. (D) Three normal-sized regular meals should be advised. No evidence justifies the use of low-roughage or bland (low-spice) feedings in patients with peptic ulcers. Such rigid dietary restrictions are unwarranted. A nighttime snack should be avoided. The ingested food will potentiate the nocturnal gastric acid secretion and may exacerbate symptoms in the early morning hours. Multiple milk and cream feedings will result in near-maximal rates of gastric acid secretion and are contraindicated. *(Cecil, p. 649; Sleisenger and Fordtran, pp. 891–893)*

7. (D) Hepatitis B antigenemia is associated with a variety of disorders presumably mediated by immune complex formation, including arthralgias, arthritis, polyarteritis, urticaria, and cryoglobulinemia. There is also a strong epidemiologic link between persistent hepatitis B antigenemia and hepatocellular carcinoma. No association between primary biliary cirrhosis and hepatitis B antigenemia has been demonstrated. *(Cecil, pp. 781–783)*

8. (C) Alpha$_1$-antitrypsin deficiency frequently presents in the neonatal period with cholestasis and then often progresses to cirrhosis, which may not become clinically apparent until later in life. Even severe (Pi^{zz}) deficiency in adults frequently is not accompanied by clinical liver dysfunction, even though the characteristic eosinophilic inclusions in periportal hepatocytes are present. Liver disease and pulmonary disease do not necessarily occur together in the same individual. *(Cecil, p. 796; Sharp)*

9. (C) Gastroesophageal reflux disease is a well-established complication of pregnancy, probably the result of diminished lower esophageal sphincter pressure caused by estrogen and progesterone. The problem typically resolves after completion of pregnancy. Virtually all asymptomatic volunteers monitored with an intraesophageal pH probe over 24 hours will have brief episodes of reflux in the upright position. Symptomatic patients tend also to have reflux at night, and it takes them longer to clear acid from the esophagus after an episode. Although mean lower esophageal sphincter pressures tend to be significantly lower in patients with esophageal reflux disease than in the normal population, there is sufficient overlap so that only the finding of very low pressures (1–2 mm Hg) is of diagnostic value, and measurement of lower esophageal sphincter pressure is not necessary in most patients. Schatzki's ring is a web of tissue occurring in the lower esophagus that can cause food impaction and dysphagia; it is not associated with gastroesophageal reflux disease. Bedtime snacks should be discouraged in patients with reflux disease because they often worsen nocturnal symptoms by stimulating postprandial gastric acid production and increasing the volume of material in the stomach that is subject to reflux. *(Cecil, pp. 622–627; Sleisenger and Fordtran, pp. 541–573)*

10. (D) This woman has the Peutz-Jeghers syndrome, an autosomal dominant disorder characterized by congenital melanin spots on lips, buccal mucosa, palms, soles, and perianal skin and polyps of the small intestine. The polyps, which occasionally may also occur in the stomach, colon, and rectum, are benign hamartomas, not adenomas, and are not premalignant. The risk of adenocarcinoma in these patients is less than 3% in contrast to those with Gardner's syndrome (familial polyposis), who have adenomas of the intestine and a greater than 95% risk of adenocarcinoma. Patients with the Peutz-Jeghers syndrome may be asymptomatic; however, the most common symptoms are abdominal pain, intestinal hemorrhage, and bowel obstruction. *(Cecil, pp. 725–726; Sleisenger and Fordtran, pp. 1219–1221)*

11. (E) This patient should undergo cholecystectomy and common duct exploration. Continued observation is inappropriate in a symptomatic patient with gallstones who is otherwise healthy, and a low-cholesterol diet is of no known benefit to such a patient. Oral administration of chenodeoxycholic acid or ursodeoxycholic acid for dissolution of cholesterol gallbladder stones continues to be evaluated in clinical trials, but is most likely to prove appropriate for asymptomatic patients or minimally symptomatic patients with gallstones whose otherwise poor health would make surgery hazardous. It has not been established that either of these acids is useful for the dissolution of common duct stones. Endoscopic sphincterotomy, which involves cutting the sphincter of Oddi, facilitates passage of common duct stones. It does not prevent continued stone formation in the gallbladder, and it appears to predispose patients with intact gallbladders to the subsequent development of acute cholecystitis. Therefore, sphincterotomy is most appropriate for previously cholecystectomized patients with retained or recurrent common duct stones. *(Cecil, pp. 754, 758, 763)*

12. (A) This patient probably has benign postoperative cholestasis. Ultrasonography is the correct answer, and is preferred to computerized tomography because of its lesser expense and the fact that it can be performed at the bedside. More invasive procedures are inappropriate in this very ill patient unless ductal dilatation is first demonstrated by ultrasound. *(Cecil, pp. 757, 774, 778)*

13. (D) Ornithine transcarbamylase deficiency is a urea cycle enzyme deficiency that causes hyperammonemia and is inherited as an X-linked dominant trait. It leads to early death in affected males, but affected females have a variable clinical picture and may not come to medical attention until adulthood. Type II glycogen storage disease is usually fatal in early infancy, and symptomatic Wilson's disease, $alpha_1$-antitrypsin deficiency, and Reye's syndrome would all be accompanied by clinical and biochemical evidence of liver dysfunction. *(Cecil, pp. 796–797, 1105; Hsia)*

14. (E) Azathioprine has been reported to cause pancreatitis that recurs with rechallenge. In addition, the National Cooperative Crohn's Disease Study showed a significantly higher incidence of pancreatitis in patients receiving only azathioprine than in patients treated with sulfasalazine, prednisone, or placebo. The other drugs listed have not been convincingly implicated in the development of pancreatitis. *(Cecil, p. 733; Mallory and Kern; Sturdevant et al.)*

15. (C) Although skin lesions are seen in patients with Crohn's disease, those described include erythema nodosum, erythema multiforme, and pyoderma gangrenosum, not generalized erythroderma. The other disorders listed are all well-recognized complications of Crohn's disease. *(Cecil, p. 716; Sleisenger and Fordtran, pp. 1052–1076)*

16. (D) All the conditions listed may be painful, but the temporal relation to defecation is most characteristic of an anal fissure *(Cecil, pp. 747–748; Sleisenger and Fordtran, pp. 1876–1882)*

17. (C) The upper gastrointestinal tract series demonstrates barium in the biliary system, proving the presence of a biliary-enteric fistula. In patients who have had choledochoduodenostomy, barium reflux may be seen on upper gastrointestinal series. A posterior penetrating duodenal bulbar ulcer may penetrate into the common bile duct, which passes posteriorly to the duodenal bulb. A perforating duodenal bulbar ulcer is invariably anterior and would not perforate into the common bile duct. In patients with chronic gallstone disease, gallstones in the common bile duct may erode through the bile duct anteriorly into the duodenal bulb producing a fistula. On occasion, large gallbladder gallstones erode into the duodenal bulb, producing a cholecystoduodenal fistula. The gallstone occasionally may also erode into the stomach or transverse colon. *(Cecil, pp. 651–652, 759, 761, 762; Sleisenger and Fordtran, pp. 921, 1310)*

18. (D) The patient's history is strongly suggestive of a partial small bowel obstruction. The increasing abdominal distention and right lower quadrant pain suggest the site of obstruction is at the terminal ileum. Since the upper gastrointestinal series suggests choledochoduodenal fistula, the symptoms of partial small bowel obstruction might be due to impaction of a passed gallstone at the ileocecal valve. Only larger gallstones would be associated with impaction in this portion of the gastrointestinal tract. *(Cecil, p. 762)*

19. (A) Subacute combined degeneration of the spinal cord results from vitamin B_{12} deficiency. Although vitamin B_{12} absorption is decreased about 50% in patients **with**

pancreatic insufficiency, it is adequate to prevent deficiency syndromes. Ingested cobalamin binds to R proteins in the stomach, which block binding of intrinsic factor. Pancreatic enzymes degrade the R proteins, allowing intrinsic factor to combine with cobalamin. Patients with pancreatic insufficiency who are receiving enzyme replacement therapy would be expected to have normal cobalamin absorption. Fat-soluble vitamins are malabsorbed in pancreatic insufficiency, and vitamin A deficiency (nyctalopia [night blindness] and keratomalacia), vitamin D deficiency (osteomalacia), and vitamin K deficiency (hypoprothrombinemia) can all be seen. Ingested calcium normally precipitates oxalate, preventing substantial absorption of oxalate by the gut. In the presence of steatorrhea, calcium binds instead to the unabsorbed fatty acids. Oxalate is hyperabsorbed and subsequently excreted by the kidneys with the production of oxalate renal stones. *(Cecil, pp. 678–703; Brugge et al.)*

20. (A) The amylase: creatinine clearance ratio is 2%, unusually low for a patient with acute pancreatitis. This finding, together with the ultrasound demonstrating a normal-sized pancreas, would tend to rule out acute pancreatitis. The air-fluid levels throughout the small bowel and the thickening of the valvulae conniventes are very suggestive of ischemic bowel disease. Considering the ultrasonographic finding, the normal amylase:creatinine clearance ratio, and the roentgenogram suggesting small bowel ischemia, the most likely diagnosis would be bowel infarction. *(Cecil, p. 721; Sleisenger and Fordtran, pp. 1899–1903)*

21. (E) Male homosexuals are at significant risk of developing a wide variety of bowel infections, including giardiasis, amebiasis, gonorrhea, salmonellosis, and shigellosis. It also appears that herpes simplex virus may be transmitted in male homosexuals. Negative stools for culture, ova, and parasites should rule out amebic colitis as well as *Salmonella* and *Shigella*. The sigmoidoscopic appearance is consistent with *Neisseria* gonorrhea. The next appropriate step is specific cultures for *Neisseria gonorrhoeae* obtained by a direct rectal swab of the rectal mucosa. *Giardia lamblia* do not produce colonic inflammatory disease such as seen in this patient. Rectal steroids are clearly contraindicated until an infectious process, specifically gonococcal infection, is excluded. *(Cecil, p. 746; Sleisenger and Fordtran, pp. 1692–1693)*

22. (B) Diverticular disease of the colon is a disease of Western civilization associated epidemiologically with a low-residue diet. In rabbits fed a low-residue diet for four months, diverticula develop in the intertenial area. The animals have raised intraluminal pressures and increased colonic responsiveness to intravenous neostigmine. In humans, the majority of colonic diverticula develop in the sigmoid colon. Approximately 40% of individuals over the age of 50 are noted to have colonic diverticula on barium enema examination. Pathologically and radiographically, diverticulitis is associated with local perforation of a diverticulum with peridiverticular and paracolonic inflammation. This perforation is rarely free into the peritoneal cavity. *(Cecil, pp. 820–822; Sleisenger and Fordtran, pp. 1745–1746; Berman and Kirsner)*

23. (B) Excessive flatus can result from lactase deficiency because the breakdown of undigested lactose in the colon yields hydrogen and carbon dioxide. The hydrogen breath test is both more sensitive and more specific than the traditional lactose tolerance test for this disorder. Because hydrogen is found in negligible quantities in the atmosphere, elevation in flatus hydrogen content could not be due to air swallowing. Vegetables such as legumes and wheat that are high in indigestible carbohydrates may cause excessive flatus. Exclusion of these foods from the diet may significantly improve the problem. Patients with gas pains usually have normal gas production; their symptoms are due to disordered intestinal motility. Methane is found in the intestinal gas of about one third of normal individuals; its absence does not signify any abnormality. *(Cecil, pp. 602–603; Sleisenger and Fordtran, pp. 387–393)*

24. (C) Obesity, which is associated with increased biliary cholesterol excretion, and ileal resection, which results in depletion of the body bile salt pool, both predispose to cholesterol cholelithiasis. Colon resection and hypercholesterolemia show no clear association with cholesterol cholelithiasis, and the patients described in (A) and (E) are most likely to have pigment gallstones. *(Cecil, p. 754)*

25. (E) Elevated levels of ammonia, false neurotransmitters, short-chain fatty acids, and mercaptans have been found in the blood and/or cerebrospinal fluid of patients with hepatic encephalopathy. Nevertheless, their role (either alone or in combination) in the pathogenesis of encephalopathy is uncertain. Branched-chain amino acids such as valine, leucine, and isoleucine are low — not elevated — in the blood of patients with chronic liver disease and encephalopathy. *(Cecil, p. 808; Schiff, pp. 474–481)*

26. (D) All the disorders listed except granuloma inguinale could produce diffuse proctitis. Granuloma inguinale is a papulovesicular and ulcerating infection of the skin, perianal area, and anus, and does not involve the mucosa of the rectum. Lymphogranuloma venereum, caused by *Chlamydia trachomatis*, causes a diffuse proctitis, often with accompanying inguinal lymphadenopathy, that heals with stricture formation. Gonococcal proctitis may be identified by Gram stain and/or culture of the rectal exudate. Radiation proctitis is often nonspecific, although mucosal telangiectasias may be seen in some patients. *(Cecil, pp. 746, 1567, 1571, 1572; Sleisenger and Fordtran, pp. 1689–1693)*

27. (E) The chest film shows a small collection of gas in the right subdiaphragmatic region. A perforation of any portion of gas-filled bowel may present with subdiaphragmatic air. An hepatic abscess may be due to gas-producing bacteria; however, the gas will be intrahepatic and not in the right subdiaphragmatic space. Acute hemorrhagic pancreatitis does not result in free intra-abdominal gas. Acute gangrenous cholecystitis may perforate but will not be associated with subdiaphragmatic air. Posterior duodenal bulbar ulcers occasionally penetrate into the retroperitoneum and/or the pancreas, but they are not associated with a free perforation into the abdominal cavity. Anterior antral ulcers may perforate freely into the peritoneum. Collections of gas resulting from these perforations will be demonstrated only on upright radiographs that include the subdiaphragmatic spaces. Radiographs taken while the patient is supine will not reliably demonstrate subdiaphragmatic gas. *(Cecil, pp. 651–652, 750–751, 820–821)*

28. (B) Ultrasonography is not indicated in this patient with evidence of acute peritonitis and a perforation of the gastrointestinal tract. Abdominal paracentesis could be done in suspicious cases to confirm the presence of blood or fecal contents in the peritoneal cavity, but in this instance, with a clear-cut demonstration of subdiaphragmatic air, no such procedure is indicated. A barium upper gastrointestinal series is contraindicated since barium could pass into the peritoneal cavity. Barium peritonitis is particularly difficult to treat surgically and may result in extensive adhesion formation and abscesses. If absolutely essential, an absorbable, water-soluble contrast agent such as Gastrografin may be used. Emergency endoscopy is contraindicated in this patient because of the perforation suspected by chest radiograph. *(Cecil, pp. 652, 819, 821; Sleisenger and Fordtran, p. 1310)*

29. (B) The most likely diagnosis in this patient is acute cholecystitis, which is generally the result of obstruction of the cystic duct by a gallstone. Neither oral cholecystography, ^{99m}Tc-HIDA scanning, nor intravenous cholangiography would be likely to visualize the gallbladder. Technetium-99m-dimethyl acetanilide iminodiacetic acid (^{99m}Tc-HIDA), like the iodinated contrast materials used for intravenous cholangiography and oral cholecystography, is taken up by hepatic parenchymal cells and enters the gallbladder in healthy adults. Failure of ^{99m}Tc-HIDA scanning to visualize the gallbladder is considered by many physicians to be sufficient evidence for a diagnosis of acute cholecystitis in the appropriate clinical setting. Ultrasonography is a sensitive and specific procedure for demonstrating gallstones, and in most patients with acute cholecystitis gallstones are present in the gallbladder as well as in the cystic duct. Computerized tomography is less accurate than ultrasonography in identifying gallstones and it exposes the patient to radiation. Like ultrasonography, CT scanning cannot reliably identify cystic duct obstruction. *(Cecil, p. 759)*

30. (E) The passage of large bloody stools is strongly suggestive of colonic bleeding. Occasionally, patients with terminal small bowel and even upper small bowel massive hemorrhage with hypotension can present with hematochezia. The patient has not passed any blood through the rectum for the past five hours and therefore gives no evidence of brisk bleeding. An angiogram done at this time would not be likely to demonstrate a precise bleeding site, because angiography requires bleeding at a rate of excess of 0.5 ml/min. Emergency colonoscopy cannot be relied on as an effective diagnostic tool. In the unprepared colon the antegrade passage of blood mixed with stool makes colonoscopy difficult. Diverticular bleeding is an extremely important cause of hematochezia. This represents the most important source of colonic bleeding, second only to hemorrhoids. A barium enema examination done immediately on the day of admission will preclude the use of emergency angiography if brisk bleeding returns. Once the patient is stabilized and gives no evidence of brisk rebleeding, an elective double-contrast barium enema examination would seem most appropriate. If brisk bleeding were to occur, angiography would be highly reliable in detecting the bleeding site. If the barium enema is completely normal, an elective arteriogram might be helpful in detecting unusual bleeding lesions, such as an angiodysplastic lesion of the cecum. *(Cecil, pp. 608–609, 816; Sleisenger and Fordtran, pp. 1757–1759; Moody)*

31. (A) Chronic pancreatitis may be complicated by periductal fibrosis causing a long smooth stricture of the common bile duct, as shown in the illustration. Clinical manifestations include painless obstructive jaundice, recurrent cholangitis, chronic abdominal pain, and secondary biliary cirrhosis. Surgical decompression of the biliary tree is required. *(Cecil, pp. 737–739; Warshaw et al., Littenberg, Afroudakis, and Kaplowitz)*

32. (C) A prospective comparison of several diagnostic tests of pancreatic cancer suggests that ultrasound should be performed first; if it is negative, a pancreatic function test is the next choice. A positive result from either test warrants endoscopic retrograde cholangiopancreatography (ERCP). CT scan can be substituted for ultrasonography, and angiography can be done if ERCP is unsuccessful or unavailable. Radioisotopic pancreatic scans are too insensitive to be useful, and visceral angiography is not appropriate as a screening test. *(Cecil, pp. 740–741; DiMagno et al.)*

33. (D) The clinical history is most compatible with acute diverticulitis of the sigmoid colon. Diverticulosis refers merely to the presence of colonic diverticula, not the inflammatory process resulting from the perforation of the diverticulum. The pneumaturia (air on urination), suggestive of a fistula between bowel and bladder, can be seen in Crohn's disease, diverticulitis, or a perforating sigmoid carcinoma. The radiograph demonstrates thickening of the sigmoid haustra and luminal narrowing most compatible with acute diverticular disease. On occasion, however, differentiation between acute diverticulitis and perforating carcinoma is not possible without colonoscopy and/or surgical exploration. *(Cecil, pp. 820–822; Sleisenger and Fordtran, pp. 1760–1763)*

34. (C) The patient should be hospitalized even though he does not appear acutely ill. Parenteral hyperalimentation or an elemental, low-residue diet given orally is indicated in this patient because of his constipation. Because of the inflammatory, infectious nature of the process and the patient's illness, broad-spectrum antibiotics, including coverage of anaerobic organisms, are indicated. Nonabsorbable antibiotics have no place in the treatment of acute diverticulitis, which is extraluminal. An intravenous pyelogram should be performed to exclude obstruction of the left ureter. If the clinical condition does not improve dramatically or if it deteriorates, a diverting colostomy is essential to prevent continued local sepsis and the development of a pelvic abscess. *(Cecil, p. 822; Sleisenger and Fordtran, pp. 1765–1766)*

35. (D) The morning vomiting of material ingested at suppertime is strongly suggestive of a gastric outlet obstruction. The fullness in the epigastrium in fact may represent a massively dilated stomach. Following the placement of a nasogastric tube to decompress the stomach, a saline infusion test with the return of more than 400 ml at the end of a 30-minute period would confirm high-grade gastric outlet obstruction. Emergency endoscopy at this point with the stomach full of retained secretions and marked edema at the peripyloric area may be extremely difficult. *(Cecil, pp. 650–651; Sleisenger and Fordtran, pp. 922–925)*

36. (D) The gastric acid secretory test with pentagastrin suggests intact gastric acid secretion. The basal serum gastrin is elevated; however, the gastrin falls in response to the intravenous injection of secretin. The elevation in basal serum gastrin, the lack of an increase with secretin, and the retained gastric acid secretory capacity following a Billroth II antrectomy and vagotomy are strongly suggestive of a retained antrum on the duodenal stump. The retained antral mucosal cells are therefore continually bathed in an alkaline medium that constantly stimulates gastrin release. Zollinger-Ellison syndrome is associated with high basal acid outputs, with basal-acid-output:peak-acid-output ratios greater than 0.6. Following the intravenous injection of secretin, patients with Zollinger-Ellison syndrome usually have an increase in gastrin levels to greater than 105 pg/ml over baseline. *(Cecil, p. 653; Sleisenger and Fordtran, pp. 864–869; Kolts, Herbst, and McGuigan)*

37. (D) The story is entirely compatible with the diagnosis of Meckel's diverticulum of the ileum. The technetium scan shown in the illustration detects the presence of gastric mucosa characteristic of many Meckel's diverticula that bleed. These remnants of the embryonic yolk sac are usually found from 50 to 100 cm proximal to the ileocecal valve. Bleeding usually is noted in younger patients: surgery is necessary. *(Cecil, p. 667; Sleisenger and Fordtran, pp. 996–997)*

38. (D) Most pancreatic carcinomas are adenocarcinomas arising from ductular cells. About 70% occur in the head of the pancreas. Selenomethionine scans of the pancreas are unreliable for diagnosing pancreatic cancer and are no longer widely used. Direct surgical biopsy does not always provide an accurate diagnosis because pancreatic carcinomas often evoke an intense fibrotic reaction, forming a hard mass in the surrounding tissue. A biopsy from the periphery of the mass may not contain malignant cells and may be interpreted as showing only chronic pancreatitis. A cytologic diagnosis of malignancy may sometimes be made after percutaneous needle aspiration of a pancreatic mass guided by sonography or computerized tomography. The considerable morbidity and mortality associated with pancreatoduodenectomy make it unacceptable as a palliative procedure. In contrast to the declining incidence of gastric cancer, the incidence of pancreatic carcinoma in the United States has been gradually increasing. *(Cecil, pp. 739–742; Sleisenger and Fordtran, pp. 1457–1467)*

39. (B) The clinical picture is entirely compatible with the diagnosis of tropical sprue. Serum folate levels will invariably be low, and the upper gastrointestinal series will show marked mucosal changes. The small bowel biopsy will show marked flattening of the villous architecture. Tetracycline produces a significant clinical response in many patients with tropical sprue, but there is no response to a gluten-free diet. B_{12} levels are commonly low in tropical sprue, but rarely so in nontropical sprue (celiac disease). *(Cecil, pp. 699–700; Sleisenger and Brandborg, pp. 222–227)*

40. (E) The report of the fear of eating because of the predictability of the onset of pain following a meal is strongly suggestive of intestinal angina. The absence of any abnormal laboratory findings or abnormal findings on the upper gastrointestinal series, endoscopy, sigmoidoscopy, and barium enema does not rule out the diagnosis of chronic intestinal ischemia. Most patients with angina are elderly and have some evidence of peripheral vascular disease. *(Cecil, p. 720; Sleisenger and Fordtran, pp. 1895–1898)*

41. (E) Only Crohn's disease shows "skip" areas of normal mucosa between segments of involved bowel. Although the rectum may appear normal by barium enema in ulcerative colitis, biopsy of the rectum essentially always shows inflammatory changes. Mucosal ulcerations, crypt abscesses, and perianal abscesses can occur in both diseases, although perianal disease is much more common in Crohn's disease. *(Cecil, pp. 704–706, 708, 712–714; Sleisenger and Fordtran, pp. 1052–1076, 1597–1653, 1658–1679)*

42. (D) The clinical picture is most compatible with cholangitis due to choledocholithiasis. Simple acute cholecystitis would not cause this much fever nor the abnormal liver function tests. Hepatic infarction and viral hepatitis are usually accompanied by more striking elevations of the SGPT and prothrombin time, and hemochromatosis typically presents in a more insidious fashion. The very high bilirubin concentration in this patient reflects markedly increased bilirubin production caused by accelerated destruction of sickled and transfused erythrocytes, as well as impaired bile flow resultant from choledocholithiasis. *(Cecil, pp. 762–763, 779–780, 797; Sheehy; Cameron, Maddrey, and Zuidema)*

43. (D) *Escherichia coli* species are enterotoxigenic or enteropathogenic. A much smaller percentage of traveler's diarrhea is due to the other agents listed. *(Cecil, pp. 676–677; Sleisenger and Fordtran, pp. 1078–1079)*

44. (D) In Crohn's disease, mesenteric lymph nodes are characteristically swollen and soft, and often contain granulomas. Aphthous ulcers of the mouth can be seen in patients with Crohn's disease, and aphthoid ulcers are thought to be the initial mucosal lesion in the bowel. The other choices are all characteristics of Crohn's disease. *(Cecil, pp. 712–714; Sleisenger and Fordtran, pp. 1052–1076)*

45. (C) Post-transfusion hepatitis is most commonly a result of "non-A–non-B" virus infection or, less commonly, hepatitis B virus infection. Either non-A–non-B or B type hepatitis may cause chronic liver disease. None of the other illnesses listed lead to chronic hepatitis. *(Cecil, pp. 783, 790)*

46. (C) Although hematochezia usually implies colonic blood loss, brisk bleeding from an upper gastrointestinal site can also result in hematochezia. Barium enema and computerized tomography will not reveal the bleeding site in either case, and colonoscopy is difficult and usually unrevealing in an unprepared colon. Although an inferior mesenteric arteriogram might reveal a colonic site of possible blood loss, it will not identify an upper GI lesion. In addition, this patient has stopped bleeding and angiography therefore is not likely to be useful at this time. Upper GI endoscopy to look for lesions in the stomach and duodenum and the presence of blood in the upper small bowel is the best initial diagnostic step. Nasogastric tube aspiration may reveal no blood in the stomach in patients who are bleeding from the duodenum or jejunum. *(Cecil, pp. 815–816)*

47. (D) Although all these lesions can result in gastrointestinal hemorrhage, villous adenomas do so rarely, and blood loss usually is not massive. Silent duodenal ulcers are a common cause of massive hemorrhage, especially in the elderly, and can present as hematochezia without hematemesis. Aortoduodenal or aortoenteric fistulas must be considered in any patient with an aortic graft. The fistulas may bleed intermittently at first and can lead to sepsis. Diagnosis is usually made by arteriography during a bleeding episode. Rarely, the source of blood loss can be seen at endoscopy if the endoscope can be passed to the area of the fistula. Therapy consists of immediate surgery, usually with bypass of the graft, followed months later by graph replacement and oversewing of the enteric fistula. Angiodysplasia of the colon can be diagnosed ón selective arteriography and is a relatively common cause of hematochezia, especially in the elderly. Bleeding diverticula are another common cause of hematochezia in the elderly; they can be diagnosed by arteriography during a bleeding episode or by fortuitous identification of the bleeding site during colonoscopy. *(Cecil, p. 816; Sleisenger and Fordtran, p. 1928; Meyer et al.)*

48. (A) Endoscopy with a small-diameter fiberoptic endoscope is safe and provides the most reliable information as to whether esophageal injury has occurred and, if so, its severity. Radiologic studies may be helpful later in determining the extent of stricture formation, but endoscopy is the procedure of choice during the initial evaluation. The absence of oropharyngeal lesions does not exclude esophageal injury. Although some authors have recommended use of a nasogastric tube or string to preserve the esophageal lumen, it would only be a consideration if endoscopy showed esophageal injury. Alkaline injury to the esophagus occurs extremely rapidly, and attempts at neutralization with acid would not be beneficial and might be harmful. *(Cecil, pp. 631–632; Sleisenger and Fordtran, pp. 600–602; Cello, Fogel, and Boland)*

49. (C) This patient has hematobilia, which results from communication of an intrahepatic vessel with the biliary tree. Blunt or penetrating trauma that fractures or lacerates hepatic parenchyma is among the most common causes of such abnormal communications, which are best diagnosed by arteriography. Other tests listed might indicate the presence but not the type of biliary disease (A and B) or would provide little useful information (D and E). *(Cecil, p. 765)*

50. (D) Although a variety of abnormalities of renal function have been demonstrated in Wilson's disease, progressive renal failure is not a mode of presentation. Wilson's disease may present with each of the other features shown, as well as with a variety of neurologic and bone abnormalities. *(Cecil, pp. 796, 1126–1128)*

51. (E) Cimetidine will block all secretagogues of gastric acid secretion. There will remain, however, some basal- and meal-stimulated acid secretion. The H-2 receptor of the gastric parietal cell is the site of action of the drug, which has documented efficacy in healing duodenal ulcers. *(Cecil, p. 647; Gardner et al.)*

52. (D) This patient has the typical history of the superior mesenteric artery syndrome, a reversible obstruction of the third portion of the duodenum as it passes between the superior mesenteric artery and the fixed retroperitoneal structures. It is seen in patients with recent substantial weight loss. Characteristically, symptoms improve with a "hands-and-knees" or prone position, as the superior mesenteric artery tends to fall away from the duodenum under the influence of gravity. Upper gastrointestinal series will often demonstrate a dilated proximal duodenum. Chronic cholecystitis can lead to postprandial symptoms, but they would not be expected to occur with the regularity seen in this patient, nor would they be relieved by a change in position. Partial obstruction with postprandial symptoms can occur with duodenal ulcer disease and pyloric channel edema or scarring in the absence of any previous history of abdominal pain or ulcer disease. Nevertheless, the obstruction caused by ulcer disease, an annular pancreas, or intestinal pseudo-obstruction is fixed and would not respond to a position change. *(Cecil, pp. 722–723)*

53. (C) The patient has delayed resolution of an acute viral hepatitis. Although it is possible that chronic hepatitis will develop, an observation period of three to six months is appropriate before the possibility is pursued further with a liver biopsy. Histopathologic changes of acute or prolonged acute viral hepatitis may mimic those of chronic active hepatitis, but do not necessarily imply the presence of chronic or progressive disease. A biopsy at this time would therefore be of limited value and might be frankly misleading. Corticosteroids have not been shown to benefit patients with severe acute viral hepatitis and should not be used here. There is no reason to advise the patient against working, if he feels able, nor is it necessary to administer gamma globulin to co-workers who have had only casual contact with the patient. In contrast, gamma globulin *would* be advisable for family members or roommates. *(Cecil, pp. 783–784)*

54. (B) *Ascaris lumbricoides* can infest the small bowel in large numbers and is well-known for its capacity to migrate into the bile duct, pancreatic duct, and appendix or through the bowel wall, resulting in obstruction or perforation. The other parasites mentioned may all reside in the gastrointestinal tract, but none is known to cause biliary obstruction. *(Cecil, p. 765; Sleisenger and Fordtran, pp. 1154–1179)*

55. (B) Although the evidence suggests a benign stricture of the distal esophagus, carcinoma cannot be excluded on the basis of either the upper gastrointestinal series or the normal CEA. Esophagoscopy with multiple esophageal mucosal biopsies must be done before any therapy can appropriately be initiated. *(Cecil, pp. 629–630; Sleisenger and Fordtran, pp. 557–559)*

56. (B) This patient has porphyria cutanea tarda. The illness is characterized by blistering of sun-exposed skin and requires both a genetic defect (deficiency of uroporphyrinogen decarboxylase) and environmental factors (hepatic dysfunction with iron overload frequently related to alcohol use or use of estrogen-containing drugs) for its full expression. The diagnosis requires demonstration of excessive urinary uroporphyrin, and the skin lesions typically respond to discontinuation of estrogen-containing compounds, phlebotomy, or both. *(Cecil, p. 1125; Kushner et al., 1975, 1976)*

57. (E) A substantial risk of malignancy exists in colonic polyps greater than 2 cm. With the advent of colonoscopic polypectomy, both polyps should be removed. The colonoscopy should not stop at the splenic flexure where the barium enema suggests the most proximal colonic polyp is located. The incidence of synchronous polyps is substantial, and a pancolonoscopy should be done. *(Cecil, p. 724; Sleisenger and Fordtran, pp. 1556–1557; 1781–1783)*

58. (E) None of the choices listed has been shown by a prospective randomized clinical trial to improve survival of patients with fulminant hepatic failure. Cimetidine has been demonstrated to decrease markedly the frequency and severity of gastrointestinal hemorrhage (which is largely due to "stress" gastritis), but not to improve survival. *(Cecil, pp. 809–810)*

59. (E) *Diphyllobothrium latum,* the fish tapeworm, can cause vitamin B_{12} deficiency and, in heavy infestations, megaloblastic anemia. The worm competes with the host for vitamin B_{12} uptake. The other parasites listed all result in iron deficiency anemia. *(Cecil, p. 1750; Sleisenger and Fordtran, pp. 1154–1179, 1705–1715)*

60. (A) When pancreatic and salivary amylase isoenzymes were evaluated in a group of alcoholics with elevated serum amylase concentrations, the elevated levels were found to be due to an increase in the salivary component in most patients. It was proposed that this was caused by a toxic effect of ethanol on the salivary glands. Other studies also indicate that chronic elevation of serum amylase in asymptomatic individuals is only infrequently associated with pancreatic disease. Determination of salivary and pancreatic amylase isoenzymes would be useful in confirming a salivary origin. The normal BUN makes renal disease unlikely. The other diagnostic tests listed are not indicated in the absence of symptoms or other evidence of disease. Oral pancreatic enzymes would not be expected to alter the serum amylase concentration. *(Cecil, pp. 734–735, 739, 740; Sleisenger and Fordtran, pp. 1423–1424; Dutta et al.)*

61. (C) The entire clinical presentation is suggestive of pseudomembranous enterocolitis related to antibiotic usage. The barium enema demonstrates shaggy, irregular mucosa, particularly in the ascending and transverse colon. The haustral folds are thickened and nodular. This film is diagnostic of an *acute* colitis. The sigmoidoscopic findings of hyperemia of the mucosa with an adherent thick mucous plaque are compatible with pseudomembranous colitis. The biopsy of the rectal mucosa shows a "volcano" lesion with a plaque of fibrin and inflammatory cells adherent to the mucosa. The lamina propria is edematous. No crypt abscesses (more compatible with ulcerative colitis) are shown. *(Cecil, p. 708; Sleisenger and Fordtran, pp. 1720–1728)*

62. (D) Pseudomembranous colitis has been reported to occur in association with a variety of orally administered and parenteral antibiotics, including clindamycin, lincomycin, ampicillin, penicillin, and tetracycline. The pathogenesis appears to be related to the overgrowth of resistant enteric flora that elaborate a heat-labile enterotoxin. The enterotoxin is neutralized by specific clostridial antitoxin, and cultures of the diarrheal stool grow a specific clostridial organism, *C. difficile*. The antibiotic probably suppresses normal enteric flora (particularly anaerobes) and allows overgrowth of these enterotoxin-producing species. *(Cecil, p. 708; Larson, Price, and Honour)*

63. (C) This patient presents the classic features of benign postoperative cholestasis, a disorder that typically follows major operations on severely ill patients who receive a number of blood transfusions. It may have a number of contributing factors, including increased bilirubin production from transfused erythrocytes and hematomas, sepsis, liver dysfunction due to intra- or postoperative hypotension, and renal failure with decreased urinary excretion of conjugated bilirubin. Jaundice of this degree resulting from halothane injury would be accompanied by marked elevations of the SGOT and prothrombin time. *(Cecil, pp. 774, 788; Schiff, pp. 1354–1361)*

64. (A) Postoperative jaundice in a severely ill patient such as this does not usually warrant invasive investigative procedures such as liver biopsy or transhepatic or retrograde cholangiography. Ultrasonography can detect the presence of dilated intrahepatic bile ducts, and thus rule in or out the possibility of extrahepatic obstruction with a high degree of reliability. Intravenous cholangiography will fail to visualize the bile ducts under these circumstances. *(Cecil, pp. 603–605, 774; Schiff, pp. 1354–1361)*

65. (E) The sonogram is suggestive of a hepatic abscess. There is a large, irregular, sonolucent (having a density less than solid tissue) defect in the midportion of the right lobe of the liver and irregular debris (darker areas) is present within the sonolucent areas. The indolent clinical course with weight loss, low-grade fever, and tender hepatomegaly is most compatible with amebic abscess due to *Entamoeba histolytica*. Suspicion should be aroused by the Mexican-American background of the patient. Diarrhea need not be present, although the portal of entry is invariably the colon. Ameba serology (indirect hemagglutination tests) will be positive. Stools may be negative for *E. histolytica* and cannot be used to exclude amebic abscess. In some centers, aspiration of the cavity is used to confirm the diagnosis. *(Cecil, pp. 794–795, 1736–1738; Sleisenger and Fordtran, pp. 1700–1705)*

66. (A) Metronidazole (Flagyl) is effective against both intestinal and hepatic amebic disease and is an acceptable drug in this situation. Large amebic abscesses, unlike pyogenic abscesses of the liver, may respond dramatically to antibiotic therapy and need not necessarily be treated with open surgical drainage. Occasionally, repeated percutaneous aspirations may be used to accelerate the rate of healing. The diagnosis of amebic abscess should always be considered because of the severity of the untreated disease, the ease of diagnosis, and the gratifying response to medical therapy. *(Cecil, pp. 794–795; Sleisenger and Fordtran, pp. 1704–1705)*

67. (D) Alcoholic hepatitis is extremely variable in its presentation and may be accompanied by marked elevations of the white blood cell count, bilirubin, and alkaline phosphatase. It has been demonstrated to progress to cirrhosis even in the absence of continued alcohol intake, and has been reproduced in primates by alcohol feeding. Although characteristic of alcoholic hepatitis, Mallory bodies (alcoholic hyaline) are seen in a variety of other disorders, including Wilson's disease and hepatocellular carcinoma, and following jejunoileal bypass. *(Cecil, pp. 800–801; Helman et al., Rubin and Lieber)*

68. (D) This patient has hereditary hemochromatosis, an autosomal recessive disorder transmitted by a locus closely linked to the HLA locus on chromosome 6. Obligate heterozygotes, particularly males such as his father, have no phenotypic expression of the disease but tend to have higher levels of liver iron and higher serum ferritin, iron, and transferrin concentrations than do age- and sex-matched controls. The sister, who is still menstruating, could be homozygous for the disorder despite the absence of obvious symptoms. Twice-weekly phlebotomy is the initial treatment of choice for all patients with hemochromatosis, as the procedure is a safe and effective way of depleting iron stores. Once iron stores are back to normal, occasional phlebotomy is still necessary to prevent reaccumulation, because hyperabsorption of dietary iron continues throughout life. In patients with anemia from some other disorder, phlebotomy is not possible, and chelation therapy with desferrioxamine may be tried. *(Cecil, p. 797; Cartwright et al.; Wright et al., pp. 793–798)*

69. (A — False; B — True; C — False; D — False; E — False) *Candida* and *Herpesvirus* are the two major pathogens involving the esophagus and are most common in immunocompromised hosts. Odynophagia is the most common presenting symptom, and dysphagia also usually occurs. These infections have no known relationship with previous reflux disease. Because appropriate therapy requires identification of the etiologic agent, and because the diagnosis frequently cannot be made on roentgenographic studies, endoscopy with biopsies and cytologic brushings should be performed if infection is suspected. There is no relationship between streptococcal pharyngitis and esophageal infection. *(Cecil, p. 631; Sleisenger and Fordtran, pp. 592–595)*

70. (A — True; B — False; C — True; D — False; E — True) Isoniazid hepatitis is a particularly troublesome form of drug-induced liver injury because it may not occur until many months after isoniazid has been begun, and it is usually indistinguishable from acute or chronic hepatitis on biopsy. Hepatitis occurs most frequently in the elderly and in patients who are rapid isoniazid acetylators; it bears no clear relationship to the mild transaminase elevations seen in many patients shortly after the drug is begun. *(Cecil, p. 788; Black et al.)*

71. (A — True; B — False; C — False; D — False; E — False) The pancreas normally secretes a much greater quantity of digestive enzymes than is needed for complete digestion. For this reason, clinically significant malabsorption does not occur until about 90% of the exocrine secretory capacity of the gland is lost. Nevertheless, 20–40% of dietary fat and protein may still be absorbed even when pancreatic enzyme secretion is less than 1% of normal. This is probably due to the presence of nonpancreatic digestive enzymes (e.g., salivary amylase, pharyngeal lipase, gastric pepsin) in the gastrointestinal tract. Vitamin B_{12} absorption is impaired in about 40% of patients with pancreatic insufficiency, but megaloblastic anemia rarely results from this. Measurement of pancreatic secretory function after injection of secretin (with or without cholecystokinin) may be useful in confirming the diagnosis, but neither secretin nor cholecystokinin has any therapeutic value. Patients with pancreatic insufficiency have not been shown to be at increased risk for intestinal parasitism. *(Cecil, pp. 678–703; Sleisenger and Fordtran, pp. 1406, 1443)*

72. (A — False; B — True; C — True; D — True; E — True) Mallory-Weiss tears of the gastroesophageal junction are most commonly seen in alcoholic patients following repetitive episodes of forceful vomiting. Patients may develop Mallory-Weiss lesions without multiple episodes of forceful vomiting, however. Even retching or coughing may occasionally cause them. Bleeding is from submucosal arterioles and usually is not torrential, but on occasion patients may require surgery to achieve hemostasis. These shallow tears are distinctly different in location and consequences from transmural tears of the esophagus, the so-called Boerhaave syndrome. Mediastinitis does not occur with Mallory-Weiss tears. Patients with hiatus hernias of the stomach may develop Mallory-Weiss tears, and these are more likely to occur on the gastric mucosal side. There is, however, no association between Mallory-Weiss lesions and hiatus hernia. *(Cecil, p. 632; Knauer)*

73. (A — False; B — False; C — True; D — False; E — False) Because of the position of the pancreas in the retroperitoneum overlying the vertebral column, apparently minor blunt abdominal trauma may damage it, resulting in pancreatitis, traumatic pseudocyst, or pancreatic ascites. If this patient is found to have a pseudocyst or pancreatic ascites requiring surgery, ERCP should be performed preoperatively to define the ductular system and locate any leaks as an aid to the surgeon. Pancreatic ascites typically does not respond to the use of diuretics because the ascites is due to leakage of fluid from a pseudocyst or disrupted duct. Anticholinergic agents are of doubtful value in the treatment of pancreatic ascites. Ultrasonography is a very reliable means of evaluating the possibility of a pseudocyst in this patient. If anything, it should be even more reliable in this setting than in alcoholic pancreatitis because this patient is less likely to have pancreatic phlegmon or an abscess, which would make identification of a pseudocyst more difficult. Treatment of symptomatic or nonresolving pseudocysts requires surgical excision or drainage. Percutaneous drainage has not been established as a safe or effective means of dealing with this problem. Traumatic pancreatic injury often occurs in the absence of damage to the spleen or liver. *(Cecil, pp. 736–737, 750; Howat and Sarles, pp. 348, 472–474; Sleisenger and Fordtran, pp. 1449–1452)*

74. (A — False; B — True; C — True; D — True; E — False) Diabetic diarrhea is seen in young, often male, insulin-dependent diabetics with a long history of diabetes. It usually occurs in patients who also have diabetic retinopathy, nephropathy, and both peripheral and autonomic neuropathy. Small bowel radiographs will show delayed gastric emptying, prolonged transit times, and dilated loops of bowel, often with thickened mucosal folds. Motor abnormalities resulting from autonomic neuropathy may be responsible for the diarrhea. Steatorrhea may also occur owing to a combination of enteric neuropathy, defective pancreatic exocrine function, bacterial overgrowth, and possibly concomitant celiac disease. Bacterial overgrowth alone is rare. Neither strict blood glucose control nor antibiotics have been shown to alleviate symptoms completely, although they may be useful in selected cases. *(Cecil, p. 1063; Sleisenger and Fordtran, pp. 454–456)*

75. (A — False; B — True; C — False; D — False; E — False) The association of psychiatric symptoms with abdominal pain has been proposed as a clue to the presence of pancreatic cancer, which is second only to colon cancer in terms of frequency of gastrointestinal cancers in the United States. Newer diagnostic techniques so far have had little impact on survival, which is only about 1–2% at five years after diagnosis. Evidence of diabetes mellitus may be seen in 25–50% of patients, but not hypoglycemia. Benign tumors of the exocrine pancreas are very rare and almost invariably are cystic adenomas. *(Cecil, pp. 739–740; Sleisenger and Fordtran, pp. 1457–1467)*

76. (A — False; B — False; C — True; D — False; E — False) All the peptide hormones listed are produced at least in part by cells of the proximal small intestine. On the basis of similarity in their amino acid sequences, gastrin and cholecystokinin represent a different family of peptides from that of the others listed. Although all the peptides affect acid secretion when administered in large doses, only gastrin is clearly established as a physiologic regulator of gastric acid output. Human diseases thought to result from peptide hypersecretion have been identified only for gastrin (Zollinger-Ellison syndrome) and vasoactive inhibitory peptide (pancreatic cholera). *(Cecil, pp. 638, 641; Sleisenger and Fordtran, pp. 107–147)*

77. (A — False; B — True; C — True; D — True; E — True) Serum gastrin is markedly elevated in certain acid hypersecretory states such as the Zollinger-Ellison syndrome, as well as in patients with pernicious anemia and achlorhydria. *(Cecil, pp. 638, 642)*

78. (A — True; B — True; C — True; D — False; E — True) Abnormal chest x-rays are found in about 20% of patients with acute pancreatitis. All the abnormalities listed except tension pneumothorax have been considered to be complications of acute pancreatitis. "Shock lung" (adult respiratory distress syndrome) usually occurs in the context of severe acute pancreatitis and is a life-threatening complication. *(Cecil, p. 736; Sleisenger and Fordtran, pp. 1420, 1425, 1426, 1434)*

79. (A — False; B — False; C — False; D — True; E — True) Smoking decreases lower esophageal sphincter pressure, as do anticholinergic drugs. Gastrin, metoclopramide, and bethanechol increase lower esophageal sphincter pressure; the last-named two agents have been used clinically to decrease gastroesophageal reflux. *(Cecil, p. 626; Sleisenger and Fordtran, pp. 541–543)*

80. (All are True) All these disorders may involve the ileocecal area. *Yersinia enterocolitica* may produce an acute ileocolitis in children and young adults, and subacute cases may mimic the barium enema findings of Crohn's disease. *(Cecil, pp. 717, 1512, 1548–1549, 1702–1703, 1736–1737; Sleisenger and Fordtran, pp. 1086–1087)*

81. (A — False; B — True; C — False; D — True; E — True) Hepatitis A is nearly always a self-limited disease, and long-term sequelae such as malignancy or chronic liver disease have not been identified. Each of the remaining factors except Wilson's disease has been linked to the development of hepatocellular carcinoma. Hepatitis B virus infection and aflatoxin ingestion are suspected on the basis of epidemiologic studies conducted largely in Africa and Southeast Asia. Moreover, hepatitis B viral DNA has been found to be incorporated into DNA isolated from some hepatocellular cancers. *(Cecil, p. 812; Wright et al., pp. 888–891)*

82. (A — True; B — True; C — True; D — False; E — False) Carcinoma of the gastric cardia can mimic achalasia both clinically and radiographically. Endoscopy is useful in the detection of gastric cancer, but is otherwise of little value in the evaluation of esophageal motor disorders. The esophageal symptoms of scleroderma are primarily the result of reflux related to a markedly hypotensive or absent lower esophageal sphincter. Pneumatic bag dilatation carries a 5–15% risk of esophageal perforation, but is still the preferred initial therapy for achalasia. Both diffuse esophageal spasm and angina may respond to sublingual nitroglycerin. *(Cecil, pp. 627–629; Sleisenger and Fordtran, pp. 513–540)*

83. (A — True, B — True; C — True; D — True; E — False) Decreased dietary intake is a significant factor in the weight loss noted in patients with subtotal gastrectomy. The mismatching of chyme from the stomach and pancreaticobiliary secretions, combined with a decrease in the effective concentrations of these secretions in the chyme, is probably the most important factor in the malabsorption following this operation. The mismatching is associated with rapid gastric emptying for both solids and liquids. Bacterial overgrowth may also be seen. Loss of antral gastrin secretion is not a factor in postgastrectomy weight loss. *(Cecil, p. 700; Sleisenger and Brandborg, pp. 206–208; MacGregor, Parent, and Meyer)*

84. (A — False; B — False; C — False; D — True; E — False) Eosinophilic gastroenteritis may involve the proximal small bowel and antral mucosa in young individuals. Postprandial abdominal pain, nausea, and vomiting are commonly seen. The weight loss is attributed to mucosal changes in the proximal small bowel. Peripheral eosinophilia is characteristic. Eosinophilic granuloma is not associated with peripheral eosinophilia. *Giardia lamblia* infestation may produce large, bulky, foul-smelling stools but is not associated with eosinophilia. Ascariasis does not produce postprandial abdominal pain, nausea, and vomiting, except in the rare condition of a large ball of adult worms. Pancreatic insufficiency does not result in peripheral eosinophilia. *(Cecil, p. 823; Sleisenger and Brandborg, pp. 180–184)*

85. (All are True) Barrett's esophagus is the term used to describe islands of columnar epithelium in the esophageal mucosa above the gastroesophageal junction. This condition may follow reflux esophagitis. Esophageal cancer is also associated with Plummer-Vinson syndrome and with hot tea consumption in certain Asian populations. *(Cecil, p. 629)*

86. (A — False; B — True; C — False; D — True; E — False) Corn and rice do not contain gluten. The other grains must be carefully avoided in patients with nontropical sprue (adult celiac disease). *(Cecil, p. 695; Sleisenger and Brandborg, pp. 166–177)*

87. (A — False; B — False; C — True; D — True; E — True) The barium enema examination will not demonstrate changes specific to irritable bowel disease, and the rectal biopsy is normal. Manometric studies can show increased motor activity to stressful situations in these patients. *(Cecil, pp. 669–670)*

88. (All are True) The manifestations of Whipple's disease are not limited to the bowel. The bowel disease may respond to long-term antibiotic administration. *(Cecil, p. 696; Sleisenger and Brandborg, pp. 174–180)*

89. (A — False; B — True; C — False; D — True; E — True) CEA levels cannot be used in inflammatory bowel disease to reliably exclude the development of a colonic carcinoma. The development of colonic malignancy does seem to correlate with prolonged active pancolonic disease. Barium enema cannot be relied on to exclude malignancy because the lesions of early carcinoma are too similar to those of ulcerative colitis for malignant change to be identified. Colonic malignancy is rarely seen in ulcerative proctitis confined to the rectum. The malignant lesions seen in association with ulcerative colitis tend to be flat and infiltrative rather than the polypoid masses typical of colon carcinoma in the absence of ulcerative colitis. *(Cecil, pp. 708, 727; Sleisenger and Fordtran, pp. 1633–1636)*

90. (A — True; B — False; C — True; D — False; E — False) *Clonorchis sinensis* and *Ascaris* may involve the biliary tract. *Giardia lamblia* infestation does not involve the biliary tree. *Schistosoma mansoni* live as adults primarily in the rectal submucosal venous channels, and deposit eggs that find their way into the inferior mesenteric venous system, ultimately lodging in the portal venules. *Trichuris* (whipworm) infection primarily involves the cecum and does not involve the biliary tree. *(Cecil, p. 793; Sleisenger and Fordtran, pp. 1322–1323)*

91. (A — False; B — True; C — False; D — True; E — True) Patients who have undergone jejunoileal bypass surgery for morbid obesity are at risk for a number of complications that range from diarrhea to protein-calorie deficiency, electrolyte imbalance, weakness, arthritis, renal oxalate stones, gallstones, skin lesions, anemia, and liver disease. Hepatic dysfunction includes fatty liver, portal fibrosis, cirrhosis, and fatal hepatic failure. Mallory bodies may also be seen on liver biopsy. Arthritis and skin lesions are usually attributed to circulating immune complexes related to bacterial overgrowth in the bypassed loop and absorption of bacterial antigens, but immune-complex glomerulonephritis has not been reported. Similarly, pancreatitis has not been recognized as a long-term complication. *(Cecil, p. 698; Sleisenger and Fordtran, pp. 31–32)*

92. (All are True) The first serologic marker of hepatitis B infection is typically the appearance of HB_sAg. HB_sAg usually disappears during the course of the clinical hepatitis, but may persist indefinitely in some patients. HB_cAb appearance usually coincides with the onset of the clinical illness and is believed to be a marker of viral replication. Since HB_cAb is found in most patients with chronic hepatitis B infection, it clearly is not protective. HB_sAb is the last marker to appear and is generally protective against future hepatitis B virus infection. Since HB_sAg may already have disappeared from the blood by the time clinical hepatitis develops, HB_cAb may occasionally be the only serologic marker of acute type B hepatitis at the time the patient first seeks medical attention. *(Cecil, pp. 781–783)*

93. (A — True; B — True; C — True; D — False; E — False) Hepatitis A virus is shed in the stool during the preicteric and early icteric phase, and hepatitis A is transmitted predominantly by the fecal-oral route. Hepatitis B virus has now been detected in a variety of body secretions, and nonparenteral transmission may occur, particularly with prolonged intimate contact. Only a small percentage of individuals who are stuck by a needle previously used in an HB_sAg-positive patient will develop clinical or biochemical evidence of hepatitis. Since the introduction of routine HB_sAg testing in blood banks, the incidence of type B post-transfusion hepatitis has been markedly reduced. Post-transfusion hepatitis is rarely, if ever, due to type A infection. Most post-transfusion hepatitis results from infection with a transmissible agent (or agents) that is neither the type A nor the type B virus. Coworkers of patients with hepatitis B are at very low risk of contracting the disease and do not require prophylaxis with hepatitis B immune globulin. *(Cecil, pp. 784–785)*

94. (A — False; B — False; C — True; D — True; E — False) The barium enema shows filling of the stomach (clearly outlining gastric rugae) from the colon near the splenic flexure, a characteristic finding in gastrocolic fistula. These lesions occur most frequently following gastric or colonic surgery or in association with chronic inflammation in either the stomach or colon. Carcinomas of the stomach, pancreas, or colon may also be associated with gastrocolic fistula. The associated diarrhea is related to the constant fecal soiling of the upper gastrointestinal tract and subsequent overgrowth by colonic flora. Many of the resident colonic flora deconjugate bile salts and interfere with normal micelle formation. Thus, steatorrhea is a common feature of this disorder. Because the fistula may be relatively small, high pressures are often necessary to visualize it on barium studies. Therefore, the most reliable means of demonstrating gastrocolic fistula is by barium enema examination rather than by low-pressure upper gastrointestinal series. *(Cecil, p. 692; Sleisenger and Fordtran, p. 977)*

95. (All are True) The clinical, biochemical, and pathologic findings of chronic active hepatitis may occur in association with ulcerative colitis and have a variety of other causes, including Wilson's disease, chronic hepatitis B virus infection, and ingestion of certain drugs (methyldopa, aspirin, oxyphenisatin, or isoniazid). Consideration of these and other causes is the most important first step in the management of patients with chronic active hepatitis. *(Cecil, p. 790; Schiff, pp. 800–803)*

96. (A — False; B — True; C — True; D — False; E — True) The patient has pancreatitis that can be assumed to be severe or hemorrhagic on the basis of the physical examination and nonspecific laboratory signs of hemoconcentration, marked leukocytosis, hyperamylasemia, and elevated serum glucose. Diabetic ketoacidosis is associated with hyperamylasemia but is not itself a cause of severe clinical pancreatitis. On the other hand, hyperglycemia is frequent in severe pancreatitis of all causes. Hemorrhagic pancreatitis typically causes hypocalcemia; thus, a normal serum calcium in this setting is a clue to previously existing hypercalcemia, such as from hyperparathyroidism. Drugs such as thiazide diuretics, azathioprine, isoniazid, corticosteroids, oral contraceptives, and methyl alcohol have been implicated as causes of pancreatitis. Thiazide diuretics can also result in hyperglycemia, hyperuricemia, and (rarely) hypercalcemia. Although "sludging" of white blood cells in small vessels occurs in acute leukemia and may be responsible for cerebral dysfunction in that disease, pancreatitis due to this mechanism has not been reported. Types I, IV, and V hyperlipoproteinemia have been associated with pancreatitis and presumably can cause pancreatitis. Most hyperlipidemia-associated pancreatitis occurs in alcoholics who have been drinking heavily before the attack or who have a pre-existing hyperlipoproteinemia, especially type V. *(Cecil, pp. 733–734; Sleisenger and Fordtran, pp. 1409–1439)*

97. (A — True; B — True; C — False; D — False; E — True) In addition to cirrhosis with portal hypertension, pancreatic pseudocyst formation from unrecognized chronic relapsing pancreatitis can lead to so-called pancreatic ascites. The development of ascites is usually gradual and removed in time from recent attacks of abdominal pain. The diagnosis is made by the finding of hyperamylasemia in association with striking amylase elevation in ascitic fluid. Alcoholism and abdominal trauma are the major etiologies. Methyl alcohol abuse is not a cause of ascites, and splenic vein thrombosis alone does not account for massive ascites. Hypothyroidism can result in ascites as well as pleural and joint effusions. The fluid is an exudate with a high protein content. *(Cecil, pp. 749–750; Donowitz, Kerstein, and Spiro; Turner and Rapoport)*

98. (A — False; B — False; C — False; D — True; E — False) The small bowel, splenic flexure, and descending colon are commonly involved in intestinal ischemia. The rectum, however, is rarely affected because of extensive collateral circulation from the iliac arteries. Occasionally a precise demarcation between normally perfused rectum and ischemic sigmoid colon can be noted on proctosigmoidoscopic exam. Nonocclusive ischemia such as in low-flow states due to cardiogenic shock, hemorrhagic shock, or sepsis is responsible for a substantial number of cases of ischemic intestinal disease. Severe intestinal ischemia usually follows if two of the three mesenteric vessels are occluded. The occlusion of one main mesenteric vessel does not inevitably result in gangrene. Vasoconstrictors will exacerbate intestinal ischemia, as they decrease mesenteric blood flow further while supporting systemic blood pressure. *(Cecil, pp. 720–722; Sleisenger and Fordtran, pp. 1889–1911)*

99. (A — True; B — False; C — True; D — True; E — False) Wedged hepatic vein pressure (WHVP) is a measure of pressure in the sinusoidal and postsinusoidal hepatic vascular tree. Disorders that cause obstruction to portal venous flow prior to the sinusoids (portal vein thrombosis, schistosomiasis, congenital hepatic fibrosis) are typically accompanied by a normal WHVP. Disorders of the hepatic parenchyma that lead to portal hypertension, such as alcoholic cirrhosis and primary biliary cirrhosis, cause obstruction to flow within the sinusoids and postsinusoidal vascular tree, and are typically accompanied by an elevated WHVP. *(Cecil, p. 804; Schiff, pp. 333–342)*

100. (A — True; B — False; C — True; D — False; E — False) Ultrasonography and computerized tomography have changed the approach to patients with acute pancreatitis and pseudocysts. Many of these pseudocysts are small and asymptomatic, and resolve spontaneously; in most cases there is no reason to intervene surgically for asymptomatic pseudocysts that are getting smaller. Infection is an infrequent complication of pseudocysts, and patients should *not* get routine antibiotic coverage. Infection may occur following ERCP, which for that reason should not be used routinely. Internal drainage of a pseudocyst into the stomach (cyst gastrostomy) or into a Roux-en-Y loop of jejunum (cyst jejunostomy) is appropriate if surgery is indicated for a symptomatic pseudocyst or one that has failed to resolve spontaneously. ERCP and antibiotic coverage may be indicated prior to surgery. *(Cecil, pp. 736–737, 750; Sleisenger and Fordtran, pp. 1449–1451; Howat and Sarles, pp. 463–478)*

101. (All are True); 102. (All are True) This patient has history and laboratory findings indicative of cholestasis. Although the overall clinical picture is very suggestive of primary biliary cirrhosis, the differential diagnosis of cholestasis includes all the disorders listed in question 101. Chronic active hepatitis may present with a cholestatic picture that can be difficult to differentiate from primary biliary cirrhosis, especially in older women without serologic evidence of previous hepatitis B virus infection. The biopsy and positive antimitochondrial antibody test establish the diagnosis of primary biliary cirrhosis, which is associated with CRST syndrome (calcinosis, Raynaud's phenomenon, sclerodactyly, telangiectasia), immunologic abnormalities such as anergy, and elevated serum IgM. Since the cholestasis associated with primary biliary cirrhosis results in malabsorption of fat-soluble vitamins, therapy usually includes vitamins A, D, and K. Finally, it is essential to visualize the biliary tree to exclude treatable lesions such as stricture or choledocholithiasis, which may be contributing to the cholestasis, particularly given this patient's history of biliary tract surgery for cholelithiasis. *(Cecil, pp. 801–802; Schiff, pp. 940–959)*

103. (A — True; B — True; C — False; D — True; E — True) The plain film shows a massively dilated transverse colon. There is also marked loss of haustral details indicative of a severe acute inflammatory process. The midtransverse colon dilatation greater than 7 cm together with the clinical course is suggestive of toxic megacolon. Toxic megacolon is commonly associated with severe acute idiopathic ulcerative colitis, and it is also seen in a variety of other acute inflammatory processes such as infections with *Shigella* and with *Entamoeba histolytica,* both of which are seen in homosexual men. Toxic megacolon can also be seen in Crohn's colitis. *Giardia lamblia* infections involve the proximal small bowel and do not produce colonic inflammatory disease. *(Cecil, pp. 705–706; Sleisenger and Fordtran, pp. 1610, 1630–1633)*

104. (A — False; B — True; C — False; D — True; E — True) In this patient with manifestations of acute toxicity and an acute toxic megacolon on radiography, the proctosigmoidoscopy is strongly suggestive of acute idiopathic ulcerative colitis. Nevertheless, friable mucosa can occasionally be seen in acute bowel infections. Although the absence of trophozoites on three successive stool examinations makes the likelihood of *E. histolytica* infection low, serologic testing should be done in the homosexual man to exclude amebic colitis definitely. Colonoscopy is distinctly contraindicated because of the danger of perforations of the large bowel in an acutely inflamed colon. The diagnosis in this patient would not depend on a barium enema, given the features of toxic megacolon on plain film and the appearance of acute ulcerative colitis on proctosigmoidoscopy. Moreover, barium enema has been implicated in exacerbating acute inflammatory bowel disease, although the association between barium enema and acute deterioration of ulcerative colitis has not been firmly established. Blood cultures are indicated, and broad-spectrum antibiotics should be started. Close follow-up of this patient is absolutely essential, and radiographs of the abdomen should be repeated within a short time. A deterioration of the clinical condition or a marked increase in colonic size would indicate the need for expeditious colectomy. *(Cecil, pp. 705–706; Sleisenger and Fordtran, pp. 1630–1633)*

105. (A — False; B — False; C — True; D — True; E — False) Because of the acute nature of the abdominal findings, the patient should be restricted from oral intake. Electrolyte abnormalities may develop very rapidly; they should be repeatedly checked for and treated aggressively. Potassium repletion is particularly important, as toxic megacolon may be caused or exacerbated by hypokalemia. A limited trial of high-dose steroids is indicated, but should be limited to 72 hours. If the patient does not improve significantly during that period, or if clinical deterioration occurs, emergency colectomy is indicated. *(Cecil, pp. 709–710; Sleisenger and Fordtran, pp. 1630–1633; Caprilli et al.)*

106. (A — True; B — True; C — True; D — False; E — True) Alcohol has a direct toxic effect on the marrow that decreases platelet production, and alcohol also decreases intestinal folate absorption. Thrombocytopenia is frequently seen in cirrhotic patients with portal hypertension and splenomegaly who are not alcoholics or who have given up drinking. Since the platelet count in these patients usually rises following splenectomy, hypersplenism probably is also a cause of their thrombocytopenia. Vitamin B_{12} deficiency is rarely present even in malnourished alcoholic cirrhotics. Disseminated intravascular coagulation (DIC) can occur in patients with severe liver disease of any etiology and can lead to thrombocytopenia. DIC may be low-grade, resulting in petechiae and laboratory abnormalities rather than massive hemorrhage. *(Cecil, pp. 982–983, 986–987)*

107. (A — True; B — False; C — False; D — True; E — True) Surgery may be necessary for control of intractable pain in patients with chronic pancreatitis. ERCP should be performed preoperatively to define ductal anatomy, which is important in the selection of the appropriate surgery. If alternating segments of narrowing and dilatation of the pancreatic duct ("chain-of-lakes") are found, longitudinal pancreaticojejunostomy (Puestow procedure), which has been reported to relieve pain in two thirds to three quarters of patients, is appropriate. Pancreatoduodenectomy (Whipple's procedure) is rarely, if ever, indicated for pain relief in chronic pancreatitis because of its formidable operative morbidity and mortality. Celiac ganglionectomy (splanchnicectomy) has been largely abandoned because most patients experience recurrence of pain within one to two years after surgery. Even after total or subtotal (95%) pancreatic resection, about 20% of patients continue to have pain. *(Cecil, pp. 737–739, 742; Sleisenger and Fordtran, pp. 1453–1455; Dutta et al.; Levitt, Ellis, and Meier)*

108. (A — False; B — False; C — False; D — True; E — True) Arthritis occurs in approximately 25% of patients with ulcerative colitis or Crohn's colitis. A substantial number of these patients will have ankylosing spondylitis, particularly if they also have the HLA-B27 phenotype. The proximal interphalangeal joints are rarely affected. Large weight-bearing joints and the large joints of the upper extremities such as shoulder and elbows are commonly involved. Treatment of the colitis does not invariably mean that the arthritis will improve; in some patients the arthritis may become worse in spite of improvement in the colitis. This is particularly evident in patients with ankylosing spondylitis and colitis. *(Cecil, p. 709; Sleisenger and Fordtran, pp. 1641–1642; Greenstein, Janowitz, and Sachar)*

109. (A — False; B — True; C — False; D — True; E — True) Increased breath hydrogen results from bacterial metabolism of carbohydrate. This can occur in the small bowel in the presence of bacterial overgrowth, or in the colon in cases of carbohydrate malabsorption such as lactase deficiency or celiac disease. Lactose metabolism remains normal during cholestyramine therapy and in pancreatic insufficiency. *(Cecil, pp. 685–687; Sleisenger and Fordtran, pp. 388–389)*

110. (A — True; B — False; C — False; D — True; E — False) The upper gastrointestinal tract radiograph shows a large ulcer on the lesser curvature of the antrum. These ulcers may be precipitated or exacerbated by long-term administration of salicylates and other nonsteroidal anti-inflammatory agents, which disrupt normal mucosal barriers in the stomach. Approximately 4% of gastric ulcers are found to be malignant on careful histologic evaluation. Although most malignant ulcers present as exophytic mass lesions with superficial ulcerations, deeply infiltrating malignancies are also encountered. The location and size of the ulcer and the presence or absence of radiating gastric folds cannot be relied on to exclude malignancy, and all patients should have histologic examination of the lesion. Although the finding of ulcers in the fundus and corpus of the stomach is more suspicious for gastric carcinoma, the antrum is the most common site for both benign and malignant gastric ulcers. Patients with benign gastric ulcers have a lower-than-normal peak acid output. Autoimmune atrophic gastritis is associated with profound achlorhydria, and benign peptic ulcers do not occur in the absence of hydrochloric acid. The incidence of gastric carcinoma, however, is increased in patients with autoimmune atrophic gastritis. *(Cecil, pp. 637, 639, 643; Sleisenger and Fordtran, pp. 876, 878–879)*

111. (A — True; B — False; C — False; D — True; E — False) Ulcerative proctitis is a benign disease with few complications. It is indistinguishable in sigmoidoscopic and histologic appearance from ulcerative colitis, except that the disease process is limited to the rectum. The age of onset and sex distribution closely parallel what is found in ulcerative colitis. Barium enema is unreliable in excluding diseases of the rectum, especially superficial mucosal diseases such as ulcerative proctitis. Thus, the barium enema is frequently normal. Systemic complications and large bowel carcinoma, which may complicate ulcerative colitis, seldom occur in ulcerative proctitis. Ulcerative proctitis, like ulcerative colitis, can result in substantial rectal bleeding, both acute and chronic. *(Cecil, p. 746; Folley)*

112. (A — False; B — False; C — False; D — True; E — False) Determination of serum lipase concentration has not been used as widely as that of amylase in the diagnosis of acute pancreatitis because of technical problems with the assays for lipase. Like amylase, lipase can also be elevated in nonpancreatic diseases; however, lipase is not found in salivary glands and therefore is not elevated in disorders of the salivary glands. Lipase tends to remain elevated longer than serum amylase. Thus, serum lipase determination may be helpful in confirming the diagnosis in a patient who has been symptomatic for three or four days and whose serum amylase is normal. Serum lipase does not provide any information about etiology or likelihood of complications and does not help in the choice of therapy. *(Cecil, p. 735; Sleisenger and Fordtran, pp. 1412, 1424)*

113. (A — True; B — True; C — False; D — True; E — True) The primary chancre of syphilis usually occurs at the anal margin or in the anal canal and only rarely in the rectal mucosa. Condylomata lata of secondary syphilis are perianal. Gonococcal proctitis is asymptomatic in up to two thirds of patients, and increased severity is not required for the complication of septicemia to develop. Lymphogranuloma venereum causes proctitis followed by rectal fibrosis and stricture formation in as many as 25% of those infected. *(Cecil, pp. 1567–1584; Catterall)*

114. (A — True; B — False; C — True; D — True; E — False) To achieve an optimal mix of enzymes and food in the small intestine, the patient should be taking two tablets before, two part-way through, and two after each meal, rather than all six before each meal. Different preparations vary widely in their potency. Increasing the dosage of the present preparation or substituting another with greater known potency may be worthwhile in this case. The presence of hypochlorhydria should increase the activity of orally administered pancreatic enzymes, many of which are easily destroyed by an acid pH. Patients with normal acid output often benefit from administration of antacid or H-2 blocking agents before each dose of pancreatic enzyme. In the absence of any significant response to pancreatic enzyme replacement in presumed chronic pancreatitis, other causes for the patient's malabsorption should be considered (e.g., primary small intestinal disease). In pancreatic insufficiency, pancreatic secretion of digestive enzymes and bicarbonate is reduced, and the total volume of pancreatic juice may also be diminished; however, this reduction in volume is not an important factor in malabsorption due to pancreatic insufficiency. *(Cecil, pp. 692, 739; Sleisenger and Fordtran, pp. 1444, 1459)*

115. (A — True; B — False; C — False; D — True; E — True) There is a strong association between hypogammaglobulinemia, especially IgA deficiency, and infection with *Giardia lamblia.* These patients may also have nodular lymphoid hyperplasia on small bowel x-ray or biopsy. Stool examination can be negative for ova and parasites, even in the presence of documented small bowel infestation. Thus, small bowel aspiration or biopsy is the standard for diagnosis, although most cases will be identified by examination of three to six stool specimens. Occult blood is rare in *Giardia* infections, and hematochezia virtually unheard of. Although steatorrhea may occur, it is rarely of sufficient severity or duration to lead to hypocalcemia. *(Cecil, pp. 1746–1747; Sleisenger and Fordtran, pp. 1154–1158)*

116. (A — False; B — True; C — False; D — True; E — True) Disease of this advanced degree would be unlikely to respond to simple measures such as sitz baths and suppositories. Incision of the hemorrhoid would probably cause severe bleeding and is clearly contraindicated. Rubber band ligation, sclerosis, or anal dilatation would all be likely to resolve this woman's problem. *(Cecil, p. 747; Sleisenger and Fordtran, p. 1876)*

117. (A — False; B — True; C — False; D — False; E — False) Asymptomatic cholelithiasis is a relatively benign condition that is estimated to be present in about 10% of Americans. Less than 25% of patients subsequently develop severe complications, and only about one half develop any symptoms at all. The chance of death due to a future complication (less than 2%) is about offset by the chance of dying at the time of elective cholecystectomy (less than 1%). Although (B) is true, the risk of gallbladder cancer in a given patient with gallstones is exceedingly small and does not constitute justification for prophylactic surgery. *(Cecil, pp. 757–758)*

118. (A — False; B — True; C — True; D — True; E — False) Patients with pancreatic insufficiency have increased iron absorption, and hemosiderosis has been reported in untreated children with cystic fibrosis. Achlorhydria can significantly decrease iron absorption, as an acid pH in the stomach is necessary for normal absorption of inorganic iron. Hemoglobin iron does not require acid for absorption, and thus patients with achlorhydria develop abnormalities of iron absorption only when meat intake is reduced. Dysphagia, angular stomatitis, and esophageal webs are seen in middle-aged women with iron deficiency anemia; this is the Plummer-Vinson syndrome. Postgastrectomy patients often develop multifactorial iron deficiency anemia as a result of recurrent ulcers, decreased gastric acidity, poor nutrition, and loss of the duodenal mucosal surface where iron absorption predominantly occurs. Phenytoin ingestion can lead to megaloblastic anemia owing to impaired folate absorption. *(Cecil, pp. 630, 685, 700, 848–849; Sleisenger and Fordtran, pp. 247–248, 291–292, 569–572; Tonz et al.)*

119. (A — True; B — True; C — False; D — False; E — True) Conjugated bile acids are normally absorbed intact in the terminal ileum. Ileal resection (A) and ileal dysfunction from disorders such as Crohn's disease (B) result in bile acid malabsorption. The bile acids are deconjugated by bacterial flora in the colon; CO_2 is released, absorbed, and then excreted in the breath. Similarly, bacterial overgrowth in the small bowel such as that seen in scleroderma (E) will result in bile acid deconjugation and excretion of CO_2. Pancreatic insufficiency (D) does not affect the normal enterohepatic circulation of bile acids. Primary biliary cirrhosis (C) causes cholestasis and decreased hepatic excretion of endogenous bile acids in bile, but does not affect normal ileal uptake of exogenously administered bile acids. *(Cecil, pp. 686–687; Sleisenger and Fordtran, pp. 277–278; Fromm, Thomas, and Hofmann)*

120–124. The pentagastrin gastric acid secretion test is performed by first collecting the basal acid output from the stomach for one hour prior to the subcutaneous injection of pentagastrin. The upper limit of normal for a young male is 5 mEq/hr. After the injection of pentagastrin, the peak acid output is determined as the sum of the two highest consecutive 15-minute collections multiplied by two. The upper limit of normal for peak acid output for a young male is 40 mEq/hr. *(Cecil, pp. 639–640; Sleisenger and Fordtran, pp. 717–726)*

120. (E) A significant basal acid output remains at 3 mEq per hour. The peak acid output is substantial and is compatible with an incomplete vagotomy. The incomplete vagotomy results from surgical error in failing to identify and transect both vagal trunks at the esophageal hiatus of the diaphragm. *(Cecil, p. 646)*

121. (A) A normal basal acid output and peak acid output is seen in this patient with a completely negative work-up. It is unlikely that peptic ulcer disease is responsible for this patient's symptoms. *(Cecil, p. 639)*

122. (D) The basal acid output is significantly above the upper limits of normal, and although the peak acid output is not excessively high, the BAO/PAO ratio is 0.8, strongly suggestive of Zollinger-Ellison syndrome. Definitive diagnosis requires an elevated serum gastrin that increases further in response to intravenous secretin. *(Cecil, pp. 641–642)*

123. (B) The marked hypochlorhydria that is unresponsive to pentagastrin stimulation is compatible with a gastric cancer. Many gastric malignancies arise in stomachs demonstrating changes of chronic atrophic gastritis. *(Cecil, p. 657; Sleisenger and Fordtran, p. 726)*

124. (C) Both the basal acid and peak acid outputs are substantially above the upper limits of normal. This may commonly be seen in patients with duodenal ulcers, although considerable overlap exists between normals and duodenal ulcer patients. *(Cecil, p. 639; Sleisenger and Fordtran, pp. 724–725)*

125. (B) This patient has idiopathic ulcerative colitis. The barium enema shows abnormal mucosa from the proximal transverse to the sigmoid colon. The granularity, shallow ulcerations, loss of haustral markings, and extent of the changes are entirely compatible with this disorder. *(Cecil, pp. 706–707)*

126. (D) The patient's family history is compatible with one of the familial colonic polyposis syndromes. The barium radiograph shows scores of small, uniform, 3- to 4-mm polypoid lesions throughout the colon. These are seen in familial polyposis or in Gardner's syndrome, both of which are associated with the development of colonic malignancy early in life. The polyps are adenomatous, and in patients with Gardner's syndrome they are accompanied by benign tumors of the skin, subcutaneous tissue, and bone. *(Cecil, pp. 723–726; Sleisenger and Fordtran, pp. 1216–1218)*

127. (A) Acute appendicitis should be strongly suspected in this patient. The barium enema shows a marked shift of the entire right colon to the midline, with a mass distorting the cecal mucosa suggestive of abscess in this area. The periappendiceal abscess may occur relatively soon after the perforation of the appendix. *(Cecil, pp. 817–820)*

128. (E) The diagnosis of intestinal tuberculosis should be strongly entertained in this patient. Tuberculosis of the gastrointestinal tract typically will involve the area of the ileocecal valve and the ascending colon. The stomach, duodenum, and other areas of the colon can also be involved in the nodular hyperplastic scarring process. This radiograph shows focal constrictions of the ascending and transverse colon with normal intervening areas. The radiographic features of intestinal tuberculosis may be difficult to distinguish from Crohn's disease, although ileal involvement alone favors the latter diagnosis. *(Cecil, pp. 717, 1548–1549)*

129. (C) The clinical features described in this patient are strongly suggestive of acute diverticulitis. The barium radiograph shows a long area of narrowing of the sigmoid colon with thickened haustra. A small amount of contrast has extended outside the lumen of the sigmoid colon and is filling the cavity of a pelvic abscess. Several diverticula are visible in the transverse and descending colon. The extent of involvement, the spasm and edema, fistulization to the pelvis, and the presence of colonic diverticula all support the diagnosis. A perforating malignancy of the sigmoid colon occasionally may present with similar clinical and radiographic features. *(Cecil, pp. 820–821)*

130. (A); 131. (D); 132. (B); 133. (C); 134. (E) Gastrin is released by antral G cells in response to a variety of stimuli, including antral distention, alkalinization of the antrum, and topical contact of the antral G cells with peptides. Most of the gut, excluding only esophagus and gastric antrum, is under the trophic influence of gastrin. Secretin stimulates pancreatic flow and increases bicarbonate concentration in the fluid. It is released in response to acidification of duodenal mucosa. Although gastric acid output is inhibited by secretin, pepsinogen secretion is stimulated. Vasoactive intestinal polypeptide (VIP) is secreted by gut endocrine cells and non-beta islet cells of the pancreas. Tumors of these cells (called VIPomas) are associated with watery diarrhea, hypokalemia, and achlorhydria, a syndrome called WDHA or pancreatic cholera.

Cholecystokinin increases pancreatic enzyme concentration and output in pancreatic juice. It also stimulates gallbladder contraction and relaxation of the sphincter of Oddi. Release of none of these hormones is blocked by cimetidine. Some studies demonstrated minor elevations in fasting serum gastrin with chronic, long-term cimetidine use. *(Cecil, pp. 639–640, 647; Sleisenger and Fordtran, pp. 904–905, 1401–1402, 1496–1497; Walsh and Grossman; Said and Faloona)*

135. (A) This man has giardiasis with mild steatorrhea. Villous atrophy can be seen in this disorder, although it is often patchy rather than diffuse. The histologic abnormalities as well as the clinical symptoms will respond to metronidazole (250 mg three times daily for ten days) or quinacrine hydrochloride. Current opinion probably favors the use of quinacrine initially, although both agents are effective. *(Cecil, p. 700; Sleisenger and Fordtran, pp. 1154–1158)*

136. (C) This man has tropical sprue with evidence of a megaloblastic anemia and severe malabsorption. Although iron deficiency anemia may occur, megaloblastic anemia is characteristically seen in cases with a duration longer than six months. It is usually due to folate deficiency, although vitamin B_{12} deficiency may also occur. Tetracycline and folic acid are curative, although prolonged treatment (for up to one year) may be required. In patients with megaloblastic anemia, vitamin B_{12} replacement is also given initially. *(Cecil, p. 700; Sleisenger and Fordtran, pp. 1143–1154; Klipstein)*

137. (D) This patient has adult celiac sprue, which will respond to a gluten-free diet. Although pancreatic insufficiency could occur in this setting, it does not result in a decreased D-xylose absorption, villous atrophy, or severe vitamin D and calcium malabsorption with osteomalacia. Kwashiorkor (protein malnutrition) can result in villous atrophy and malabsorption, but requires a severely deficient diet and is most common in young children in developing countries. *(Cecil, p. 695; Sleisenger and Fordtran, pp. 1029–1051)*

138–142 *(Cecil, pp. 786–789)*

138. (G) This patient has fulminant hepatic failure. For oral ingestion of the drugs listed, this effect has been clearly associated only with acetaminophen in a dose of 10 gm or more. Lower doses of acetaminophen have occasionally been associated with severe hepatic damage, particularly in malnourished alcoholic patients.

139. (I) This patient has hepatocellular carcinoma, which has been clearly linked to prolonged administration of androgenic-anabolic steroids. An association with oral contraceptives has been suggested, but not clearly established.

140. (D) This patient has intra-abdominal rupture of an hepatocellular adenoma. This histologically benign tumor occurs with increased frequency in women taking oral contraceptives.

141. (C) The pathologic findings are characteristic of chronic active hepatitis. Of the drugs listed, only methyldopa has been clearly linked to this disorder.

142. (B) Tetracycline, particularly when administered intravenously in doses exceeding 2 gm per day, can produce fulminant hepatic failure and characteristic microvesicular fatty changes.

143. (D) This patient's history is very suggestive of idiopathic inflammatory bowel disease, specifically Crohn's disease. The colonic biopsy shows diffuse mucosal and submucosal inflammation, with two submucosal granulomas in the center of the field. Although not essential for the histologic diagnosis, submucosal granulomas without caseation are strongly suggestive of Crohn's disease. Additional histologic features that may be encountered are transmural inflammation and fibrosis. Multiple affected areas of the small and large bowel may be separated by areas of uninvolved bowel ("skip" lesions). *(Cecil, pp. 712–714)*

144. (C) Schistosomiasis commonly presents with complications of portal hypertension. Hepatocellular function is largely preserved. The rectal biopsy shows numerous submucosal, darkly stained foreign bodies strongly suggestive of the ova of *Schistosoma mansoni*. The adult females, which may live for decades, reside in the inferior mesenteric venules around the rectosigmoid. Eggs deposited by the female erode through the submucosa to the mucosa and then are deposited in the stool. Colonic mucosal appearance ranges from normal to chronically inflamed with pseudopolypoid appearance. Rectal valve biopsy is a highly accurate means of diagnosis. *(Cecil, pp. 1758–1759)*

145. (F) Frequent short-lived episodes of abdominal cramps with mucous and bloody stools in a young or middle-aged patient suggest ulcerative colitis. The biopsy shows submucosal inflammation and one large colonic crypt filled with polymorphonuclear leukocytes. This is a classic crypt abscess of acute ulcerative colitis. Crypt abscesses are occasionally seen in other conditions such as shigellosis, ischemia, toxin exposure, and other acute inflammatory diseases of the colon. In ulcerative colitis the crypt abscesses coalesce to form larger abscesses that ulcerate. *(Cecil, pp. 704–705)*

146. (A) Clindamycin and other broad-spectrum antibiotics have been associated with the overgrowth of clostridial species such as *C. difficile*. These organisms elaborate a heat-labile enterotoxin that produces pseudomembranous damage throughout the colon, usually involving the rectosigmoid. The biopsy shows submucosal inflammation and focal areas of attachment of a superficial necrotic membrane consisting of polymorphonuclear leukocytes and fibrin, strongly suggestive of pseudomembranous colitis. *(Bartlett et al., Sleisenger and Fordtran, pp. 1720–1728)*

147. (E) Amebic colitis commonly occurs in travelers to underdeveloped areas of the world. Its signs and symptoms mimic those of ulcerative colitis. The biopsy shows a foreign population of large ovoid cells, some with multiple nuclei, surrounded by necrotic debris. These cells are trophozoites of *Entamoeba histolytica*. Grossly, the mucosa in these patients may range from near normal to diffusely ulcerative. The organisms are best demonstrated by microscopy of mucus aspirated from the base of the ulcerations. *(Cecil, pp. 707, 736–739; Sleisenger and Fordtran, pp. 1695–1696)*

148. (B) Intermittent hematochezia and/or iron deficiency anemia without altered bowel habits is the common clinical presentation of an adenomatous colonic polyp. The biopsy shows a small adenomatous polyp with characteristic branching glands in the polyp head and a sizeable stalk. The vast majority of colorectal polyps are adenomatous and benign; however, with increasing size, foci of carcinoma in situ can be demonstrated. Larger polyps (> 2-cm diameter) have a higher rate of malignancy and are associated with superficial mucosal ulceration and iron deficiency anemia. In general, polyps larger than 1 cm in diameter should be removed, preferably by sigmoidoscopic or colonoscopic means. *(Cecil, p. 724)*

149–152. *(Cecil, p. 737; Sleisenger and Fordtran, pp. 350, 1476.*
149. (C) Kwashiorkor can result in reduced pancreatic enzyme secretion, which returns to normal on an adequate diet unless extensive pancreatic fibrosis has already occurred.

150. (B) While gallstone disease accounts for about 40% of cases of *acute* pancreatitis seen in the United States, it rarely results in chronic pancreatitis.

151. (A) Alcoholism is involved in about 75% of patients with chronic pancreatitis in the United States. Irreversible structural changes are usually present in the pancreas prior to the first clinical episode of pancreatitis.

152. (D) The finding of reduced stool trypsin activity in infants or small children is suggestive of cystic fibrosis.

153–156. *(Cecil, pp. 626, 627, 629, 630; Sleisenger and Fordtran, pp. 557–565, 575)*
153. (C) Columnar epithelium can result from chronic reflux esophagitis and is a predisposing factor for adenocarcinoma of the esophagus.

154. (B) Untreated or inadequately treated achalasia appears to be a predisposing factor for esophageal cancer. Achalasia is not associated with reflux esophagitis.

155. (C) Strictures may result from either disease. Strictures of both types may respond to careful dilatation, although great care must be exercised in dilating malignant strictures. (It should be done over a guidewire under fluoroscopic guidance.)

156. (A) Cimetidine has been shown to provide symptomatic relief in reflux esophagitis. It has no proven role in the treatment of carcinoma of the esophagus.

157. (F) The Crigler-Najjar syndrome (congenital nonhemolytic jaundice) is characterized by unconjugated hyperbilirubinemia and occurs in two forms. Type I results from the congenital absence of bilirubin glucuronyl transferase and is characterized by severe unconjugated hyperbilirubinemia (20–40 mg/dl), usually leading to kernicterus and death in early infancy. Type II presumably results from a partial enzyme deficiency and is characterized by milder (6–25 mg/dl) unconjugated hyperbilirubinemia, usually without symptoms. These cases may not come to medical attention until early adulthood. *(Cecil, pp. 773, 774; Arias et al.)*

158. (D) The Dubin-Johnson syndrome results from defective excretion of conjugated bilirubin and is characterized by variable, predominantly conjugated, hyperbilirubinemia. Because these patients also exhibit defective excretion of biliary contrast media, the oral cholecystogram typically fails to visualize the gallbladder, often leading to the incorrect diagnosis of biliary tract disease. These patients have an abnormality in urinary coproporphyrin excretion and do not itch because hepatic secretion of bile salts and most other biliary substances is not impaired. Rotor's syndrome is similar to the Dubin-Johnson, but the oral cholecystogram is typically normal, total coproporphyrins as well as type I isomer are increased in the urine, and the plasma BSP disappearance curve does not show a secondary rise. *(Cecil, pp. 773, 774; Wolkoff, Cohen, and Arias)*

159. (B) Benign recurrent cholestasis is a disorder of unknown etiology that involves recurrent, self-limited episodes of cholestasis characterized by predominantly conjugated hyperbilirubinemia, elevated alkaline phosphatase, clay-colored stools, and icterus. It is frequently familial and, despite numerous episodes of cholestasis, the long-term prognosis is good. *(Cecil, p. 773; Schiff, pp. 1384–1388)*

160. (A) Gilbert's syndrome is characterized by mild unconjugated hyperbilirubinemia that is typically exacerbated by fasting or a low-fat diet. Although the exact cause of this disorder is unknown, defects in both the hepatic uptake and conjugation of bilirubin have been detected. *(Cecil, pp. 773, 774; Schiff, p. 301)*

161. (B) This series of tests for malabsorption demonstrates substantial steatorrhea with excellent preservation of B_{12} absorption in the terminal ileum. Absorption of D-xylose in the proximal small bowel is normal. The massive steatorrhea in the absence of mucosal disease is suggestive of pancreatic exocrine insufficiency. *(Cecil, pp. 685–690)*

162. (D) Nontropical sprue is a severe proximal small bowel mucosal disease. There is significant steatorrhea with 30 gm of fat in a 24-hour fecal collection (normal would be less than 6 gm per day on a 100-gm per day intake). The 1 gm of D-xylose in the five-hour urine specimen is strongly suggestive of severe proximal mucosal disease. The low serum albumin also suggests significant malnutrition or protein loss. The normal Schilling test indicates normal distal ileal function. *(Cecil, pp. 685–690)*

163. (C) There is significant steatorrhea with modest depression in D-xylose and serum albumin levels. The Schilling test is markedly abnormal, which in patients with scleroderma is commonly related to small bowel overgrowth. The presence of unconjugated bile salts in the duodenum may be attributed to small bowel overgrowth with colonic flora that deconjugate bile salts. The increase in small bowel colonic flora relates to the hypomotility in patients with severe sclerodermatous involvement of the bowel. *(Cecil, pp. 685–690)*

164. (E) The extensive resection of 100 cm of the terminal ileum would be expected to cause impaired absorption of bile salts in addition to a marked decrease in the absorptive ability for B_{12}. The significant steatorrhea of 12 gm per day and the markedly abnormal Schilling test are compatible with extensive ileal resection. *(Cecil, pp. 685–690)*

165. (A) The patient with nontropical sprue in remission usually has normal tests of absorptive function as long as his diet remains free of gluten. Reversion to a state of abnormal absorptive function may occur promptly after ingesting gluten. *(Cecil, pp. 688, 694–696)*

166. (F) A severe protein-losing enteropathy is usually noted in intestinal lymphangiectasia. Severe hypoalbuminemia and mild steatorrhea may also be seen. B_{12} and carbohydrate absorption are normal. *(Cecil, pp. 685–690; Sleisenger and Brandborg, pp. 200–204)*

167. (C); 168. (D); 169. (D); 170. (A) Both procedures clearly reduce the incidence of recurrent variceal hemorrhage. Neither has clearly been shown to prolong useful life in patients who have bled from varices. Even a combined analysis of all prospective trials of standard portacaval shunt surgery has yielded equivocal results. The distal splenorenal shunt is less often accompanied by hepatic encephalopathy than is the standard shunt, but this patient's previous episode of encephalopathy would not necessarily preclude the use of either operation. The likelihood of intractable and disabling encephalopathy in this patient following a standard portacaval shunt is 20% or less. Postoperatively, impairment of liver function correlates with loss of liver blood flow, and occurs to a significant extent in many patients who receive a standard shunt. The distal splenorenal shunt preserves both hepatic blood flow and liver function in all patients in the immediate postoperative period. Although hepatic blood flow eventually falls in many patients with a distal splenorenal shunt, liver function remains better preserved. *(Cecil, p. 806; Conn; Rikkers et al., Nabseth)*

171. (D) While considerable work is being done in this area, an infectious etiology has not been established for either disease. A number of possible etiologies have been proposed (infectious, immunologic, psychogenic, and so forth), but none have been proved. *(Cecil, pp. 704, 712; Sleisenger and Fordtran, pp. 1059–1061, 1599–1601, 1659)*

172. (C) Ankylosing spondylitis is 20 times more frequent in patients with inflammatory bowel disease than in the general population. It can accompany either ulcerative colitis or Crohn's disease and often persists after total colectomy (unlike the arthritis of inflammatory bowel disease, which generally disappears after total colectomy). About 75% of patients with ankylosing spondylitis and inflammatory bowel disease have the HLA-B27 histocompatibility antigen. *(Cecil, pp. 709, 716; Sleisenger and Fordtran, pp. 1064, 1641–1642)*

173. (B) Perianal abscess and fistula formation is commonly seen in Crohn's disease, but is not usually an important aspect of ulcerative colitis. *(Cecil, p. 715; Sleisenger and Fordtran, pp. 1063, 1661)*

174. (A) This patient may have partial biliary obstruction from a stone or tumor, and percutaneous transhepatic cholangiography is the procedure of choice. Endoscopic retrograde cholangiography is technically difficult in a patient with a Billroth II anastomosis. Ultrasonography has already demonstrated dilated ducts, so that computed tomography would be superfluous. Intravenous cholangiography, although it might visualize the biliary tree at this bilirubin concentration, does not provide the resolution obtainable with percutaneous or retrograde cholangiography. Moreover, intravenous cholangiography has an unacceptably high false-negative rate and cannot be depended on to exclude biliary disease. ^{99m}Tc-HIDA scan and oral cholecystography are useful primarily for detecting gallbladder disease, which is not the principal concern in this patient. *(Cecil, pp. 756–757, 763, 778)*

175. (B) Endoscopic retrograde cholangiography is the correct answer. Because the clinical picture is so strongly suggestive of biliary obstruction, direct visualization of the biliary tree is mandatory and should be carried out regardless of the findings of noninvasive studies. Repeat sonographic examination, computerized tomography and the remaining procedures are not essential, therefore. Percutaneous transhepatic cholangiography is contraindicated because of hypothrombinemia. Intrahepatic ducts sometimes fail to dilate in patients with cirrhosis and biliary obstruction, presumably because of the poor distensibility of the surrounding hepatic parenchyma. This may explain the negative sonographic findings in this patient. *(Cecil, pp. 756–757, 802)*

176. (E) A normal study with normal peristaltic activity is seen. The history is strongly suggestive of globus hystericus. *(Sleisenger and Fordtran, pp. 8, 196)*

177. (A) The motility/manometry study demonstrates a hypotensive lower esophageal sphincter with preservation of peristaltic activity. The hypotensive lower esophageal sphincter is correlated with significant gastroesophageal reflux. *(Cecil, pp. 622–623; Sleisenger and Fordtran, pp. 547–548)*

178. (D) The motility/manometry study shows an absence of a lower esophageal sphincter and essentially no peristaltic activity. This is compatible with the diagnosis of scleroderma, which tends to involve severely the smooth muscle portion (distal two thirds) of the esophagus. *(Cecil, pp. 628–629; Sleisenger and Fordtran, pp. 535–537)*

179. (B) Diffuse esophageal spasm is seen. Extremely hot or cold drinks may exacerbate the pain of diffuse esophageal spasm. There may be dramatic relief of pain with sublingual nitroglycerin, which suppresses the chaotic repetitive contractions throughout the esophagus. *(Cecil, pp. 628–630; Sleisenger and Fordtran, p. 532)*

180. (C) The motility/manometry study shows a hypertensive lower esophageal sphincter with failure of complete relaxation on swallowing. These findings indicate a persistent barrier to the passage of food from the esophagus into the stomach. In addition, there is poor peristaltic activity. The finding of a hypertensive lower esophageal sphincter that fails to relax promptly with deglutition, together with a peristaltic defect in motility, is compatible with the diagnosis of achalasia. *(Cecil, pp. 628–630; Sleisenger and Fordtran, p. 524)*

181. (D) This man has Crohn's disease with a persistent stricture of the terminal ileum causing intermittent small bowel obstruction. *(Cecil, pp. 714–715)*

182. (B) This man has the carcinoid syndrome. Diarrhea and flushing generally appear after the tumor has spread to the liver and substances such as serotonin are released into the systemic circulation. Ileal carcinoids often cause a dense fibrotic reaction in adjacent small bowel loops, resulting in angulated fixed loops as seen on the small bowel film. *(Cecil, pp. 731–732, 1312–1317)*

183. (A) This man has a primary intestinal lymphoma with a mass displacing multiple loops of bowel. Steatorrhea and malabsorption owing to submucosal infiltration or intestinal lymphatic obstruction can occur in these patients, especially in those from the middle East who have α-chain lymphoma. *(Cecil, p. 699; Sleisenger and Fordtran, pp. 1115–1124)*

184. (E) This woman has multiple jejunal diverticula resulting in bacterial overgrowth and malabsorption. *(Cecil, p. 692)*

185. (C) This boy has juvenile hamartomatous polyps of the small bowel with recurrent hemorrhage and iron deficiency anemia. Small bowel polyps may bleed intermittently, or cause small bowel obstruction and/or intussusception. If only a few polyps are present, surgery is curative. *(Cecil, p. 726; Sleisenger and Fordtran, pp. 1211–1222)*

186. (C); 187. (B); 188. (A); 189. (D) Although the ascitic fluid may vary considerably in a given disorder, certain characteristics are generally present. Chylous ascites (A), characterized by its grossly milky appearance and very high triglyceride content, frequently results from traumatic disruption of intestinal lymphatics, and is also associated with abdominal neoplasms and congenital lymphatic disorders. Ascites due to the nephrotic syndrome (B) is typically a transudate. Spontaneous bacterial peritonitis (C) is a serious complication of advanced liver disease, and its presence should be strongly suspected when the white blood cell count in the ascitic fluid exceeds 1000/cu mm.

Intra-abdominal neoplasms such as hepatocellular carcinoma (D) are frequently accompanied by frankly bloody ascitic fluid. *(Cecil, pp. 749–750)*

190. (C) Both duodenal and gastric ulcers are more common in men than in women. In some studies, sex ratios as high as 5 to 1 have been reported. Peptic ulcer disease is extremely prevalent, with lifetime incidence rates of 8% among male physicians, for example. High autopsy incidence rates are likewise reported, with 27% of men and 15% of women having ulcers, scarring, or both at necropsy. *(Cecil, p. 636; Sleisenger and Fordtran, pp. 875–876)*

191. (A) Gastric ulcer disease is associated with lower-than-normal peak acid output, and correspondingly higher fasting and postprandial serum gastrin. Duodenal ulcers are associated with high peak acid outputs; basal serum gastrin level is normal and postprandial serum gastrin is modestly elevated. *(Cecil, pp. 638–639; Sleisenger and Fordtran, p. 796)*

192. (C) Gastric ulcers most commonly occur at the junction of fundic gland and antral pyloric gland mucosa. Duodenal ulcers most commonly occur in the postpyloric channel area at the junction between pyloric and duodenal mucosa. The mechanisms responsible for the development of mucosal ulcerations at these sites are poorly defined; however, altered mucosal defense mechanisms and the presence of gastric acid clearly play important roles. *(Cecil, pp. 635–636, 643)*

193. (D) Most patients with duodenal ulcers have higher-than-normal peak acid output, increased acid delivery to the duodenum, and a consistently lower duodenal pH. Although often postulated, neither impaired release of secretin nor impaired pancreatic bicarbonate secretion has been convincingly demonstrated for either duodenal or gastric ulcers. *(Cecil, pp. 638–639; Sleisenger and Fordtran, pp. 794–796)*

194. (B) Elevated serum group I pepsinogen concentration, probably transmitted as an autosomal dominant trait, has been demonstrated in families with a high prevalence of duodenal ulcer disease. Abnormal frequencies of blood group O, secretory status of blood group antigens, and certain HLA antigens have likewise been noted in patients with duodenal ulcers. *(Cecil, pp. 636–637; Rotter et al.)*

195. (E) The film shows large thick gastric rugae. The low basal acid output and peak acid output are strongly compatible with the diagnosis of Menetrier's disease. Definitive diagnosis usually requires full-thickness mucosal biopsy. *(Cecil, pp. 634–635; Scharschmidt)*

196. (B) The film shows a large duodenal bulbar ulcer and a distal duodenal ulcer strongly suggestive of a marked gastric acid hypersecretory state. The large liver may suggest the presence of hepatic metastases. This patient most likely has Zollinger-Ellison syndrome resulting from a gastrinoma. *(Cecil, pp. 641–642)*

197. (C) Pernicious anemia is associated with a higher-than-normal incidence of gastric malignancy. The film shows a large nodular gastric mass on the greater curvature in the antrum. Cytology or endoscopic biopsy will confirm the diagnosis. *(Cecil, pp. 656–657)*

198. (D) The film shows a benign gastric ulcer on the lesser curvature with a Hampton line. Aspirin ingestion is associated with a higher-than-normal incidence of gastric ulceration. *(Cecil, pp. 637, 643)*

199. (A) The film shows a Billroth II anastomosis with a stomal ulceration. These ulcerations are extremely difficult to demonstrate radiographically. Often the diagnosis of a recurrent ulcer adjacent to a gastrojejunostomy requires endoscopy. Typically, these ulcers are resistant to medical management, and an additional gastric resection or search for a nontransected vagal branch must be undertaken. *(Cecil, p. 653)*

200. (D); 201. (B) Alcoholic cirrhosis is characteristically monolobular (micronodular) in type, whereas postnecrotic cirrhosis due to chronic hepatitis, Wilson's disease, or hemochromatosis is characteristically multilobular (macronodular), such as that shown in Figure B. *(Cecil, pp. 790, 801; Ishak)*

202. (E) This biopsy shows the characteristic early lesion of primary biliary cirrhosis, in which intact and partially degenerating interlobular bile ducts are surrounded by a mononuclear infiltrate. *(Cecil, p. 801)*

203. (F) The presence of polymorphonuclear leukocytes inside the interlobular bile ducts is characteristic of acute cholangitis. *(Wright et al., pp. 314–315)*

204. (A) Figure A shows an egg of *Schistosoma mansoni* surrounded by several giant cells and epithelial cells *(Cecil, pp. 793, 1758–1759)*

205. (C) Figure C shows a sharply defined granuloma composed almost entirely of epithelioid cells in a patient with hepatic sarcoidosis. *(Cecil, p. 797)*

206. (D) This woman has classic *Salmonella* gastroenteritis, probably acquired from contaminated eggs or poultry. The organism is noninvasive in this localized form of salmonellosis; blood cultures will be negative, although stool cultures will be positive. The clinical course is usually one to four days, and antibiotics are not necessary for a simple case. *(Cecil, pp. 1510–1513; Sleisenger and Fordtran, pp. 1079–1082)*

207. (E) This man has cholera, a profuse secretory diarrhea caused by the enterotoxin produced by *Vibrio cholerae* after it infects the small intestine. The toxin elicits massive electrolyte and water secretion, and death can occur from rapid dehydration. Therapy includes intravenous administration of fluids and electrolytes and oral administration of glucose, electrolyte solutions, and tetracycline. *(Cecil, pp. 1519–1521)*

208. (A) This child has a *Yersinia* infection of the distal small bowel and cecum that can mimic acute appendicitis or Crohn's disease. Pathologically, acute and chronic mucosal inflammation can be seen, occasionally with small mucosal ulcers. Diarrhea can persist for weeks to months, even after a course of tetracycline. *(Cecil, p. 717; Sleisenger and Fordtran, pp. 1086–1087; Vantrappen et al.)*

209. (C) This woman has become infected with *Giardia lamblia*, probably from drinking contaminated stream water. *Giardia* can cause a malabsorption syndrome as well as diarrhea, and the patient should be treated with metronidazole or quinacrine hydrochloride. Duodenal aspiration or small bowel biopsy may be necessary to visualize the organisms if stool examination is negative. *(Cecil, pp. 1746–1747; Sleisenger and Fordtran, pp. 1152–1158; Brandborg et al.)*

210. (B) This man has an acute colitis caused by infection with *Campylobacter fetus*, probably acquired from animal exposure. The organism can be cultured from the stool and generally responds to erythromycin therapy. *C. fetus* may cause illness ranging from mild diarrhea to severe colitis, and can mimic acute ulcerative colitis. *(Cecil, p. 707; Blaser, Parsons, and Wang)*

BIBLIOGRAPHY

Arias, I. M., Gartner, L. M., Cohen, M., et al.: Chronic nonhemolytic unconjugated hyperbilirubinemia with glucuronyl transferase deficiency. Clinical, biochemical, pharmacologic and genetic evidence for heterogeneity. Am. J. Med., *47*:395, 1969.

Bartlett, J. G., Moon, N., Chang, T. W., et al.: Role of *Clostridium difficile* in antibiotic-associated pseudomembranous colitis. Gastroenterology, *75*:778, 1978.

Berman, P. M., and Kirsner, J. B.: Current knowledge of diverticular disease of the colon. Am. J. Dig. Dis., *17*:741, 1972.

Black, M., Mitchell, J. R., Zimmerman, H. J., et al.: Isoniazid-associated hepatitis in 114 patients. Gastroenterology, *69*:289, 1975.

Blaser, M. J., Parsons, R. B., and Wang, W.-L. L.: Acute colitis caused by *Campylobacter fetus* ss. *jejuni.* Gastroenterology, *78*:448, 1980.

Brandborg, L. L., Owen, R., Fogel, R., et al.: Giardiasis and traveler's diarrhea. Gastroenterology, *78*:1602, 1980.

Brugge, W. R., Goff, J. S., Allen, N. G., et al.: Development of a dual label Schilling test for pancreatic exocrine function based on the differential absorption of cobalamin bound to intrinsic factor and R protein. Gastroenterology, *78*:937, 1980.

Cameron, J. L., Maddrey, W. C., and Zuidema, G. D.: Biliary tract disease in sickle cell anemia. Ann. Surg., *174*:702, 1971.

Caprilli, R., Verma, P., Colaneri, O., et al.: Risk factors in toxic megacolon. Dig. Dis. Sci., *25*:817, 1980.

Cartwright, G. E., Edwards, C. Q., Kravitz, K., et al.: Hereditary hemochromatosis: phenotypic expression of the disease. N. Engl. J. Med., *301*:175, 1979.

Catterall, R. D.: Sexually transmitted diseases of the anus and rectum. Clin. Gastroenterol., *4*:659, 1975.

Cello, J. P., Fogel, R. P., and Boland, R.: Liquid caustic ingestion. Spectrum of injury. Arch. Intern. Med., *140*:501, 1980.

Conn, H. O.: Therapeutic portacaval anastomosis; to shunt or not to shunt. Gastroenterology, *67*:1065, 1974.

DiMagno, E. P., Malagelada, J. R., Taylor, W. F., et al.: A prospective comparison of current diagnostic tests for pancreatic cancer. N. Engl. J. Med., *297*:737, 1977.

Donowitz, M., Kerstein, M. D., and Spiro, H. M.: Pancreatic ascites. Medicine, *53*:183, 1974.

Dutta, S., Douglas, W., Smalls, U. A., et al.: Prevalence and nature of hyperamylasemia in acute alcoholism. Dig. Dis. Sci., *26*:136, 1981.

Folley, J. H.: Ulcerative proctitis. N. Engl. J. Med., *282*:1362, 1970.

Fromm, H., Thomas, P. J., and Hofmann, A. F.: Sensitivity and specificity in tests of distal ileal function: prospective comparison of bile acid and vitamin B_{12} absorption in ileal resection patients. Gastroenterology, *64*:1077, 1973.

Gardner, J. D., Jackson, M. J., Batzsi, S., et al.: Potential mechanisms of interaction among secretagogues. Gastroenterology, *74*:348, 1978.

Greenstein, A. J., Janowitz, H. D., and Sachar, D. B.: The extra-intestinal complications of Crohn's disease and ulcerative colitis; a study of 700 patients. Medicine, *55*:401, 1976.

Helman, R. A., Tempko, M. H., Nye, S. W., et al.: Alcoholic hepatitis. Natural history and evaluation of prednisolone therapy. Ann. Intern. Med., *74*:311, 1971.

Howat, H. T., and Sarles, H. (eds.): The Exocrine Pancreas. London, W. B. Saunders Company, 1979.

Hsia, Y. E.: Inherited hyperammonemic syndromes. Gastroenterology, *67*:347, 1974.

Ishak, K. G.: Laboratory Medicine. Hagerstown, Md, Harper & Row, 1973, pp. 1–48.

Klipstein, F. A.: Tropical sprue in travelers and expatriates living abroad. Gastroenterology, *80*:590, 1981.

Knauer, C. M.: Mallory-Weiss syndrome. Gastroenterology, *71*:5, 1976.

Kolts, B. E., Herbst, C. A., and McGuigan, J. E.: Calcium and secretin-stimulated gastrin release in the Zollinger-Ellison syndrome. Ann. Intern. Med., *81*:758, 1974.

Kushner, J. P., Barbuto, A. J., and Lee, G. R.: An inherited enzymatic defect in porphyria cutanea tarda. Decreased uroporphyrinogen decarboxylase activity. J. Clin. Invest., *58*:1089, 1976.

Kushner, J. P., Steinmuller, D. P., and Lee, G. R.: The role of iron in the pathogenesis of porphyria cutanea tarda. II. Inhibition of uroporphyrinogen decarboxylase. J. Clin. Invest., *56*:661, 1975.

Larson, H. E., Price, A. B., and Honour, P.: *Clostridium difficile* and the aetiology of pseudomembranous colitis. Lancet, *1*:1063, 1978.

Levitt, M. D., Ellis, C. V., and Meier, P. B.: Extrapancreatic origin of chronic unexplained hyperamylasemia. N. Engl. J. Med., *302*:670, 1980.

Littenberg, G., Afroudakis, A., and Kaplowitz, N.: Common bile duct stenosis from chronic pancreatitis: a clinico-pathologic spectrum identified by serum alkaline phosphatase elevation. Medicine, *58*:385, 1979.

MacGregor, I., Parent, J., and Meyer, J. H.: Gastric emptying of liquid meals and pancreatic and biliary secretion after subtotal gastrectomy or truncal vagotomy and pyloroplasty in man. Gastroenterology, *72*:195, 206, 1977.

Mallory, A., and Kern, F.: Drug-induced pancreatitis: a critical review. Gastroenterology, *78*:813, 1980.

Meyer, C. T., Troncale, F. J., Galloway, S., and Sheahan, D. G.: Arteriovenous malformations of the bowel: an analysis of 22 cases and a review of the literature. Medicine, *60*:36, 1981.

Meyers, M. A., Alonso, D. R., Gray, G. F., et al.: Pathogenesis of bleeding colonic diverticulosis. Gastroenterology, *71*:577, 1976.

Moody, F. G.: Current concepts — rectal bleeding. N. Engl. J. Med., *290*:839, 1974.

Nabseth, D. C.: The distal splenorenal shunt: an enigma. Am. J. Surg., *141*:579, 1981.

Rikkers, L. F., Rudman, D., Galambos, J. T., et al.: A randomized controlled trial of the distal splenorenal shunt. Ann. Surg., *188*:271, 1978.

Rotter, J. I., Sones, J. Q., Samloff, I. M., et al.: Duodenal ulcer disease associated with elevated serum pepsinogen I. N. Engl. J. Med., *300*:63, 1979.

Rubin, E., and Lieber, C. S.: Fatty liver, alcoholic hepatitis and cirrhosis produced by alcohol in primates. N. Engl. J. Med., *290*:128, 1974.

Said, S. I., and Faloona, G. R.: Elevated plasma and tissue levels of vasoactive intestinal polypeptide in the watery-diarrhea syndrome due to pancreatic, bronchogenic and other tumors. N. Engl. J. Med., *293*:155, 1975.

Salt, W. B., II, and Schenker, S.: Amylase — its clinical significance: a review of the literature. Medicine, *55*:269, 1976.

Scharschmidt, B. F.: The natural history of hypertrophic gastropathy (Menetrier's disease). Am. J. Med., *63*:644, 1978.

Schiff, L. (ed.): Diseases of the Liver. Philadelphia, J. B. Lippincott Company, 1975.

Sharp, H. L.: The current status of α-1-antitrypsin, a protease inhibitor, in gastrointestinal disease. Gastroenterology, *70*:611, 1976.

Sheehy, T. W.: Sickle cell hepatopathy. South. Med. J., *70*:533, 1977.

Silvoso, G. R., Ivey, K. J., Butt, J. H., et al.: Incidence of gastric lesions in patients with rheumatic disease on chronic aspirin therapy. Ann. Intern. Med., *91*:517, 1979.

Sleisenger, M. H., and Brandborg, L. L.: Malabsorption. Philadelphia, W. B. Saunders Company, 1977.

Sleisenger, M. H., and Fordtran, J. S. (eds.): Gastrointestinal Disease. 2nd ed. Philadelphia, W. B. Saunders Company, 1978.

Sturdevant, R. A. L., Singleton, J. W., Derer, J. J., et al.: Azathioprine-related pancreatitis in patients with Crohn's disease. Gastroenterology, *77*:883, 1979.

Tonz, O., Weiss, S., Strahm, H. W., and Rossi, E.: Iron absorption in cystic fibrosis. Lancet, *2*:1096, 1965.

Turner, J. A., and Rapoport, J.: Myxoedema ascites. Postgrad. Med. J., *53*:343, 1977.

Vantrappen, G., Agg, H. O., Ponette, E., et al.: *Yersinia* enteritis and enterocolitis: gastroenterological aspects. Gastroenterology, *72*:220, 1977.

Walsh, J. H., and Grossman, M. I.: Gastrin. N. Engl. J. Med., *292*:1324, 1975.

Warshaw, A. L., Schapiro, R. H., Ferrucci, J. T., Jr., et al.: Persistent obstructive jaundice, cholangitis, and biliary cirrhosis due to common bile duct stenosis in chronic pancreatitis. Gastroenterology, *70*:562, 1976.

Wolkoff, A. W., Cohen, L. E., and Arias, I. M.: Inheritance of the Dubin-Johnson syndrome. N. Engl. J. Med., *288*:113, 1972.

Wright, R., Alberti, K. G. M. M., Karran, S., and Millward-Sadler, G. H.: Liver and Biliary Disease. Philadelphia, W. B. Saunders Company, 1979.

PART 5

HEMATOLOGY AND ONCOLOGY

Gerald Logue

DIRECTIONS: For questions 1 to 28, choose the ONE BEST answer to each question.

1. The prognosis of patients with beta-thalassemia major is determined primarily by which one of the following factors?

A. Amount of hemoglobin F in peripheral blood
B. Degree of hepatic dysfunction
C. Degree of endocrine dysfunction
D. Degree of cardiac disease

2. Which one of the following facilitates oxygen release at the tissues, and thus shifts the oxygen-hemoglobin dissociation curve to the right?

A. Fall in temperature
B. Fall in intraerythrocyte 2,3-diphosphoglycerate (DPG) concentration
C. Increase in carbon dioxide concentration
D. Increase in pH

3. Which of the following would be LEAST important during the initial evaluation of a patient with anemia and hemoglobinuria?

A. Detailed drug history
B. Microscopic examination of peripheral blood
C. Examination of urine sediment
D. Examination of bone marrow
E. Coombs' test (antiglobulin test)

4. Which of the following would be LEAST important during the initial evaluation of a patient with erythrocytosis?

A. Arterial blood gases
B. Liver-spleen scan
C. ^{51}Cr measurement of red cell mass
D. Bone marrow aspiration and biopsy

5. Which of the following statements regarding chronic myelogenous leukemia (CML) is correct?

A. The disease usually follows an indolent course, and patients frequently survive eight to ten years or longer from the time of diagnosis
B. Anemia, if present at disease onset, usually persists for the duration of disease whether or not chemotherapy is given
C. Virtually any agent that can cause leukopenia can be used in the initial treatment of CML
D. The survival rate of patients with CML has improved remarkably with the advent of chemotherapy

6. Which of the following is characteristic of *both* childhood (acute) idiopathic thrombocytopenic purpura (ITP) *and* adult (chronic) ITP?

A. Most patients will respond to high-dose corticosteroid therapy
B. Splenectomy is usually required
C. Frequently seen following viral illness
D. Increased incidence in patients with lymphoproliferative diseases

7. Which of the following is an indication for splenectomy in a patient with Felty's syndrome?

A. Neutrophil count less than 0.5×10^9/liter
B. Recurrent bacterial infection
C. Thrombocytopenia
D. Worsening of the arthritis

8. Which one of the following would EXCLUDE a diagnosis of iron deficiency?

A. Normal mean corpuscular volume (MCV)
B. Normal percentage saturation of serum iron-binding capacity
C. Normal serum ferritin
D. Normal bone marrow iron stores

9. Which one of the following findings would be useful in differentiating infectious mononucleosis from cytomegalovirus infection?

A. Abnormal liver function studies
B. Splenomegaly
C. Pharyngitis
D. Atypical mononuclear cells in the peripheral blood

10. Which of the following statements regarding the hemorrhagic diathesis of diffuse liver disease is correct?

A. Vitamin K is usually beneficial
B. The euglobulin lysis time is usually normal
C. Qualitative or quantitative platelet defects are common
D. Vitamin K–dependent clotting factor concentrates are useful in treatment

QUESTIONS 11–15

A 36-year-old woman has a left breast mass, which she discovered by self-examination. She is relatively certain that the nodule was not present two months ago. She is otherwise without symptoms. On physical examination, a firm 2 × 2–cm nodule is present in the upper outer quadrant of the left breast.

11. Which of the following groups of diagnostic procedures is most appropriate in the initial preoperative evaluation?

A. Roentgenograms of the chest and skeleton, serum alkaline phosphatase

B. Roentgenograms of the chest and skeleton, radionuclide bone scan
C. Roentgenogram of the chest, radionuclide bone scan, serum alkaline phosphatase
D. Roentgenogram of the chest, radionuclide bone scan, bone marrow biopsy

12. Biopsy of the lesion reveals moderately well-differentiated carcinoma, and the tumor is found to be estrogen receptor–positive. The patient undergoes mastectomy but refuses further therapy; eight months later she begins to have rib pain. Bone scan is positive in multiple areas, and biopsy of the rib lesion reveals metastatic adenocarcinoma. Which one of the following forms of therapy would you choose?

A. Surgical oophorectomy alone
B. Chemotherapy alone
C. Surgical oophorectomy and chemotherapy
D. Local radiation therapy to painful bone lesions alone

13. The patient receives appropriate therapy but continues to have pain, which is well controlled with Percodan. Two weeks later she develops gastrointestinal bleeding requiring multiple red cell transfusions. Which of the following statements regarding gastrointestinal bleeding in this patient is correct?

A. Breast cancer rarely metastasizes to the gastrointestinal tract
B. Since the pain is well controlled with Percodan, this medication should be continued
C. Platelet function studies will probably be normal
D. Stress ulcers are common in this type of patient

14. The patient's gastrointestinal bleeding stops. She refuses further chemotherapy. Which of the following courses of action is most appropriate?

A. Advise her that an adequate trial of chemotherapy has not been completed and that you will be unable to treat her further unless she agrees to follow your instructions
B. Although an adequate trial of chemotherapy has not been completed, you should agree to continue to provide her with symptomatic care, and the possibility of subsequent chemotherapy should not be discussed further
C. You should agree to withhold chemotherapy but provide whatever supportive care seems appropriate; it is also appropriate to discuss the possibility of continuing chemotherapy on subsequent visits
D. Obtain a psychiatric consultation

15. Which of the following statements regarding estrogen receptors in breast tumors is correct?

A. Measurement of estrogen receptors in human breast tumors is principally a research tool with, as yet, little clinical application
B. Lack of estrogen receptors in tumors of premenopausal women means that hormone manipulation will have a less than 10% chance of being beneficial
C. The presence of estrogen receptors in tumors of premenopausal women means that hormonal manipulation has a greater than 90% chance of being beneficial
D. If a primary tumor has estrogen receptors, metastatic tumors can also be expected to have them

16. Which of the following statements regarding histopathologic diagnosis and classification of Hodgkin's disease is correct?

A. Older patients with systemic symptoms are likely to have lymphocyte-predominant type
B. Patients between the ages of 15 and 35 years who have predominantly mediastinal involvement are likely to have nodular sclerosis type
C. Although Reed-Sternberg cells are characteristic of Hodgkin's disease, they need not be identified to establish this diagnosis
D. The histopathologic subclassifications of lymphocyte-predominant type, nodular sclerosis type, mixed cellularity type, and lymphocyte-depletion type are clearly different clinical entities

17. Which of the following statements regarding staging laparotomy with splenectomy in a patient with Hodgkin's disease is correct?

A. Splenic involvement with Hodgkin's disease represents stage IV disease
B. Liver biopsy is not indicated if the spleen is enlarged
C. Splenectomy will allow the patient to tolerate larger doses of chemotherapy or radiation therapy
D. Splenectomy increases the risk of systemic bacterial infections

18. Which of the following is a complication of coumarin therapy?

A. Necrotic skin ulcers
B. Thrombocytopenia
C. Bone marrow depression
D. Hepatocellular dysfunction

19. Which one of the following is associated with chronic aplastic anemia?

A. Hereditary spherocytosis
B. Paroxysmal nocturnal hemoglobinuria
C. Glucose-6-phosphate dehydrogenase (G6PD) deficiency
D. Sickle cell disease

20. Which of the following is a characteristic of megaloblastic cell maturation?

A. Tritiated thymidine incorporation into DNA is markedly diminished
B. RNA synthesis is normal or increased
C. Protein synthesis is decreased
D. Impairment of DNA synthesis is restricted to erythroid precursors

21. Severe hypophosphatemia causes which one of the following hematologic abnormalities?

A. Hemolytic anemia
B. Disseminated intravascular coagulation
C. Granulocyte dysfunction
D. Bone marrow suppression

22. Which one of the following best describes the sequence of changes observed as iron deficiency develops?

A. Decreased plasma iron concentration, mobilization and depletion of marrow iron stores, anemia, hypochromia
B. Decreased plasma iron concentration, anemia, mobilization and depletion of marrow iron stores, hypochromia

C. Mobilization and depletion of marrow iron stores, anemia, hypochromia, decreased plasma iron concentration
D. Mobilization and depletion of marrow iron stores, decreased plasma iron concentration, anemia, hypochromia
E. Mobilization and depletion of marrow iron stores, decreased plasma iron concentration, hypochromia, anemia

23. The presence of which one of the following abnormalities would eliminate the need for staging laparotomy in a patient with Hodgkin's disease?

A. Pleural effusion
B. Abnormal lymphangiogram
C. Reed-Sternberg cells on bone marrow biopsy
D. Splenic enlargement

24. Which of the following is NOT associated with an increased incidence of breast cancer?

A. Obesity
B. Early pregnancy
C. Previous history of breast cancer
D. Family history of breast cancer

25. Which of the following is the primary treatment for hemolysis in patients with cold agglutinin disease?

A. Splenectomy
B. Corticosteroids
C. Avoidance of cold exposure
D. Chlorambucil

26. All the following historical findings are useful in distinguishing thrombocytopenia due to decreased production of platelets from thrombocytopenia due to shortened platelet survival EXCEPT

A. multiple congenital skeletal abnormalities
B. quinine ingestion
C. blood transfusion within the previous week
D. photosensitive dermatitis
E. thiazide diuretic therapy

27. Which of the following is the most common cause of immediate hemolytic transfusion reaction?

A. Improper temperature control during blood storage
B. Improper identification of blood samples, donor bags, or patients
C. Improper identification of minor blood group antigens
D. Transfusion of whole blood rather than packed red cells

28. Which of the following procedures establishes the diagnosis of chronic lymphocytic leukemia?

A. Lymph node biopsy
B. Microscopic examination of peripheral blood
C. Bone marrow aspiration and biopsy
D. Serum protein electrophoresis

DIRECTIONS: For questions 29 to 86, you are to decide whether EACH choice is true or false. Any combination of answers, from all true to all false, may be present. Mark the answer sheet "T" or "F" in the space provided.

29. In which of the following diseases would the serum folate level be expected to be low?

A. Aplastic anemia
B. Iron deficiency
C. Pyruvate kinase deficiency
D. Vitamin B_{12} deficiency
E. Acute leukemia

30. The mean corpuscular volume (MCV) would usually be increased in which of the following diseases?

A. Chronic anemia of renal disease
B. Pernicious anemia
C. Aplastic anemia
D. Chronic anemia of liver disease
E. Thalassemia

31. Which of the following statements regarding the treatment of acute leukemia is/are correct?

A. For both acute lymphoblastic and acute myelogenous leukemia, initial chemotherapy (induction therapy) is intended to produce an abrupt lowering of the number of leukemic cells in the blood and bone marrow
B. "Prophylactic" platelet transfusions every two to three days are indicated when the platelet count falls below 20,000/cu mm
C. Following successful initial treatment (induction therapy) of acute leukemia, prophylactic central nervous system therapy is indicated in both acute myelogenous and acute lymphoblastic leukemia
D. Immunization of patients in remission with killed leukemic cells or with BCG appears to be useful in prolonging remission of both acute myelogenous and acute lymphoblastic leukemia

32. Which of the following statements regarding cancer of the prostate is/are correct?

A. Every reasonable measure should be taken to eradicate a tumor that is localized to the pelvis
B. Serum acid phosphatase is elevated in more than 90% of patients with distant metastatic disease
C. Estrogen therapy usually prolongs life in patients with prostatic cancer
D. Estrogen therapy or orchiectomy provides palliation in more than 50% of patients with metastatic disease

33. Which of the following statements regarding human chorionic gonadotropin (HCG) is/are correct?

A. HCG measurements are extremely important in the management of patients with trophoblastic tumors
B. Specific sensitive assays for this glycoprotein require antisera directed against the beta subunit of the molecule
C. HCG and alpha-fetoprotein always rise and fall simultaneously in the plasma of patients with trophoblastic tumors
D. HCG may be detected in patients with gastric or pulmonary cancer

34. An increase in the proportion of fetal hemoglobin in peripheral blood occurs in which of the following conditions?

A. Beta-thalassemia
B. Myelofibrosis
C. Acute leukemia
D. Severe anemia from blood loss

35. Which of the following statements regarding vitamin K deficiency is/are correct?

A. It impairs the synthesis of the polypeptide precursors of factors II, VII, IX, and X
B. It is usually attributable to an inadequate diet
C. It is common in malabsorption syndromes such as sprue or celiac disease
D. A significantly prolonged prothrombin time establishes the diagnosis

36. Which of the following statements regarding untoward effects of coumarin is/are correct?

A. Salicylates decrease the effects of coumarin upon the clotting system
B. Subarachnoid bleeding is a frequent complication of coumarin overdose
C. Only vitamin K_1 is effective in reversing the effects of the coumarin derivatives
D. Infusion of fresh-frozen plasma or vitamin K–dependent factor concentrates is the most rapid means of correcting the coagulation abnormalities

37. Which of the following immune abnormalities is/are associated with Hodgkin's disease?

A. Impaired mitogen-induced lymphocyte transformation
B. Autoimmune hemolytic anemia
C. Immune thrombocytopenic purpura
D. Hypergammaglobulinemia

38. Which of the following statements concerning immune hemolytic anemia resulting from methyldopa is/are correct?

A. The antibodies formed usually have specificity for Rh red cell antigens
B. Antiglobulin testing (Coombs' test) will reveal IgG without complement on the red cells
C. Severe hemolysis is common
D. The direct antiglobulin test (direct Coombs' test) usually becomes negative within one month of discontinuing the drug

39. Which of the following statements regarding immunologic function in patients with Hodgkin's disease is/are correct?

A. These patients have a higher frequency of cutaneous anergy than do normal individuals
B. Loss of immunologic function is more severe with advanced or extensive disease
C. Absolute lymphopenia in the peripheral blood is common
D. The immunologic deficiency usually worsens with chemotherapy

QUESTIONS 40–42

A 56-year-old man who had a subtotal gastrectomy and Billroth II procedure nine years ago now has fatigue and dyspnea on exertion; he is found to be anemic.

40. Which of the following physical findings would be helpful in differentiating iron deficiency from vitamin B_{12} deficiency in this patient?

A. Papilledema
B. Glossitis
C. Dysphagia
D. Splenomegaly

41. Which of the following laboratory findings would be helpful in differentiating iron deficiency from vitamin B_{12} deficiency in this patient?

A. Thrombocytopenia
B. Thrombocytosis
C. Elevated serum lactic dehydrogenase
D. Elevated blood urea nitrogen

42. Which of the following statements regarding iron therapy for iron deficiency is/are correct?

A. Since the patient has had a gastrectomy, initial therapy should include parenteral iron
B. Enteric-coated iron preparations are often useful in this clinical setting
C. Iron therapy may be discontinued as soon as the red blood count has returned to normal
D. Symptomatic improvement is often observed within 48 hours of initiation of iron therapy

---

43. Which of the following laboratory tests is/are characteristically *abnormal* in chronic myelogenous leukemia and polycythemia vera?

A. Basophil count
B. Red cell osmotic fragility
C. Serum vitamin B_{12} level
D. Serum iron concentration

44. Which of the following is/are characteristic of an immediate hemolytic transfusion reaction?

A. Chills, fever, and severe abdominal pain, back pain, or headache
B. Inability to maintain hemostasis during surgery
C. Dark brown appearance of plasma (methemoglobinemia) 12 to 24 hours after transfusion
D. Urticaria

45. Which of the following immunologic complications is/are associated with chronic lymphocytic leukemia?

A. Autoimmune hemolytic anemia
B. Autoimmune thrombocytopenia
C. Hypogammaglobulinemia
D. Monoclonal immunoglobulinopathy

46. Which of the following statements regarding hairy cell leukemia is/are true?

A. Splenic enlargement and pancytopenia are the most common presenting features
B. Alkylating agents and corticosteroids are usually beneficial
C. Splenectomy will benefit most patients, but relapse is frequent
D. Intensive leukapheresis is beneficial in patients with a large number of circulating hairy cells

QUESTIONS 47–48

A 56-year-old man is found to be anemic during a routine physical examination. Red cell rouleaux are identified on peripheral blood film; serum protein electrophoresis reveals a homogeneous monoclonal serum protein.

47. Which of the following clinical findings would be useful in differentiating multiple myeloma from other plasma cell dyscrasias in this patient?

A. Generalized osteoporosis on skeletal films
B. Long history of biliary tract disease
C. Hypercalcemia
D. Renal insufficiency

48. The patient is found to have an IgG paraprotein in the serum, and bone marrow examination shows 40% atypical-appearing plasma cells. Which of the following statements regarding these plasma cells is/are correct?

A. They synthesize an IgG paraprotein of only one light-chain type
B. Their numbers will be proportional to the amount of abnormal protein in the serum or urine
C. They may produce an antibody directed against a specific antigen
D. The diagnosis of multiple myeloma can be established by the morphology of these cells alone

---

49. Which of the following statements regarding the treatment of chronic lymphocytic leukemia is/are correct?

A. Asymptomatic patients should not be treated until the disease progresses
B. Corticosteroids are most effective for acute immune complications
C. Extended field radiation therapy is beneficial
D. Administration of gamma globulin is useful for patients with hypogammaglobulinemia and recurrent infections

50. Side effects of busulfan include which of the following?

A. Gonadal failure and hyperpigmentation
B. Cardiac toxicity
C. Progressive pulmonary fibrosis
D. Prolonged profound thrombocytopenia

51. Which of the following is/are likely to be useful in predicting relapse in patients with previously treated Hodgkin's disease?

A. Serum protein electrophoresis
B. Erythrocyte sedimentation rate
C. Leukocyte alkaline phosphatase
D. Serum copper
E. Urinary lysozyme

52. Which of the following statements regarding iron absorption is/are correct?

A. Ferrous salts are absorbed better than ferric compounds
B. Ascorbic acid enhances iron absorption
C. Food substances such as phytates and phosphates interfere with iron absorption
D. Iron absorption is enhanced when intestinal luminal contents are at acid or neutral pH

53. Which of the following statements regarding patients with an unstable hemoglobin variant is/are true?

A. Hemolysis often follows ingestion of drugs
B. Hemoglobin electrophoresis is frequently normal
C. Heinz bodies are often found in the peripheral blood
D. Inheritance is autosomal recessive

QUESTIONS 54–55

A 26-year-old woman has noted painless swelling in the left neck and axilla. On physical examination, enlarged, painless, discrete lymph nodes are palpable in the left cervical, supraclavicular, and axillary regions

54. Which of the following findings would be useful in distinguishing Hodgkin's disease from non-Hodgkin's lymphoma in this patient?

A. Involvement of the oropharynx or nasopharynx
B. Spinal cord compression from extradural tumor
C. Involvement of mesenteric lymph nodes
D. Autoimmune hemolytic anemia

55. Which of the following diagnostic procedures would be useful in determining the extent of Hodgkin's disease in this patient?

A. Lymphangiogram
B. Bone marrow biopsy
C. Brain scan
D. Liver-spleen scan

---

56. Causes of acute intravascular hemolysis include which of the following?

A. Clostridial toxins
B. Copper
C. Certain poisonous mushrooms
D. Arsenic

57. Which of the following mechanisms is/are important in the pathogenesis of the anemia of chronic systemic disease?

A. Shortened red cell lifespan
B. Ineffective erythropoiesis
C. Failure of bone marrow to increase erythropoiesis to compensate for anemia
D. Impaired release of iron from reticuloendothelial cells

58. Which of the following is/are associated with vitamin B_{12} deficiency?

A. Paresthesias
B. Paranoid ideation
C. Loss of vibratory sense
D. Difficulty in swallowing

59. Schistocytes are usually seen in the peripheral blood of patients with which of the following disorders?

A. Malignant hypertension
B. Rocky Mountain spotted fever
C. Periarteritis nodosa
D. March hemoglobinuria

60. Which of the following statements regarding hereditary elliptocytosis is/are true?

A. Most affected individuals manifest hemolysis
B. Splenectomy is usually required
C. Hypersplenism and mild thrombocytopenia are common
D. It is associated with hereditary spherocytosis in some families

61. Which of the following should be done if a hemolytic transfusion reaction is suspected?

A. Immediately stop transfusion and send samples of donor and recipient blood to the blood bank for further studies
B. Initiate procedures to maintain urinary flow at or above 100 ml/hour
C. Initiate procedures to maintain systolic blood pressure at or above 100 mm Hg
D. If oliguria persists beyond 24 hours, maintain fluid intake above 2000 ml/day

62. Thalassemic syndromes include which of the following?

A. Diamond-Blackfan syndrome
B. Hemoglobin Constant Spring
C. Hemoglobin Kempsey
D. Hemoglobin H disease

63. Which of the following statements regarding sideroblastic anemia is/are true?

A. Hereditary forms are usually X-linked
B. Various antituberculous agents cause sideroblastic anemia
C. Acute leukemia occurs in about 10% of patients with primary disease
D. It is frequently associated with hemochromatosis
E. It can be induced by acute alcohol intoxication

64. Which of the following statements regarding hypercalcemia of neoplastic disease is/are correct?

A. Hypercalcemia in association with neoplasms of the lung indicates metastatic disease
B. Polyuria and polydipsia are common early symptoms of hypercalcemia
C. Metabolically active tumor products such as prostaglandins cause the hypercalcemia in some patients
D. Urinary and serum phosphate levels in patients with hypercalcemia of neoplastic disease are similar to those of patients with primary hyperparathyroidism

65. Which of the following statements regarding idiopathic thrombocytopenic purpura (ITP) is/are correct?

A. Platelet survival time is decreased in patients with ITP
B. Infants born to women with ITP are frequently thrombocytopenic
C. Infusion of plasma from patients with ITP produces severe thrombocytopenia in normal subjects
D. Cultured splenic cells of patients with ITP produce antiplatelet antibodies

66. Clinical features of the anemia of chronic disease include which of the following?

A. Reticulocytopenia
B. Reduced serum ferritin
C. Increased bone marrow cellularity
D. Thrombocytopenia

67. Which of the following statements regarding glucose-6-phosphate dehydrogenase (G6PD) is/are correct?

A. Type B G6PD is considered to be the normal form of the enzyme and is found in approximately 70% of blacks and nearly all whites
B. Type A G6PD is a rapidly moving electrophoretic variant seen in approximately 30% of blacks
C. Most blacks with G6PD deficiency have electrophoretic type B enzyme
D. Inheritance of G6PD deficiency is autosomal recessive

68. Which of the following statements concerning chloramphenicol is/are correct?

A. Even brief exposure to chloramphenicol can induce aplastic anemia
B. It is the drug most commonly associated with aplastic anemia
C. The dose-related bone marrow toxicity of chloramphenicol is reversible
D. Chloramphenicol-induced aplastic anemia is usually milder than other forms of aplastic anemia

69. Causes of methemoglobinemia (oxidation of the iron in heme to the ferric form) include which of the following?

A. Prolonged inspiration of high concentrations of oxygen
B. Exposure to potent oxidizing chemicals
C. Amino acid substitutions in the heme pocket of the globin chain
D. Inherited red cell enzyme deficiency

70. Stomatocytosis is seen in which of the following clinical settings?

A. Autoimmune hemolytic anemia
B. As an autosomal dominant inherited disorder
C. Following splenectomy
D. Alcoholic liver disease

71. Which of the following laboratory abnormalities is/are associated with thalassemia trait?

A. Decreased mean corpuscular volume (MCV)
B. Increased hemoglobin A_2 or hemoglobin F
C. Low reticulocyte count
D. Thrombocytopenia

72. Which of the following statements regarding the Schilling test is/are correct?

A. Abnormal Schilling test documents vitamin B_{12} deficiency
B. Vitamin B_{12} deficiency can cause reversible abnormalities in the second part of the Schilling test (with intrinsic factor)
C. It is seldom necessary to repeat an abnormal Schilling test obtained when a patient is anemic
D. The Schilling test itself will alter serum vitamin B_{12} levels

73. Which of the following statements regarding adults with homozygous hemoglobin SS disease is/are correct?

A. Splenomegaly is common
B. Chronic, nonhealing leg ulcers are a common complication
C. Pregnancy is seldom concluded successfully
D. Hepatomegaly is common

74. Which of the following findings is/are useful in distinguishing acute myelogenous leukemia from acute lymphoblastic leukemia?

A. Positive staining of the leukemic cells with peroxidase and Sudan black
B. Presence of terminal deoxyribose transferase (TDT) in the leukemic cells
C. The morphologic finding of Auer rods on blood smear
D. Severe anemia and thrombocytopenia

75. Which of the following diseases can be expected to respond favorably to splenectomy?

A. Warm-reacting IgG autoimmune hemolytic anemia
B. Cold agglutinin disease
C. Immune thrombocytopenic purpura
D. Hairy cell leukemia

76. Which of the following statements concerning the differentiation of myoglobinuria from hemoglobinuria is/are correct?

A. Benzidine reagents will give a negative reaction in a patient with myoglobinuria
B. Simple chemical procedures differentiate myoglobin from hemoglobin on the basis of their molecular size
C. Syndromes that cause myoglobinuria are usually asymptomatic
D. Myoglobinuria can often be distinguished from hemoglobinuria by examining the color of the patient's plasma

77. Which of the following findings would be useful in differentiating polycythemia vera from secondary polycythemia?

A. Normal hemoglobin electrophoretic pattern
B. Elevated erythropoietin activity in serum or urine
C. Elevated serum uric acid level
D. Family history of polycythemia

78. Which of the following findings would be useful in differentiating a leukemoid reaction from chronic myelogenous leukemia?

A. Anemia
B. Elevated leukocyte alkaline phosphatase
C. Splenic enlargement
D. Bone marrow hypercellularity with an increase in granulocyte precursors

79. Which of the following is/are associated with pure red cell aplasia?

A. Acute leukemia
B. Thymoma
C. Low serum erythropoietin levels
D. Serum antibodies directed against red cell precursors

80. Which of the following statements regarding the Philadelphia chromosome (Ph^1 chromosome) is/are correct?

A. It is found in a variety of hematologic disorders in addition to chronic myelogenous leukemia
B. Ph^1-positive marrow cells often persist during chemotherapy-induced remission of chronic myelogenous leukemia
C. Patients without the Philadelphia chromosome, who otherwise appear to have chronic leukemia,

have a better prognosis than patients with this chromosomal abnormality
D. It is caused by translocation of a portion of chromosome 22, usually to chromosome 9

81. Which of the following statements about nodular non-Hodgkin's lymphoma is/are true?

A. Chemotherapy frequently produces complete remission
B. Five-year survival is greater than for diffuse non-Hodgkin's lymphoma
C. It is frequently localized to one lymph node area (stage I)
D. It frequently involves mesenteric lymph nodes

82. Characteristics of hereditary spherocytosis include which of the following?

A. Autosomal recessive inheritance
B. Diagnosis usually established by examination of the peripheral blood smear
C. Usually detected in childhood
D. Splenectomy benefits patients with severe hemolysis or massive splenomegaly

83. Which of the following statements regarding histiocytic lymphoma is/are true?

A. Complete response to chemotherapy with a prolonged, disease-free interval occurs in approximately 50% of patients
B. When it is isolated to one anatomic area, radiation therapy is indicated
C. It may present with signs and symptoms of gastric carcinoma
D. It frequently progresses to a leukemic phase late in the course of disease

84. Which of the following statements regarding eosinophilia is/are correct?

A. Eosinophilic leukemoid reactions are often seen in allergic drug reactions
B. Benign eosinophilic leukemoid reactions are usually associated with proliferation of immature eosinophilic precursors in the bone marrow
C. Eosinophilia, in conjunction with an elevated white blood cell count, is usually indicative of some type of leukemia
D. Measurement of leukocyte alkaline phosphatase activity is useful in distinguishing chronic eosinophilic leukemia from an eosinophilic leukemoid reaction

85. Which of the following statements regarding the treatment of chronic idiopathic thrombocytopenic purpura (ITP) is/are correct?

A. Empiric therapy with vincristine will produce remission of thrombocytopenia in some patients
B. Prophylactic platelet transfusions are useful to prevent major bleeding episodes
C. Recurrent hemorrhage during the menses should be treated by hysterectomy
D. Approximately 20% of patients do not respond to splenectomy

86. Which of the following statements regarding polycythemia vera is/are true?

A. Progression to acute leukemia is unrelated to the form of therapy used to control the early phase of the illness
B. It is extremely rare for polycythemia vera to transform into myelofibrosis
C. Upper gastrointestinal hemorrhage occurs in approximately 10% of patients with polycythemia vera
D. Hyperuricemia associated with polycythemia vera does not require therapy with allopurinol unless overt clinical gout is present

DIRECTIONS: Questions 87 to 166 are matching questions. For each numbered item, choose the most likely associated lettered item from those provided. Each numbered item has ONLY ONE answer. Within each group, each lettered item may be the answer to one, more than one, or none of the numbered items.

QUESTIONS 87–94

For each of the following diseases, select the drug, used either alone or in combination with other drugs, that is most appropriate for initial treatment.

A. *Cis*-platinum
B. Hydroxyurea
C. Methotrexate
D. Cytosine arabinoside
E. Procarbazine (Matulane)
F. Doxorubicin (Adriamycin)
G. Melphalan
H. Chlorambucil

87. Hodgkin's disease

88. Multiple myeloma

89. Diffuse histiocytic lymphoma

90. Chronic lymphocytic leukemia

91. Macroglobulinemia

92. Acute myelogenous leukemia

93. Osteogenic sarcoma

94. Testicular carcinoma

QUESTIONS 95–101

For each of the following diseases, select the most likely type of neoplastic cell proliferation.

A. Proliferation of B lymphocytes
B. Proliferation of T lymphocytes
C. Proliferation of both B and T lymphocytes
D. Proliferation of neither B nor T lymphocytes

95. Histiocytic lymphoma

96. Mycosis fungoides

97. Hairy cell leukemia

98. Chronic lymphocytic leukemia

99. Nodular, poorly differentiated lymphocytic lymphoma

100. Sézary syndrome

101. Waldenström's macroglobulinemia

QUESTIONS 102–107

For each of the following characteristics, select the most likely type of lung cancer.

A. Oat cell carcinoma of the lung
B. Epidermoid carcinoma of the lung
C. Associated approximately equally with both of these
D. Not associated with either of these

102. Hypercalcemia

103. Carcinomatous meningitis

104. One-year history of positive sputum cytology without localization of primary tumor

105. Overall five-year survival rate of 10–15%

106. Postobstructive pneumonia

107. Greater than 50% objective response rate to cytotoxic chemotherapy

QUESTIONS 108–112

Select the type of transfusion reaction best described by each statement.

A. Post-transfusion purpura
B. Urticarial transfusion reaction
C. Febrile transfusion reaction
D. Delayed hemolytic transfusion reaction
E. Anaphylactic reaction to transfused blood

108. Usually caused by incompatibilities of minor blood group antigens

109. Frequently caused by sensitivity to donor leukocytes

110. Caused by anti-IgA antibodies

111. Patients who have had this form of reaction can be safely transfused only with red cells that have been extensively washed, such as those that have been stored frozen and repeatedly washed during thawing

112. A rare reaction that may be seen in women who have not had previous transfusion

QUESTIONS 113–117

For each of the following statements, select the most likely associated type of hemoglobinopathy.

A. Hemoglobin S–beta-thalassemia (sickle cell–thalassemia)
B. Hemoglobin SC
C. Hemoglobin SD–Punjab
D. Hemoglobin CC

113. Second most frequent symptomatic hemoglobinopathy found in blacks

114. Commonly associated with asymptomatic splenomegaly

115. Associated with important ophthalmologic complications that require periodic evaluation

116. Occurs frequently in nonblacks

117. Patients often have detectable hemoglobin A

QUESTIONS 118–124

For each of the following, select the best classification

A. Pluripotent bone marrow stem cell disorder
B. Committed bone marrow stem cell disorder
C. Not a disorder of bone marrow stem cells

118. Paroxysmal nocturnal hemoglobinuria

119. Chronic granulocytic leukemia

120. Fanconi's anemia

121. Acquired pure red cell aplasia of adults

122. Diamond-Blackfan syndrome

123. Cyclic neutropenia

124. Neonatal neutropenia

QUESTIONS 125–128

For each of the following findings, select the most commonly associated type of immunoprotein abnormality.

A. Light chain (Bence Jones protein)
B. IgA heavy chain (alpha-chain disease)
C. Monoclonal IgA
D. Monoclonal IgM
E. Monoclonal IgG

125. Hyperviscosity

126. Lymphadenopathy and splenomegaly

127. Chronic diarrhea and malabsorption

128. Renal failure

QUESTIONS 129–133

For each of the following statements, select the type of glucose-6-phosphate dehydrogenase (G6PD) deficiency it best describes.

A. G6PD deficiency seen in black patients
B. G6PD deficiency seen in white patients
C. G6PD deficiency seen in both black and white patients

129. Young red cells have normal G6PD activity

130. Chronic hemolytic anemia occurs in the absence of drug exposure

131. Sex-linked disorder

132. Brisk hemolytic anemia occurs upon ingestion of fava beans

133. Heinz bodies are seen

QUESTIONS 134–138

For each of the following characteristics, select the type of deficiency it best describes.

A. Vitamin B_{12} deficiency
B. Folate deficiency
C. *Both* vitamin B_{12} *and* folate deficiency
D. *Neither* vitamin B_{12} *nor* folate deficiency

134. Commonly results from dietary deficiency

135. Frequently associated with autoantibodies

136. Therapeutic trial is useful to document the deficiency

137. Complication of hemolytic anemia

138. A number of drugs interfere with absorption and produce deficiency

QUESTIONS 139–143

For each of the following, select the coagulation abnormality it best describes.

A. Congenital dysfibrinogenemia
B. Congenital deficiency of fibrinogen
C. Factor VII deficiency
D. Factor IX deficiency
E. Factor XII deficiency
F. Factor XIII deficiency

139. Treatment requires frequent large-dose factor replacement

140. Slow wound healing is a common manifestation

141. Usually asymptomatic

142. Sex-linked inheritance

143. Associated with platelet function abnormalities

QUESTIONS 144–147

For each of the following, select the red cell enzyme deficiency it best describes.

A. Lactate dehydrogenase deficiency
B. Phosphoglycerate kinase deficiency
C. Pyruvate kinase deficiency
D. Triosephosphate isomerase deficiency

144. Adult patients with enlarged spleens and crenated red cells in the peripheral blood

145. The most common glycolytic pathway enzyme deficiency

146. Sex-linked inherited disorder

147. Patients usually die in childhood of a progressive neurologic disease

QUESTIONS 148–152

For each of the following statements, select the abnormality it best describes.

A. Factor VIII deficiency (classic hemophilia)
B. von Willebrand's disease
C. Both factor VIII deficiency and von Willebrand's disease
D. Neither factor VIII deficiency nor von Willebrand's disease

148. Low factor VIII antigen in plasma

149. Platelet function abnormalities

150. Abnormal prothrombin time

151. Autosomal dominant inheritance

152. Patients should avoid salicylates

QUESTIONS 153–156

Immune hemolytic anemia is associated with each of the following disorders. For each disorder, select the immunoprotein that is usually found on the patient's red cells when immune hemolysis is present. (Direct antiglobulin [Coombs'] test is positive in each case.)

A. Immunoglobulin G (IgG) only
B. Complement components only
C. IgG *and* complement components
D. Neither IgG nor complement components

153. Systemic lupus erythematosus

154. Methyldopa-induced autoimmune hemolytic anemia

155. "Innocent bystander" immune hemolytic anemia caused by quinidine

156. Cold agglutinin syndrome

QUESTIONS 157–166

For each of the following adverse reactions, select the drug *most* likely to have caused it.

A. *Cis*-platinum
B. Prednisone
C. Bleomycin
D. Doxorubicin (Adriamycin)
E. Methotrexate
F. Vincristine
G. BCNU
H. Chlorambucil
I. Cyclophosphamide (Cytoxan)

157. Pulmonary toxicity

158. Cardiac toxicity

159. Mucositis

160. Bone marrow suppression four to six weeks after drug administration

161. Hemorrhagic cystitis

162. Neuropathy

163. Bone demineralization

164. Obstipation

165. Cutaneous toxicity

166. Renal failure

PART 5

HEMATOLOGY AND ONCOLOGY

ANSWERS

1. (D) Patients with beta-thalassemia major have a severe defect of hemoglobin production. The result is severe anemia, usually with large proportions of hemoglobin F in the small amount of blood they are able to produce. Before the use of regular blood transfusions, patients with this disorder usually died at an early age. With the use of hypertransfusion, early growth and development may be normal, but severe iron overload virtually always ensues. The secondary hemochromatosis produces liver and endocrine dysfunction, but these abnormalities do not usually cause death. Cardiac dysfunction, as the result of iron overload, is the most common cause of death, usually in the second or third decade of life. New approaches to therapy include efforts to circumvent iron overload. *(Cecil, p. 883)*

2. (C) The binding and release of oxygen by intraerythrocyte hemoglobin, as manifested by the oxygen-hemoglobin dissociation curve, is altered by a variety of physiologic changes. Rise in temperature, increased intracellular DPG, increased CO_2, or increased hydrogen ions (decreased pH) facilitate oxygen release, and thus oxygen delivery to tissues. *(Cecil, p. 830)*

3. (D) Hemoglobinuria is a manifestation of severe intravascular hemolysis. Examination of the urine sediment is helpful in differentiating hematuria (the presence of intact red cells in the urine) from hemoglobinuria. Since severe hemoglobinuria may occur with the "innocent bystander" form of drug-induced immune hemolytic anemia, such as seen with quinidine, the patient's drug and chemical exposure history should be rapidly reviewed. Coombs' test will usually be positive in this situation. Microscopic examination of the peripheral blood is useful to screen for forms of red cell destruction such as schistocytic hemolytic anemia or the cold agglutinin syndrome. Bone marrow examination can usually be delayed until the initial evaluation is complete. *(Cecil, pp. 872–874, 875, 896–898)*

4. (D) Erythrocytosis is an interesting diagnostic problem. First, true erythrocytosis must be differentiated from the relative form, in which contraction of plasma volume leads to elevation of peripheral red cell count. Since arterial hypoxemia is a frequent cause of polycythemia, arterial blood gases should be measured initially. Some 75% of patients with polycythemia vera have enlarged spleens; thus, radionuclide liver-spleen scans are useful. Bone marrow examination is of limited usefulness in the differential diagnosis in a patient with erythrocytosis. *(Cecil, pp. 937–940)*

5. (C) Chronic myelogenous leukemia has two distinct phases. During the first phase, virtually any agent that can produce leukopenia is effective, and the parameters of disease, including fatigue, bone pain, abdominal fullness, splenic enlargement, leukocytosis, anemia, and thrombocytosis, will usually be corrected. Despite this ease of control, most patients with CML will enter an accelerated or "blast" phase after two to four years. Survival in the accelerated phase is quite limited. Interestingly, overall survival of patients with CML has not changed significantly with the advent of chemotherapy, and ten-year survivors are uncommon. *(Cecil, pp. 929–930)*

6. (A) The clinical associations, prognosis, and approach to therapy for childhood or acute ITP are considerably different from those for adult or chronic ITP. Although both childhood and adult ITP usually respond to high-dose corticosteroid therapy, such treatment is usually unnecessary in the former. Childhood ITP is a self-limited disease that is often seen following viral illnesses. In contrast, adult ITP is often associated with other diseases, such as systemic lupus erythematosus or malignant lymphoma. In the adult form, relapse of thrombocytopenia with tapering of corticosteroids is the rule, and splenectomy is usually required. Approximately 70% of patients with chronic ITP will maintain long-term remissions following splenectomy. *(Cecil, pp. 984–985)*

7. (B) Splenectomy benefits approximately two thirds of patients with Felty's syndrome, but the indications for this therapy are somewhat controversial. Patients with severe neutropenia are more prone to serious infections, but it is not unusual for patients with Felty's syndrome and severe neutropenia to avoid infections for months or even years. Thus, the absolute neutrophil count cannot be used as an indication for therapy. Thrombocytopenia usually is not severe and is not predictive of benefit from splenectomy. The most clear-cut indications for therapy are recurrent bacterial infections or chronic nonhealing skin ulcers. *(Cecil, pp. 915–916, 1851; Blumfelder, Logue, and Shimm)*

8. (D) Although all these laboratory parameters are characteristically reduced in iron deficiency, examination of the bone marrow for iron stores remains the single most accurate way to document iron deficiency. *(Cecil, pp. 849–850; Williams et al., pp. 370–372)*

9. (C) Cytomegalovirus (CMV) infection may occur in healthy individuals or in patients who have received massive transfusions. Many of the manifestations of CMV are similar to those of infectious mononucleosis, such as splenomegaly, atypical mononuclear cells in the peripheral blood, and liver abnormalities. Pharyngitis, however, is not commonly seen with CMV infection, as it is in infectious mononucleosis. *(Cecil, pp. 1649–1651)*

10. (C) The bleeding tendency of liver disease is caused by multiple factors, including hypoprothrombinemia and deficiency of vitamin K–dependent clotting factors as well as both quantitative and qualitative platelet abnormalities. Although the vitamin K–dependent factors are depressed, vitamin K is usually of little benefit. A variety of other laboratory abnormalities are also present, including abnormalities often seen in association with disseminated intravascular coagulation. These include shortened euglobulin lysis time and increased fibrin degradation products in the plasma. Although transfusion of fresh-frozen plasma temporarily corrects some of the coagulation defects, vitamin K–dependent clotting factor concentrates are potentially dangerous, since fibrinolytic reactions often occur with their use. *(Cecil, pp. 989, 1003–1004)*

11. (C) The first step in planning treatment of suspected breast cancer is to define the extent of the disease. If disseminated disease is present at the outset, extensive surgical procedures are unwarranted. Roentgenogram of the chest, radionuclide bone scans, and serum alkaline phosphatase are useful preliminary staging procedures. Skeletal films and bone marrow biopsies are not useful if the bone scan is normal. *(Cecil, pp. 1032–1033)*

12. (A) In a premenopausal patient with estrogen receptor–positive tumor, the likelihood of response to surgical oophorectomy is at least 50%. It is useful to know whether such a response occurs, because if it does and relapse ensues, the patient may again respond to second-line endocrine therapy. The role of chemotherapy in this disease is changing; some clinicians would treat with both chemotherapy and oophorectomy initially. The response to chemotherapy is generally at least as good as to hormonal manipulation, but skeletal metastases do not respond as well to chemotherapy. Thus, remission is more likely with oophorectomy than with chemotherapy in this patient. Chemotherapy would be indicated if she failed to respond to oophorectomy. Local radiotherapy to painful lesions is indicated if the disease is unresponsive to oophorectomy and chemotherapy. *(Cecil, pp. 1282–1286; Legha, Davis, and Muggia)*

13. (D) Gastrointestinal bleeding is common in patients with cancer and may be due to a variety of causes. Metastases to the gastrointestinal tract should be considered. Stress ulcers are also common and may be exacerbated by gastric irritants such as aspirin, as contained in Percodan. Aspirin also produces platelet function abnormalities. Adequate pain management should be possible with other analgesics that do not contain aspirin. *(Cecil, pp. 983–984, 1017–1019)*

14. (C) The care of patients with terminal diseases often presents moral dilemmas. What seems to the physician to be a rational therapeutic plan may be unacceptable to the patient. In this situation, continued supportive care should be offered. It must be remembered that patients' emotional responses to their illnesses will vary with time. A decision to stop suggested forms of therapy is not irrevocable, and at different times, under different circumstances, these decisions may change. A patient's decision to stop therapy is not an indication of psychiatric illness. *(Cecil, pp. 1017–1019)*

15. (B) The measurement of estrogen receptors in breast tumors is of benefit in predicting response to hormonal manipulation. If tumors of premenopausal women lack estrogen receptors, hormonal manipulations will be of benefit in less than 10% of patients; in the presence of known metastatic disease, such hormonal manipulations are probably unwarranted. Unfortunately, only about 60% of premenopausal patients whose tumors are estrogen receptor–positive will respond to hormonal manipulation such as castration. Interestingly, in some patients the primary tumor will possess estrogen receptors, but metastatic tumor cells will not. Thus, it is of benefit to measure estrogen receptors in metastatic tumors as well as in the primary tumor if the primary is positive for estrogen receptors. *(Cecil, pp. 1283–1284)*

16. (B) Young patients with mediastinal disease often have a nodular sclerosis variety of Hodgkin's disease. In contrast, older patients with systemic symptoms usually show the histologic variety of mixed cellularity or lymphocyte depletion. Lymphocyte-predominant Hodgkin's disease is relatively uncommon. Reed-Sternberg cells in an appropriate histopathologic setting are required to establish the diagnosis of Hodgkin's disease. Histopathologic subclassification of Hodgkin's disease is generally useful, but different clinical features may be seen with any histopathologic type. *(Cecil, pp. 954–955)*

17. (D) The risk of serious infection, such as gram-positive bacteremia, increases following splenectomy. This complication, however, is most likely to occur in patients who have also received radiation therapy and chemotherapy. There is no evidence to suggest that these therapies will be better tolerated following splenectomy. Although the likelihood of liver involvement is increased when Hodgkin's disease is present in the spleen, splenic involvement alone does not represent stage IV disease. *(Cecil, pp. 958–959; Williams et al., pp. 1045–1047)*

18. (A) The most common side effects of the coumarins are caused by the anticoagulation produced. In addition to coagulation toxicity, as manifested by gastrointestinal bleeding and hematuria, the coumarins may cause a peculiar idiosyncratic reaction characterized by necrotic skin ulcers. These lesions do not resemble most other types of drug-induced skin diseases and, if unrecognized, may produce severe disability. Thrombocytopenia, a relatively common untoward effect of heparin anticoagulation, does not occur with coumarin. Bone marrow suppression or hepatocellular defects are not typical complications. *(Cecil, pp. 330, 1003–1004)*

19. (B) Patients with a variety of types of hemolytic anemias may suffer from transient episodes of reduced bone marrow activity, often caused by folic acid deficiency. Thus, patients with hereditary spherocytosis, G6PD deficiency, and sickle cell disease may have transient "aplastic crisis," but do not develop prolonged, profound bone marrow aplasia. In contrast, patients with paroxysmal nocturnal hemoglobinuria have not only hemolytic anemia but also a more basic defect in bone marrow stem cells. This latter defect is often associated with bone marrow hypoplasia and, in some instances, aplastic anemia. *(Cecil, pp. 835–836)*

20. (B) Megaloblastic anemia is the result of impaired synthesis of thymidylate. DNA synthesis can occur if thymidine is provided but, in the absence of synthesis of thymidylate, DNA synthesis is impaired despite continuing RNA and protein production. The DNA-RNA imbalance leads to decreased production of cells and ultimately to premature cell destruction in the marrow (ineffective erythropoiesis). Although this process is more severe in erythroid precursors, it occurs in other marrow cells and can produce pancytopenia. *(Cecil, pp. 853–854)*

21. (A) Hemolytic anemia may occur in patients with severe hypophosphatemia (serum phosphate less than 1.0 mg/dl). Depletion of red cell phosphate leads to reduction in ATP, which causes marked changes in red cell deformability. This type of hemolytic anemia usually occurs in severely malnourished patients such as those with severe alcoholism. The red cell defect and hemolysis may continue one to two weeks after the serum phosphate is corrected. *(Jacob and Amsden)*

22. (D) The sequence of changes that occur as iron deficiency develops is predictable and involves initial mobilization of iron stores, followed by a decrease of plasma iron concentration with an increase in the plasma transferrin. If these changes, along with increased intestinal iron absorption, are inadequate to meet erythroid demands, anemia ensues. Finally, iron-deficient hematopoiesis ultimately results in hypochromic red cells. *(Cecil, p. 849)*

23. (C) The staging laparotomy is useful to determine the extent of the disease *if* the results of this diagnostic procedure would change the therapy plan. Stage IV disease with bone marrow involvement (as evidenced by the Reed-Sternberg cell) would indicate that chemotherapy without radiation therapy was appropriate. Thus, the staging laparotomy would not change the approach to therapy of Hodgkin's disease in a patient with proved bone marrow involvement. Splenic enlargement and abnormal abdominal lymph nodes do not indicate disease that cannot be treated by radiation therapy. Pleural effusion may be the result of lymphatic obstruction without extralymphatic Hodgkin's disease. Thus, with these three abnormalities, the staging laparotomy may be useful in determining the extent of disease in order that therapy may be planned. *(Cecil, pp. 958–959)*

24. (B) Early sexual activity and early pregnancy are associated with an increased incidence of cancer of the cervix but, in contrast, cancer of the breast is decreased in such individuals. Childless women, on the other hand, are at considerably greater risk for development of breast cancer. For reasons that are unclear, familial clustering of breast cancer is evident. Breast cancer is bilateral in 4 to 10% of women when first seen, and women with a history of breast cancer should be strongly encouraged to have regular examinations. Again for unclear reasons, the incidence of breast cancer is increased in obese women. *(Cecil, pp. 1282–1283)*

25. (C) Hemolysis in the cold agglutinin syndrome is due predominantly to complement activation by an antibody that binds to cells at reduced temperatures. Splenectomy does not alter this process and, in fact, can be quite dangerous because of reduction of the patient's temperature during surgery. The beneficial effect of corticosteroids is controversial. Although some patients with antibodies of high thermal amplitude may be helped by corticosteroids, in general this therapy is not of benefit. The primary treatment of this disorder is the avoidance of cold exposure. With the onset of rapid hemolysis, every effort should be made to raise the patient's surrounding temperature to 37°C. For patients with chronic cold agglutinin syndrome, great care must be taken to avoid exposure of the extremities, and many such patients who live in colder climates find it necessary to move to warmer areas during the winter months. For patients with cold agglutinin disease in whom hemolysis cannot be adequately controlled by avoidance of cold exposure, chlorambucil may be indicated in an attempt to reduce the rate of production of the pathologic immunoglobulin. This therapy is not uniformly successful. *(Cecil, p. 873; Logue and Kurlander)*

26. (E) The thiazide diuretics can cause thrombocytopenia. The mechanism, however, varies from patient to patient. Immunologic drug purpura of the sort seen with quinine occurs in some patients, but in others the thiazide diuretics appear to cause thrombocytopenia by producing bone marrow injury. Familial aplastic anemia (Fanconi's anemia) is a rare congenital disorder in which multiple skeletal abnormalities are present. In the first or second decade of life, these patients develop progressive, usually fatal, aplastic anemia with severe thrombocytopenia caused by lack of production of platelets. Drug ingestion is a frequent cause of thrombocytopenic purpura in adults. For drugs such as quinine or quinidine, an immunologic reaction occurs with the rapid destruction of circulating platelets. Thus, these patients may develop profound thrombocytopenia after a brief exposure to the offending agent. Post-transfusion purpura is a rare form of immunologic purpura that can occur in patients lacking the PL^{A1} platelet antigen. Following blood transfusion there is a sudden onset of severe destructive thrombocytopenia, which is somehow self-perpetuating for up to six weeks. Post-transfusion purpura should be suspected in any patient who develops sudden purpura within a few days after blood transfusion. Autoimmune thrombocytopenic purpura is often associated with collagen vascular disease. Idiopathic thrombocytopenic purpura occurs in approximately 10% of patients with systemic lupus erythematosus, and thrombocytopenia may herald disease onset when such minimal other symptoms as photosensitive dermatitis have been present. *(Cecil, pp. 982–983, 985–986; Budman and Steinberg)*

27. (B) Immediate hemolytic transfusion reactions are life-threatening reactions almost uniformly caused by the patient's receiving ABO-incompatible blood. This is usually due to a breakdown of identification procedures outside the blood bank. *(Cecil, p. 900; Mollison)*

28. (B) The diagnosis of chronic lymphocytic leukemia is established by microscopic examination of the peripheral blood. Bone marrow examination is often helpful to establish the extent of disease, but lymphocytic infiltration of the marrow is not necessary to establish this diagnosis. Lymph node enlargement is characteristic of chronic lymphocytic leukemia, and biopsy will often be interpreted as well-differentiated lymphocytic lymphoma. Some consider chronic lymphocytic leukemia a leukemic phase of this lymphoma. Hypogammaglobulinemia is common in chronic lymphocytic leukemia, but is neither specific for this disease nor required to establish the diagnosis. *(Cecil, pp. 932–933)*

29. (A — False; B — False; C — True; D — False; E — False) Body stores of folate are only sufficient to supply several months' need. Folate requirement increases in patients with hemolytic anemia, and folate deficiency with decreased serum folate levels can occur. When the rate of production of red cells is decreased, as in aplastic anemia, iron deficiency, or acute leukemia, serum folate level is usually normal or somewhat elevated. In vitamin B_{12} deficiency the serum folate level is usually normal or elevated. *(Cecil, pp. 857, 858–860)*

30. (A — False; B — True; C — False; D — True; E — False) With the advent of automated cell counting, the reproducibility and accuracy of the red cell indices have increased remarkably. Thus, these indices are much more frequently detected as abnormal and often provide abnormal laboratory data that need to be explained. In some diseases, large red cells are produced by the bone marrow, as for instance in pernicious anemia in which a decreased number of nuclear divisions leads to egress of cells with markedly increased MCV. In other disorders such as liver disease, the MCV may be increased after release of cells from the bone marrow. In liver disease, alterations in plasma lipids lead to increased lipid accumulation on the red cell membrane, and thus an increase in MCV. These two different types of processes that produce elevated

MCV are easily distinguishable by microscopic examination of the peripheral blood. In aplastic anemia and the anemia of chronic disease, the MCV is usually normal; in thalassemia it is typically decreased. *(Cecil, pp. 829, 843; Williams et al., pp. 14–15)*

31. (A — True; B — True; C — False; D — False) The therapy of acute leukemia is divided into phases of induction, consolidation, and maintenance. The point of induction therapy is to reduce the number of leukemic cells so that they are no longer detectable by routine clinical examination. Consolidation therapy is an attempt to reduce this leukemic cell population further in the patient who has achieved disease remission. Finally, the maintenance phase is the chronic therapy given in the attempt to prevent disease relapse. Survival during induction and consolidation therapy depends heavily on general supportive measures such as prophylactic platelet transfusions. Since the possibility of cure in acute lymphoblastic leukemia has become reasonable, empiric therapy of leukemic cells in sanctuaries such as the central nervous system is beneficial. For acute myelogenous leukemia, unfortunately, systemic disease relapse is the rule and, with current therapy, there is no proved benefit in such empiric CNS therapy. Despite early reports, immunotherapy does not appear to prolong remission in acute leukemia. *(Cecil, pp. 924–926)*

32. (A — True; B — False; C — False; D — True) After the diagnosis of prostatic cancer is established, clinical staging to determine the extent of the disease is necessary before appropriate therapy can be outlined. Clinical stage 3 or less represents disease confined to the pelvis or the prostate itself and should be treated by local measures such as surgery, radiation therapy, or both. The serum acid phosphatase is a useful laboratory test in such staging evaluations, but it will be elevated in only approximately two thirds of patients with distant metastatic disease. When distant metastatic disease is present, hormonal manipulation, either with orchiectomy or exogenous estrogens, will produce objective improvement in more than one half of patients. The clinical course of metastatic prostatic cancer, however, can be quite variable, and neither castration nor estrogen therapy can be shown to prolong life in such patients. *(Cecil, pp. 1022, 1257–1258)*

33. (A — True; B — True; C — False; D — True) Human chorionic gonadotropin (HCG) is a hormone molecule secreted by placental trophoblastic cells. It is increased in plasma during pregnancy, but in addition it is produced by germ cell neoplasms of the ovary or testes as well as by trophoblastic tumors. Serial measurement of HCG in patients with these diseases is an effective way to measure response to therapy. HCG has alpha and beta subunits. The structure of the alpha subunit is similar to that of other hormones and thus may cross-react with them. Radioimmunoassays for HCG use antisera produced to the specific beta subunit. Although HCG and alpha-fetoprotein often rise and fall simultaneously in the plasma of patients with these neoplasms, discordant behavior of these two marker substances may be seen in some patients. Discordance in the level of these two substances suggests that different clones of neoplastic cells exist within the same tumor. HCG has been detected in the plasma of patients with non–germ cell tumors such as gastric or pancreatic carcinoma. *(Cecil, p. 1021)*

34. (All are True) The percentage of fetal hemoglobin in the peripheral blood may be increased in a variety of diseases. In some, such as beta-thalassemia, increases may be due to a specific disorder in the regulation of synthesis of globin genes. In other diseases, such as severe anemia from blood loss, the increased proportion of fetal hemoglobin is due to rapid proliferation of erythroid progenitor cells and to premature egress of erythroid cells from the marrow. Finally, in diseases such as acute leukemia and myelofibrosis, the proportion of fetal hemoglobin may be increased as the result of more generalized marrow dysplasia. *(Cecil, p. 825; Williams et al., p. 1602)*

35. (A — False; B — False; C — True; D — False) Vitamin K is required to convert the polypeptide precursors of factors II, VII, IX, and X into active clot-promoting substances: i.e., these polypeptide chains are formed in the absence of vitamin K, but this vitamin appears to transform them into functional clotting units. The normal diet contains an abundance of vitamin K and, in addition, intestinal bacteria are able to synthesize it; thus, inadequate diet alone is rarely a cause of vitamin K deficiency. Vitamin K deficiency is commonly seen in malabsorption syndromes. A prolonged prothrombin time is seen with vitamin K deficiency, but to establish the diagnosis the prothrombin time should significantly shorten within a few hours after administration of this vitamin. *(Cecil, p. 1003)*

36. (A — False; B — False; C — True; D — True) Many patients with thromboembolic diseases are treated for extended times with coumarin derivatives. A variety of drugs can complicate this therapy. Salicylates, in addition to a large number of other drugs including sulfonamides, indomethacin, and allopurinol, potentiate the anticoagulant actions of the coumarins. Bleeding is a common manifestation when the clotting factor deficiencies become too great, and hematuria and gastrointestinal bleeding are frequent. More severe bleeding, such as into the subarachnoid space, is much less common. Only vitamin K_1 is effective in overcoming the effects of coumarin therapy. Immediate, but transient, correction of many of these drugs' effects may be provided in life-threatening situations by transfusion of plasma or concentrates of vitamin K–dependent factors. *(Cecil, pp. 1003–1004; Brozović)*

37. (All are True) All patients with Hodgkin's disease have a variety of immune abnormalities that do not appear to be caused by therapy. Altered T-lymphocyte function, as evidenced by impaired lymphocyte transformation to mitogens, appears to be primary. In some patients, altered humoral immune function appears to be the result of disordered regulatory T-lymphocyte activity; autoimmune hemolytic anemia, immune thrombocytopenic purpura, and hyper- or hypogammaglobulinemia may occur. *(Cecil, pp. 957–958)*

38. (A — True; B — True; C — False; D — False) The antihypertensive agent methyldopa (Aldomet) causes a form of hemolytic anemia in approximately 10% of patients taking the drug. This is an "autoimmune" drug-induced hemolysis in that the antibody produced bears no relationship to methyldopa as an antigen. The antibodies usually have specificity for Rh antigens, do not fix complement, and generally do not produce severe hemolysis. Although the antiglobulin tests usually become negative after discontinuing the drug, the immune reaction often persists for from two to three months after drug cessation. Positive Coombs' tests have persisted for as long as one year. *(Cecil, pp. 873–874; Petz and Fudenberg)*

39. (A — True; B — True; C — True; D — False) Patients with Hodgkin's disease have a variety of cellular immune defects, first recognized as cutaneous anergy in patients with Hodgkin's disease and acute tuberculosis. The loss of immunologic function, in general, is more easily detected by more sensitive tests of immunologic function, and this loss tends to be more severe with advanced disease. Recovery of parameters of delayed hypersensitivity is sometimes seen when disease is adequately controlled with chemotherapy, despite the general immunosuppressive effects of such agents, but most patients with Hodgkin's disease are lymphopenic. *(Cecil, pp. 957–958)*

40. (A — True; B — False; C — True; D — False) Papilledema is an extremely rare but very dramatic complication of iron deficiency. Increased cerebrospinal fluid pressure is associated; if it is unrecognized and untreated, blindness is likely to follow. Although a smooth or sore tongue is characteristic of vitamin B_{12} deficiency, it is also seen with severe iron deficiency. Glossitis in the former is due to megaloblastic changes in the papillary surface cells and in the latter to iron requirements of proliferating epithelial cells. A variety of epithelial changes in addition to glossitis are seen in patients with iron deficiency. Esophageal webs, or the so-called Paterson-Kelly or Plummer-Vinson syndrome, can cause dysphagia. Other epithelial changes in iron deficiency include spoon nails and gastritis. Splenomegaly, caused by unknown mechanisms, is seen in approximately 5 to 10% of patients with iron deficiency and in 5 to 10% of patients with vitamin B_{12} deficiency. Splenic enlargement will regress with therapy. *(Cecil, pp. 849, 856; Sullivan; Wintrobe et al., p. 653)*

41. (A — True; B — True; C — True; D — False) Vitamin B_{12} deficiency causes defective DNA synthesis in all proliferating cells, including red cells, white cells, and platelet precursors. Thus, leukopenia and thrombocytopenia frequently accompany anemia. Thrombocytopenia is associated with iron deficiency in children. Thrombocytosis, with platelet counts in the range of 0.5 to 1.0 $\times$ 10^6/cu mm, is frequently observed with iron deficiency. Although quite rare, platelet elevations to the range of 2 to 3 $\times$ 10^6 have been described. The mechanism producing this abnormality is unknown, but thrombocytosis will be corrected with iron therapy. Defective maturation of red cell precursors caused by vitamin B_{12} deficiency produces ineffective erythropoiesis characterized by the production and destruction of red cells within the marrow space. Because of this intramedullary hemolysis, the serum LDH will most likely be markedly elevated in vitamin B_{12} deficiency. Severe anemia caused by deficiency of iron or vitamin B_{12} may lead to high-output heart failure and prerenal azotemia. *(Cecil, pp. 849–850, 856–857; Williams et al., p. 370)*

42. (A — False; B — False; C — False; D — True) Orally administered iron should be attempted first in all patients unless the daily rate of iron loss is known to exceed the capacity to absorb iron from the gastrointestinal tract. Some patients, such as those with gastrectomy, may prove unable to absorb iron by mouth and require parenteral iron therapy, but such therapeutic requirements should be documented for each patient. Enteric-coated iron preparations generally are poorly absorbed. If orally administered iron is effective, it should be given for at least six months in order to replenish iron stores. An initial sense of well-being is observed within 48 hours of successful iron therapy in many patients. This effect will be observed before objective changes in red cells can be measured. *(Cecil, pp. 850–851)*

43. (A — True; B — False; C — True; D — False) Polycythemia vera and chronic myelogenous leukemia are characterized by autonomous bone marrow proliferation. Basophilia and elevated serum vitamin B_{12} levels are frequent laboratory abnormalities resulting from increased granulocyte turnover. There are no characteristic changes in red cell osmotic fragility or in serum iron concentration in either of these disorders. *(Cecil, pp. 928, 939; Williams et al., p. 626)*

44. (A — True; B — True; C — True; D — False) In an unanesthetized patient, immediate hemolytic transfusion reactions are usually heralded by chills, fever, and some variety of severe pain. It is difficult to distinguish the chills and fever of an immediate hemolytic transfusion reaction from other less serious types of febrile transfusion reactions. In the anesthetized patient, an increased bleeding tendency due to accompanying thrombocytopenia, diffuse intravascular coagulation, or both, may be the first sign of the transfusion of ABO-incompatible blood. With intravascular hemolysis following such a transfusion reaction, some plasma hemoglobin will become bound to albumin and be oxidized to methemoglobin, forming the compound methemalbumin, which gives plasma a characteristic muddy brown appearance. Urticarial transfusion reactions do not result in hemolysis. *(Cecil, p. 900)*

45. (All are True) Chronic lymphocytic leukemia is characterized by the accumulation of immunoincompetent lymphocytes. A variety of associated immunologic complications are seen, including autoimmune disorders directed against platelets or red cells, hypogammaglobulinemia, and, in approximately 5% of patients, a monoclonal gammopathy. *(Cecil, pp. 931–934)*

46. (A — True; B — False; C — True; D — True) It is extremely important to recognize hairy cell leukemia since it usually does not respond favorably to the types of chemotherapy used for other types of chronic leukemia. The most common presentation is splenomegaly and pancytopenia in a middle-aged or elderly patient. Bone marrow biopsy will usually show replacement of the marrow architecture by these peculiar leukemic cells. Splenectomy is beneficial in many patients, despite the extensive bone marrow involvement, but relapse of the pancytopenia is frequent. Most patients have a small number of circulating leukemic cells, but in those patients with more than 10,000 hairy cells per cu mm, intensive leukapheresis is beneficial. *(Cecil, pp. 935–936)*

47. (A — True; B — True; C — True; D — False) The diagnosis of multiple myeloma is established by finding a distinct clinical pattern primarily characterized by widespread bone destruction. This may be recognized as discrete osteolytic lesions or by generalized osteoporosis. In addition to the bone findings, a variety of other manifestations such as leukopenia or thrombocytopenia may be evident. These abnormalities may correct with successful cytotoxic chemotherapy.

Monoclonal protein disorders are seen in a variety of clinical situations in which overt multiple myeloma is not present. This protein abnormality can be seen in patients with chronic infection, and has been described in patients with chronic biliary tract disease. Monoclonal proteins are also seen in association with nonreticular malignancies such as cancer of the colon or breast, and in asymptomatic elderly individuals. The likelihood of these patients developing overt multiple myeloma remains controversial.

The clinical pattern of multiple myeloma often includes hypercalcemia as the result of bone destruction and cytopenia as a result of the neoplastic process involving the bone marrow. Renal insufficiency is common in patients with multiple myeloma, but it is also characteristic of patients with amyloidosis who otherwise do not have overt skeletal multiple myeloma. The difficulty lies in differentiating patients with "primary" amyloidosis, since many will have monoclonal serum proteins. In addition, patients with multiple myeloma often develop "secondary" amyloidosis. *(Cecil, pp. 965–967, 972–973; Kyle)*

48. (A — True; B — True; C — True; D — False) Multiple myeloma is caused by infiltration of the bone marrow by neoplastic plasma cells. These cells often produce homogenous immunoglobulin of one light-chain type. The amount of immunoglobulin produced is proportional to the number of malignant plasma cells. In a significant number of patients, these immunoglobulins are found to have apparent antibody specificity against defined antigens. The plasma cells often appear atypical on microscopic examination, but the diagnosis of multiple myeloma cannot be established on these grounds alone. *(Cecil, pp. 965–966; Williams et al., pp. 1103–1105)*

49. (A — True; B — True; C — False; D — False) The treatment of chronic lymphocytic leukemia is controversial, but most experienced hematologists would not treat asymptomatic patients. When treatment is necessary, alkylating agents such as chlorambucil are usually used. Corticosteroids augment the antileukemic effect of alkylating agents, but they are most useful to control acute immune complications such as immune thrombocytopenic purpura or autoimmune hemolytic anemia. Extended field radiation therapy generally is not of benefit in these patients. Although hypogammaglobulinemia and recurrent bacterial infections are frequent in patients with chronic lymphocytic leukemia, prophylactic gamma globulin has not been shown to be effective. *(Cecil, pp. 933–934)*

50. (A — True; B — False; C — True; D — True) Busulfan (Myleran) is a sulfonyl ester, used to treat chronic myelogenous leukemia, that shares many effects with alkylating agents. In addition to the usual transient bone marrow suppressive effects of alkylating agents, busulfan has several unusual side effects, including a rare syndrome characterized by skin hyperpigmentation and gonadal failure, a syndrome of progressive pulmonary fibrosis, and, in some patients, prolonged thrombocytopenia after therapy. *(Cecil, p. 929)*

51. (A — False; B — True; C — True; D — True; E — True) Documentation of relapse of Hodgkin's disease in previously treated patients is often difficult. Bone or liver involvement often occurs without overt lymph node enlargement. A variety of laboratory tests have been suggested to be useful in screening patients in presumed disease remission in order to predict imminent relapse. Abnormal elevations of all the laboratory tests described here except serum protein electrophoresis have been correlated with disease activity. Although hypo- and hypergammaglobulinemia occur in Hodgkin's disease, these findings are not predictive of relapse. *(Cecil, p. 957)*

52. (All are True) Iron is absorbed in the ferrous state, and absorption occurs more readily at neutral or acid pH. Ascorbic acid increases absorption, but oral elemental iron therapy is usually sufficient to combat iron deficiency, and the added cost of the ascorbic acid–containing iron preparations is not warranted. Although some foods such as leafy green vegetables are relatively high in iron content, substances such as phytates in these foods greatly interfere with iron absorption. *(Cecil, pp. 850–851; Wintrobe et al., pp. 650–656)*

53. (A — True; B — True; C — True; D — False) Patients with an unstable hemoglobin may have varying degrees of clinical hemolysis, but exposure to oxidant drugs will either produce or exacerbate red cell destruction. Hemoglobin electrophoresis is often normal, either because the amino acid substitution does not involve a change in charge or because the unstable hemoglobin is preferentially destroyed in the circulation. Diagnosis is established by documenting precipitation of the abnormal hemoglobin by one of several *in vitro* incubation procedures. Heinz bodies are often seen in supravital stains of the peripheral blood, especially during hemolysis. Clinical disease occurs in the heterozygous state; homozygous patients have not been described. *(Cecil, pp. 892–893)*

54. (A — True; B — False; C — True; D — False) Oropharyngeal or nasopharyngeal involvement occurs in approximately 20% of patients with non-Hodgkin's lymphoma. These lymph nodes are rarely involved with Hodgkin's disease. Spinal cord compression from extradural tumor occurs in patients with Hodgkin's disease as well as in those with non-Hodgkin's lymphoma. This medical emergency must be recognized early and appropriate therapy instituted in order to prevent irreversible neurologic damage in patients who otherwise might respond well to therapy. In contrast to Hodgkin's disease, which often appears to have a unicentric origin in lymph nodes above the diaphragm, other forms of malignant lymphoma frequently involve lymph tissue outside the axial skeleton lymph node areas. Mesenteric lymph node involvement is common in non-Hodgkin's lymphoma, and it frequently invades the gastrointestinal tract. Autoimmune hemolytic anemia is associated with both Hodgkin's disease and non-Hodgkin's lymphoma. Nevertheless, the most common cause of anemia in both these disorders is bone marrow involvement by lymphoma. *(Cecil, pp. 949–950, 955–958; Williams et al., p. 1042)*

55. (A — True; B — True; C — False; D — True) The clinical staging of Hodgkin's disease is extremely important in determining appropriate therapy. Radiologic visualization of abdominal lymph nodes to determine the extent of disease and bone marrow biopsy to ascertain whether stage IV disease of bone exists are both very important and useful diagnostic procedures. Involvement of the brain with Hodgkin's disease is extremely rare. Radionuclide liver-spleen scan, although of less diagnostic specificity, is also generally useful. *(Cecil, p. 958)*

56. (All are True) Acute hemolysis may occur following exposure to a variety of substances. Clostridial toxins, toxins from certain poisonous mushrooms, and arsenic or copper poisoning may be associated with hemolysis, presumably as a result of deleterious membrane changes. Hemolysis from copper poisoning has occurred in patients undergoing hemodialysis when dialysis solutions became very alkaline. Some patients with Wilson's disease undergo hemolytic episodes early in the course of the disease. *(Cecil, p. 874)*

57. (A — True; B — False; C — True; D — True) Anemia is a common finding in a variety of diseases, including infection, renal insufficiency, collagen vascular diseases, and chronic hepatic disorders. Although primary causes of anemia such as iron deficiency should be excluded, chronic nonprogressive anemia is the rule in these systemic disorders. The causes of the anemia are many, including mild hemolysis, lack of appropriate bone marrow response, and inadequate release of iron from the reticuloendothelial system. Ineffective erythropoiesis is not an element of the anemia of chronic disorders. *(Cecil, pp. 842–843)*

58. (A — True; B — True; C — True; D — False) Subacute combined degeneration is associated with vitamin B_{12}

deficiency. This may produce peripheral neuropathy; degeneration of the dorsal and lateral columns of the spinal cord; or cerebral cortical dysfunction including restlessness, loss of memory, or (in some situations) frank psychosis. Cranial nerve involvement is not associated with vitamin B_{12} deficiency. *(Cecil, p. 856)*

59. (A — True; B — True; C — True; D — False) Fragmentation hemolytic anemia occurs in all these disorders. In malignant hypertension, Rocky Mountain spotted fever, or periarteritis nodosa, this process is described as microangiopathic in that there are microvascular abnormalities that lead to red cell fragmentation. In march hemoglobinuria, red cell fragmentation occurs upon repeated trauma to a body part. In that setting, red cells appear either to be completely destroyed or to survive unharmed, and schistocytes are rarely seen. *(Cecil, p. 875)*

60. (A — False; B — False; C — False; D — True) Hereditary elliptocytosis is characterized by red blood cells that are elliptic rather than spheroidal. This shape change has no pathologic sequelae in the vast majority of affected individuals. Hemolysis, splenomegaly, and other blood cell disorders are infrequent, and splenectomy is rarely required. Hereditary elliptocytosis is similar in some respects to hereditary spherocytosis, and these two disorders have been observed concomitantly in some families. *(Cecil, p. 865; Lessin)*

61. (A — True; B — True; C — True; D — False) Successful treatment of immediate hemolytic transfusion reactions requires rapid diagnosis, including serologic confirmation by the blood bank. Therapy should be directed at maintaining renal perfusion and urinary flow. This may require the monitoring of central venous pressure and the use of diuretics. If oliguria occurs despite such therapy, however, fluid should be restricted to 500 ml plus visible output per day, and the patient should be treated for acute renal failure. *(Cecil, p. 900)*

62. (A — False; B — True; C — False; D — True) The thalassemic syndromes are a heterogeneous group of disorders characterized by retarded production of globin chains. In some instances, secondary accumulation of unpaired globin chains may lead to abnormal molecules such as hemoglobin H (four beta globin chains) or Bart's hemoglobin (four gamma globin chains). In other instances, a thalassemic defect is characterized by the production of a hemoglobin that is the result of the failure of a DNA termination codon (hemoglobin Constant Spring). Hemoglobin Kempsey is not a thalassemic defect, but a hemoglobin produced by an amino acid substitution that causes polycythemia because of altered oxygen affinity. Diamond-Blackfan syndrome is an acquired disorder of red cell production in children. *(Cecil, pp. 882, 884–885, 893)*

63. (A — True; B — True; C — True; D — False; E — True) Sideroblastic anemia is a descriptive term for a group of disorders characterized by perinuclear deposition of iron within developing red cell precursors. Sideroblastic anemia occurs in a variety of situations. It may be an X-linked hereditary disorder; acquired forms are associated with exposure to drugs, toxins, or alcohol, such as with antituberculous therapy or lead poisoning. Idiopathic sideroblastic anemia can transform to acute leukemia. Hemochromatosis, although associated with marked accumulation of iron in tissues, is not usually associated with sideroblastic anemia. *(Cecil, pp. 852–853)*

64. (A — False; B — True; C — True; D — True) Hypercalcemia is a relatively common metabolic abnormality in cancer patients. The earliest symptoms include polyuria and polydipsia resulting from nephrogenic diabetes insipidus. With progressive hypercalcemia, mental obtundation and coma may ensue. There are a variety of causes for hypercalcemia in cancer patients, including ectopic production of parathyroid hormone–like materials or other tumor products such as prostaglandins. Laboratory findings usually associated with hyperparathyroidism, namely hyperphosphaturia and hypophosphatemia, are seen in patients who have ectopic production of substances with parathyroid hormone–like activity. *(Cecil, pp. 1023–1024; Mazzaferri, Odorisio, and LoBuglio)*

65. (All are True) ITP can be classified as a thrombocytopenia of decreased platelet survival. There is strong evidence to suggest that ITP is in fact autoimmune thrombocytopenic purpura. Plasma transfusion experiments with whole plasma or with 7S gamma globulin fractions, and observations concerning placental transfer of the disease, strongly implicate IgG antibodies as the cause of this disorder. Tests for antiplatelet antibodies *in vitro*, although technically difficult, reveal such antibodies in the majority of patients with ITP. These antiplatelet antibodies also have been shown to be produced *in vitro* by spleen cells of patients with ITP. *(Cecil, p. 98; Williams et al., pp. 1345–1346)*

66. (A — True; B — False; C — False; D —False) Although the anemia of chronic disorders such as renal disease, liver disease, or chronic inflammatory disease has a varied pathophysiology, the predominant clinical effect is that of bone marrow failure. Reticulocytopenia is common; the bone marrow cellularity is usually normal or decreased. Normal to increased iron stores are usually present, resulting in normal to increased serum ferritin. Leukocyte and platelet counts usually are not depressed. *(Cecil, p. 844)*

67. (A — True; B — True; C — False; D — False) G6PD is an enzyme of the hexose monophosphate shunt pathway, which is of major importance in protecting red cells from oxidation. Because G6PD has several electrophoretic variants, it has proved a useful genetic marker. Type B is the most common form of the enzyme; type A, which moves rapidly on electrophoresis, is seen in approximately 30% of blacks. The type A variant has normal enzyme activity in most individuals. G6PD deficiency in blacks occurs in a subgroup with type A enzyme that is defective in its enzyme activity. Inheritance is sex-linked. *(Cecil, pp. 867–869)*

68. (A — True; B — True; C — True; D — False) Chloramphenicol produces two types of bone marrow damage, one that is dose-related and reversible, and a second that is non–dose-related, severe, and irreversible. Chloramphenicol is the drug most associated with severe aplastic anemia, and this complication may occur with only brief drug exposure. Chloramphenicol-induced aplastic anemia is usually severe and often fatal. *(Cecil, p. 836; Williams et al., pp. 259–260)*

69. (A — False; B — True; C — True; D — True) The iron in the heme of hemoglobin normally exists in the reduced or ferrous form. This iron is normally resistant to oxidation, including that caused by high inspired partial pressures of oxygen. Methemoglobinemia may occur on exposure to chemicals with high oxidizing potential or in patients with several different inherited disorders. Deficiencies of the red cell enzyme methemoglobin reductase and certain hemoglobinopathies (the "M" hemoglobins) cause congenital methemoglobinemia. The M hemoglobins are characterized by amino acid substitutions, in the heme pocket of globin, that allow the formation of methemoglobin. *(Cecil, pp. 894–896)*

70. (A — False; B — True; C — False; D — True) Stomatocytosis is characterized by red cells that have linear mouthlike areas of central pallor as seen on stained peripheral blood films. This can be seen as a rare type of autosomal dominantly inherited hemolytic anemia or in patients with alcoholic liver disease. *(Cecil, p. 865; Williams et al., p. 125)*

71. (A — True; B — True; C — False; D — False) Thalassemia trait is the heterozygous form of an inherited defect in the regulation of the production of beta globin chains. Because of relative overproduction of alpha globin chains, mild hemolytic anemia occurs, often with modest reticulocytosis. Characteristically, the MCV is low, and there is elevation of either hemoglobin A_2 or F. If hemolysis is relatively severe, thrombocytosis may be present; however, thrombocytopenia is not seen. *(Cecil, p. 884; Williams et al., pp. 396–397)*

72. (A — False; B — True; C — False; D — True) The Schilling test is very useful in discovering an inability to absorb oral vitamin B_{12}. Since normal B_{12} stores are sufficient for many years, B_{12} malabsorption and tissue B_{12} deficiency are not synonymous. Serum B_{12} levels should be ascertained before a Schilling test is made, since a peripheral loading dose of unlabeled vitamin B_{12} is given prior to the study of intestinal absorption of radioactive B_{12}. Since vitamin B_{12} deficiency can cause megaloblastosis in gastrointestinal tract cells, a patient with severe B_{12} deficiency due to lack of production of intrinsic factor may not absorb B_{12} with exogenous intrinsic factor until the tissue B_{12} deficiency has been corrected. For this reason, Schilling tests that are abnormal in both parts 1 and 2 should be repeated after parenteral B_{12} therapy. The vitamin B_{12} itself may correct the vicious cycle of intestinal malabsorption in such patients. *(Cecil, p. 857)*

73. (A — False; B — True; C — False; D — True) With improved nutrition and preventive care, many more patients with hemoglobin SS are able to live relatively normal lives. Types of complications that occur in adults differ from those of childhood. Although splenomegaly is common in early childhood, splenic atrophy is the rule in the adult. This splenic atrophy is presumably caused by repeated splenic infarctions. Chronic nonhealing leg ulcers, a relatively uncommon complication in children, are much more frequent in adults. Pregnancy can be concluded safely, although special care must be taken during the prenatal period. Hepatomegaly is common in adult patients with hemoglobin SS and is frequently associated with abnormal liver function studies. *(Cecil, pp. 891–892)*

74. (A — True; B — True; C — True; D — False) The differentiation of acute lymphoblastic leukemia (ALL) from other forms of acute leukemia, including acute myelogenous leukemia (AML), is essential, since therapies are remarkably different. Histochemical reactions are useful in differentiating these forms of leukemia. Myeloblasts of AML usually have positive-staining reactions with peroxidase and Sudan black, whereas lymphoblasts of ALL do not stain with these reagents. In contrast, lymphoblasts usually have coarse cytoplasmic staining with periodic acid-Schiff (PAS) reagents, whereas myeloblasts will not. Esterase stains are also useful in this regard. TDT is found in high concentrations in the cells of many patients with ALL, but is not present in myeloblasts. This enzyme is also found experimentally in some types of thymic lymphocytes. Its role in the pathogenesis of leukemia is unknown. Auer rods are highly refractile cytoplasmic rods that appear to derive from coalescence of azurophilic granules. They are present in only approximately one third of patients with AML, but when seen are pathognomonic for this disease. Both ALL and AML are usually detected when the patient is anemic and thrombocytopenic. *(Cecil, pp. 922–923; Gralnick et al., Kung et al.)*

75. (A — True; B — False; C — True; D — True) Splenectomy is beneficial for patients with a variety of hematologic diseases. In some diseases such as warm-reacting IgG autoimmune hemolytic anemia, the beneficial effect of splenectomy is due to removal of a site of specific immune-mediated cell destruction. In other diseases such as immune thrombocytopenic purpura, decreased rate of destruction of antibody-coated cells, as well as decreased production of antibody, appears to result from splenectomy. The beneficial effect of splenectomy in hairy cell leukemia is well described but the pathophysiology is obscure. Clinical improvement in this disease may be due to either reduction of "hypersplenism" or the removal of a large number of slowly dividing leukemic cells. In contrast, splenectomy does not benefit patients with the cold agglutinin syndrome, and in fact the risk of rapid hemolysis caused by reduction in body temperature during surgery is great. *(Cecil, pp. 871–872, 873, 936, 985)*

76. (A — False; B — True; C — False; D — True) Myoglobinuria is usually seen in association with severe forms of muscle cell lysis, and reviewing the clinical history is valuable. When pigmenturia is seen after crush injuries, extreme exercise, or heavy alcohol intake, myoglobinuria should be suspected. Myoglobin is smaller than hemoglobin (17,500 vs. 66,000 molecular weight) and, because of this molecular difference, myoglobin is rapidly filtered and excreted in the urine. With myoglobinuria, myoglobinemia usually is not detected by visual inspection. Plasma hemoglobin, on the other hand, is not excreted rapidly and is actively reabsorbed by the renal tubular cells. Thus, for sufficient hemoglobin to be excreted in the urine, plasma hemoglobin levels are usually quite high and discoloration of plasma easily seen. Both hemoglobin and myoglobin react with benzidine reagents. Myoglobinuria can be differentiated from hemoglobinuria by simple chemical procedures such as ammonium sulfate precipitation. *(Cecil, pp. 896–898)*

77. (A — False; B — True; C — False; D — True) Many of the abnormal hemoglobins with altered oxygen dissociation do not have electrical charge differences from normal hemoglobin. Thus, if a polycythemia-producing hemoglobinopathy is suspected, oxygen dissociation studies should be done. In addition to arterial hypoxemia, a variety of other conditions produce secondary polycythemia. In most of these diseases the bone marrow reacts normally to erythropoietin activity, but this activity remains high despite elevated red cell counts. For arterial hypoxemic states and with hemoglobins of altered oxygen affinity, tissue distribution of oxygen is inadequate, and erythropoietin production continues. In some diseases such as renal or brain tumors, or in nonmalignant renal diseases such as medullary cystic disease, nonphysiologic erythropoietin production is seen. In both primary and secondary polycythemia, the serum uric acid concentration may be greatly elevated: this is due to the rapid turnover of bone marrow erythroid cells in both disorders. Although there are rare instances in which polycythemia vera apparently has occurred as a familial disease, the most common cause of familial polycythemia is a genetically transmitted hemoglobin abnormality. Such abnormalities are transmitted as autosomal dominant characteristics, and these hemoglobins of altered oxygen affinity produce polycythemia by the mechanism described above. *(Cecil, pp. 893–894, 939, 941–943; Williams et al., p. 647)*

78. (A — False; B — True; C — True; D — False) Differentiation of chronic myelogenous leukemia (CML) from a secondary leukemoid reaction involves the sequential evaluation of clinical and laboratory data. Characteristically, patients with untreated CML are anemic, but diseases that cause leukemoid reactions also cause anemia. For reasons that are unclear, leukocyte alkaline phosphatase (determined by histochemical staining) is characteristically decreased or absent in CML, whereas the concentration of this enzyme is usually elevated in secondary leukemoid reactions. Splenic enlargement is characteristic of CML. Although a marked increase in cellularity and in granulocyte precursors in the bone marrow is characteristic of CML, these bone marrow findings are also seen in leukemoid reactions. Thus, morphologic examination of the blood and bone marrow does not usually aid in this differentiation. Short of bone marrow karyotype analysis, the combination of a low leukocyte alkaline phosphatase and splenomegaly makes the diagnosis of CML quite likely. *(Cecil, pp. 917–918, 928–929)*

79. (A — False; B — True; C — False; D — True) Pure red cell aplasia appears to be an autoimmune disease in which antibodies are directed against red cell precursors. It is frequently associated with thymic tumors, and sometimes can be successfully treated by removal of a thymoma or by immunosuppressive agents. Bone marrow elements other than the red cells are normal and thus, in contrast to primary myeloproliferative syndromes, transformation to acute leukemia does not occur. In response to the anemia, serum erythropoietin levels are high. *(Cecil, pp. 837–840; Krantz)*

80. (A — False; B — True; C — False; D — True) The Philadelphia chromosome is an acquired marker chromosome that is present in bone marrow stem cells but not in other somatic cells of patients with chronic myelogenous leukemia (CML). It is rarely, if ever, seen in any disease except CML. Patients who appear to have CML, but lack the chromosomal abnormality, generally have a much poorer prognosis, with less predictable response to chemotherapy. *(Cecil, p. 919)*

81. (A — False; B — True; C — False; D — True) The classification of non-Hodgkin's lymphoma into two general groups, nodular and diffuse, has proved useful for predicting response to therapy and disease prognosis. The nodular lymphomas are usually disseminated at diagnosis, and often involve lymph node areas not treated by standard radiation therapy ports. These diseases usually respond favorably to chemotherapy, but a complete response or remission is infrequently observed. Thus, extremely aggressive chemotherapy does not seem beneficial. Despite the foregoing, patients often have a rather indolent clinical course, and the five-year survival rates for nodular lymphoma are usually greater than for patients with the diffuse varieties. *(Cecil, pp. 945–947, 952–953)*

82. (A — False; B — True; C — False; D — True) Hereditary spherocytosis is an autosomal dominant disorder that occurs in as many as one in 5000 individuals of northern European descent. The disease is characterized by abnormally shaped red cells, mild anemia, splenomegaly, and mild jaundice. It is often undetected until adulthood. Indeed, when a patient with hereditary spherocytosis is discovered, family members of all ages should be screened for the defect by microscopic examination of the peripheral blood. Although the indications for splenectomy are somewhat controversial, most hematologists advise splenectomy in patients of more than 6 years of age. Splenectomy lessens hemolysis in virtually all patients. *(Cecil, pp. 864–865)*

83. (A — True; B — True; C — True; D — False) Aggressive chemotherapy is beneficial in disseminated diffuse histiocytic lymphoma. Complete remission occurs in somewhat more than half the patients so treated. Patients who do not achieve complete remission usually do quite poorly, and rapid, chemotherapy-resistant tumor growth often ensues. A number of patients with histiocytic lymphoma may present with the disease localized to one anatomic area. It is not unusual, for instance, for histiocytic lymphoma to be localized in the gastrointestinal tract, e.g., in the stomach. For patients with localized disease, radiation therapy may be curative. Progression of histiocytic lymphoma to a leukemic phase with circulating lymphoma cells is rarely seen. *(Cecil, pp. 949–952)*

84. (A — True; B — True; C — False; D — False) Eosinophilic leukemoid reactions occur in a variety of conditions including drug reactions, parasitic infection, and dermatologic disease. In contrast, eosinophilic leukemia is extremely rare. Thus, eosinophilia with or without an elevated white blood cell count is most likely due to a benign condition. Since eosinophils normally do not have leukocyte alkaline phosphatase activity, the leukocyte alkaline phosphatase score will not identify eosinophilic leukemia. Eosinophilia of any sort, including eosinophilic leukemoid reactions, will be associated with proliferation of immature eosinophilic precursors in the marrow. *(Cecil, p. 918)*

85. (A — True; B — False; C — False; D — True) Some patients with ITP will remain refractory to corticosteroids and splenectomy; some of these will benefit from vincristine. Prophylactic platelet transfusion is not useful, since the platelets will be destroyed rapidly by circulating antiplatelet antibodies. Platelet infusions are beneficial in life-threatening hemorrhage, however. Patients with chronic ITP who experience heavy bleeding with menses are often remarkably improved by suppression of ovarian function with hormonal agents. *(Cecil, p. 985; Ahn et al.)*

86. (A — False; B — False; C — True; D — False) Polycythemia vera is a chronic disease, and patients often live more than a decade after the onset. Approximately half of these patients will die as a direct result of the hematologic disorder. Acute leukemia is a major complication in patients who have received previous bone marrow suppressive therapy, but without such suppressive therapy early bleeding or clotting deaths occur. A significant percentage of polycythemia vera patients develop a terminal "spent" phase, which clinically and pathologically is indistinguishable from myelofibrosis. It is unclear whether this complication is related to previous therapy. The incidence of gastrointestinal hemorrhage is high, especially if thrombocytosis persists. The hyperuricemia of polycythemia vera is due to massive overproduction of uric acid, and most authors agree that allopurinol is indicated *(Cecil, pp. 940–941)*

87. (E); 88. (G); 89. (F); 90. (H); 91. (H) Although cytotoxic chemotherapy is, in large part, empiric, controlled studies of multiple agents have shown different forms of cytotoxic chemotherapy to be useful in different diseases. In some disorders, such as chronic lymphocytic leukemia and macroglobulinemia, single-agent chemotherapy is often effective; in other diseases, such as histiocytic lymphoma and Hodgkin's disease, multiple agents are used. With aggressive cytotoxic chemotherapy, initial complete remission rates in these diseases are high and prolonged disease-free intervals are seen. It is of interest that some agents of the same drug class, e.g., alkylating agents, are of differential usefulness in different diseases. For instance, chlorambucil appears to be most effective in chronic lymphocytic leukemia, whereas melphalan is not as effective; in contrast, melphalan appears to be more useful in multiple myeloma. *(Cecil, pp. 934, 951–952, 959, 968, 971; Burchenol)*

92. (D) The antimetabolite cytosine arabinoside has proved useful in inducing disease remissions in acute myelogenous leukemia. *(Cecil, pp. 924–925)*

93. (C) Methotrexate, especially when given in high doses with Leucovorin rescue, appears to be useful in some patients with osteogenic sarcoma. *(Cecil, pp. 1038–1039)*

94. (A) Aggressive cytotoxic chemotherapy with multiple agents, including *cis*-platinum, has proved very beneficial in patients with testicular carcinoma other than seminoma. This chemotherapy not only produces more than 50% remission rates, but also significantly prolongs life in responding patients. *(Cecil, pp. 1042, 1254)*

95. (A) The term "histiocytic" lymphoma is, in most instances, a misnomer; i.e., the neoplastic cell of origin of this type of lymphoma appears to be a B lymphocyte. *(Cecil, pp. 945–947)*

96. (B) Mycosis fungoides, in contrast, appears to be due to proliferation of T lymphocytes. In some instances, these T lymphocytes are found to be modulators of B-lymphocyte function. These functional similarities are sometimes shared with the malignant T lymphocytes seen in the Sézary syndrome. *(Cecil, pp. 945–947)*

97. (A) The origin of the proliferating cell in patients with hairy cell leukemia is somewhat controversial. Although some evidence has suggested that these cells derive from a monocyte precursor, the weight of current experimental evidence suggests that this cell with very peculiar cytoplasmic characteristics is most closely related to B lymphocytes. *(Cecil, p. 934)*

98. (A) The vast majority of patients with chronic lymphocytic leukemia (CLL) have a neoplastic proliferation and/or accumulation of abnormal B lymphocytes. A small percentage of those with chronic lymphocytic leukemia are found to have accumulation of T lymphocytes. These patients with "T-cell" CLL differ somewhat in clinical presentation, having an increased likelihood of skin infiltration, marked liver infiltration, and decreased survival. In patients in whom a clinical diagnosis of CLL seems likely, it is quite useful to obtain cell surface markers in order to better predict the course of the disease. *(Cecil, pp. 931–932)*

99. (A) Most forms of nodular lymphomas, including nodular, poorly differentiated lymphocytic lymphoma, appear to arise from the malignant proliferation of B lymphocytes. *(Cecil, pp. 945–947, 949)*

100. (B) Sézary syndrome is characterized by a generalized erythroderma in association with a peculiar type of malignant lymphocyte that, on examination by electron microscopy, usually has a distinctive cerebriform nucleus. These lymphocytes appear to have T-lymphocyte surface characteristics. *(Cecil, p. 933)*

101. (A) Waldenström's macroglobulinemia is due to a proliferation of cells in the B-lymphoid line, somewhat intermediate between B lymphocytes and plasma cells. These malignant cells produce IgM immunoglobulin, and thus cause many of the clinical characteristics of this disorder, including a variety of manifestations of hyperviscosity. *(Cecil, pp. 970–971)*

102. (B); 103. (A); 104. (B); 105. (B); 106. (C); 107. (A) *(Cecil, pp. 415–418; Sarna, Holmes, and Petrovich; Weiss)*

102. Hypercalcemia may occur as the result of a variety of pathophysiologic processes, including extensive bone marrow metastases and production of an ectopic hormone with parathyroid hormone–like activity. Hypercalcemia is much more commonly associated with epidermoid carcinoma of the lung and is often due to production of ectopic hormone activity. In contrast, hypercalcemia is a very unusual complication of patients with oat cell carcinoma of the lung, despite the high incidence of bone marrow metastases. **103.** Small cell or oat cell carcinoma of the lung is usually a rapidly progressive tumor with a high propensity for metastatic disease. Without prophylactic cranial irradiation, most patients will develop symptomatic CNS metastases. Even with prophylactic cranial irradiation, some patients with small cell carcinoma of the lung develop leptomeningeal metastases. This complication seems to occur most frequently in patients who have marrow involvement by tumor at the time of diagnosis. **104.** In contrast to small cell carcinoma of the lung, epidermoid carcinoma of the lung sometimes appears to develop more slowly. With the more widespread use of cytologic testing, some patients have been found to shed malignant squamous epithelial cells from the lower respiratory tract, although testing, including bronchoscopy, is unable to localize a specific tumor site. **105.** Early diagnosis of epidermoid carcinoma of the lung, either by x-ray or cytologic screening, allows a subgroup of patients to achieve a cure by surgery. In contrast, the more rapidly progressive small cell carcinoma of the lung, with its higher metastatic potential, is seldom cured by surgery. Despite the advances in chemotherapy of small cell carcinoma of the lung described below, a significant five-year survival in this disease has not yet been achieved. **106.** Both types of lung cancer often begin in the perihilar area, and bronchial obstruction is relatively common in either disease. The response of this complication to either chemotherapy or radiation therapy is significantly greater in patients with small cell carcinoma. **107.** With combination chemotherapy, including alkylating agents and/or anthracyclines, more than half of patients with small cell carcinoma of the lung have an objective response to chemotherapy. This chemotherapeutic response seems to increase with increasing drug doses, but it is not clear whether it will be associated with increased survival.

108. (D) Delayed hemolytic transfusion reactions are caused by antibodies directed against minor blood group antigens to which the patient has previously been exposed. These antibodies are not detected during the crossmatch procedure. Nevertheless, antibody response occurs following transfusion, so that hemolysis occurs three to ten days after transfusion. *(Cecil, p. 900)*

109. (C) Febrile transfusion reactions are usually due to the transfusion of incompatible leukocytes or platelets to which the patient has developed antibodies. These reactions usually are self-limited and can be treated symptomatically. The primary problem is differentiating this type of transfusion reaction from the more serious immediate hemolytic transfusion reaction. *(Cecil, pp. 900–901)*

110. (E) IgA deficiency occurs in approximately one out of every 200 normal individuals. On occasion, these IgA-deficient people produce antibodies to IgA, which can cause severe anaphylactic reactions upon transfusion of any blood product. *(Cecil, p. 901)*

111. (E) The anaphylactic reaction seen in patients with antibodies against IgA can be prevented by extensively washing red cells prior to transfusion. If a patient who requires transfusion has a history of anaphylactic reaction to blood products, his own IgA level should be immediately studied; if found to be deficient in this immunoglobulin, the patient should receive only thawed, previously frozen red cells. *(Cecil, p. 901)*

112. (A) In rare situations, patients who are lacking the common platelet antigen PL^{A1} will develop profound thrombocytopenic purpura upon transfusion with blood products containing platelets with this antigen. This reaction is frequently seen in women with multiple previous pregnancies. The mechanism of thrombocytopenia is unclear, since the patient subsequently destroys her own platelets; this form of platelet destruction can persist for up to six weeks following transfusion. *(Cecil, p. 901; Williams et al., pp. 1341–1342)*

113. (B); 114. (D); 115. (B); 116. (C); 117. (A) There are a variety of hemoglobinopathies that may produce clinical abnormalities. These include double heterozygote conditions or syndromes in which patients are homozygous for the significant types of polymerizing hemoglobins, hemoglobins S or C. Patients who are homozygous for hemoglobin C are usually asymptomatic and do not manifest hemolytic anemia, but they usually have splenic enlargement. Hemoglobin C occurs as a heterozygous state in approximately 2 to 3% of American blacks. Patients with hemoglobin SC often have a peculiar form of retinovascular occlusion that can cause neovascular proliferation or retinal detachment. Hemoglobin SD-Punjab has many features of sickle cell anemia except that it is often seen in whites. Patients homozygous for hemoglobins S or C or doubly heterozygous for hemoglobins S, C, or D will have no detectable hemoglobin A, whereas patients with sickle cell–thalassemia may have hemoglobin A that is detectable by electrophoresis. *(Cecil, pp. 887–892; Orkin and Nathan; Williams et al., pp. 507–511)*

118. (A); 119. (A); 120. (A); 121.(B); 122. (B); 123. (B); 124. (C) Bone marrow culture techniques have allowed better classification of blood diseases caused by defective production of cellular elements. For some diseases such as paroxysmal nocturnal hemoglobinuria, chronic granulocytic leukemia, and Fanconi's anemia, the disorder affects pleuripotent stem cells, and thus granulocytes, red cells, and platelets are abnormal. For other diseases, such as pure red cell aplasia in adults and the childhood equivalent, Diamond-Blackfan syndrome, and cyclic neutropenia, the defect appears to reside with committed stem cells. In these disorders, there is a lack of production of a single cellular element. In pure red cell aplasia of adults, this isolated cellular defect is the result of an autoimmune process in which antibodies that react with the committed stem cell precursor are produced. Neonatal neutropenia is due to transplacental passage of maternal antibodies directed against the neonate's neutrophils, and thus neutropenia appears to be the result of peripheral cellular destruction. *(Cecil, pp. 834–835)*

125. (D) IgM paraproteins, because of their high molecular weight, are frequently associated with hyperviscosity syndromes. This hyperviscosity can lead to circulatory impairment, especially of the central nervous system. *(Cecil, pp. 970–971)*

126. (D) The neoplastic proliferation of IgM paraprotein-producing cells is most often associated with Waldenström's macroglobulinemia. This disease has many characteristics of a malignant lymphoma rather than multiple myeloma. Lymphadenopathy and liver and splenic enlargement are common; skeletal lesions are rare. *(Cecil, pp. 970–971)*

127. (B) IgA heavy chain (alpha-chain) disease produces a clinical pattern sometimes referred to as Mediterranean-type abdominal lymphoma. Lymphoid infiltration of the gastrointestinal tract in this disease produces chronic diarrhea and a malabsorption syndrome. *(Cecil, p. 971)*

128. (A) The etiology of renal failure in multiple myeloma is controversial. Factors such as hypercalcemia or chronic infection undoubtedly contribute to the renal disease, but Bence Jones proteinuria is a major etiologic factor in the renal failure of multiple myeloma. *(Cecil, p. 965; Williams et al., pp. 1107–1108)*

129. (A) A major cause of adverse drug reactions is the ingestion of an oxidizing drug by patients who have a latent red cell enzyme deficiency. In black patients with G6PD deficiency, the red cells, although deficient in this enzyme, have a normal lifespan in the absence of drug exposure or severe metabolic stress. However, following exposure to oxidizing drugs such as nitrofurans or antimalarials, hemolysis will occur. Older red cells will be preferentially destroyed, since enzyme activity decreases as cells age. *(Cecil, pp. 867–868)*

130. (B) In contrast to G6PD deficiency in blacks, red cells of all ages are affected in whites with G6PD deficiency. Thus, G6PD deficiency in whites is often associated with chronic hemolytic anemia in the absence of drug exposure. The incidence of this defect varies considerably in different populations. The gene frequency in northern Europeans is less than 0.1%, whereas it is as high as 50% in some Mediterranean Caucasian populations. *(Cecil, pp. 867–868)*

131. (C) Although G6PD deficiency is due to a wide range of genetic defects, all these variations are sex-linked. *(Cecil, p. 867)*

132. (B) A large number of oxidant drugs produce hemolysis in both blacks and whites with G6PD deficiency. Interestingly, however, favism (severe hemolysis following ingestion of fava beans) occurs only in patients with the Caucasian variety of G6PD deficiency. Blacks with G6PD deficiency are unaffected by this agent. An inherited mechanism in addition to the enzyme deficiency may be active here. *(Cecil, pp. 867–868)*

133. (C) During hemolytic episodes, intracellular oxidation of hemoglobin occurs. Thus, methemoglobinemia and/or Heinz bodies may be present in patients with either type of deficiency. *(Cecil, pp. 867–868)*

134. (B); 135. (A); 136. (C); 137. (B); 138. (B) Megaloblastic anemia is usually caused by either vitamin B_{12} or folate deficiency. Body stores of folate will last for only three to six months, whereas B_{12} stores are sufficient for many years. Thus, folate deficiency is more often seen in association with inadequate diet or with increased folate requirements, such as in pregnancy or hemolytic anemia. Dietary folate must be deconjugated prior to absorption, and a variety of drugs, including phenytoin sodium (Dilantin) and oral contraceptives, interfere with this process. Vitamin B_{12} deficiency is commonly caused by decreased intrinsic factor secretion, and in this setting autoimmune antibodies against parietal cells are frequently observed. *(Cecil, pp. 852–860; Sullivan)*

139. (C) Management of inherited coagulation factor deficiency requires knowledge of the form of replacement that contains active factors and the plasma half-life of the infused factor. Factor VII is quite stable during storage, and stored plasma or vitamin K–dependent factor concentrates may be used. On the other hand, this factor has a very short biologic half-life after transfusion, and thus repeated large infusions are required. *(Cecil, p. 1001)*

140. (F) Patients with factor XIII deficiency will appear normal by routine coagulation assays, including partial thromboplastin time, prothrombin time, and thrombin clotting time; however, they usually have neonatal umbilical bleeding and abnormal wound healing. Thus, minor surgical procedures or trauma may produce large hypertrophic scarring in these patients. *(Cecil, pp. 1002–1003)*

141. (E) Patients with factor XII (Hageman factor) deficiency characteristically have prolonged whole blood clotting times. Despite striking laboratory abnormalities, the patients usually have no symptoms of abnormal bleeding and require no specific therapy. *(Cecil, p. 1000)*

142. (D) Factor IX deficiency or Christmas disease is clinically indistinguishable from classic hemophilia (factor VIII deficiency). That is, both these disorders are sex-linked, and disease severity varies from family to family. The major difference between these two disorders relates to therapy, in that cryoprecipitates of plasma lack factor IX. *(Cecil, p. 1001)*

143. (A) Patients with congenital dysfibrinogenemia have fibrinogen present in normal amounts, but the activity of this precursor substance is abnormal. In some patients with this disorder, platelet function will be abnormal, presumably because of the interaction between the abnormal fibrinogen and the platelet membrane. *(Cecil, p. 1002; Williams et al., pp. 1424–1429)*

144. (C); 145. (C); 146. (B); 147. (D) 144 and 145. A variety of inherited enzyme deficiencies of the Embden-Meyerhof pathway affect red cells, producing hemolytic anemia. The disease most frequently encountered is pyruvate kinase deficiency. Adult patients with this disorder present with splenomegaly, mild-to-moderate degrees of hemolytic anemia, and irregularly contracted or crenated red cells in the peripheral blood. Patients with this intrinsic red cell defect usually receive partial benefit from splenectomy. **146.** All the disorders of the Embden-Meyerhof pathway are inherited as autosomal recessive traits except for phosphoglycerate kinase deficiency, which is sex-linked. **147.** In triosephosphate isomerase deficiency, enzyme activity is low in somatic cells as well as in red cells. Thus, these patients succumb to failure of other organs. A progressive neurologic disorder is the usual cause of death in children with this type of hemolytic anemia. *(Cecil, pp. 866–867; Valentine; Williams et al., pp. 485–486)*

148. (B) In both classic hemophilia and von Willebrand's disease, factor VIII coagulation activity may be decreased. In the former this is usually associated with normal or increased factor VIII antigen activity in the plasma, whereas in the latter factor VIII antigen activity correlates with coagulation activity. *(Cecil, pp. 994, 999–1000)*

149. (B) Patients with von Willebrand's disease have abnormal platelet function as well as deficient fluid phase coagulation activity. Thus, they often have abnormal bleeding time and usually have abnormal platelet aggregation to the antimicrobial agent ristocetin. *(Cecil, pp. 999–1000)*

150. (D) Prothrombin time is not affected by deficiencies in factor VIII, and the platelet abnormalities associated with von Willebrand's disease do not alter this test. *(Cecil, p. 996)*

151. (B) The clinical presentation of von Willebrand's disease is different from that of classic hemophilia. The latter is a sex-linked disorder in which males are predominantly affected. In contrast, von Willebrand's disease has relatively equal frequency in men and women. In patients with von Willebrand's disease, bleeding symptoms vary considerably among affected members of the same family. *(Cecil, pp. 999–1000)*

152. (C) Salicylates will alter platelets in patients with either disorder, causing increased risk of serious bleeding. Salicylate-containing analgesics should be avoided in patients with either classic hemophilia or von Willebrand's disease. *(Cecil, p. 999)*

153. (C) Patients with systemic lupus erythematosus often develop autoimmune hemolytic anemia owing to warm-reacting IgG autoantibodies. Direct antiglobulin testing on these patients' red cells often shows both IgG and complement components. The complement components are attached to the red cells, presumably through activation of the complement cascade by the autoantibody. *(Cecil, pp. 871–872; Logue and Kurlander)*

154. (A) Autoimmune drug-induced hemolytic reactions due to methyldopa are caused by antibodies directed against the Rh antigens of red cells. Since these antibodies are unable to activate complement, IgG only is detected on red cells. *(Cecil, pp. 873–874)*

155. (B) In the so-called "innocent bystander" form of drug-induced immune hemolytic anemia, the drug functions as a haptene, and the antibodies are removed when red cells are washed prior to antiglobulin testing. Thus, only complement components are detected on the patient's red cells. *(Cecil, pp. 873–874)*

156. (B) The cold-reactive IgM autoantibodies responsible for hemolysis in the cold agglutinin syndrome activate components producing intravascular hemolysis. Upon warming, the antibody disassociates from the cell. Thus, only complement components are detected on the patient's red cells. *(Cecil, pp. 872–873)*

157. (C) The most serious side effect of bleomycin is pulmonary toxicity. This toxicity may begin as pneumonitis and progress to pulmonary fibrosis. Because of this reaction, the total dose of bleomycin given must be limited. Methotrexate has been reported, in rare instances, to produce pulmonary toxicity. *(Cecil, pp. 1042–1043; Friedman and Carter)*

158. (D) Cardiac toxicity, particularly cardiomyopathy, occurs with total doses of doxorubicin (Adriamycin) in excess of 550 mg/m^2. Thus, this reaction limits the total dose of Adriamycin that may be administered to individual patients. *(Cecil, p. 1043)*

159. (E) In addition to myelotoxicity, ulcerative stomatitis and gastrointestinal toxicity regularly occur with increasing doses of methotrexate. Although a somewhat less common reaction, stomatitis is also produced by bleomycin in some patients. *(Cecil, pp. 1038–1039)*

160. (G) The nitrosourea compounds such as BCNU produce delayed marrow toxicity with a nadir at four to six weeks. *(Cecil, pp. 1041–1042)*

161. (I) Sterile hemorrhagic cystitis caused by the accumulation of cyclophosphamide (Cytoxan) metabolites in the bladder is a preventable complication of this therapy. Patients receiving this drug should be instructed to maintain ample fluid intake and empty their bladders frequently. *(Cecil, p. 1041)*

162. (F) Vinca alkaloids produce dose-dependent neurotoxicity manifested predominantly as peripheral neuropathy. Autonomic or cranial nerve damage can also occur. *(Cecil, pp. 1043–1044)*

163. (B) Corticosteroids, because of their lack of bone marrow toxicity, are used in a variety of combination chemotherapy protocols. These agents are far from harmless, however, and complications such as bone demineralization, exacerbation of diabetes mellitus, and susceptibility to infections should be considered when they are used. *(Cecil, pp. 1045–1046)*

164. (F) Severe neurogenic constipation can occur with vincristine therapy, especially in children and young adults. Appropriate prophylactic treatment should be given with this agent. *(Cecil, pp. 1043–1044)*

165. (C) Bleomycin-produced dermatologic side effects include hyperpigmentation, hyperkeratosis, and ulceration, especially of the hands and feet. *(Cecil, pp. 1042–1043)*

166. (A) *Cis*-platinum has been found to be effective in a variety of neoplastic diseases such as testicular carcinoma. The major toxicity is renal damage, which can usually be prevented by maintaining high urine flow. *(Cecil, p. 1042)*

BIBLIOGRAPHY

Ahn, Y. S., Harrington, W. S., Seelman, R. C., et al.: Vincristine therapy of idiopathic and secondary thrombocytopenias. N. Engl. J. Med. *291*:376, 1974.

Blumfelder, T. M., Logue, G. L., and Shimm, D. S.: Felty's syndrome: effects of splenectomy upon granulocyte count and granulocyte-associated IgG. Ann. Intern. Med., *94*:623, 1981.

Brozović, M.: Oral anticoagulants in clinical practice. Semin. Hematol., *15*:27, 1978.

Budman, D. R., and Steinberg, A. D.: Hematologic aspects of systemic lupus erythematosus. Ann. Intern. Med., *86*:220, 1977.

Burchenol, J. H.: The historical development of cancer chemotherapy. Semin. Oncol., *4*:135, 1977.

Friedman, M. A., and Carter, S. B.: Serious toxicities associated with chemotherapy. Semin. Oncol., *5*:193, 1978.

Gralnick, H. R., Galton, D. A. G., Catovsky, D., et al.: Acute leukemia. Ann. Intern. Med., *87*:740, 1977.

Jacob, H., and Amsden, T.: Acute hemolytic anemia with rigid red cells in hypophosphatemia. N. Engl. J. Med., *285*:1446, 1971.

Krantz, S. B.: Pure red cell aplasia. Br. J. Haematol., *25*:1, 1973.

Kung, P. C., Long, J. C., McCaffrey, R. P., et al.: Terminal deoxynucleotidyl transferase in the diagnosis of leukemia and malignant lymphoma. Am. J. Med., *64*:788, 1978.

Kyle, R. A.: Monoclonal gammopathy of undetermined significance. Natural history of 241 cases. Am. J. Med., *64*:814, 1978.

Legha, S. S., Davis, H. L., and Muggia, F. M.: Hormonal therapy of breast cancer. Ann. Intern. Med., *88*:69, 1978.

Lessin, L.: Clinical implications of red cell shape. Adv. Intern. Med., *21*:451, 1976.

Logue, G. L., and Kurlander, R.: Immunologic mechanism of hemolysis in autoimmune hemolytic anemia. *In* Ioachim, H. L. (ed.): Pathobiology Annual. New York, Raven Press, 1978, p. 61.

Mazzaferri, E., Odorisio, T. M., and LoBuglio, A. F.: Hypercalcemia associated with malignancy. Semin. Oncol., *5*:141, 1978.

Mollison, P.: Blood Transfusion in Clinical Medicine. London, Blackwell Scientific Publications, Ltd., 1974.

Orkin, S. H., and Nathan, D. G.: The thalassemias. N. Engl. J. Med., *295*:710, 1977.

Petz, L., and Fudenberg, H.: Immunologic mechanisms in drug-induced cytopenias. Prog. Hematol., *9*:185, 1975.

Sarna, G. P., Holmes, E. C., and Petrovich, Z.: Lung cancer. *In* Haskell, C. M. (ed.): Cancer Treatment. Philadelphia, W. B. Saunders Company, 1980, pp. 197–226.

Sullivan, L. W.: Differential diagnosis and management of the patient with megaloblastic anemia. Am. J. Med., *48*:609, 1970.

Valentine, W. N.: Hemolytic anemia and inborn errors of metabolism. Blood, *54*:549, 1979.

Weiss, R. B.: Small cell carcinoma of the lung: therapeutic management. Ann. Intern. Med., *88*:522, 1978.

Williams, W. J., Beutler, E. L., Erslev, A. J., and Rundles, R. W.: Hematology. 2nd ed. New York, McGraw-Hill Book Company, 1977.

Wintrobe, M. W., Lee, E. G. R., Boggs, D. R., et al.: Clinical Hematology. 7th ed. Philadelphia, Lea & Febiger, 1974.

PART 6

GENETICS AND METABOLIC DISEASE

Guy Weinberg

DIRECTIONS: For questions 1 to 37, choose the ONE BEST answer to each question.

1. The transmission of a genetic disorder from father to son automatically EXCLUDES which pattern of inheritance?

A. Autosomal dominant
B. Autosomal recessive
C. X-linked
D. Chromosomal
E. None of the above

2. Your evaluation of a 3-year-old girl reveals a previously undescribed malformation syndrome. None of her three brothers and neither parent is affected. Which one of the following patterns of inheritance can be EXCLUDED on the basis of this family history ALONE?

A. Autosomal dominant
B. Autosomal recessive
C. X-linked
D. Chromosomal
E. None of the above

3. The gene coding for Tay-Sachs disease has a high frequency among Jews of Eastern European ancestry. This phenomenon is best explained by

A. Hardy-Weinberg equilibrium
B. genetic drift
C. pleiotropy
D. consanguinity

4. The most frequent initial manifestation of renal involvement in Alport's syndrome (chronic hereditary nephritis) is

A. proteinuria
B. acute renal failure
C. hematuria
D. hypertension
E. renal tubular acidosis

5. The biochemical abnormality that is most reproducibly found in the cells of patients with classic xeroderma pigmentosum is

A. inability to excise ultraviolet-induced cyclobutane thymine dimers in DNA
B. accelerated formation of ultraviolet-induced DNA crosslinks
C. increased susceptibility to ultraviolet-induced depurination in DNA
D. abnormal ultraviolet absorption spectrum of melanin

6. All the following disorders have been associated with neurofibromatosis EXCEPT

A. facial asymmetry
B. precocious puberty
C. pheochromocytoma
D. mental retardation
E. gastrinoma

7. Clinical concomitants of myotonic muscular dystrophy include all the following EXCEPT

A. cataracts
B. testicular atrophy
C. mental retardation
D. increased weakness in warm weather

8. The clinical feature of Duchenne muscular dystrophy that most reliably distinguishes it from other childhood muscular dystrophies is

A. massively elevated serum creatine phosphokinase
B. "Duchenne-pattern" electromyogram
C. age at onset and rate of progression
D. pseudohypertrophy of the calves

9. A man with oculocutaneous albinism and his albino spouse have five normally pigmented children. This pedigree demonstrates the principle/phenomenon of

A. genetic heterogeneity
B. pleiotropy
C. spontaneous mutation
D. variable expressivity
E. sister chromatid exchange

10. A boy and his maternal aunt have what percentage of autosomal genes in common?

A. 5%
B. 12½%
C. 25%
D. 33⅓%

11. The frequency of a recessive disorder in the general population is 36%. Assuming a Hardy-Weinberg equilibrium, what is the frequency of the single alternative allele that codes for the corresponding dominant trait?

A. 16%
B. 24%
C. 30%
D. 40%
E. 64%

12. All these globin molecules are coded for by genes linked to the γ-globin gene EXCEPT

A. δ
B. β
C. ϵ
D. α

13. The deletion of a specific gene as reflected in amniotic fluid cells can best be detected by the technique of

A. cellular hybridization and cloning
B. molecular hybridization with a complementary DNA
C. restriction endonuclease mapping
D. quantifying the activity of the gene product

14. An asymptomatic 20-year-old woman has one brother with cystic fibrosis. Neither of her parents is affected. The chance that she is a carrier is

A. 25%
B. 33⅓%
C. 50%
D. 66⅔%
E. 75%

15. The only child of a 22-year-old woman has died of Menkes' syndrome, a lethal X-linked recessive disorder of copper metabolism. The chance that the mother is a carrier of the gene coding for Menkes' syndrome is

A. 25%
B. 50%
C. 66⅔%
D. 75%
E. 100%

16. Initial or presenting clinical manifestations of Wilson's disease include all the following EXCEPT

A. psychosis
B. hemolytic anemia
C. hepatitis
D. acute tubular necrosis

17. The abnormality in iron metabolism characteristic of hemochromatosis is

A. increased gastrointestinal absorption
B. decreased biliary excretion
C. deficiency in serum apoferritin synthetase
D. increased affinity of transferrin for iron

18. Analysis of the karyotype in patients with Turner's syndrome reveals which one of the following?

A. Abnormal chromosomal banding pattern
B. Deletion of a chromosome
C. Presence of an extra chromosome
D. Normal karyotype

19. "Codons" are composed of how many nucleotide bases?

A. One
B. Two
C. Three
D. Four

20. A male patient has an unusual clinical disorder. On questioning you discover that his father had the same disorder and one of his two daughters has a similar illness. This pattern of inheritance is most likely

A. autosomal recessive
B. autosomal dominant
C. X-linked recessive
D. X-linked dominant

21. A young female immigrant to this country presents with an undiagnosed symptom complex. On taking a family history you find that both her mother and father are from a small isolated village in the Swiss Alps that has had a very stable population for the last 1000 years. Although the parents are both normal, two of the patient's six siblings, a brother and a sister, are also affected with this disorder. The patient's three children are normal. Assuming that this is an inherited disorder, which of the following is the most likely pattern of transmission?

A. Autosomal recessive
B. Autosomal dominant
C. X-linked recessive
D. X-linked dominant

22. The pedigree shown below is most consistent with which one of the following patterns of inheritance?

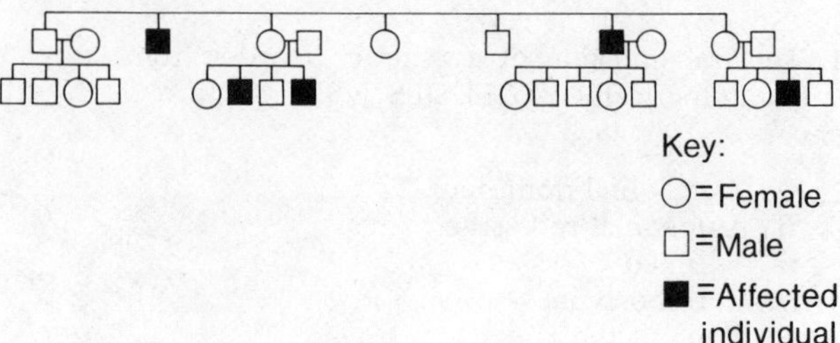

A. Autosomal recessive
B. Autosomal dominant
C. X-linked recessive
D. X-linked dominant

23. The association between a given disorder and the HLA type of the patient may be described by which one of the following genetic phenomena?

A. Pleiotropy
B. Independent assortment
C. Genetic or linkage disequilibrium
D. Lyon hypothesis

24. The frequency of chromosomal abnormalities in spontaneous abortuses is approximately

A. 5%
B. 10%
C. 20%
D. 50%

25. Which of the following corresponds to the karyotype 47,XX,+21?

A. Down's syndrome
B. Turner's syndrome
C. Klinefelter's syndrome
D. Bloom's syndrome

26. Mosaicism is usually caused by which of the following abnormalities?

A. Chromosome rearrangement
B. Chromosome deletion
C. Chromosome nondisjunction
D. Chromosome breakage

27. Which of the following is the most reliable means for differentiating between classic galactosemia (due to a deficiency of galactose-1-phosphate uridyl transferase) and the galactosemia that occurs with galactokinase deficiency?

A. Blood galactose levels
B. Mode of inheritance
C. Presence of cataracts
D. Presence of mental retardation and liver disease

28. The clinical presentation of hereditary fructose intolerance is most similar to that of which one of the following inborn errors of metabolism?

A. Type I glycogen storage disease
B. Type II glycogen storage disease
C. Classic galactosemia
D. Essential fructosuria

29. A bone marrow aspirate examined under phase microscopy appears as shown in the illustration.

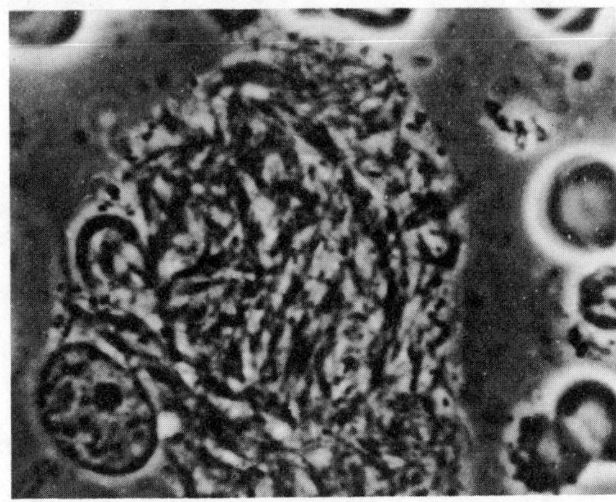

What is the most likely diagnosis?

A. Hunter's syndrome
B. Hurler's syndrome
C. Gaucher's disease
D. Niemann-Pick disease

30. Clinical gout, defined as arthritis, tophi, renal failure, or renal calculi, occurs in what percentage of hyperuricemic subjects?

A. 10–20%
B. 20–30%
C. 30–40%
D. 40–50%

31. A patient consults you because of acute pain in the left knee. Arthrocentesis reveals a synovial fluid with a white blood cell count of 70,000/cu mm. Examination of this fluid under compensated, polarized light microscopy reveals the findings shown in the illustrations opposite.

What is the most likely diagnosis?

A. Gout
B. Pseudogout
C. Reiter's syndrome
D. Infection

32. In patients with severe neurologic or neuromuscular dysfunction, it may be necessary to treat an attack of acute intermittent porphyria with intravenous hematin. Which of the following mechanisms is thought to be responsible for the rapid response observed following hematin infusion?

A. Reversal of the neurotoxic effects of porphobilinogen
B. Stimulation of uroporphyrinogen synthetase activity
C. Suppression of delta-aminolevulinic acid (ALA) synthetase activity
D. Increase in urinary porphyrin excretion

33. Which of the following findings is most consistent with a diagnosis of protoporphyria?

A. Severe scarring and mutilation of hands and face
B. Blister formation after trivial trauma
C. Solar urticaria or eczema
D. Hypertrichosis

34. A neurologist asks for your opinion regarding a mentally retarded 7-year-old boy who has passed many radiolucent renal calculi. The child has choreoathetosis, spasticity, and dysarthria, and recently has begun to bite his fingers and lips. Measurement of which of the following substances would be most likely to yield a diagnosis?

A. PP-ribose-P synthetase
B. Glucose-6-phosphatase
C. Hypoxanthine-guanine phosphoribosyltransferase
D. Xanthine oxidase

35. Which of the following clinical or laboratory findings is most characteristic of essential pentosuria?

A. Positive reaction of urine with glucose oxidase reagent on dip sticks
B. Positive reaction of urine with reagents used to detect reducing sugar
C. Early cataract formation
D. Retinopathy similar to that seen in patients with diabetes

36. Familial dysbetalipoproteinemia (broad-beta disease) may be distinguished from the other inborn errors of lipoprotein metabolism by which of the following findings?

A. Premature atherosclerosis
B. Corneal arcus
C. Tendon xanthomas
D. Planar xanthomas in palmar and digital creases

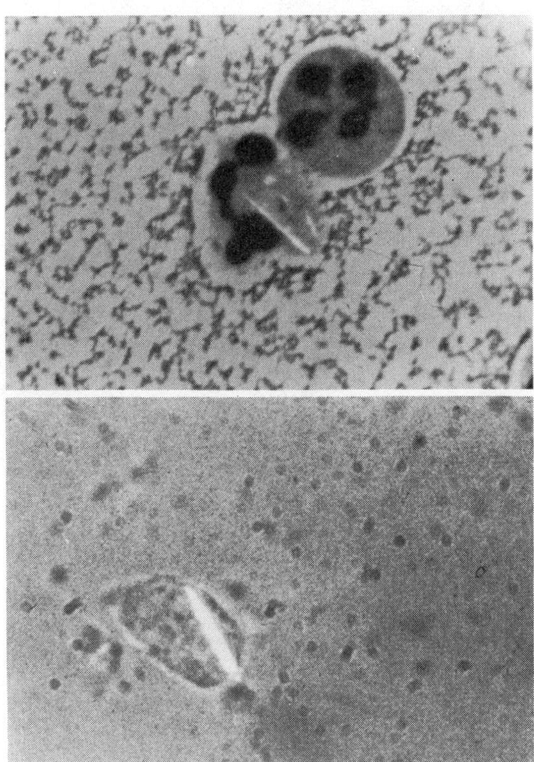

37. Maple syrup urine disease is characterized by excessive renal excretion of leucine, isoleucine, alloisoleucine, and valine caused by

A. a defect in decarboxylation of branched-chain alpha-ketoacids
B. a defect in renal transport of branched-chain alpha-ketoacids
C. increased intestinal absorption of branched-chain alpha-ketoacids
D. increased metabolic production of branched-chain alpha-ketoacids

DIRECTIONS: For questions 38 to 57, you are to decide whether EACH choice is true or false. Any combination of answers, from all true to all false, may be present. Mark the answer sheet "T" or "F" in the space provided.

38. Which of the following statements regarding cystic fibrosis is/are true?

A. Sweat sodium concentration is decreased
B. Carrier frequency in whites is approximately 4%
C. Aspermia is common in affected males
D. A defect in the receptor–adenyl cyclase membrane coupling protein "N" is found in cells of patients with cystic fibrosis

39. Which of the following statements regarding the slow hepatic isoniazid transacetylation phenotype is/are true?

A. Prevalence is approximately 5% in whites
B. Patients have increased susceptibility to isoniazid hepatotoxicity
C. The inheritance pattern is autosomal dominant
D. The enzymatic abnormality can be diagnosed by measuring the "dibucaine number"

40. Which of the following statements regarding copper metabolism is/are true?

A. Serum transport of copper is mainly by ceruloplasmin
B. The major excretory route for copper is the biliary system
C. There is increased serum concentration of copper in Wilson's disease
D. There is increased urinary excretion of copper in Wilson's disease

41. A 30-year-old man has a single café au lait spot and one 2 × 2–mm subcutaneous nodule that is shown by biopsy to be a neurofibroma. The patient's brother has moderately short stature, severe scoliosis, a malignant glioma, and large numbers of pedunculated cutaneous neurofibromas. The principles demonstrated by this sibship include which of the following?

A. Diminished penetrance
B. Variable expressivity
C. Pleiotropy
D. Sex-limited inheritance

42. Which of the following statements regarding glucose-6-phosphate dehydrogenase deficiency (G6PD) is/are true?

A. Inheritance is X-linked
B. Administration of sulfa drugs induces hemolysis in these patients
C. It is associated with neurologic deterioration
D. Enzyme deficiency is most easily documented immediately following an episode of hemolysis

43. A patient is referred to you by an ophthalmologist because a diagnosis of Marfan's syndrome or homocystinuria is suggested from the finding of ectopia lentis. Although these two disorders are phenotypically similar, a specific diagnosis is required, since the management of patients with these two disorders differs in which of the following categories?

A. Genetic counseling
B. Prognosis
C. Treatment
D. Associated clinical abnormalities

44. For which of the following disorders is it appropriate to screen the family members of an affected person for the heterozygous or carrier state?

A. Marfan's syndrome
B. Tay-Sachs disease
C. Translocation Down's syndrome
D. Lesch-Nyhan syndrome

45. Amniocentesis is useful in intrauterine diagnosis of which of the following types of disorders?

A. Chromosomal aberrations
B. Inborn errors of metabolism
C. Neural tube defects
D. Teratogenic abnormalities

46. Characteristic findings in familial lipoprotein lipase deficiency (type 1 hyperlipoproteinemia) include which of the following?

A. Lipemia retinalis
B. Eruptive xanthomas
C. Recurrent bouts of pancreatitis
D. Premature atherosclerosis

47. Abetalipoproteinemia is characterized by which of the following?

A. Premature atherosclerosis
B. Ataxia and peripheral neuropathy
C. Obesity
D. Acanthocytes

48. Hyperuricemia results from which of the following?

A. Increased purine absorption
B. Decreased uric acid excretion
C. Increased purine synthesis
D. Decreased uric acid catabolism

49. Which of the following clinical manifestations of gout is/are due to the deposition of monosodium urate crystals?

A. Renal calculi
B. Acute arthritis
C. Tophi
D. Gouty kidney

50. A clinical diagnosis of gout may be suspected from which of the following historical points?

A. Rapid onset of pain
B. Severe pain with little or no inflammation
C. Monarticular pain
D. Failure of the pain to resolve in a period of one month

51. Uric acid calculi are associated with which of the following abnormalities?

A. Increased uric acid excretion
B. Persistently alkaline urine
C. Highly concentrated urine
D. Renal tubular acidosis

52. Orotic aciduria is seen in which of the following conditions?

A. Deficiencies of orotate phosphoribosyltransferase and orotidine 5′-phosphate decarboxylase
B. Therapy with allopurinol
C. Ornithine transcarbamylase deficiency
D. Carbamyl phosphate synthetase deficiency

53. Acute intermittent porphyria is associated with which of the following findings?

A. Cutaneous photosensitivity with scarring
B. Excretion of red urine
C. Central nervous system dysfunctions
D. Severe abdominal pain

54. Which of the following drugs is/are contraindicated in patients with acute intermittent porphyria, variegate porphyria, and hereditary coproporphyria?

A. Phenothiazines
B. Barbiturates
C. Sulfonamides
D. Intravenous glucose

55. Porphyria cutanea tarda is associated with which of the following findings?

A. Cutaneous lesions
B. Abdominal pain
C. Neurologic dysfunction
D. Hepatic dysfunction

56. Laurence-Moon-Biedl syndrome is associated with which of the following findings?

A. Obesity
B. Retinitis pigmentosa
C. Hypogonadism
D. Polydactyly

57. Which of the following statements regarding familial Mediterranean fever is/are correct?

A. It is inherited in an autosomal dominant manner
B. It is more common in people of Mediterranean or Middle Eastern origin living in the United States
C. There is no effective therapy
D. Amyloidosis is a rare complication of this disorder in patients living in the United States

DIRECTIONS: Questions 58 to 119 are matching questions. For each numbered item, choose the most likely associated lettered item from those provided. Each numbered item has ONLY ONE answer. Within each group, each lettered item may be the answer to one, more than one, or none of the numbered items.

QUESTIONS 58–61

For each of the following abnormalities, select the specific type of genetic alteration responsible for it.

A. Mispairing and unequal crossing over
B. Integration of transposable elements
C. Non-sense mutation
D. Mis-sense mutation
E. Mutation of the initiator codon
F. Mutation in the terminator codon

58. Hemoglobin Lepore

59. Hemoglobin Constant Spring

60. β^0 thalassemia (certain forms)

61. Sickle cell hemoglobin

QUESTIONS 62–64

For each developmental phenomenon, select the agent most closely correlated with its induction.

A. H-Y antigen
B. Testosterone
C. Dihydrotestosterone
D. Desoxycorticosterone

62. Appearance of pubic hair, enlargement of phallus, lowering of voice

63. Formation of penis and scrotum

64. Differentiation of testes

QUESTIONS 65–72

For each of the following hereditary disorders, select the manifestation that is most likely to influence adversely the prognosis of an affected individual.

A. Renal failure
B. Respiratory failure
C. Arterial rupture
D. Aortic root dilatation
E. Adverse reaction to medication, particularly during surgery
F. Neurologic deterioration
G. Malignant transformation

65. Marfan's syndrome

66. Malignant hyperthermia

67. Ehlers-Danlos syndrome, type IV

68. Pseudocholinesterase deficiency

69. Duchenne muscular dystrophy

70. Hyperkeratosis of palms and soles

71. Gardner's syndrome

72. Homozygous deficiency of α_1-antitrypsin

QUESTIONS 73–76

For each of these congenital conditions, select whether an increased incidence is associated with advancing age of the mother, the father, or neither parent.

A. Mother
B. Father
C. Neither

73. Trisomy 18

74. Sporadic Marfan's syndrome (i.e., new mutation)

75. Sporadic achondroplasia (i.e., new mutation)

76. Dizygotic twinning

QUESTIONS 77–81

For each patient described below, select the most appropriate therapy for the genetic disease.

A. Phlebotomy
B. Penicillamine
C. Androgens
D. Castration
E. Hematin
F. Progesterone

77. A 20-year-old woman with a one-year history of schizophrenia. Her psychosis has become worse in spite of phenothiazine therapy, and she has a movement disorder that began at the same time that phenothiazine was started

78. A 40-year-old man with impotence, hypogonadism, mildly elevated SGOT, and symmetric arthritis affecting the second and third metacarpophalangeal joints

79. A 20-year-old woman with episodic abdominal pain, often associated with generalized nonpitting edema

80. A 9-year-old girl with short stature and a webbed neck. Karyotype reveals a 40, XO/46, XY mosaicism

81. A 20-year-old woman with abdominal pain and acute psychosis that began 36 hours after she started taking oral contraceptives. Serum sodium is 120 mEq/L

QUESTIONS 82–85

For each of the following patients, select the most likely associated malformation.

A. Aortic stenosis
B. Coarctation of the aorta
C. Atrioventricular canal
D. Pulmonic stenosis
E. Patent ductus arteriosus

82. An infant with hypotonia, brachydactyly, and trisomy for a small acrocentric autosome

83. A 10-year-old boy with hypertelorism, downward eye slant, mild mental retardation, pectus excavatum, and a webbed neck

84. A 15-year-old girl with a webbed neck, cubitus valgus, gonadal dysgenesis, short stature, normal intelligence, and 45 chromosomes; as a newborn, she was noted to have pedal edema

85. A 20-year-old man with a coarse voice, thickened lips, stellate iris, and mental retardation; he has a history of neonatal hypercalcemia

QUESTIONS 86–87

The following abnormal hemoglobins are commonly associated with a specific form of α-thalassemia. For each of them, select the number of functioning α-globin genes characteristic of the corresponding α-thalassemia.

A. None
B. One
C. Two
D. Three

86. γ_4 (Hb Bart's)

87. β_4 (Hb H)

QUESTIONS 88–91

For each clinical description, select the most likely associated enzyme deficiency.

A. Glucose-6-phosphatase deficiency (type I glycogen storage disease)
B. α-1,4-glucosidase deficiency (type II glycogen storage disease)
C. Phosphorylase deficiency (type V glycogen storage disease)
D. Glucocerebrosidase deficiency (Gaucher's disease)
E. Hexosaminidase A deficiency (Tay-Sachs disease)

88. Adult with muscle cramping and myoglobinuria after strenuous exercise

89. Adult with hepatosplenomegaly, bone pain, and lipid-laden, PAS-positive histiocytes in bone marrow aspirate

90. Infant with severe hypotonia, cardiomegaly, and congestive heart failure

91. Infant with hepatosplenomegaly, neurologic deterioration, and PAS-positive lipid-laden histiocytes in bone marrow aspirate

QUESTIONS 92–95

For each phenotype, select the most likely associated biochemical abnormality.

A. Deficiency of serum high-density lipoprotein
B. Deficiency of cell surface low-density lipoprotein (LDL)
C. Uroporphyrinogen synthetase deficiency
D. Unresponsiveness to parathyroid hormone
E. Cystathionine synthetase deficiency
F. Accumulation of phytanic acid
G. α-galactosidase deficiency

92. Ectopia lentis, venous thrombosis, seizures, osteoporosis

93. Retinitis pigmentosa, ataxia, ichthyosis, peripheral neuropathy, short fourth metatarsals

94. Yellow hyperplastic tonsils

95. Painful dysesthesias, diffuse telangiectases, renal failure

QUESTIONS 96–99

For each characteristic, select the enzyme deficiency responsible for the corresponding adrenogenital syndrome.

A. 21-hydroxylase deficiency
B. 17α-hydroxylase deficiency
C. 11β-hydroxylase deficiency
D. None of the above

96. The most common adrenogenital syndrome

97. Sexual infantilism

98. Salt wasting

99. Autosomal dominant inheritance

QUESTIONS 100–102

Match the following statements with the most appropriate type of glycogen storage disease.

A. Type I (glucose-6-phosphatase deficiency)
B. Type III (amylo-1,6-glucosidase deficiency)
C. Type IV (amylo-1,4 $\rightarrow$ 1,6-transglucosylase deficiency)
D. Type V (phosphorylase deficiency)

100. Associated with the development of gout

101. Associated with both hepatic and muscle manifestations

102. Associated with splenomegaly

QUESTIONS 103–106

Match each of the following lipoprotein classes with the type of lipid it transports in the serum.

A. Triglyceride
B. Cholesterol
C. Both triglyceride and cholesterol

103. Chylomicrons

104. Very-low-density lipoproteins (VLDL)

105. High-density lipoproteins (HDL)

106. Low-density lipoproteins (LDL)

QUESTIONS 107–111

Match the biochemical deficiencies with the appropriate disorder of lipoprotein metabolism.

A. Type I hyperlipoproteinemia
B. Familial dysbetalipoproteinemia

C. Tangier disease
D. Familial hypercholesterolemia
E. Abetalipoproteinemia

107. Deficiency of the apo E-3 component of the arginine-rich apoprotein

108. Deficiency of the high-affinity receptor for low-density lipoprotein

109. Deficiency of lipoprotein lipase

110. Deficiency of B-apoprotein

111. Deficiency of A-apoprotein

QUESTIONS 112–115

Match the following clinical disorders with the appropriate inborn error of purine metabolism.

A. Myoadenylate deaminase deficiency
B. Adenosine deaminase deficiency
C. Xanthine oxidase deficiency
D. Purine nucleoside phosphorylase deficiency

112. Combined immunodeficiency disease with severe T- and B-lymphocyte dysfunction

113. Immunodeficiency disease with a predominant T-lymphocyte dysfunction

114. Nonprogressive myopathy with normal lactate production but decreased ammonia production

115. Myopathy due to crystal deposition

QUESTIONS 116–119

Match the clinical descriptions with the appropriate syndrome.

A. Hunter's syndrome
B. Hurler's syndrome
C. Morquio's syndrome
D. Maroteaux-Lamy syndrome
E. Scheie's syndrome
F. Sanfilippo's syndrome

116. Severe mental retardation, early corneal clouding, severe skeletal changes, valvular heart disease, death before age 10

117. Normal intelligence, corneal clouding, dwarfism and skeletal changes, cervical myelopathy, aortic disease, death before age 55

118. Slow mental deterioration, no corneal clouding, mild-to-severe skeletal changes, X-linked inheritance, death before age 15

119. Normal intelligence, corneal clouding, stiff joints, aortic disease, normal lifespan

PART 6

GENETICS AND METABOLIC DISEASE

ANSWERS

1. (C) In humans the male is the heterogametic sex, and the sex of the offspring is determined by the sex chromosome inherited from the father. Thus, any offspring inheriting an X-linked trait from the father must by definition have inherited the X chromosome and therefore be a female. In disorders (such as pseudohypoparathyroidism) in which the available pedigrees do not allow a clear distinction between autosomal dominant and X-linked dominant transmission, examples of father-to-son transmission confirm autosomal inheritance. *(Cecil, p. 4; Jackson and Schimke, pp. 22–23)*

2. (E) A common error is that a negative family history precludes the possibility of a hereditary disease. This disorder, if it is genetic, could represent: (1) a spontaneous mutation of an autosomal dominant disorder; (2) a recessive disorder, in which case it is expected that neither parent would be affected; (3) an X-linked disorder inherited from a subclinically affected mother; or (4) a spontaneous mutation of an X-linked condition. Alternatively, the child could possess chromosomal aneuploidy on the basis of either maternal or paternal gametic nondisjunction or the inheritance of an imbalanced translocation from a balanced carrier parent. A useful summary of basic aspects of genetic counseling is found in *Smith, pp. 416–431.*

3. (B) Genetic drift is defined as the random fluctuation of gene frequencies in small populations. A special case of genetic drift occurs when a new colony is established in isolation from a parent population, and the gene pool of the derived population differs from that of the parent population; this is referred to as the *founder principle*. Thus, a gene, such as that coding for Tay-Sachs disease, that had a very low frequency in the parent population may have an extraordinarily high frequency in the derived population.

The Hardy-Weinberg equilibrium refers to an idealized population in which the observed frequency of genotypes will be in the proportions expected from the Hardy-Weinberg law. These proportions will remain constant over succeeding generations provided that there are no new mutations, that there is no difference in the biologic fitness of any of the genotypes, and that mating is random.

Pleiotropy refers to the multiple phenotypic effects produced by one mutant gene. The vast majority of genetic disorders are pleiotropic.

Although the frequency of recessive disorders is much greater among the offspring of consanguineous matings, consanguinity is not in itself a cause for the high frequency of a particular mutant allele in a given population. *(Cecil, pp. 1, 2, 5; Jackson and Schimke, pp. 20–21, 622; Vogel and Motulsky, pp. 102, 435)*

4. (C) Alport's syndrome is a hereditary disorder resulting in chronic nephritis and progressive sensorineural deafness; it accounts for approximately 1% of hereditary deafness. The disease is generally more severe in males, and there is controversy regarding the mode of inheritance (X-linked dominant versus autosomal dominant). Approximately 50% of congenital deafness is hereditary, and most of these cases represent recessive disorders. *(Cecil, p. 568; Jackson and Schimke, pp. 443–448)*

5. (A) Xeroderma pigmentosum is an autosomal recessive disorder in which there is a defect in DNA repair resulting in increased susceptibility to UV-induced damage of the DNA. The increased frequency of skin cancers among patients with xeroderma pigmentosum may be due to somatic mutations caused by this damage. Ultraviolet radiation, although non-ionizing, is capable of exciting the electrons in the double bonds of adjacent thymine nucleotides, resulting in cyclobutane thymine dimers. If not excised prior to DNA synthesis, these dimers result in reduced fidelity of DNA replication and concomitant mutation. *(Cecil, p. 2274; Stanbury, Wyngaarden, and Fredrickson, pp. 1073–1095; Jackson and Schimke, p. 76)*

6. (E) Neurofibromatosis is one of the most pleiotropic of all genetic disorders; it can affect, primarily or secondarily, virtually any organ system. It is also characterized by widely variable severity and expressivity. A proliferation of skin and subcutaneous tissues may lead to asymmetric hypertrophy, including that of the face. Precocious puberty may result from neurologic abnormalities that release inhibitory effects of the hypothalamus on gonadotropin release. Focal gliosis and ectopic islands of gray matter in the cerebral cortex may lead to mental retardation. Pheochromocytomas are found with increased frequency in neurofibromatosis, but gastrinomas are not. *(Cecil, pp. 2043–2044; Smith, pp. 302–303; Jackson and Schimke, pp. 99, 335, 394, 450, 503, 557)*

7. (D) The muscular dystrophies are extraordinarily heterogeneous (different disorders with common characteristics, different genotypes with similar phenotypes), and myotonic muscular dystrophy is exceptionally pleiotropic (one genotype with many phenotypic consequences). Myotonia (not weakness) increases in *cold* weather. Premature cataracts, frontal baldness in men, testicular atrophy, and mental retardation are characteristic findings in this disorder. *(Cecil, p. 2172; Smith, pp. 114–115; Stanbury, Wyngaarden, and Fredrickson, pp. 1265–1269)*

8. (C) The underlying genetic defect has yet to be defined for most of the muscular dystrophies. Thus, accurate diagnosis is generally made on the basis of a combination of clinical and laboratory features. CPK elevations, myopathic electromyograms, and muscle biopsies are often useful in separating the muscular dystrophies from other disorders of muscle (e.g., congenital myopathy, glycogen storage diseases); however, these tests frequently do not allow clear separation of the various forms of muscular dystrophy. This often requires examination of specific clinical features such as the pattern of muscle involvement. The most characteristic clinical features of Duchenne muscular dystrophy are the age of onset (age 2 to 4 years) and the rate of progression (rapid with loss of ambulation by early adolescence and death in the late teens or early 20s). *(Cecil, pp. 2171–2172; Dubowitz, pp. 1–18)*

9. (A) Generally, when two people with the same recessive disorder mate, it is expected that all their offspring will be similarly affected since there are no normal alleles among the available gametes. In an instance such as this in which the offspring are all normal, it must be postulated that disorders that appear to be the same are in fact different genotypically (genetic heterogeneity). The offspring are therefore a consequence of genetic complementation in which the normal allele of each parent offsets the missing allele of the other parent. *(Cecil, pp. 15–16; Vogel and Motulsky, pp. 116–117)*

10. (C) The percentage of autosomal genes shared by any two relatives is a direct function of their degree of relation, i.e., as given by the equation

$$C = 0.5^n$$

where n is the degree of relation and C is the percentage of genes in common. Thus, first-degree relatives (e.g., sibling-sibling, parent-offspring) share 50% of their genes and second-degree relatives (e.g., nephew-aunt) share 25% of their autosomal genes. Calculations of this sort are important in determining the increased risk for a deleterious recessive disorder among the offspring of a consanguineous mating. A more rigorous explanation and derivation of the "coefficient of kinship" is found in *Vogel and Motulsky, pp. 414–416.*

11. (D) The Hardy-Weinberg equation is

$$p^2 + 2pq + q^2 = 1$$

where p is the frequency of the dominant gene and q is the frequency of the corresponding recessive gene ($p + q = 1$). For a population in Hardy-Weinberg equilibrium, p^2 is the frequency of the homozygous dominant genotype, q^2 is the frequency of the homozygous recessive genotype, and 2pq is the frequency of the heterozygote. Therefore, in this problem where $q^2 = 0.36$,

$$p = 1 - \sqrt{0.36} = 1 - 0.6 = 0.4$$

(Cecil, pp. 5–6; Vogel and Motulsky, pp. 102, 372, 381)

12. (D) Recent technical advances in molecular biology have allowed detailed mapping and, in certain instances, sequencing of the globin genes. The ζ and α globin genes are linked and located on chromosome number 16. The coding genes in the "β-globin system" are linked and on chromosome number 11; these include (in a 5′ to 3′ direction) epsilon, G-gamma-, A-gamma-, delta-, and beta-globin genes. Note that these progress in the same order in which they appear during embryonic and fetal development! This relationship may reflect or parallel the evolutionary development of these related genes. *(Cecil, pp. 11–12; Jackson and Schimke, pp. 349–350)*

13. (B) The presence or absence of a gene is best demonstrated by the ability of the DNA in question to hybridize to an appropriate complementary DNA (cDNA). *Cellular* hybridization and cloning has a wide variety of applications including the mapping of a gene to a particular chromosome or chromosomal segment. The absence of a gene product does not necessarily imply absence of the gene, which may be present but not expressed. *(Cecil, pp. 11–12; Kan et al.; Taylor et al.)*

14. (D) Assuming that both the woman's parents are carriers for the cystic fibrosis gene, the expected phenotypic ratios among their offspring would be 1:2:1 (homozygous normal:carrier (asymptomatic):affected). Since any asyptomatic offspring is known not to be affected, it follows that an unaffected offspring has a one-third chance of being homozygous normal and a two-thirds chance of being a carrier. *(Cecil, p. 3)*

15. (C) It is difficult to counsel a woman who has a single male child affected by a lethal X-linked disorder for which there is no good method for carrier detection. The major issue is whether the child represents a new mutation (with risk to subsequent offspring being effectively zero) or whether the mother is a carrier (with a 50–50 risk to subsequent male offspring). If the mutation rates are the same in males and females, it is possible to form a complex Bayesian statistical calculation that defines a two-thirds probability that the mother is a carrier and a one-third probability that the singleton male is a new mutation. An easy way to remember this is that there are three X chromosomes involved here: the mother has two of them, and therefore her probability for having the X chromosome with the mutation on it is two thirds. The offspring has only one of the X chromosomes, and his probability of being a sporadic mutation is therefore one third. *(Stanbury, Wyngaarden, and Fredrickson, p. 1116; Vogel and Motulsky, pp. 294–295)*

16. (D) Wilson's disease is an autosomal recessive disorder characterized by excessive accumulation of copper and inadequate synthesis of ceruloplasmin. Hemolytic anemia in Wilson's disease is presumably a consequence of abrupt release of hepatic stores of copper. The renal involvement may be detectable as a mild Fanconi syndrome; however, acute renal failure is exceedingly uncommon. *(Cecil, pp. 1126–1128; Stanbury, Wyngaarden, and Fredrickson, pp. 1098–1102)*

17. (A) Hemochromatosis is characterized by an excessive accumulation of iron owing to increased gastrointestinal absorption of iron. It is a genetic disorder that has recently been demonstrated to be transmitted as an autosomal recessive trait. The heterozygote frequency has been estimated to be as high as 10 to 11% in studies in Utah and Brittany, which establish hemochromatosis as being one of the most common human genetic disorders. *(Cecil, pp. 1128–1131; Cartwright et al.)*

18. (B) Deletion of an entire chromosome (e.g., the X chromosome in Turner's syndrome) or the presence of an extra chromosome (e.g., trisomy 21 in Down's syndrome) is easily detected on karyotypic analysis. In addition, much more subtle changes to chromosome structure can now be detected with special staining techniques called "banding." *(Cecil, pp. 19, 20; Sutton, Ch. 4)*

19. (C) Proteins are composed of 20 different amino acids, yet DNA is composed of only four different nucleotide bases. The translation of the genetic information in DNA into the synthesis of a protein is accomplished by arranging the nucleotides in units called "codons" composed of three nucleotide bases. *(Cecil, p. 8; Stanbury, Wyngaarden, and Fredrickson, pp. 47–49)*

20. (B) This is most likely to be an autosomal dominant trait. Since it occurs in three successive generations, autosomal recessive inheritance is unlikely. Father-to-son transmission excludes an X-linked disorder. *(Cecil, pp. 2–4; Sutton, Ch. 1–3)*

21. (A) This is most likely an autosomal recessive disorder, since both males and females are affected, affected individuals occur in only one generation, and the geographic isolation of the population suggests consanguinity. *(Cecil, p. 3; Sutton, Ch. 1–3)*

22. (C) This is most likely an X-linked recessive trait, since only males are affected, transmission is through females who are normal, and there is no evidence of father-to-son transmission. *(Cecil, p. 4; Sutton, Ch. 1–3)*

23. (C) There is a strong association between a number of disorders (e.g., ankylosing spondylitis) and the HLA type of the individual. The explanation for these associations is not known at present, but they may represent examples of genetic or linkage disequilibrium. *(Cecil, p. 5)*

24. (C) Nearly all cytogenetic aberrations among spontaneous abortions are numerical abnormalities. The most common specific defect is X monosomy (25% of abnormals); autosomal monosomies (45%) and polyploidies (20%) account for most of the remaining abnormalities. Among live-born infants, six of 1000 have a chromosomal defect sufficient to cause disability at some time in their lives. *(Cecil, p. 17; Hassold et al.)*

25. (A) By conventional nomenclature this shorthand notation describes a female XX with 47 chromosomes, including an extra chromosome 21. The clinical diagnosis is Down's syndrome. *(Cecil, p. 19; Stanbury, Wyngaarden, and Fredrickson, pp. 54–59)*

26. (C) Mosaicism typically results from mitotic nondisjunction, the failure of a set of paired chromosomes to separate during mitotic division. *(Cecil, pp. 19–20)*

27. (D) Mental retardation and cirrhosis are thought to be the consequence of galactose-1-phosphate accumulation in patients with the transferase deficiency. *(Cecil, pp. 1079–1080; Stanbury, Wyngaarden, and Fredrickson, pp. 160–182)*

28. (C) Hereditary fructose intolerance (deficiency of phosphofructoaldolase B) may be confused with classic galactosemia because the liver abnormalities and other metabolic derangements are similar in these two conditions. One potential explanation is that a phosphorylated hexose, i.e., galactose-1-phosphate and fructose-1-phosphate, accumulates in the liver and other organs. *(Cecil, pp. 1082–1083; Stanbury, Wyngaarden, and Fredrickson, pp. 121–137)*

29. (C) Cells from patients with Gaucher's disease have this characteristic appearance. Cells from patients with Hurler's syndrome have characteristic granules in the cytoplasm called Reilly bodies. Foam cells are found in the marrow of children with Niemann-Pick disease. *(Cecil, pp. 1093–1094; Stanbury, Wyngaarden, and Fredrickson, pp. 731–747)*

30. (A) Hyperuricemia cannot be equated with clinical gout. Although all patients with gout have hyperuricemia, only 10 to 20% of individuals with hyperuricemia will develop one of the clinical manifestations listed. *(Cecil, p. 1107; Wyngaarden and Kelley, pp. 21–38)*

31. (A) These slides show intracellular, negatively birefringent, needle-shaped crystals, i.e., monosodium urate. Demonstration of these crystals is the most reliable method for diagnosing gouty arthritis. Similar crystals may be obtained upon aspiration of liquefied tophi in gout. *(Cecil, pp. 1115–1116; Wyngaarden and Kelley, pp. 177–192)*

32. (C) The increased activity of ALA synthetase in patients with acute intermittent porphyria is thought to be secondary to decreased feedback inhibition and/or derepression due to the primary block in heme synthesis, i.e., uroporphyrinogen synthetase deficiency. Following the administration of hematin there is immediate feedback inhibition and later repression of ALA synthetase, with subsequent decrease in ALA and porphobilinogen synthesis. *(Cecil, p. 1124–1125; Dhar et al.)*

33. (C) The skin lesions in protoporphyria are distinct from those seen in other types of porphyria in that they do not heal with scarring, and there is no associated hypertrichosis. *(Cecil, p. 1123; Stanbury, Wyngaarden, and Fredrickson, pp. 1166–1221)*

34. (C) The neurologic history and self-destructive behavior are typical of the Lesch-Nyhan syndrome. The radiolucent calculi are most likely the result of uric acid stones. The diagnosis can be established by quantification of hypoxanthine-guanine phosphoribosyltransferase activity in erythrocyte lysate. *(Cecil, p. 1119; Stanbury, Wyngaarden, and Fredrickson, pp. 1011–1037)*

35. (B) Hereditary pentosuria is a benign condition without clinical consequences. It may be mistaken for diabetes mellitus because the xylulose excreted in the urine will react with reducing agents used in qualitative tests for urine glucose. Xylulose does not react with glucose oxidase. *(Cecil, p. 1082; Stanbury, Wyngaarden, and Fredrickson, pp. 110–121)*

36. (D) Presence of the characteristic planar xanthomas in palmar and digital creases is pathognomonic for this disorder if obstructive disease of the biliary tract has been excluded. *(Cecil, p. 1087; Stanbury, Wyngaarden, and Fredrickson, pp. 633–641)*

37. (A) This branched-chain aminoaciduria is not due to a defect in the renal transport system; rather, it is an example of "overflow" aminoaciduria caused by a defect in decarboxylation of branched-chain alpha-ketoacids. *(Cecil, pp. 1105–1106)*

38. (A — False; B — True; C — True; D — False) The specific molecular defect in this lethal autosomal recessive disorder remains unknown, and there is as yet no therapy specific for it. Recent increases in survival are a consequence of the availability of better therapy for chronic and intercurrent complications of this disorder. A 50% reduction in the activity of a membrane protein responsible for coupling the receptor for hormones and guanine nucleotides to adenyl cyclase has recently been described in the red cells of patients with pseudohypoparathyroidism, not cystic fibrosis. *(Cecil, pp. 387–388; Farfel et al.)*

39. (All are False) Slow inactivators of INH have a diminished activity of hepatic *N*-acetyl transferase, and this phenotype is inherited in an autosomal recessive fashion. The frequency of homozygotes for the slow variant allele is 50% among European populations. The frequency of INH-induced polyneuropathy (and systemic lupus erythematosus) is higher among *slow* inactivators, whereas the hepatic toxicity of INH is more frequent among *rapid* inactivators. Other genetic disorders that illustrate the application of pharmacogenetics to general internal medicine include G6PD deficiency and pseudocholinesterase deficiency. The "dibucaine number" is used to diagnose the common pseudocholinesterase variant associated with increased sensitivity to drugs such as succinylcholine. It is defined as the percentage inhibition of pseudocholinesterase activity by 10^{-5}M dibucaine, and is *lower* in patients with the variant pseudocholinesterase than in those with the normal enzyme. *(Cecil, pp. 63–64; Vogel and Motulsky, pp. 257–258; Jackson and Schimke, pp. 249–250)*

40. (A — False; B — True; C — False; D — True) Ceruloplasmin is *not* the copper serum transport molecule, but is an enzyme (functioning as a ferroxidase) in which copper is a covalently bound and non–freely dissociable component.

The underlying defect in Wilson's disease is unknown. It adversely affects biliary excretion of copper, resulting in accumulation of total body copper and subsequent deposition in various tissues (liver, eye, brain, bone, and kidney). Hepatic synthesis of ceruloplasmin is also adversely affected, since copper cannot be effectively incorporated into the ceruloplasmin molecule. As a consequence serum ceruloplasmin and total serum copper levels are *decreased;* however, owing to the excess of total body copper, the free serum copper is elevated significantly so that the urinary copper excretion is actually *increased* in Wilson's disease. *(Cecil, pp. 1126–1128; Stanbury, Wyngaarden, and Fredrickson, pp. 1098–1102)*

41. (A — False; B — True; C — True; D — False) Penetrance refers to the likelihood that a person with a given genotype will express the corresponding phenotype. This is calculated by determining the percentage of obligate carriers for any specific genetic disorder that have some clinical manifestations of it. The penetrance in neurofibromatosis is greater than 95%; however, this is not related to the expressivity (severity), which is quite variable within and between families with the neurofibromatosis gene. *(Cecil, p. 2; Smith, pp. 302–303; Vogel and Motulsky, pp. 84, 89)*

42. (A — True; B — True; C — False; D — False) The gene coding for human G6PD is X-linked. There are more than 80 defined variants of this enzyme. The two most clinically significant forms of G6PD deficiency are those associated with either the African variant (which affects 10% of black American males) or the Mediterranean variant (frequency among white males approximately one in 1000). Hemolysis following exposure to any of a variety of oxidizing drugs (including sulfas) is characteristic of these disorders. Hemolysis in the Mediterranean form is much more severe and is elicited by a larger number of drugs. The disorder common among blacks is due primarily to enzyme instability, and since the hemolysis affects only older red cells it is functionally self-limited. Younger erythrocytes possess sufficient enzyme activity to avoid drug-induced hemolysis, and patients frequently have *increased* G6PD activity (per red cell) after a hemolytic episode. Neurologic deterioration is not a feature of this disorder. *(Cecil, pp. 867–868; Vogel and Motulsky, pp. 201–204, 257)*

43. (All are True) A comparison of these two phenotypically similar disorders illustrates many of the principles basic to caring for individuals with genetic diseases. Similar-appearing diseases may have different modes of transmission (heterogeneity). Marfan's syndrome is an autosomal dominant disorder, whereas homocystinuria is autosomal recessive. Thus, family history may be useful in arriving at the correct diagnosis. The estimates of recurrence risk in the children of an affected parent are quite different: in a dominant trait, 50% of the offspring will be affected; in a rare recessive trait, none of the offspring will be affected unless the affected person marries a heterozygote. Thus, careful diagnosis of genetic disorders is the first step, since counseling and therapy are dependent upon a specific diagnosis. *(Cecil, pp. 23–24; Sutton, Ch. 25, 26)*

44. (All are True) Although "heterozygote detection" is traditionally an issue associated with recessive disorders, carrier detection is critical in any situation in which a family member may carry an abnormal gene or chromosomal abnormality that is not expressed, but which could represent a risk to offspring. Thus, for example, when one is confronted by apparently normal parents with a single child affected by Marfan's syndrome it is important to establish (as best as possible) the "carrier status" of the parents. If one parent is very mildly affected, the risk to the offspring is 50 to 50, whereas it is negligible if both parents are noncarriers. *(Cecil, p. 25)*

45. (A — True; B — True; C — True; D — False) Teratogenic abnormalities are not detected by amniocentesis. Inborn errors of metabolism and chromosomal aberrations may be detected *in utero.* Neural tube defects may be suspected from an elevated alpha-fetoprotein level (either in amniotic fluid or maternal serum) or elevated amniotic acetylcholinesterase levels. *(Cecil, pp. 24–25; Omenn)*

46. (A — True; B — True; C — True; D — False) All these physical findings can be explained by the high levels of chylomicrons found in the serum of these patients following the ingestion of a fatty meal. However, there is no increased incidence of atherosclerosis. *(Cecil, pp. 1087–1088; Stanbury, Wyngaarden, and Fredrickson, pp. 608–617)*

47. (A — False; B — True; C — False; D — True) The neurologic disease results from demyelination of axons, and the acanthocytes are caused by changes in the red cell membrane. Both are direct consequences of the abnormalities in lipid transport that result from the deficiency of beta-lipoproteins. Obesity is not observed because of the severe malabsorption seen in these patients, and there is no increased incidence of atherosclerosis. *(Cecil, p. 1089; Stanbury, Wyngaarden, and Fredrickson, pp. 553–565)*

48. (A — False; B — True; C — True; D — False) Although mechanisms A and D are potential causes of hyperuricemia, they have not been shown to produce hyperuricemia. Decreased renal clearance of urate and increased purine synthesis are both well-documented causes of hyperuricemia. Both pathogenic mechanisms may be operative in the same patient. *(Cecil, pp. 1109–1111; Wyngaarden and Kelley, pp. 133–158)*

49. (A — False; B — True; C — True; D — True) The renal calculi found in gouty patients contain uric acid, not monosodium urate. *(Cecil, pp. 1111–1112; Wyngaarden and Kelley, pp. 177–210)*

50. (A — True; B — False; C — True; D — False) Gouty arthritis is typically rapid in onset, severely painful, highly inflammatory, and often associated with systemic symptoms. In early cases it usually is monarticular. Characteristically, the acute attack completely subsides, and the patient enters a symptom-free interval one to two weeks after the acute attack. *(Cecil, pp. 1112–1113; Wyngaarden and Kelley, pp. 213–226)*

51. (A — True; B — False; C — True; D — False) Uric acid stones are most likely to occur in patients with excessive purine biosynthesis and increased uric acid excretion, in individuals with persistently acid urine, and in patients who excrete highly concentrated urine. There is no association between renal tubular acidosis and uric acid calculi. *(Cecil, p. 1114; Stanbury, Wyngaarden, and Fredrickson, pp. 268, 283)*

52. (A — True; B — True; C — True; D — False) Deficiencies of orotate phosphoribosyltransferase and orotidine 5′-phosphate decarboxylase lead to hereditary orotic aciduria — a disorder characterized by megaloblastic anemia, leukopenia, and growth retardation. Ornithine transcarbamylase deficiency is a urea cycle defect that produces orotic aciduria owing to overflow of carbamyl phosphate from the urea cycle into the pyrimidine pathway. Carbamyl phosphate synthetase deficiency, another urea cycle defect, leads to decreased carbamyl phosphate synthesis and does not result in orotic aciduria. Allopurinol therapy produces orotic aciduria by inhibiting orotidine 5'-decarboxylase activity. *(Cecil, p. 1121; Stanbury, Wyngaarden, and Fredrickson, pp. 1045–1072)*

53. (A — False; B — False; C — True; D — True) Acute intermittent porphyria is not associated with photosensitivity or scarring, and the freshly voided urine is usually normal in color. Urine turns dark only on standing, following the conversion of porphobilinogen to porphyrins and porphobilin. The striking neurologic disease and bouts of abdominal pain are characteristic, and during the acute attack the Watson-Schwartz test is strongly positive. *(Cecil, pp. 1122–1125; Stanbury, Wyngaarden, and Fredrickson, pp. 1166–1221)*

54. (A — False; B — True; C — True; D — False) These types of hepatic porphyria may be exacerbated following the administration of barbiturates or sulfonamides, as well as many other types of drugs. Intravenous glucose may abort an attack, and phenothiazines are the preferred treatment for pain. *(Cecil, pp. 1124–1125; Stanbury, Wyngaarden, and Fredrickson, pp. 1166–1221)*

55. (A — True; B — False; C — False; D — True) Porphyria cutanea tarda patients do not exhibit the abdominal crises or neurologic disease found in those with acute intermittent porphyria or variegate porphyria. However, these patients do exhibit skin lesions, as do those with variegate porphyria. Hepatic dysfunction that is often caused by chronic alcoholism is an acquired abnormality, but appears to be necessary for the clinical expression of the underlying genetic disorder in porphyric metabolism. *(Cecil, p. 1125; Stanbury, Wyngaarden, and Fredrickson, pp. 1166–1221)*

56. (All are True) This autosomal recessive disorder is also associated with mental retardation. The condition must be distinguished from Fröhlich's syndrome in which there are clear-cut abnormalities in the hypothalamic-pituitary axis. *(Cecil, p. 1140)*

57. (A — False; B — True; C — False; D — True) Familial Mediterranean fever is an autosomal recessive disorder. For unexplained reasons, amyloidosis is rarely seen in patients with familial Mediterranean fever living in the United States, although these patients develop the characteristic acute inflammatory episodes. Patients from the same ethnic background exhibit a high incidence of amyloidosis in Israel and the Middle East. Colchicine has been reported to be effective in diminishing the frequency of acute inflammatory episodes. *(Cecil, pp. 1904–1905)*

58. (A); 59. (F); 60. (C); 61. (D) Many aspects of the molecular biology of globin gene expression are relatively well understood. Clinical abnormalities that result from abnormal globin molecules or defective globin gene expression can now be shown to be the consequence of demonstrable alterations in the coding or intervening sequences of globin genes. **58.** The hemoglobin Lepore molecule, which is a fusion between δ- and β-globin segments, is the consequence of unequal crossing over between homologous sections of the δ- and β-globin genes on homologous chromosomes. **59.** Hemoglobin Constant Spring results from a mutation in the terminator codon of β-globin. **60.** Certain forms of β^0-thalassemia have been shown to be due to non-sense mutations in which there is a base replacement that results in premature termination in the synthesis of the β-globin molecule. **61.** Sickle cell hemoglobin results from a mis-sense mutation in which a base change alters the codon for a glutamic acid residue to that of valine. *(Cecil, pp. 9–10, 14; Stanbury, Wyngaarden, and Fredrickson, pp. 1465–1523)*

62. (B); 63. (C); 64. (A) Testosterone is important in the development of secondary sex characteristics. Dihydrotestosterone functions during the embryonal and fetal periods to induce the male external primary sex characteristics. The presence of H-Y antigen (independent of the Y chromosome) will result in the formation of testes from an undifferentiated gonad. The autosomal recessive disorder characterized by deficiency of 5-alpha testosterone reductase activity results in children with primary sex characteristics of females (owing to deficiency of dihydrotestosterone) who subsequently develop male sexual characteristics at the time of puberty (owing to normal testosterone levels). *(Cecil, p. 1252; Jackson and Schimke, p. 315; Vogel and Motulsky, pp. 276–277)*

65. (D) Marfan's syndrome is an autosomal dominant disorder that primarily affects three organ systems: (1) the eye with ectopia lentis, myopia, and cataracts; (2) the cardiovascular system with aortic root dilatation or dissection, and mitral prolapse; and (3) the skeleton with "marfanoid" body habitus (arachnodactyly, abnormal upper to lower body segment ratio) and associated changes including scoliosis and chest wall deformity. The ectopia can be very subtle, often requiring a slit lamp examination to confirm redundant suspensory ligaments. The aortic root abnormalities significantly limit the prognosis and longevity of patients. *(Cecil, p. 1138)*

66. (E) Malignant hyperthermia is a dominant disorder in which affected individuals develop marked hyperpyrexia, muscle rigidity, massively elevated serum creatine phosphokinase, and hyperkalemia during anesthesia. These episodes are often fatal. Affected individuals often have constitutionally elevated serum CPK levels, and it is important to screen family members for the presence of this potentially lethal genotype. *(Cecil, pp. 2174–2175; Jackson and Schimke, pp. 383–384)*

67. (C) The Ehlers-Danlos syndromes are a heterogeneous group of disorders that are genetically distinct but share certain phenotypic characteristics, including joint laxity, easy bruisability, poorly healing tissue, and hyperelastic skin. There are at least eight forms, and more are being defined as time goes by. Type IV is usually inherited in a dominant fashion. It is clinically significant because of the frequency of sudden death among affected individuals, which usually is due to rupture of a large artery. *(Cecil, pp. 1138–1140; Stanbury, Wyngaarden, and Fredrickson, p. 1377)*

68. (E) Deficiency of pseudocholinesterase is associated with prolonged paralysis and apnea following exposure to succinylcholine. *(Stanbury, Wyngaarden, and Fredrickson, p. 1721)*

69. (B) Children with Duchenne muscular dystrophy now commonly live into their early 20s, so that internists are more often confronted with the problems of managing them. Respiratory failure, with or without intercurrent infection, is a frequent cause of death. *(Cecil, pp. 2171–2172; Jackson and Schimke, pp. 374–375; Stanbury, Wyngaarden, and Fredrickson, p. 1377)*

70. (G) The Howell-Evans syndrome is an autosomal dominant disorder characterized by hyperkeratosis of the palms and soles and age-dependent penetrance (roughly 95% by age 50) of esophageal carcinoma. Frequent esophagoscopy is indicated, with consideration of prophylactic esophagectomy when squamous dysplasia occurs. *(Cecil, pp. 1029–1032; Jackson and Schimke, pp. 102–103)*

71. (G) Each of the common familial gastrointestinal polyposis syndromes is dominant; however, not all of them carry an increased risk for malignant transformation. Gardner's syndrome is similar to the classic familial colonic polyposis syndrome, but has additional features of osseous and soft tissue tumors and cysts. The colonic polyps of these two syndromes are prone to malignant transformation. *(Cecil, p. 725)*

72. (B) There are at least 20 different α_1-antitrypsin variant proteins. The most clinically significant forms can often be detected by a decreased α_1 peak in the standard serum protein electrophoresis (α_1-antitrypsin is normally the major component of this peak). The precise mechanism of lung injury is unknown, but homozygotes are at a greatly increased risk for the early onset and rapid progression of emphysema; furthermore, cigarette smoking appears to accelerate this process substantially. The homozygote α_1-antitrypsin deficiency genotypes may also be associated with neonatal hepatitis and cirrhosis. *(Cecil, pp. 14–15, 367; Stanbury, Wyngaarden, and Fredrickson, pp. 1719–1720)*

73. (A); 74. (B); 75. (B); 76. (A) Maternal age has a significant influence on the incidence of chromosomal aneuploidies. The frequency of certain autosomal dominant disorders is correlated with paternal age. The former is presumably due to increased susceptibility to chromosomal nondisjunction among older gametes, whereas the latter is presumably due to an increased frequency of mutations in "older" DNA, which has undergone a large number of replications; each replication carries a finite probability of mutation at any specific locus. The probability of dizygotic twinning increases with maternal age. *(Cecil, p. 2; Vogel and Motulsky, pp. 176, 284, 301–307)*

77–81. It is important to recognize that many genetic disorders (including those that mimic other, more common diseases) are amenable to therapeutic intervention, often with dramatically beneficial results.

77. (B) This patient has Wilson's disease and should be treated with penicillamine. Wilson's disease frequently presents with abnormalities of either hepatic function or the central nervous system. The latter are often manifested as psychiatric abnormalities in place of or in addition to the more classic movement disorders. Thus, the tardive dyskinesia in this patient was *not* a consequence of phenothiazine therapy, and an appropriate diagnosis could not be made until this is recognized. This point is particularly important since Wilson's disease represents one of the few treatable and reversible forms of progressive neurologic deterioration. *(Cecil, pp. 1126–1128; Stanbury, Wyngaarden, and Fredrickson, pp. 1098–1116)*

78. (A) Deposition of iron in hemochromatosis can result in hypofunction of the anterior pituitary with consequent hypogonadotropic hypogonadism, which is often apparent long before clinically overt signs of hepatic or pancreatic dysfunction appear. Thus, organic impotence and/or hypogonadism in a middle-aged man should raise the suspicion of hemochromatosis. Interestingly, one of the few clinical consequences of hemochromatosis that does not respond to phlebotomy is the arthritis that characteristically affects the second and third metacarpophalangeal joints and is often associated with positive rheumatoid factor. *(Cecil, pp. 1128–1131; Stanbury, Wyngaarden, and Fredrickson, pp. 1127–1159)*

79. (C) This patient has hereditary angioedema, which is due to C1 inhibitor deficiency. Androgens have been found not only to prevent attacks of edema and abdominal pain, but to cause a reversal of the biochemical defect. There is a rapid reappearance of the functional form of the serum C1 esterase inhibitor. *(Cecil, p. 1798; Stanbury, Wyngaarden, and Fredrickson, pp. 1745–1749)*

80. (D) The characteristic karyotype of Turner's syndrome is 45, XO; however, it should be noted that the Turner's phenotype is associated specifically with deletion of the short arm of the X chromosome, whereas gonadal dysgenesis *per se* is due to deletion of the long arm of the X chromosome. Frequently, patients with Turner's syndrome have a mosaic karyotype, the most common of which is 45, XO/46, XX. Patients with mosaic karyotypes that include a cell line possessing the Y chromosome are at extreme risk for a neoplastic transformation in a dysgenetic gonad. Thus, the gonads should be removed as soon as this diagnosis is made. *(Cecil, pp. 20, 1267; Jackson and Schimke, pp. 46–50)*

81. (E) This patient has acute intermittent porphyria. Exacerbations of this syndrome sometimes correlate with the menstrual cycle, and in many patients an attack may be precipitated by the use of oral contraceptives. The neurologic consequences of an acute exacerbation of acute intermittent porphyria include abnormalities of the neurohypophysis, such as the syndrome of inappropriate ADH secretion. *(Cecil, pp. 1123–1125; Stanbury, Wyngaarden, and Fredrickson, pp. 1166–1209)*

82–85. Dysmorphic syndromes are often associated with abnormalities of major organ systems, and the pattern of involvement can be specific for a particular syndrome. Adequate medical care requires awareness and anticipation of the affiliated organ abnormalities and the potential medical complications characteristic of the disorder.

82. (C) The major cause of early death in trisomy 21 is cardiovascular malformation; nearly half of those with cardiac abnormalities die in infancy. *(Cecil, pp. 20, 169; Smith, pp. 6–9)*

83. (D) Often called "male Turner's syndrome," Noonan's syndrome is actually autosomal dominant and occurs in both sexes with equal frequency. Mild mental retardation is characteristic. *(Cecil, p. 1141; Smith, pp. 50–51)*

84. (B) Turner's syndrome is usually associated with normal intelligence. Neonatal lymphedema (responsible for webbing of the neck and other phenotypic traits) is characteristic. *(Cecil, pp. 20, 1267; Smith, pp. 46–49)*

85. (A) Supravalvular aortic stenosis is characteristic of Williams' syndrome (idiopathic hypercalcemia of pregnancy), which is not hereditary. *(Smith, pp. 54–55)*

86. (A); 87. (B) Molecular hybridization studies utilizing radio-labeled DNA complementary to the genomic globin DNA (cDNA) have shown that the α-thalassemia syndromes are usually due to deletion or absence of α-globin genes. This is in distinction to the β-thalassemias, in which the β-globin genes are generally present, but there is a defect at any one of the multiple levels of gene expression (transcription, RNA processing, or translation). The α-thalassemia characterized by a complete absence of

α-globin genes (hydrops fetalis) results in the presence of hemoglobin Bart's (γ_4). Hemoglobin H disease occurs when there is a single copy of the α-globin gene, and these patients are therefore capable of generating hemoglobin A, which constitutes the major component of their hemoglobin. The β_4 hemoglobin generally constitutes from 5 to 30% of total hemoglobin in these patients. *(Cecil, p. 885; Stanbury, Wyngaarden, and Fredrickson, pp. 1515–1518; Kan et al.; Taylor et al.)*

88. (C) This patient has McArdle's disease (glycogen storage disease type V). The symptoms are rather mild, particularly in comparison with the muscular involvement of glycogen storage disease type II. Nevertheless, it is important when counseling patients to remember that their perception of the severity of a disorder is not necessarily in agreement with that of the physician. *(Cecil, pp. 1081–1082; Stanbury, Wyngaarden, and Fredrickson, pp. 151–153)*

89. (D); 91. (D) Gaucher's disease is an example of heterogeneity of phenotypes in a disease resulting from a single enzyme deficiency. Thus, Gaucher's disease can be divided into an adult form (this is the most common), an acute neonatal neuronopathic form with progressive neurologic deterioration, and a juvenile or subacute form with an intermediate prognosis. There are several other examples of varying but specific clinical phenotypes associated with a single, well-defined enzyme deficiency. These include Scheie's syndrome and Hurler's syndrome, various forms of Nieman-Pick disease, and type II glycogen storage disease. *(Cecil, pp. 1093–1094)*

90. (B) The α-1, 4-glucosidase deficiency (type II glycogen storage disease or Pompe's disease) most commonly results in profound neonatal hypotonia and congestive heart failure with early demise. There are, however, two other groups of patients in which the symptom complex presents in either a subacute or chronic fashion in adolescence or adulthood. *(Cecil, p. 1081; Stanbury, Wyngaarden, and Fredrickson, pp. 146–147)*

92. (E) Although the organ systems involved in homocystinuria overlap somewhat with those affected by Marfan's syndrome, the specific patterns of involvement in the two disorders are distinct. In contrast to the ectopia lentis of Marfan's syndrome, the ectopia found in over 90% of patients with homocystinuria is usually downward. These individuals may be tall and slender, but osteoporosis is the most prominent skeletal feature of homocystinuria. Cardiovascular abnormalities account for significant morbidity and mortality in both Marfan's syndrome and homocystinuria, although the latter is characterized by thromboembolism rather than aortic root or mitral valve pathology. Mental retardation is seen in more than 50% of patients with homocystinuria. It is one of the few autosomal recessive disorders that exhibit marked variability in expression. Approximately 50% of patients respond (improvement in biochemical abnormalities) to pyridoxine therapy. *(Cecil, pp. 1106–1107, 1138; Stanbury, Wyngaarden, and Fredrickson, pp. 467–472)*

93. (F) Refsum's disease is an autosomal recessive disorder characterized by the ineffective disposition and secondary accumulation of phytanic acid. Phytanic acid is obtained exclusively from the diet, and dietary restriction results in biochemical and symptomatic improvement. *(Cecil, p. 16; Stanbury, Wyngaarden, and Fredrickson, p. 688)*

94. (A) Tangier disease is a rare recessive disorder that often results in peripheral neuropathy. If the tonsils have been removed, the diagnosis can be made by the characteristic appearance of the rectum on sigmoidoscopy (multiple orange spots). Hypocholesterolemia (40–120 mg/dl) is also characteristic. *(Cecil, pp. 1089–1090; Stanbury, Wyngaarden, and Fredrickson, pp. 570–575)*

95. (G) Central nervous system disorders (e.g., seizures) and superficial cataracts are additional features of Fabry's disease. Female carriers of this X-linked disorder may show mild phenotypic expression. *(Cecil, pp. 1092–1093; Smith, p. 360)*

96. (A); 97. (B); 98. (A); 99. (D) 21-hydroxylase deficiency accounts for 95% of the congenital adrenal hyperplasia syndromes. Of the defects listed, only 21-hydroxylase deficiency results in salt wasting. Sexual infantilism is a consequence of a deficiency of 17α-hydroxylase, which is required for synthesis of both estrogens and androgens. An associated increase in mineralocorticoids leads to hypertension, which is reversed by treatment with glucocorticoids to suppress ACTH. Deficiency of 11β-hydroxylase is the second most common variety of congenital adrenal hyperplasia. Its clinical manifestations are hypertension and virilism. All the adrenogenital syndromes are autosomal recessive. *(Cecil, pp. 1240–1241; Jackson and Schimke, pp. 303–305; Stanbury, Wyngaarden, and Fredrickson, pp. 869–883)*

100. (A); 101. (B); 102. (C) *(Cecil, pp. 1080–1082; Stanbury, Wyngaarden, and Fredrickson, pp. 137–160)*

103. (A); 104. (C); 105. (B); 106. (B) *(Cecil, pp. 1084–1085; Stanbury, Wyngaarden, and Fredrickson, pp. 544–548, 601–608)*

107. (B); 108. (D); 109. (A); 110. (E); 111. (C) *(Cecil, pp. 1086–1090; Stanbury, Wyngaarden, and Fredrickson, pp. 544–589, 604–656)*

112. (B); 113. (D); 114. (A); 115. (C) *(Cecil, pp. 1118, 1120–1121)*

116. (B); 117. (C); 118. (A); 119. (E) *(Cecil, p. 1135; Stanbury, Wyngaarden, and Fredrickson, pp. 1282–1308)*

BIBLIOGRAPHY

Cartwright, G. E., Edwards, C. Q., Kravitz, K., et al.: Hereditary hemochromatosis: phenotypic expression of the disease. N. Engl. J. Med., *301*:175, 1979.

Dhar, G. J., Bossenmaier, I., Petryka, Z. J., et al.: Effects of hematin in hepatic porphyria. Ann. Intern. Med., *83*:20, 1975.

Dubowitz, V.: Muscle Disorders in Childhood. Philadelphia, W. B. Saunders Company, 1978.

Farfel, Z., Brickman, A. S., Kaslow, H. R., et al.: Defect of receptor-cyclase coupling protein in pseudohypoparathyroidism. N. Engl. J. Med., *303*:237, 1980.

Hassold, T. J., Matsuyama, A., Newlands, I. M., et al.: A cytogenetic study of spontaneous abortions in Hawaii. Ann. Hum. Genet., *41*:443, 1978.

Jackson, L. G., and Schimke, R. M.: Clinical Genetics: A Sourcebook for Physicians. New York, John Wiley & Sons, 1979.

Kan, Y. W., Dozy, A. M., Trecartin, R., and Todd, D.: Identification of a nondeletion defect in α-thalassemia. N. Engl. J. Med., *297*:1081, 1977.

Omenn, G. S.: Prenatal diagnosis of genetic disorders. Science, *200*:952, 1978.

Smith, D. W.: Recognizable patterns of human malformation. Philadelphia, W. B. Saunders Company, 1976.

Stanbury, J. B., Wyngaarden, J. B., and Fredrickson, D. F. (eds.): The Metabolic Basis of Inherited Disease. 4th ed. New York, McGraw-Hill Book Company, 1978.

Sutton, E. H.: An Introduction to Human Genetics. 2nd ed. New York, Holt, Rinehart & Winston, 1975.

Taylor, J. M., Dozy, A., Kan, Y. W., et al.: Genetic lesion in homozygous α-thalassemia (hydrops fetalis). Nature, *251*:392, 1974.

Vogel F., and Motulsky, A. G.: Human Genetics: Problems and Approaches. New York, Springer-Verlag, 1979.

Watson, J. D.: Molecular Biology of the Gene. 3rd ed. Menlo Park, CA, Benjamin-Cummings Publishing Company, 1976.

Wyngaarden, J. B., and Kelley, W. N.: Gout and Hyperuricemia. New York, Grune & Stratton, 1976.

PART 7

ENDOCRINOLOGY AND DIABETES MELLITUS

Francis A. Neelon and George J. Ellis

DIRECTIONS: For questions 1 to 80, choose the ONE BEST answer to each question.

1. A 17-year-old girl consults you because of amenorrhea. Menarche was spontaneous at age 12, and she has had cyclic menses until two months ago when menses ceased. She denies all other symptoms and denies any recent sexual exposure. Physical examination is unrevealing. Which one of the following would you do next?

A. Measure chorionic gonadotropin in urine or blood
B. Assess pituitary function including skull radiographs
C. Measure serum estrogen and gonadotropins
D. Assess vaginal cytology and cervical mucus for estrogen effects
E. Administer progesterone in oil, 100 mg intramuscularly, and observe for menses

2. Effective strategies for dealing with patients having idiopathic reactive hypoglycemia include all the following EXCEPT

A. using sugar or candy to treat symptoms
B. five to six feedings daily
C. weight reduction
D. carbohydrate restriction
E. psychotherapy

3. Which of the following is LEAST likely to result from intramuscular testosterone enanthate injections?

A. Gynecomastia
B. Acceleration in the growth of a prostatic carcinoma
C. An increase in serum hemoglobin concentration
D. Intrahepatic cholestasis
E. Decreased spermatogenesis

4. Estrogen produces all the following effects EXCEPT

A. a predominance of superficial cells in the vaginal epithelium
B. the "thermogenic shift" — a rise of more than 0.3°C in basal body temperature
C. "ferning" in dried cervical mucus
D. thickening of the endometrial mucosa
E. vaginal bleeding after administration of progesterone

5. A 55-year-old obese man presents with typical symptoms of diabetes mellitus. Urine shows 5% sugar and small ketones. Serum bicarbonate is 22 mEq/L. Plasma glucose is 475 mg/dl. After aggressive dietary and transient insulin therapy, plasma glucose levels are normal even without insulin. The glucose tolerance test still meets the criteria for diabetes. Factors contributing to this excellent result may include all EXCEPT

A. improved insulin secretion
B. loss of anti-islet cell antibodies
C. improved insulin sensitivity
D. lowered levels of hormones antagonistic to insulin

6. The 15-year-old girl shown below is 137 cm (54 inches) tall, and has a low hairline; widely spaced, poorly developed breasts; and primary amenorrhea. Evaluation shows gonadotropins to be in the menopausal range. The karyotype would most likely be

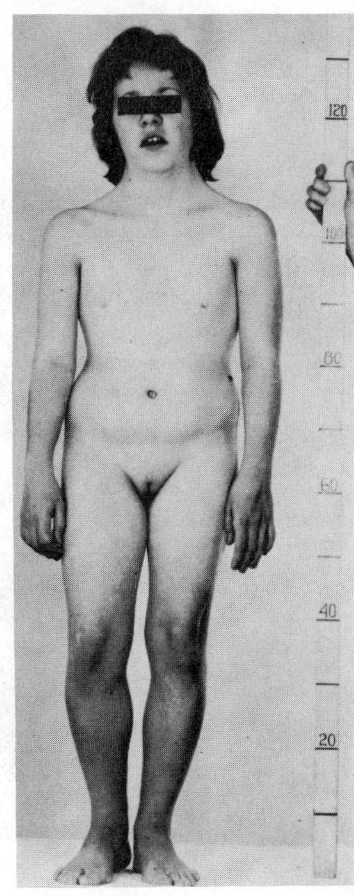

A. 45, X
B. 47, XXX
C. 47, XXY
D. 45, X/46, XX
E. 46, XY

7. Predisposition to bacterial infection in patients with insulin-dependent diabetes may result from all the following EXCEPT

A. abnormal immune responsiveness
B. hyperglycemia
C. ischemia
D. sluggish macrophages

QUESTIONS 8–9

8. A 24-year-old man has experienced a 15-pound weight loss, poor appetite, loss of interest in his job and hobbies, and increasing pigmentation of the skin and buccal mucosa. Evaluation of this patient would probably reveal all the following EXCEPT

A. low diastolic blood pressure
B. elevated serum potassium
C. small cardiac silhouette
D. hypoglycemia during prolonged fasting
E. fever

9. The patient described in question 8 requires laboratory studies to confirm the diagnosis. Which one of the following would be sufficient to allow a certain diagnosis?

A. Fasting plasma cortisol
B. Urinary 17-hydroxycorticoids
C. Plasma cortisol 30 minutes after intravenous administration of cosyntropin (0.25 mg)
D. Plasma cortisol after eight hours of constant intravenous infusion of 50 units of adrenocorticotropic hormone (ACTH)
E. Computerized tomography of the abdomen

---

10. Which of the following is the LEAST common clinical manifestation of the endocrine disorder that produces purplish striae as pictured?

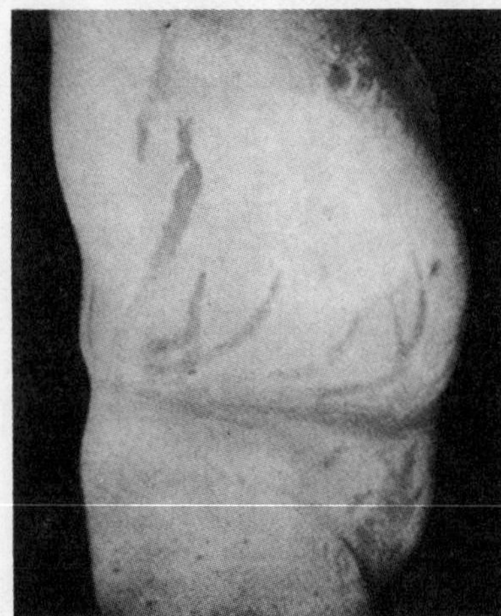

A. Obesity
B. Oligomenorrhea
C. Impaired glucose tolerance
D. Kidney stones
E. Hypertension

11. A patient whose diabetes has been well controlled by diet and 40 units of NPH insulin each morning (rare urinary sugar levels above ½%) displays a urine record that shows negative sugar but large acetone before breakfast. By lunch the sugar is 5% with small acetone; ketonuria and glycosuria clears by the next afternoon without change of regimen. Which of the following is the most likely cause of the loss of control in this patient?

A. Infection
B. Starvation
C. Insulin deficiency
D. Hypoglycemia
E. Incorrect testing technique

12. Hypertension with elevated secretion of 11-deoxycorticosterone is typical of congenital adrenal hyperplasia secondary to a deficiency of

A. 11β-hydroxylase
B. 21-hydroxylase
C. 20α-hydroxylase
D. 18-hydroxysteroid dehydrogenase
E. 17α-hydroxylase

13. Which of the following is NOT characteristic of the potassium depletion of primary aldosteronism?

A. Potassium wasting that is exaggerated by high sodium intake
B. Very low urinary potassium excretion (<1.0 mEq/day)
C. Hypertensive complications
D. Electrocardiographic abnormalities
E. Impaired renal concentrating ability that is not corrected by vasopressin

14. In the evaluation of a woman for hirsutism, which of the following findings is most likely to indicate a benign cause?

A. Clitoral enlargement
B. Onset at the time of puberty
C. Abdominal or flank mass
D. Laryngeal enlargement
E. Plasma testosterone greater than 0.20 μg/dl (N <0.08)

15. Improved vision may result from treatment of all the following manifestations of diabetes EXCEPT

A. fluctuating hyperglycemia
B. lipemia retinalis
C. cataracts
D. proliferative retinopathy
E. background retinopathy

16. A 13-year-old girl with insulin-dependent diabetes is taking six units of regular and 28 units of lente insulin each morning. She reports all negative urines with no hypoglycemia. Her parents are having difficulty getting her to comply with her diet and urine-testing requirements because control is so smooth. Physical examination, complete blood count, and renal function studies are normal. Plasma glucose two hours after lunch is 210 mg/dl. Hemoglobin A_1 is 16% (N = 6–9%). This clinical picture is consistent with any of the following EXCEPT

A. high renal threshold
B. fraudulent urine results
C. inactive urine test reagents
D. denial of diabetes
E. optimal control of diabetes

17. Which of the following is the most common cause of Addison's disease in the United States?

A. Tuberculosis of the adrenal cortex
B. Idiopathic adrenal atrophy
C. Amyloidosis of the adrenal
D. Adrenal destruction by metastatic tumor
E. Adrenal apoplexy

18. Appropriate management of patients with adrenal insufficiency secondary to hypopituitarism includes all the following EXCEPT

A. glucocorticoid replacement
B. mineralocorticoid therapy
C. steroid coverage for surgical procedures
D. instructions in self-injection of soluble glucocorticoid
E. wearing of an identification bracelet bearing medical information

19. An obese child should be evaluated for Cushing's disease if there is concomitant

A. premature puberty
B. growth arrest
C. eosinophilia
D. muscular hypertrophy
E. polycythemia

20. In a patient with lung cancer, which of the following is most suggestive of hypercortisolism?

A. Unprovoked hypokalemia
B. Cutaneous striae
C. Muscular weakness
D. Osteoporosis
E. Erythrocytosis

21. The "fed" state is characterized by all the following EXCEPT

A. high plasma insulin and low plasma glucagon levels
B. glycogen synthesis
C. fat synthesis
D. amino acid incorporation into protein
E. enhanced ketone synthesis

22. A 36-year-old man consults you because of polyuria and a 15-pound weight loss. He is 70 inches tall and weighs 225 pounds. Urinalysis shows 5% glycosuria and negative ketones. Plasma glucose is 375 mg/dl. Serum bicarbonate is 24 mEq/L. The most appropriate initial therapy is

A. intermittent intramuscular insulin or intravenous insulin infusion until stable
B. NPH or lente insulin, 20–30 units daily, with a diabetic diet
C. sulfonylurea plus a diabetic diet
D. diabetic diet alone

23. A 32-year-old obese woman has hypertension and easy bruisability. She smokes 1½ packs of cigarettes daily; her only medication is an oral contraceptive that she has taken for four years. She is 66 inches tall and weighs 214 pounds. Blood pressure is 160/105 mm Hg. Plasma cortisol is 62 μg/dl at 8:00 AM (N = 8–25) and 57 μg/dl at 5:00 PM (N <8). Which of the following is the most appropriate diagnostic procedure?

A. Roentgenogram of the chest to rule out lung cancer
B. Measurement of plasma adrenocorticotropic hormone (ACTH)
C. Measurement of plasma cortisol at 8:00 AM after giving 1 mg dexamethasone at midnight
D. Measurement of urinary 17-OH corticoids after two days of small doses of dexamethasone (0.5 mg every six hours)
E. Measurement of urinary 17-OH corticoids after two days of high doses of dexamethasone (2.0 mg every six hours)

24. In adult patients with Cushing's disease due to excessive secretion of pituitary adrenocorticotropic hormone (ACTH), the present treatment of choice (in the absence of contraindications) is

A. pituitary irradiation with 4000–5000 rads
B. pituitary suppression by cyproheptadine
C. trans-sphenoidal pituitary microdissection and adenomectomy
D. bilateral adrenalectomy
E. adrenocortical destruction by mitotane

25. Enlarged breasts in an adult man may be due to any of the following EXCEPT

A. primary testicular atrophy
B. Graves' disease
C. cocaine inhalation
D. Klinefelter's syndrome
E. oat cell carcinoma

26. All the following statements about cortisol are true EXCEPT

A. It circulates bound to an α_2-globulin
B. It increases fat deposition
C. It increases glucose uptake by muscle cells
D. It increases water excretion
E. It increases protein catabolism

27. An 11-year-old girl being treated appropriately for diabetic ketoacidosis follows her meal plan carefully. Her insulin requirement falls from 1 unit/kg to 0.4 unit/kg four months later. All urine tests are free of sugar, and hemoglobin A_1 is 9% (N=6–9%). All the following are likely to be true EXCEPT

A. C-peptide reactivity by immunoassay probably increases after meals
B. Diet alone should now suffice for adequate control
C. Insulin sensitivity is normal
D. Increasing insulin requirements are likely in the future

28. A jogger with diabetes uses a mixture of regular and lente insulin before breakfast and supper, rotates injection sites methodically, and runs just before his afternoon injection. He complains of occasional hypoglycemic symptoms during and after his daily exercise. Glycosuria follows a slight reduction in the morning dose of lente. You should have him change his

A. injection site
B. eating pattern
C. insulin dose
D. time of exercise
E. source of insulin

29. A 24-year-old woman is brought to the emergency room hypotensive and in coma. Plasma glucose is 60 mg/dl, serum sodium 120 mEq/L, and serum potassium 4.4

mEq/L. Two years ago the patient developed galactorrhea and amenorrhea, and underwent pituitary irradiation for a prolactinoma. Although galactorrhea ceased, amenorrhea has persisted. Three days ago she began taking L-thyroxine, 0.3 mg daily, which her gynecologist had prescribed for symptoms typical of hypothyroidism. Which of the following is the most appropriate emergency therapy for this patient?

A. Methimazole, 100 mg by nasogastric tube, followed by saturated solution of potassium iodide, ten drops every eight hours
B. Hydrocortisone, 100 mg intravenously every six hours, with normal saline sufficient to replace 10 to 20% of the extracellular volume
C. 50% dextrose in water, 50-ml bolus intravenously
D. L-thyroxine, 300 μg intravenously
E. 3% saline solution, 2 liters intravenously over two hours

30. You are called in consultation to see a Caucasian patient of English descent with uncontrolled diabetes. Despite dietary compliance, urinary sugars are over 2% four times daily with a renal threshold of 200 mg/dl. Hemoglobin A_1, a measure of integrated blood glucose control, is 7.8% (N = 6–9%). Complete blood count and reticulocyte count are normal. What is the most likely explanation for this patient's problem?

A. Renal glycosuria
B. Unrecognized hypoglycemia
C. Nonglucose melituria
D. Insulin deficiency

31. The 52-year-old woman pictured has had progressive enlargement of the hands and feet, thickening of the tongue, mild headaches, and increased sweating for the last 15 years. Fasting serum growth hormone level is 23 ng/ml (N <5). Which one of the following should be done next to confirm the diagnosis?

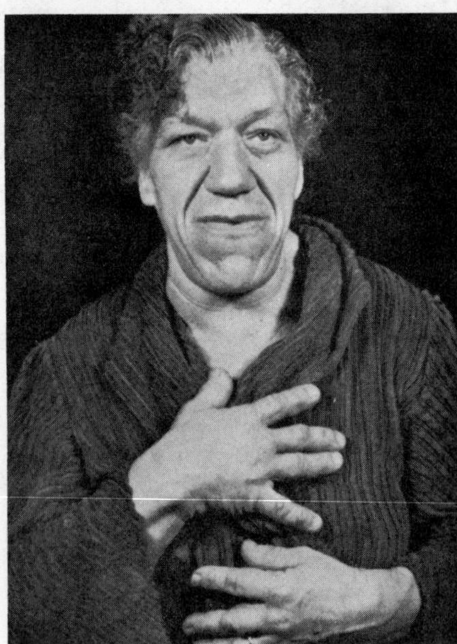

A. Perform a visual field examination
B. Perform an insulin tolerance test
C. Measure serum growth hormone level after exercise
D. Measure serum growth hormone during an oral glucose tolerance test
E. Computed tomography of the skull including the sella turcica

32. Effective stimulators of insulin release include all the following EXCEPT

A. sulfonylureas
B. alpha-adrenergic stimulation
C. some gut hormones
D. amino acids
E. potassium ions

33. Which of the following is the most common *laboratory* abnormality in adult patients with hypopituitarism?

A. Plasma growth hormone less than 5 ng/ml after insulin-induced hypoglycemia
B. Plasma prolactin greater than 50 ng/ml (N = 5–25)
C. Serum testosterone less than 0.3 μg/dl in men or serum estrogen less than 0.2 μg/dl in women.
D. A rise in serum thyroid-stimulating hormone (TSH) of less than 5 μU/ml after administration of thyrotropin-releasing hormone (TRH)
E. Fasting morning cortisol less than 5 μg/dl (N = 8–25)

34. A previously undiagnosed patient is found to have ketoacidosis after five weeks of polyuria. Plasma glucose is 485 mg/dl; blood urea nitrogen is 29 mg/dl; serum electrolytes show sodium 142, potassium 3.9, chloride 98, and bicarbonate 12 mEq/L. After therapy with saline, intermittent intramuscular insulin, and bicarbonate, the patient develops generalized weakness, hypoventilation, and cardiac irritability. What is the most likely cause of this complication?

A. Hypoglycemia
B. Hyponatremia
C. Magnesium depletion
D. Hypokalemia
E. Hypophosphatemia

35. The metabolic actions of growth hormone include all the following EXCEPT

A. osteogenesis and chondrogenesis
B. production of somatomedin (sulfation factor)
C. fat deposition
D. insulin resistance
E. nitrogen retention

36. Hypothalamic disease (as opposed to hypophysectomy) may result in loss of all the following anterior pituitary hormone secretions EXCEPT

A. thyroid-stimulating hormone (TSH)
B. prolactin
C. growth hormone
D. gonadotropins (LH, FSH)
E. adrenocorticotropic hormone (ACTH)

37. A 57-year-old woman with diabetes is following her meal plan carefully and is approaching her ideal weight at the rate of 1 pound per week. Plasma glucose levels are 200–300 mg/dl. She has asymptomatic peripheral neuropathy, background retinopathy, and proteinuria. Blood urea nitrogen is 37 mg/dl. Any of the following oral agents would be acceptable treatment for this patient EXCEPT

A. tolbutamide
B. tolazamide
C. acetohexamide
D. chlorpropamide

38. Although not always the complaint that brings the patient to the doctor, the *earliest* symptom of pituitary tumor is usually

A. visual disturbance (e.g., bitemporal hemianopia)
B. gonadal insufficiency
C. headache
D. extraocular muscle paresis
E. diabetes insipidus

39. In achieving the steady state that obtains in a patient taking drugs such as estrogens, which raise the serum concentration of thyroxine-binding globulin (TBG), all the following occur EXCEPT

A. The concentration of unoccupied TBG increases
B. Thyroxine synthesis increases
C. The concentration of free thyroxine is restored to normal
D. Thyroxine metabolism increases
E. The concentration of thyroxine bound to TBG increases

40. All of the following medications can precipitate diabetes in certain patients EXCEPT

A. hydrochlorothiazide
B. phenytoin
C. prednisolone
D. estrogenic oral contraceptives
E. clofibrate

41. All the following statements regarding chronic lymphocytic thyroiditis (Hashimito's thyroiditis) are true EXCEPT

A. It is a common cause of goiter in adolescents
B. It is more common in women than in men
C. It is more common in young women than in old women
D. It is found in association with pernicious anemia
E. Antithyroid antibodies are usually present

42. A 23-year-old woman who has been taking insulin for control of diabetes mellitus for seven years is found during a routine examination to have a firm nodule in the left lobe of the thyroid gland. The right lobe is easily palpable and possibly enlarged. Serum thyroxine is 6.2 μg/dl (N = 5–11); resin T_3 uptake, 0.60 (N = 0.85–1.15); and serum thyroid-stimulating hormone (TSH) 42 μU/ml (N = 0–6). Thyroidal uptake of radioiodine at 24 hours is 40% (N = 5–30); radioisotope thyroid scan shows all uptake confined to the palpable nodule (reported as a "hot nodule"). What is the most appropriate action?

A. Administration of L-thyroxine to suppress the nodule
B. Measurement of serum triiodothyronine (T_3) to detect "T_3 toxicosis"
C. Radioiodine ablation of the nodule
D. Administration of propylthiouracil
E. Needle aspiration of the nodule

43. Elevated insulin levels after glucose characterize the diabetes secondary to each of the following EXCEPT

A. acromegaly
B. pancreatitis
C. Cushing's syndrome
D. obesity
E. lipoatrophy

44. A 55-year-old man noted a mass in his neck while shaving. Physical examination is normal except for a firm, 5-cm oval nodule in the left lobe of the thyroid gland. The right lobe cannot be felt. Serum thyroxine is 8.4 μg/dl (N= 5–11); resin T_3 uptake, 1.04 (N= 0.85–1.15); free thyroxine index, 8.7 (N= 4.7–10.5); and thyroid-stimulating hormone (TSH), 1.9 μU/ml (N=0–6). Radioisotope thyroidal scan is shown in the accompanying illustration. Which of the following actions is most appropriate?

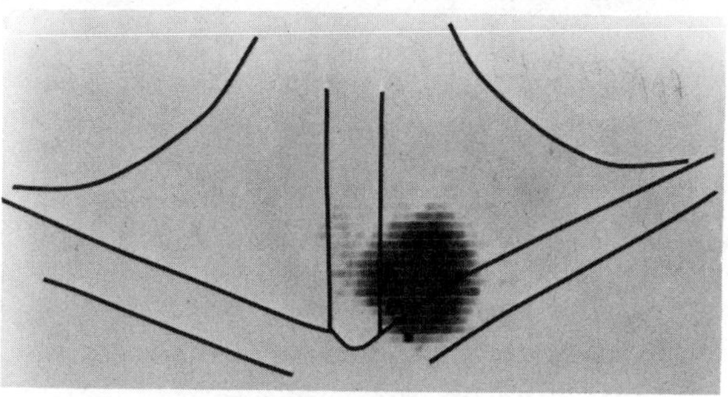

A. Measurement of antithyroid antibodies
B. Measurement of serum triiodothyronine (T_3)
C. Aspiration biopsy of nodule
D. Radioiodine ablation of nodule
E. Surgical excision of nodule after propylthiouracil treatment

45. In a patient with symptomatic hyperthyroidism as a result of subacute thyroiditis, which one of the following therapeutic measures would be most appropriate for the hyperthyroidism?

A. Subtotal thyroidectomy
B. Propranolol, 20 mg four times daily
C. Propylthiouracil, 200 mg three times daily, and propranolol, 20 mg four times daily
D. Radioiodine therapy
E. Saturated solution of potassium iodide, three drops three times daily

46. Your diet-compliant patient takes 42 units of lente insulin each morning. Urinary sugar is usually negative except in the double-voided bedtime specimen, which is trace to 3%. Fasting plasma glucose is 94 mg/dl. Renal threshold is 180 mg/dl. Which one of the following would you do?

A. Add regular insulin in the morning injection
B. Increase morning lente insulin
C. Increase evening exercise
D. Give divided insulin dose
E. Omit the bedtime snack

47. An 18-year-old woman is referred for evaluation of a large goiter. She is euthyroid clinically and by laboratory tests. She has had moderate nerve deafness since early childhood. Her mother and younger brother also have goiters and partial deafness. The thyroid radioiodine uptake is 30% at two hours, and this value is reduced to 10% two hours after the administration of potassium perchlorate, orally. Which one of the following conditions does the patient have?

A. Iodide-trapping defect
B. Iodide-organification defect
C. Iodotyrosine-deiodinase defect
D. Iodotyrosine-coupling defect
E. None of the above

48. Hypothyroidism in the adult is associated with all the following EXCEPT

A. weakness and lethargy
B. impaired memory
C. muscle and joint pain
D. loss of hair
E. systemic hypotension

49. The clinical manifestations of Graves' disease include all the following EXCEPT

A. unilateral exophthalmos
B. finger clubbing
C. lymphadenopathy and splenomegaly
D. paralysis of eye muscles
E. gynecomastia in males

50. The identical twin of a 20-year-old man who has had insulin-dependent diabetes mellitus for five years has normal glucose tolerance tests. The risk of this twin developing diabetes in the future is

A. over 90%
B. 30–60%
C. 10–20%
D. Under 2%

51. Under normal conditions the percentage of thyroid hormone that is *not* bound to protein (i.e., the percentage that is free in solution) is

A. less than 1%
B. about 10%
C. about 25%
D. about 50%
E. about 75%

52. A 55-year-old woman with diabetes mellitus of 20 years' duration suddenly develops diplopia. Examination of extraocular movements reveals paresis of external rotation of her left eye, as illustrated below. You also discover a symmetric, stocking-type of anesthesia in the lower extremities. You find no other abnormalities on neurologic examination. Which one of the following should you do?

A. Advise the patient that her double vision will probably resolve spontaneously in several weeks
B. Obtain a computerized tomography (CT) scan of the brain to rule out a mass lesion
C. Consider this a potential neurosurgical emergency and arrange for immediate hospitalization
D. Obtain a neurology consultation to rule out a systemic demyelinating disease
E. Advise the patient that she has had a small stroke and that her double vision is probably permanent

53. A 47-year-old nurse was advised 25 years ago to take two grains of desiccated thyroid daily because of "fatigue." She has taken the medication faithfully since that time and has had no other symptoms of endocrine dysfunction. You are skeptical of the need for thyroid hormone replacement and advise the patient to discontinue the medication. She returns in three weeks complaining of mild constipation, increased lethargy, and a 2-pound weight gain. Thyroid studies show the serum thyroxine to be 5.7 μg/dl (N = 5–11); resin T_3 uptake, 0.9 (N = 0.85–1.15); and thyroid-stimulating hormone (TSH), 2.8 μU/ml (N = 0–6). Which of the following statements is correct?

A. The findings indicate hypothalamic failure
B. The patient should have complete evaluation of anterior pituitary function
C. The patient probably has normal thyroid function, and should return in three weeks for further testing
D. The patient has primary thyroid disease and will become symptomatic unless thyroxine replacement is reinstituted immediately
E. The patient has been surreptitiously taking triiodothyronine (Cytomel)

54. Which of the following statements concerning vascular disease in patients with diabetes mellitus is FALSE?

A. In the absence of a demonstrable circulating lipid abnormality, people with diabetes are not more susceptible to premature atherosclerosis than nondiabetics
B. Coronary insufficiency in premenopausal diabetic women is 20 times more common than in premenopausal nondiabetic women
C. Gangrene of the feet caused by ischemia is 70 times more frequent in diabetics than in nondiabetics
D. Over 50% of all diabetics die of myocardial infarction
E. The five-year survival rate after myocardial infarction in a diabetic patient is half that of the nondiabetic

55. Subacute (nonsuppurative) thyroiditis may cause all the following EXCEPT

A. symptomatic hyperthyroidism
B. elevated thyroidal radioiodine uptake
C. elevated erythrocyte sedimentation rate
D. ear pain
E. fever, malaise, and chills

56. A 59-year-old man has gradually withdrawn from daily activities. His weight has gradually increased despite a poor appetite. His thinking seems slowed, and his hearing is diminished. Pulse rate is 58 per minute. The skin is dry and sallow. The thyroid gland is palpable but not definitely enlarged. Deep tendon reflexes are symmetric but

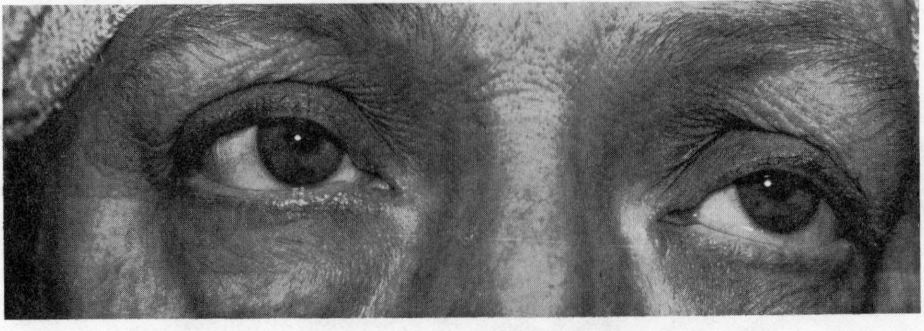

slow to relax. Serum thyroxine concentration is 3.1 μg/dl (N = 5–11) and resin T_3 uptake is 0.67 (N = 0.85 –1.15). Which one of the following should be done next?

A. Measure serum triiodothyronine (T_3)
B. Measure serum thyroid-stimulating hormone (TSH)
C. Perform thyrotropin-releasing hormone (TRH) infusion test
D. Begin thyroxine replacement therapy
E. Begin cortisol replacement followed by thyroxine therapy

57. A 23-year-old woman has Graves' disease with mild exophthalmos (22 mm bilaterally). She is treated with propylthiouracil, 150 mg three times daily, and after two months both free thyroxine index and serum triiodothyronine (T_3) are within the normal range. Six weeks later the thyroid gland is found to be enlarged. The patient has been taking her medication as usual. In addition to measuring free thyroxine index and serum T_3, you should

A. measure serum thyroid-stimulating hormone (TSH)
B. perform thyrotropin-releasing hormone (TRH) infusion test
C. discontinue propylthiouracil in favor of methimazole to block thyroid function more completely
D. add propranolol to block T_4 to T_3 conversion
E. double the dose of propylthiouracil

58. A 21-year-old woman complains of increasing neck size over a 12-month period. The swelling is not painful, but she is disturbed by its cosmetic appearance and can no longer wear some of her necklaces. She has no symptoms suggestive of either hyper- or hypothyroidism. The thyroid gland is diffusely enlarged to approximately four times normal size. Serum values are as follows: thyroxine, 6.2 μg/dl (N = 5–11); free thyroxine index, 6.4 (N = 4.7–10.5); triiodothyronine, 120 ng/dl (N = 80–220); thyroid-stimulating hormone, 15 μU/ml (N = 0–6). The antithyroglobulin antibody titer is very high (1:64,000). Which of the following is most appropriate for this patient?

A. No therapy
B. Subtotal thyroidectomy
C. L-thyroxine, 0.15 mg daily
D. Radioiodine therapy
E. Saturated solution of potassium iodide, three drops three times daily

59. A 40-year-old obese woman with diabetes mellitus of ten years' duration is hospitalized with diabetic ketoacidosis. She has been using insulin and oral hypoglycemic agents intermittently. The ketoacidosis does not respond to intravenous insulin and fluids. On the third hospital day, despite several hundred units of insulin per day, the patient remains ketoacidotic (plasma glucose, 550 mg/dl; plasma ketones, positive [1:32]; serum sodium, 140 mEq/L; and serum chloride, 113 mEq/L). As a consultant, you would correctly advise all the following EXCEPT

A. She has developed insulin resistance, probably as a consequence of excessive circulating antibodies to insulin
B. High-dose steroid therapy (30 to 60 mg prednisone daily) would be appropriate
C. She should receive only pure pork insulin because it is less immunogenic
D. The biologic effect of fish insulin would be neutralized by excessive antibody titers against conventional commercial insulins
E. Large intravenous boluses of insulin should be avoided

60. A 47-year-old man undergoes elective abdominal surgery. On the first postoperative day he becomes restless, tremulous, and disoriented. Pulse rate is 160 per minute with many ectopic beats; temperature is 40°C, and the skin is warm and moist. A small, diffuse goiter with a pyramidal lobe is noted. The patient's wife describes a family history suggestive of hyperthyroidism and tells you that the patient has lost weight recently despite a good appetite. Samples of sputum, urine, and blood are taken for bacteriologic cultures, and measurement of serum thyroxine is ordered. Roentgenogram of the chest is normal. Which of the following courses of action is indicated?

A. Begin propranolol, high-dose salicylates, and digoxin
B. Begin propylthiouracil, potassium iodide drops, propranolol, hydrocortisone, and use of a cooling blanket
C. Administer gentamicin and penicillin
D. Administer large doses of radioiodine to ablate the thyroid gland
E. Withhold therapy until the serum thyroxine value is obtained.

61. A 27-year-old white woman with Graves' disease is treated with radioiodine for hyperthyroidism. One year later she becomes hypothyroid and is subsequently maintained on L-thyroxine, 150 μg daily. Three months ago she began to experience eye irritation, particularly on awakening in the morning. She is now clinically euthyroid with serum thyroxine and thyroid-stimulating hormone (TSH) values within the normal range. Visual acuity is normal and there is no diplopia. Conjunctival injection and chemosis are present, as well as mild exopthalmos (front of cornea 22 mm anterior to the lateral orbital ridge). All the following may be of therapeutic value for this patient EXCEPT

A. six-inch elevation of the head of the bed
B. methylcellulose eyedrops
C. a thiazide diuretic at bedtime
D. reduction of the L-thyroxine to 50 μg daily
E. taping the eyelids closed during sleep

62. A 70-year-old boardinghouse tenant is found stuporous in his room by fellow lodgers. The label on an empty bottle in his room indicates that it once contained thyroxine. On examination in the hospital the patient is comatose; pulse rate is 52 per minute; rectal temperature is 30° C. There is a midline, transverse scar in the lower neck. Rales are heard at the base of the left lung. Emergency management of this patient should include all the following EXCEPT

A. L-thyroxine, 2 μg per kg intravenously
B. raising body temperature rapidly with a heating blanket
C. evaluation and treatment of infection
D. measurement of arterial blood Po_2 and Pco_2
E. monitoring serum sodium levels

63. The effects of parathyroid hormone (PTH) on the kidney include all the following EXCEPT

A. increased tubular reabsorption of magnesium
B. increased production of cyclic 3′5′-AMP

C. increased tubular reabsorption of bicarbonate
D. increased activation of 25-hydroxycholecalciferol
E. increased tubular reabsorption of calcium

64. Which of the following is the most common presentation of primary hyperparathyroidism?

A. Muscular weakness
B. Renal stone formation
C. Central nervous system impairment
D. Bone pain
E. No symptoms

65. A patient who is being evaluated for hypoglycemia has a glucose tolerance test after appropriate preparation. Plasma glucose rises from 58 mg/dl fasting to 130 mg/dl at 30 minutes; 215 mg/dl at one hour; and 119, 113, 65, and 51 mg/dl at subsequent hours. Insulin levels and other studies are pending. These glucose tolerance test results are most consistent with

A. idiopathic reactive hypoglycemia
B. early diabetes mellitus
C. islet cell tumor
D. hypopituitarism
E. alimentary hypoglycemia

66. Radiographs of the hand on fine-grain, industrial film are sometimes indicated in the evaluation of hypercalcemic patients for which one of the following reasons?

A. Even tiny metastases may be noted, confirming paraneoplastic hypercalcemia
B. The finding of subperiosteal bone resorption is diagnostic of hyperparathyroidism
C. These are useful as a gauge of response to treatment
D. Abnormal metacarpal length indicates familial hypocalciuric hypercalcemia
E. The finding of metastatic soft tissue calcification indicates vitamin D intoxication

67. A 49-year-old woman has weakness and hypertension. Serum calcium is 12.8 mg/dl (N = 8.9–10.1); serum phosphate, 1.9 mg/dl (N = 2.5–4.5); serum chloride, 111 mEq/L (N = 98–108); serum parathyroid hormone concentration, 478 pg/ml (N = 10–150). On physical examination a 2-cm nodule can be felt in the left lobe of the thyroid gland. This nodule most likely represents which one of the following?

A. A palpable parathyroid adenoma
B. Metastatic cancer of the lung
C. A parathyroid carcinoma
D. A thyroid adenoma
E. A lymphoma arising from the thyroid gland

68. A 55-year-old house painter has had mild hypercalcemia (serum calcium approximately 10.8 mg/dl) for several years. He has declined surgery, and therefore a program of periodic surveillance is undertaken. Urgent recommendation of surgery should follow the occurrence of any of the following EXCEPT

A. radiographic evidence of metabolic bone disease
B. increasing serum creatinine
C. serum phosphate below 1.7 mg/dl
D. serum calcium above 11.0 mg/dl
E. passage of kidney stones

69. Characteristic findings in hypocalcemia include all the following EXCEPT

A. numbness and tingling of the lips and mouth
B. flaccidity of muscles
C. calcification of basal ganglia
D. lens cataracts
E. epileptiform seizures

70. During a prolonged fast a male patient's plasma glucose level falls steadily from 70 mg/dl to 34 mg/dl in 24 hours. Insulin levels fall steadily from 20 μU/ml to 16 μU/ml. Which of the following would be LEAST appropriate?

A. Abdominal surgery
B. Localization studies
C. A trial of diazoxide
D. Tolbutamide test

71. A 45-year-old woman has recurrent episodes of severe flank pain. Physical examination is unremarkable, and she is taking no medications. Serum values are as follows: calcium, 11.9 mg/dl (N = 8.9–10.1); phosphate, 1.8 mg/dl (N = 2.5–4.5); and chloride, 108 mEq/L (N = 98–108). Complete blood count, erythrocyte sedimentation rate, blood urea nitrogen, and serum creatinine are all within normal limits. A representative film from an intravenous urogram is illustrated. Roentgenogram of the chest is normal. Serum parathyroid hormone (PTH) concentration, reported by a commercial laboratory using an aminoterminal assay, is normal. In evaluating this patient further, which one of the following measurements would be of most diagnostic value?

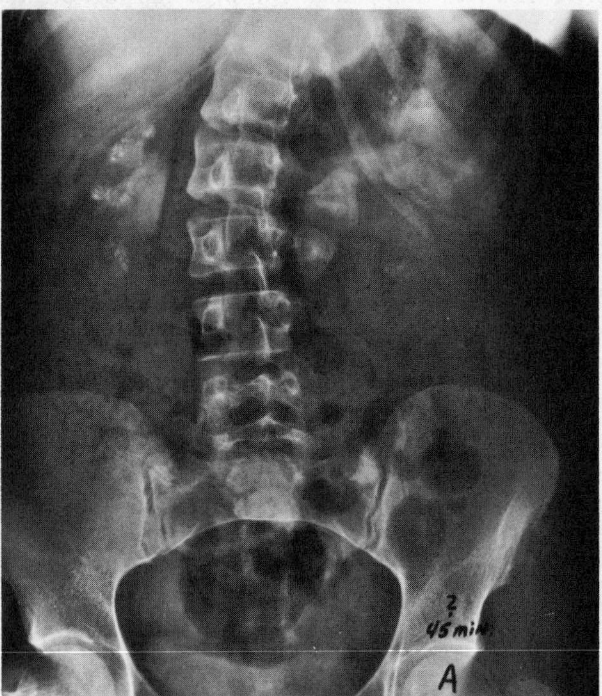

A. Serum alkaline phosphatase
B. 24-hour urinary calcium excretion
C. Serum PTH determination using a carboxylterminal assay
D. Serum magnesium concentration
E. Serum calcitonin

72. A 20-year-old man has polyuria and polydipsia. He has taken no medications. Water deprivation and vasopressin therapy both fail to concentrate the urine. Others in his family have a similar problem. All laboratory tests, including serum glucose, calcium, and potassium, urinalysis, and hemoglobin, are normal. Which of the following is most likely to be effective?

A. Chlorpropamide
B. Lithium carbonate
C. Nicotine
D. Hydrochlorothiazide
E. Clofibrate

73. Which of the following is LEAST likely to cause polyuria that is relatively resistant to antidiuretic hormone (ADH)?

A. Hypercalcemia
B. Hypernatremia
C. Lithium administration
D. Sickle cell disease
E. Hypokalemia

74. In central (hypothalamic) diabetes insipidus requiring vasopressin therapy, which of the following forms of vasopressin is the drug of choice, in terms of duration of action, route of administration, and absence of side effects?

A. 1-Deamino, 8-D-arginine vasopressin (dDAVP)
B. Lysine vasopressin
C. Vasopressin tannate in oil
D. Aqueous vasopressin
E. Posterior pituitary extract

75. A 34-year-old man is referred to you because of infertility. Libido and potency are normal. There is no history of drug or radiation therapy. Routine physical examination is unremarkable. Serum testosterone is 0.57 μg/dl (N = 0.3–1.2); serum luteinizing hormone (LH), 9 mIU/ml (N = 4–19); and follicle-stimulating hormone (FSH), 75 mIU/ml (N = 4–27). Which of the following is correct?

A. Complete pituitary evaluation is indicated
B. Gonadotropin-releasing hormone (Gn/RH) will improve fertility
C. Prolonged testosterone enanthate therapy will improve fertility
D. The infertility is almost certainly irreversible
E. Testicular biopsy should be performed to establish the diagnosis

76. A 15-year-old girl presents because of failure to begin menses and insufficient sexual development, which has caused her to withdraw from social contacts. In contrast to her peers she has had no breast enlargement, and she is acutely embarrassed by her "abnormality." Physical examination shows a few fine strands of pubic hair, which she had not noticed, and small islands of breast tissue below the areolae. The remainder of the examination reveals no abnormalities. Which one of the following would you order next?

A. Karyotyping
B. Full pituitary evaluation
C. Pelvic ultrasound to detect the presence of ovaries
D. Serum gonadotropin and estrogen measurements
E. None of the above

77. Hypersecretion of which of the following hormones is LEAST likely in hyperpituitarism?

A. Follicle-stimulating hormone (FSH)
B. Prolactin
C. Growth hormone
D. Adrenocorticotropic hormone (ACTH)

78. The appropriate treatment of an intrathyroidal papillary carcinoma always includes which one of the following?

A. Total thyroidectomy, preserving parathyroid glands if at all possible
B. Ablation of residual thyroid tissue and metastatic cancer with radioiodine
C. Radical, bilateral neck dissection to detect and remove lymph node metastases
D. Total suppression of thyroid-stimulating hormone (TSH) by exogenous thyroxine
E. External radiation therapy

79. A 52-year-old woman undergoes evaluation for unexplained weight loss and poor appetite. An upper gastrointestinal series, barium enema, and oral cholecystogram are normal. Subsequent thyroid function studies show a resin T_3 uptake of 0.95 (N = 0.85–1.15); serum thyroxine (T_4) concentration, 12.3 μg/dl (N = 5–11); and serum triiodothyronine (T_3) concentration, 85 ng/dl (N = 80–220). Which of the following is the most likely diagnosis?

A. Hyperthyroidism
B. Hypothyroidism
C. Subacute thyroiditis
D. Abnormality of serum TBG concentration
E. None of the above

80. You are asked to examine an 8-year-old boy who has several close relatives who have had surgically proved medullary carcinoma of the thyroid and hyperparathyroidism. Routine examination reveals no abnormalities. Which of the following is appropriate?

A. Measurement of serum calcitonin after pentagastrin infusion
B. Radioisotope thyroid scan
C. Aspiration biopsy of the thyroid gland
D. Subtotal thyroidectomy
E. Thyroid suppression with L-thyroxine

DIRECTIONS: For questions 81 to 118, you are to decide whether EACH choice is true or false. Any combination of answers, from all true to all false, may be present. Mark the answer sheet "T" or "F" in the space provided.

81. A 24-year-old woman who has had diabetes for six years becomes pregnant. Variables affecting choice of delivery date include which of the following?

A. Estrogen levels
B. Amniotic fluid lecithin and sphingomyelin
C. Results of an oxytocin challenge test
D. Excessive weight gain

82. A 5-year-old boy has pubic and axillary hair growth, an enlarged phallus, and testes that measure 1.5 × 3.0 cm bilaterally. Possible causes include which of the following?

A. Adrenal 21α-hydroxylase deficiency
B. Aberrant pinealoma
C. Adrenal 11β-hydroxylase deficiency
D. Hepatoblastoma

83. Maintenance therapy for Addison's disease generally includes which of the following?

A. Glucocorticoid replacement equivalent to 20 mg of cortisol daily
B. A low-sodium, low-potassium diet
C. Fludrocortisone, 0.1 mg once daily
D. Supplemental carbohydrate feedings

84. The use of sodium bicarbonate in patients with diabetic ketoacidosis contributes to which of the following undesirable effects?

A. Insulin resistance
B. Hypokalemia
C. Obtundation
D. Tissue hypoxia

85. Patients with adrenal insufficiency secondary to hypopituitarism usually show which of the following manifestations of Addison's disease?

A. Mucocutaneous hyperpigmentation
B. Hyperkalemia
C. Axillary hair loss in the female
D. General debilitation and weakness
E. Peripheral vascular collapse with severe stress

86. A 23-year-old female nurse is brought to the emergency room in coma. Plasma glucose is 16 mg/dl, and insulin 86 μU/ml. After resuscitation she responds normally to a 100-gm glucose tolerance test. After a 72-hour fast, the plasma insulin is less than 2 μU/ml and glucose is 49 mg/dl. Which of the following tests would be appropriate now?

A. Pancreatic angiography
B. Assay for C-peptide in the original blood sample
C. Leucine tolerance test
D. Assay for anti-insulin antibodies

87. The nitrogen-sparing effect of intravenous glucose is mediated by which of the following?

A. A slight increase in insulin secretion
B. Enhanced glucose transport into muscle
C. Suppression of glycogenolysis
D. Suppression of gluconeogenesis

88. The young woman illustrated consults you because of primary amenorrhea. Other members of her family have had a similar problem. On examination the secondary sexual characteristics are well developed; however, the vagina is shallow and ends blindly in a pouch. No uterus is present. The karyotype is XY. Which of the following statements about this condition is/are correct?

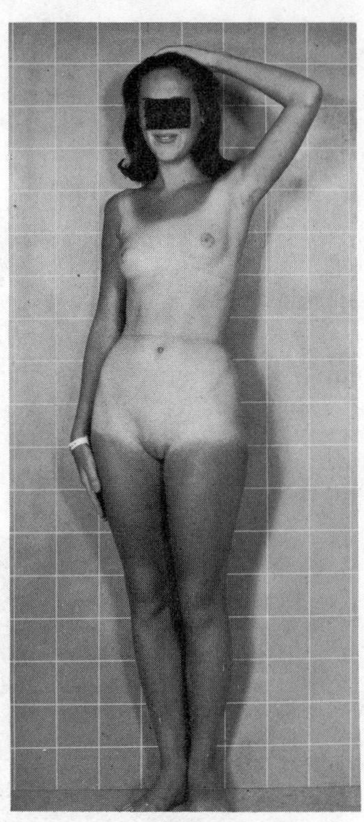

A. The biochemical defect in this condition is the absence of cytoplasmic receptors for testosterone
B. The serum testosterone is likely to be undetectable
C. Therapy should include administration of high doses of testosterone to establish normal male secondary sexual characteristics
D. There is a significant risk of cancer developing in the gonads, which should be removed surgically

89. Complications of oral contraceptive medications include which of the following?

A. Hypertension
B. Increased incidence of gallstones
C. Hypoglycemia
D. Hemorrhage from hepatic adenomas
E. Thromboembolism

90. Clinical states associated with congenital adrenal hyperplasia include which of the following?

A. Excessive mineralocorticoid production
B. Deficient mineralocorticoid production
C. Excessive androgen production
D. Deficient androgen production

91. Conditions for performing a diagnostic glucose tolerance test should include which of the following?

A. Fasting plasma glucose consistently over 140 mg/dl
B. Absence of severe physical or emotional stress
C. Avoidance of sweets for three days
D. Correction of any hypokalemia

92. Abnormally high concentrations of cortisol impair the bodily responses to injury or infection through which of the following mechanisms?

A. Decreased accumulation of leukocytes at the site of tissue injury
B. Impaired migration of leukocytes through tissues
C. Diminished antibody production
D. Inhibited lymphocyte proliferation

93. The secretion of adrenocorticotropic hormone (ACTH) is controlled by which of the following?

A. The level of cortisol
B. The level of 11-deoxycortisol
C. Production of tetrahydrocortisol
D. The sleep-wake cycle
E. Physiologic stress

94. Which of the following statements concerning the measurement of urinary glucose is/are true?

A. Clinitest tablets quantify glycosuria
B. Paper enzyme strips that detect glycosuria (Diastix, TesTape, Clinistix) are less sensitive for glucose than Clinitest tablets
C. The normal renal threshold for glucose is approximately 100 mg/dl
D. Clinitest tablets will detect factitious sucrosuria (e.g., table sugar added to urine samples)
E. High doses of vitamin C interfere with glycosuria determination by both Clinitest tablets and paper enzyme strips

95. Pharmacologic agents that induce prolactin secretion include

A. ergot alkaloids
B. phenothiazines (e.g., chlorpromazine)
C. thyrotropin-releasing hormone (TRH)
D. estrogens
E. dopamine

96. Psychologic stimuli (including depression, anxiety, and deprivation of maternal nurturing) can alter the secretion of which of the following pituitary hormones?

A. Growth hormone (GH)
B. Luteinizing hormone (LH)
C. Thyroid-stimulating hormone (TSH)
D. Adrenocorticotropic hormone (ACTH)

97. Improved endogenous insulin secretion contributes to improved diabetes control after which of the following?

A. Aggressive treatment of ketoacidosis
B. Sulfonylurea therapy
C. Diet therapy
D. Insulin therapy

98. A patient with diabetes is referred to you for evaluation of refractory hyperglycemia. He is 69 inches tall and weighs 205 pounds. His physician has monitored fasting plasma glucose levels to determine the current insulin dose of 130 units of NPH U100 insulin daily. Which of the following is/are likely to give insight into the mechanism of this patient's diabetic instability?

A. Urine checks four times daily
B. Timing of hypoglycemic symptoms in the past
C. History of sleep problems
D. History of weight changes

99. In a patient with a solitary thyroid nodule, which of the following is/are associated with an increased likelihood of malignancy?

A. History of neck irradiation in childhood
B. Lack of radioisotope uptake in the nodule
C. Young, male patient
D. Presence of hypothyroidism with increased serum concentration of thyroid-stimulating hormone (TSH)

100. A 67-year-old woman has had a multinodular goiter for many years without noticeable change. Recently she has noted weight loss and shortness of breath, and she has been taking digoxin prescribed for atrial fibrillation four weeks ago. Serum thyroxine (T_4) is 10.1 μg/dl (N = 5–11); resin T_3 uptake, 1.08 (N = 0.85–1.15); free thyroxine index, 10.9 (N = 4.7–10.5). Appropriate action includes which of the following?

A. Measure serum triiodothyronine (T_3)
B. Perform thyrotropin-releasing hormone (TRH) infusion test
C. Initiate treatment with prophylthiouracil
D. Initiate treatment with L-thyroxine to suppress goiter

101. Insulin therapy may reasonably be delayed in a patient with ketoacidosis who presents with which of the following?

A. Evidence of an acute abdomen
B. Lipemia retinalis
C. Oliguria and a blood pressure of 70/40 mm Hg
D. Flat T waves, prolonged Q-T interval, and U waves on the electrocardiogram

102. Which of the following statements concerning diabetic nephropathy is/are true?

A. Proteinuria develops in approximately two thirds of patients who have had diabetes for 20 years or more
B. The average diabetic patient developing proteinuria will develop uremia in five years
C. The proteinuria associated with diabetic nephropathy diminishes with progressive renal failure
D. 40% of patients with juvenile-onset diabetes die from renal failure
E. Normal kidneys transplanted into patients with diabetes have developed the pathologic changes of diabetic nephropathy

103. A 30-year-old man with diabetes mellitus has recently developed uremia. Laboratory studies reveal: blood urea nitrogen, 90 mg/dl; serum creatinine, 10.3 mg/dl; and urinary protein, 4+. Which of the following statements concerning this patient's future course is/are true?

A. He will probably require less insulin now than he did before he developed uremia
B. His renal threshold for glycosuria is likely to be lower now than before he developed uremia

C. He will probably fare worse on chronic hemodialysis than would a nondiabetic patient of similar age
D. His chance of dying from renal transplantation is higher than that of a nondiabetic patient of similar age
E. His chances of survival are better with renal transplantation than with chronic hemodialysis

104. A 27-year-old mother of two children has noted two months of weight loss without dieting, irritability with her husband and children, sleeplessness, increased sweating, and frequent palpitations. Pulse is 120 per minute. She has stare and lid lag and a firm diffuse goiter. There is a tremor of the outstretched hand. The skin is moist. Serum thyroxine is 17.8 μg/dl (N = 5–11), and resin T_3 uptake is 1.56 (N = 0.85–1.15). Which of the following studies should be ordered?

A. Measurement of serum triiodothyronine (T_3)
B. Thyrotropin-releasing hormone (TRH) infusion test
C. Radioisotope thyroid scan
D. Radioiodine uptake

105. The short plasma half-life for insulin (3–10 minutes) may be explained by which of the following?

A. Its rapid removal from blood by the liver
B. Binding of insulin to proteins in the circulation
C. Its low molecular weight
D. Hepatic receptors recognizing the carbohydrate moiety of the insulin molecule

106. Reduction of the free thyroxine index *without* elevation of serum thyroid-stimulating hormone (TSH) may be encountered in which of these patients?

A. A young man with epilepsy
B. An overweight woman attending a "weight loss" clinic
C. A middle-aged woman with severe rheumatoid arthritis
D. A businessman with impotence, fatigue, and bitemporal hemianopia

107. A patient who has had insulin-dependent diabetes mellitus for 15 years now has a blood urea nitrogen of 50 mg/dl, and a serum creatinine of 3 mg/dl. Plasma glucose is in the range of 100 to 200 mg/dl around the clock. Urinalysis shows a specific gravity of 1.018, 1/2% glucose, negative protein, 4 white cells/high power field, and no red cell casts. Which of the following is/are correct?

A. The duration of diabetes is consistent with the impairment in renal function
B. Diabetic retinopathy is almost certainly present
C. There is some other cause of renal impairment besides diabetes
D. Severe renal failure will probably occur in about five years

108. A 33-year-old woman with Graves' disease has been receiving propylthiouracil for eight months. Her symptoms have been well controlled. The drug is discontinued, and her symptoms (heat intolerance, hyperdefecation, tachycardia, and weight loss) reappear. Serum thyroxine (T_4) is 16.8 μg/dl (N = 5–11) and resin T_3 uptake is 1.4 (N = 0.85–1.15). Which of the following statements regarding the use of radioiodine therapy in this patient is/are true?

A. The risk of subsequent hypothyroidism is slight (approximately 10%)
B. Because of the gonadal irradiation, the risk of her having malformed offspring in the future is markedly increased
C. The risk of radiation-induced malignancy is very low
D. The treatment should be avoided in pregnancy

109. Parathyroid hormone (PTH) maintains serum calcium by which of the following mechanisms?

A. Increased release of calcium from bone
B. Decreased excretion of calcium by the kidney
C. Increased absorption of calcium from the gut
D. Decreased excretion of phosphate in the urine

110. A 53-year-old woman complains of excessive itching, weakness, constipation, polyuria, and difficulty in mental concentration. Serum calcium is 11.9 mg/dl (N = 8.9–10.1). In assessing the diagnosis, the physician should pay particular attention to which of the following?

A. Use of thiazide diuretics by the patient
B. Evidence of coexisting malignancies
C. Use of excessive vitamin D or vitamin A
D. Coexisting hyperthyroidism

111. Which of the following is/are indicated as routine diagnostic tests before parathyroid surgery?

A. Esophagography
B. Ultrasonography
C. Computerized tomography
D. Vascular radiography
E. Radioimmunoassay for parathyroid hormone (PTH)

112. A 2-year-old child with earache and fever of 104° F wakes her parents crying in the night. They plan to take her to the emergency room after lowering her temperature, but before they leave home the child becomes unconscious. On arrival at the hospital ten minutes later the child is unresponsive, but wakes quickly with intravenous glucose. Plasma glucose before treatment was 18 mg/dl. Which of the following would you do to evaluate the hypoglycemia?

A. Obtain more history
B. Measure plasma insulin
C. Measure plasma C-peptide level
D. Measure blood alcohol

113. A 27-year-old woman develops persistent acral paresthesias and tetany following a thyroidectomy for Graves' disease. Representative serum calcium is 6.4 mg/dl (N = 8.9–10.1) and serum phosphate 5.7 mg/dl (N = 2.5–4.5). Appropriate initial therapy consists of which of the following?

A. Oral calcium as the gluconate or chloride salt
B. 10% calcium gluconate solution by slow intravenous infusion
C. Intramuscular parathyroid hormone (PTH), 200 U intramuscularly every six hours
D. Dihydrotachysterol, 4 mg per day

114. Corticosteroids frequently decrease the hypercalcemia associated with which of the following?

A. Sarcoidosis
B. Multiple myeloma
C. Vitamin D intoxication
D. Primary hyperparathyroidism

115. An adolescent girl has muscular weakness. She is short and obese, and has a round face and ocular strabismus. Roentgenogram of the hands is shown. Serum calcium is 7.5 mg/dl (N = 8.9–10.1), and serum phosphate is 5.5 mg/dl (N = 2.5–4.5). Which of the following is/are likely in this patient?

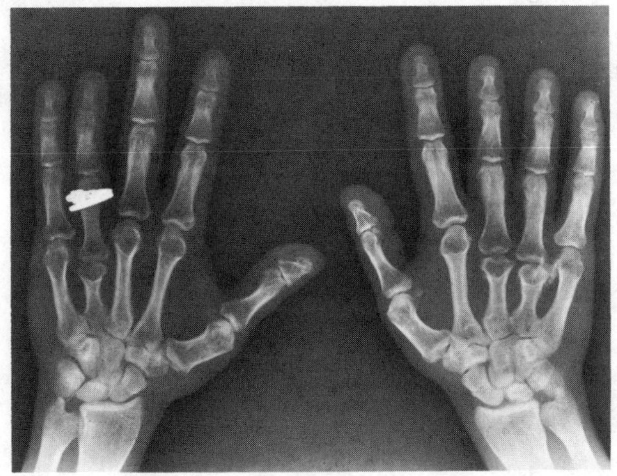

A. Increased serum parathyroid hormone (PTH) concentration
B. Basal ganglia calcification on skull film
C. A normal urinary cyclic AMP response to PTH
D. Subnormal intelligence
E. Family members of the same phenotype

116. A marked rise in plasma glucose after 1 mg of glucagon given intravenously during fasting hypoglycemia is compatible with which of the following?

A. Islet cell tumor
B. Adrenal insufficiency
C. Retroperitoneal tumor with nonsuppressible, insulin-like activity
D. Alcohol hypoglycemia

117. Thirst is mediated by which of the following factors?

A. Direct stimulation of "thirst center" by antidiuretic hormone (ADH)
B. Hyperosmolality of cells in the "thirst center"
C. The accumulation of "idiopathic dipsogens" in "thirst center" neurons
D. Actions of angiotensin II on the "thirst center"

118. Which of the following result(s) in release of antidiuretic hormone (ADH)?

A. Increased intrathoracic pressure
B. Systemic arterial hypotension
C. Pain
D. Physical stress (e.g., surgery)

DIRECTIONS: Questions 119 to 171 are matching questions. For each numbered item, choose the most likely associated lettered item from those provided. Each numbered item has ONLY ONE answer. Within each group, each lettered item may be the answer to one, more than one, or none of the numbered items.

QUESTIONS 119–122

For each of the following diseases, select the most likely mechanism of hypoglycemia.

A. Insufficient cofactors for hepatic glucose production
B. Suppression of hepatic glucose release
C. Impaired nutrient-stimulated insulin release
D. Lack of substrate for glyconeogenesis

119. Islet cell tumor

120. Adrenal insufficiency

121. Alcohol excess

122. Early diabetes mellitus

QUESTIONS 123–126

For each of the following sets of laboratory and clinical features, select the most likely associated hypogonadal condition.

A. Sertoli cell–only syndrome (germinal cell aplasia)
B. Klinefelter's syndrome
C. Hypogonadotropic hypogonadism
D. Myotonic muscular dystrophy

	Testes		Serum		
	Size (Long Axis: cm)	*Consistency*	*LH*	*FSH*	Additional Features
123.	3	normal	normal	high	
124.	1.5	firm	high	high	
125.	1.5	soft	high	high	Lens cataracts, frontal baldness
126.	2	soft	low-normal	low-normal	Hyposmia

QUESTIONS 127–131

For each of the following sets of laboratory values, choose the most closely associated group of conditions.

A. Anovulation, hirsutism, acne, multiple follicular cysts
B. Amenorrhea following septic abortion
C. Amenorrhea, hot flashes, atrophic vaginitis
D. Amenorrhea, galactorrhea, headaches
E. Amenorrhea, infantile genitalia, anosmia

	LH (mIU/ml; N=4–19)	FSH (mIU/ml; N=4–27)	Prolactin (ng/ml; N=5–25)
127.	6	6	250
128.	120	50	18
129.	12	14	10
130.	30	20	20
131.	1	2	10

QUESTIONS 132–137

For each of the following patients who are being evaluated for the possibility of Cushing's syndrome, select the most likely associated set of laboratory values (see below).

132. A 41-year-old woman with amenorrhea, acne, beard growth, deep voice, and a palpable mass in the left flank

133. An overweight 26-year-old woman receiving oral contraceptives

134. A 52-year-old woman with a basophilic pituitary adenoma

135. A 55-year-old man with cough, weakness, hypokalemia, and a lung mass on roentgenogram of the chest

136. A 5-year-old boy with phallic enlargement, accelerated growth, and high blood pressure

137. A 24-year-woman with sleep disturbance, easy fatigability, central obesity, abdominal striae, and an adrenal mass on computerized tomography

	Plasma Cortisol 8:00 AM	Plasma Cortisol 5:00 PM	Plasma ACTH 8:00 AM	Urinary 17-OH Corticoids	Urinary 17-Keto-steroids	Urinary 17-OH Corticoids After Dexamethasone	
						0.5 mg every 6 hr	*2.0 mg every 6 hr*
(normal)	*(8–25 μg/dl)*	*(5–10 μg/dl)*	*(<80 pg/ml)*	*(3–7 mg/gcr*)*	*(<20 mg/day)*	*(<2 mg/gcr*)*	*(<2 mg/gcr*)*
A.	27	25	65	19	27	15	6
B.	15	21	20	14	10	15	16
C.	12	8	92	15	25	<2	<2
D.	25	23	20	18	343	16	23
E.	55	42	250	45	114	47	48
F.	35	30	75	6	12	<2	<2

*gcr = gram of creatinine.

QUESTIONS 138–143

For each of the following thyroid conditions, select the most appropriate therapy.

A. Thyroidectomy and maximal-dose radioiodine treatment
B. Total (bilateral) thyroidectomy
C. Palliative thyroidectomy
D. Calcitonin replacement therapy
E. Subtotal thyroidectomy

138. A "hot" nodule in a thyrotoxic patient

139. Familial medullary carcinoma

140. Metastatic follicular carcinoma

141. Intrathyroidal papillary carcinoma

142. Giant cell anaplastic thyroid carcinoma

143. A solitary, functionless ("cold") nodule in a young man

QUESTIONS 144–152

For each of the following patients, select the most likely associated laboratory values:

	Serum thyroxine (μg/dl; N=5–11)	Resin T_3 uptake (N=0.85–1.15)	Serum TSH (μu/ml; N=0–6)	24-hour radioiodine uptake (N=5–30)
A.	17.0	1.17	0.8	44%
B.	15.3	0.66	1.8	21%
C.	5.8	0.73	3.9	6%
D.	3.7	0.91	38.2	14%
E.	16.3	1.09	0.9	1%

144. A pregnant woman

145. A patient with hypothalamic-pituitary sarcoidosis

146. A young woman with Graves' disease

147. A patient with goiter caused by Hashimoto's thyroiditis, detected on routine examination

148. A patient with fever due to subacute thyroiditis

149. A patient surreptitiously ingesting triiodothyronine in excess

150. A man receiving diethylstilbestrol for prostatic carcinoma

151. A woman who develops atrial fibrillation while taking thyroxine, 0.1 mg daily, to suppress a multinodular goiter

152. A patient two weeks after stopping unnecessary thyroxine treatment

QUESTIONS 153–157

For each of the following clinical conditions, select the most appropriate laboratory values.

	Serum Calcium (mg/dl; N=8.9–10.1)	Serum Phosphate (mg/dl; N=2.5–4.5)	Serum PTH (pg/ml; N=10–150)	Urinary Cyclic AMP Response to PTH
A.	7.1	4.9	8	Increased
B.	7.4	5.3	300	Decreased
C.	7.3	4.3	35	Normal or decreased
D.	7.9	2.1	195	Normal
E.	6.9	2.3	4	Normal

153. A 15-year-old girl with Addison's disease and *Candida* infection of the nails

154. A 42-year-old man two days after successful resection of a single parathyroid adenoma

155. A short, stocky, round-faced brother and sister with mental retardation

156. A 24-year-old man with persistent tetany following total thyroidectomy for follicular thyroid carcinoma

157. A 15-year-old boy with vitamin D deficiency rickets

QUESTIONS 158–161

For each of the following problems with insulin injection, select the most appropriate response.

A. Use a less antigenic insulin
B. Inject a less antigenic insulin at the edge of the lesion
C. Avoid this site; rotate sites so that repeat injections occur in not less than two to four weeks
D. Check the injection technique and continue the same insulin

158. Lipoatrophy

159. Slight redness at some injection sites

160. Lipohypertrophy

161. A red, hot nodule at the injection site lasting 1–2 days

QUESTIONS 162–166

For each patient, select the most likely associated set of laboratory values from the table below.

162. A member of a large family with asymptomatic hypercalcemia unresponsive to parathyroidectomy

163. A 49-year-old cigarette smoker with a nodule on chest radiography

164. A 56-year-old woman with constipation, confusion, and kidney stones

165. A hypertensive man treated with thiazide diuretics

166. A health faddist taking large doses of vitamin D

	Serum Calcium (mg/dl; N=8.9–10.1)	Serum Phosphate (mg/dl; N=2.5–4.5)	Serum Chloride (mEq/L; N=98–108)	Serum PTH (pg/ml; N=10–150)	24-hour urinary Calcium (mg; N=100–300)
A.	11.5	2.2	109	175	297
B.	12.7	2.5	103	137	424
C.	10.9	3.7	94	14	250
D.	11.1	2.7	105	75	43
E.	12.4	4.1	105	8	582

QUESTIONS 167–171

A group of subjects undergo a water-deprivation test. Water is withheld for 14 to 16 hours, during which time urinary osmolality is monitored on an hourly basis until this value no longer increases. At this point the serum osmolality is measured, 5 units of aqueous vasopressin are injected subcutaneously, and urinary osmolality is again measured one hour later. Although this test does not discriminate absolutely between the different conditions listed below, select the conditions *most* consistent with each of the following sets of data.

A. Partial antidiuretic hormone (ADH) deficiency
B. Complete ADH deficiency
C. Congenital nephrogenic diabetes insipidus
D. Primary polydipsia (compulsive water drinking)
E. Normal subject

	Maximal Urinary Osmolality (after dehydration, mOsm/kg)		**Maximal Serum Osmolality (after dehydration; before vasopressin injection) (mOsm/kg; N=285–295)**
	Before Vasopressin	***After Vasopressin***	
167.	150	450	310
168.	1000	980	288
169.	100	140	315
170.	400	500	295
171.	550	570	289

PART 7

ENDOCRINOLOGY AND DIABETES MELLITUS

ANSWERS

1. (A) Despite the patient's denial of sexual activity, pregnancy cannot be discounted. It remains the chief cause of "secondary amenorrhea" and should *always* be excluded before other expensive (and even contraindicated) procedures are undertaken. *(Cecil, p. 1271)*

2. (A) Ingestion of substantial amounts of free carbohydrate simply triggers insulin release again, leading to further symptoms in a short while. Multiple feedings are helpful in warding off between-meal hypoglycemia. Weight reduction may correct insulin resistance, leading to a lag in insulin peak. Carbohydrate restriction reduces insulin sensitivity and reduces the amount of insulin released per feeding. Psychotherapy may be appropriate for the associated emotional distress that many of these patients have. *(Cecil, p. 1074)*

3. (D) Testosterone, particularly if administered at much greater than physiologic doses, may cause gynecomastia. Testosterone may stimulate the growth of prostatic carcinoma, and this diagnosis should be considered before therapy is begun. Androgens stimulate erythropoiesis and thereby increase the serum hemoglobin concentration. Although intrahepatic cholestasis may rarely occur with testosterone administration, this is more likely to happen with methyltestosterone than with testosterone enanthate injections. Testosterone markedly inhibits spermatogenesis, possibly by inhibiting pituitary gonadotropin output even though intratesticular testosterone concentrations are less than normal. *(Cecil, p. 1248)*

4. (B) Although absolute quantification of hormonal adequacy depends on laboratory measures, certain clinical observations allow accurate inference of estrogen status in mature women. All the items noted are effects of estrogen except the rise in basal body temperature. This thermogenic shift is caused by the progesterone produced from the corpus luteum following ovulation. Although its measurement is tedious, the temperature rise provides an index of presumptive ovulation and can be used to determine the time of likely fertility. *(Cecil, pp. 1261–1262)*

5. (B) Anti-islet cell antibodies are of importance in the pathogenesis of the insulin-dependent diabetes typically seen in younger and thinner patients, but even in these patients they do not fall in titer to account for the "honeymoon." In the older, obese patient, insulin secretion may be improved once compensation takes place. Insulin sensitivity is improved by weight loss and carbohydrate restriction by virtue of increased numbers of insulin receptors. During the acute decompensation, elevated levels of counter-regulatory hormones may also have played a role. *(Cecil, pp. 1058–1066)*

6. (A) This patient has Turner's syndrome with a single X chromosome. *(Cecil, p. 1267)*

7. (A) Although abnormal immune responsiveness may be related to the original development of diabetes, the susceptibility to bacterial infections is thought to be related to excessive substrate availability, poor tissue oxygen supply, and the fact that many cells perform poorly in high tonicity. *(Cecil, p. 1064)*

8. (E) These symptoms are typical of adrenal failure. Associated with this may be hypotension, hypovolemia (producing a small heart silhouette), elevated serum potassium (if mineralocorticoid secretion is lost) and an inability to maintain serum glucose during prolonged fasting. Infection may precipitate addisonian crisis but, in general, fever is not a feature of uncomplicated hypoadrenalism. *(Cecil, pp. 1228–1229)*

9. (D) In establishing a diagnosis of glandular hypofunction, provocative testing is essential to prove lack of reserve. Fasting plasma cortisol or urinary 17-hydroxycorticoid excretion may well be low, but these are insufficient to establish the diagnosis. A brisk cortisol response to cosyntropin excludes adrenal insufficiency, but a subnormal response is not diagnostic. Only if there is no cortisol response to prolonged ACTH (or cosyntropin) infusion can the diagnosis of Addison's disease, with its requirement for lifelong medical attention, be safely assigned. Prolonged infusion of ACTH can further distinguish primary adrenal insufficiency (no response after 48 hours of continuous infusion) from secondary hypoadrenalism due to ACTH deficit (return of cortisol secretion to normal by 48 hours). Computerized tomography is not sensitive enough to detect functional abnormalities. *(Cecil, pp. 1228–1229)*

10. (D) The patient pictured has Cushing's syndrome. Kidney stones occur in only 12% of such patients; the other findings are present in more than 70%. *(Cecil, p. 1233)*

11. (D) Infection, in addition to specific symptoms, will generally give a more prolonged loss of control. Starvation will give ketosis without glycosuria. Insulin deficiency would be surprising in a patient whose control was very stable and whose requirement had not changed. Nocturnal hypoglycemia (Somogyi effect) can best account for an abrupt shift from negative to positive sugars, particularly if acetone is present. *(Cecil, pp. 1069–1070)*

12. (A) 11β-hydroxylase deficiency is the second most common form of congenital adrenal hyperplasia. Because 11-hydroxylation is needed in the formation of both cortisol and aldosterone, large quantities of their precursors accumulate. 11-deoxycortisol, which is biologically inactive, can be measured to aid in making the diagnosis. 11-deoxycorticosterone (DOC), an aldosterone precursor, is a weak mineralocorticoid, but levels are so high that hypertension results. *(Cecil, pp. 1241–1242)*

13. (B) Continued loss of potassium in the urine despite very low serum potassium concentrations is the hallmark of hypersecretion of aldosterone. The urinary potassium excretion usually exceeds 30 mEq/day. *(Cecil, pp. 1237–1238; Ehrlich)*

14. (B) Benign forms of hirsutism often have their onset at the time of puberty. Slowly progressive, they are characterized chiefly by excessive hair growth and sometimes by menstrual irregularity. Ominous forms of hirsutism often have signs of virilization (clitoromegaly, voice change, Adam's apple enlargement, masculine body habitus). Plasma testosterone in excess of 0.20 μg/dl is uncommon in benign hirsutism. A palpable flank mass in a hirsute patient must raise a question of adrenal tumor. *(Cecil, pp. 1276–1278)*

15. (B) Visual instability is a common presenting complaint of diabetes and is readily corrected when the osmotic shifts in the lens can be arrested. Lipemia retinalis, although it may be associated with fluctuating blood sugars, does not in itself affect vision. Cataracts can be removed. Photocoagulation can arrest the recurrent hemorrhages of proliferative retinopathy. Background retinopathy may impair vision because of the extreme permeability associated with it, and it may respond to photocoagulation. *(Cecil, pp. 1061–1062)*

16. (E) The most likely answer is fraudulent urine results. Denial is a prominent mechanism in such children. Without the hemoglobin A_1 result, which reflects the average blood sugar over a period of several weeks, the elevated blood sugar might simply be attributed to the stress of the visit to the physician. This is a prime use of the glycosylated hemoglobin assay in estimating the average plasma glucose. The hemoglobin A_1 fails to provide any insight into the diurnal pattern of glucose utilization, which is provided by urine and blood glucose monitoring throughout the day. Non–insulin-dependent patients in particular are able to normalize blood glucose with a day or two of dieting before clinic visits in order to please the physician, but they shouldn't be able to fool the hemoglobin A_1 assay! *(Citrin, Ellis, and Skyler)*

17. (B) Addison's original description attributed adrenal failure to tuberculous destruction. In some countries tuberculosis still accounts for most adrenal hypofunction, but in the United States idiopathic adrenal atrophy is the prime cause. An autoimmune etiology is suspected for this condition, which may occur in association with failure of any of several other organs (including thyroid, parathyroid, pancreatic islets, gonads, skin melanocytes, and gastric parietal cells). Amyloidosis, tumor infiltration, and adrenal apoplexy are extraordinarily rare causes of adrenal failure. *(Cecil, p. 1228; Hall and Evered)*

18. (B) Because aldosterone secretion is largely, if not totally, mediated via angiotensin II stimulation of the zona glomerulosa of the adrenal cortex, this function is preserved in patients with ACTH deficiency. Mineralocorticoid replacement therefore is not necessary. Glucocorticoid replacement, preparation for surgery, the wearing of an identification bracelet, and knowledge of self-injection of steroids are as important in patients with ACTH deficiency as they are in patients with primary adrenal failure. *(Cecil, p. 1232; Ehrlich)*

19. (B) Obesity in childhood is a serious problem, but not all such patients need to be evaluated for Cushing's disease. An important clue that glucocorticoid excess may be involved is the failure to grow normally, especially if the growth pattern was previously normal. Most obese children grow more, not less, rapidly than children of normal weight, and growth failure should raise the question of hyperadrenocorticism. Premature puberty, eosinophilia, and muscular hypertrophy may require evaluation, but they are not caused by Cushing's disease. Polycythemia can be seen with cortisol excess, but it not sufficient *per se* to suggest Cushing's disease. *(Cecil, p. 1234)*

20. (A) The rapidly progressive and profound hypercortisolism of the "ectopic ACTH" syndrome often induces serious biochemical disturbance long before there are obvious changes in fat deposition or protein catabolism, which produce the typical clinical picture of Cushing's syndrome. Thus, hypokalemia, unprovoked by vomiting, diarrhea, or diuretics, may be the earliest clue of this syndrome in a cancer patient, and warrants measurement of cortisol. Cutaneous striae and osteoporosis are not usually seen or are unrelated. Muscular weakness is so common in patients with cancer that it cannot serve as a "clue" to the presence of ectopic ACTH secretion. Likewise, erythrocytosis is much more likely to be caused by associated lung disease than by Cushing's syndrome, and does not warrant cortisol studies. *(Cecil, pp. 1234–1235, 1236–1237; Sherwood and Gould)*

21. (E) High insulin and low glucagon levels characterize the fed state and are responsible for the production of energy storage compounds, glycogen and fat. In addition, structural protein can be synthesized. Ketones are synthesized during dietary deprivation and represent a transformation of stored fat into a more utilizable form. *(Cecil, pp. 1054–1055)*

22. (D) Although insulin or oral agents may be required to achieve normal plasma glucose control, there are several advantages to beginning with diet alone. The patient will be impressed by the symptomatic improvement, and 80% of patients will become aglycosuric. Such improvement might be attributed to medications if they were provided. Once on stable diet therapy, as many as one third of patients may have improved insulin release with recovery from islet cell decompensation. *(Cecil, p. 1066; Doar et al., Perkins et al.)*

23. (D) It is important to remember that estrogens (oral contraceptives, pregnancy) increase the serum concentration of transcortin. Measurement of total plasma cortisol will give very high values that will appear not to suppress with dexamethasone. To rule out Cushing's syndrome we must rely on measurement of urinary 17-OH corticoids (or cortisol); since we are concerned about adrenal hyperfunction, a suppression test is called for. High-dose dexamethasone (2.0 mg every six hours) is *not* a diagnostic test for Cushing's syndrome — it is used to distinguish Cushing's *disease* from other forms of the syndrome. We do not yet have a diagnosis, so a low-dose dexamethasone suppression test (0.5 mg every six hours) is in order. If 17-OH corticoids or cortisol levels are not suppressed on this test, a high-dose suppression test, measurement of plasma ACTH, roentgenogram of the chest, and a number of other procedures would be indicated, but not before. *(Cecil, p. 1235)*

24. (C) Trans-sphenoidal removal of a pituitary microadenoma can cure Cushing's disease and leave pituitary function intact. Since this procedure attacks the root of the disorder, it is the best available choice. Pituitary irradiation by conventional x-ray is slow to take effect and is too often unsuccessful (cyclotron irradiation does cure about 80 to 90% of patients but is rarely available.) Bilateral adrenalectomy almost always cures the cortisol excess, but creates Addison's disease and makes the patient susceptible to Nelson's syndrome (enlarging pituitary tumor and cutaneous hyperpigmentation). Mitotane is used only for patients who cannot be treated with other means. It is slow to act, difficult to tolerate, and not always effective. Cyproheptadine has been proposed, but it is rarely effective as the sole therapy. *(Cecil, pp. 1235–1236; Tyrrell et al.)*

25. (C) Breast enlargement frequently occurs in Graves' disease. Although it is often minimal and unrecognized, it occasionally is the presenting complaint. Likewise, gynecomastia may occur in testicular failure (with elevated pituitary gonadotropins) or in oat cell carcinomas (or other tumors) because of their elaboration of ectopic chorionic gonadotropin. Patients with Klinefelter's syndrome typically have enlarged breasts and tiny testes. Breast hypertrophy in men is seen with drugs (e.g., estrogens, digoxin, spironolactone). Marijuana and alcohol have been implicated in gonadal failure; however, cocaine has not been reported to cause gynecomastia. *(Cecil, pp. 1280–1282)*

26. (C) Cortisol is the most important product of the human adrenal cortex. Under normal conditions most of the cortisol in serum is bound to transcortin, an α_2-globulin. Alterations in transcortin concentration can change total cortisol values while free cortisol remains normal (analogous to thyroxine-TBG relationships). Free cortisol is the metabolically active fraction; it promotes protein breakdown, gluconeogenesis, and increased fat deposition and *impairs* glucose uptake by muscle. In addition, cortisol is necessary for effective renal water excretion. Hyponatremia can occur when cortisol-deficient patients receive more water than they can excrete. *(Cecil, p. 1225)*

27. (B) The mechanism of the "honeymoon" is thought to relate to endogenous insulin secretion for which C-peptide (connecting peptide) is a marker. Insulin sensitivity is generally normal in an insulin-dependent patient at normal weight. After the "honeymoon," dependence on exogenous insulin increases, and dose requirements generally increase also. Although some patients may remain asymptomatic for a period on a diabetic diet alone, many authorities feel it unwise to interrupt insulin. The risk of insulin allergy on resumption may be increased, and it may be difficult for the patient to adapt psychologically to a need to resume insulin therapy. It is possible that continued therapy with the highest dose of insulin tolerated without hypoglycemia may contribute to the protection of endogenous insulin reserve for a somewhat longer period than usual. *(Cecil, p. 1058; Jackson and Guthrie)*

28. (A) If the patient's hypoglycemia were a regular occurrence, anticipatory changes in diet or insulin might be appropriate. The irregularity of hypoglycemic symptoms suggests that he may be injecting his exercising extremity before some jogging bouts. Insulin absorption from an exercising extremity is markedly facilitated. It is best to use abdominal sites before vigorous exercise, and rotate injections not associated with exercise among other sites. The patient should rotate a given injection (e.g., the morning or afternoon injection when no exercise is planned) only within a certain region of the body, since absorption characteristics vary remarkably between regions. *(Koivisto and Felig)*

29. (B) Vigorous thyroid replacement therapy in a patient with panhypopituitarism can precipitate an adrenal crisis. Before replacing thyroid hormone in such a patient, secondary adrenal insufficiency should always be ruled out, and the replacement dosage of thyroxine should be initially small and increased gradually. If treatment is begun before cortisol secretory status is known, prophylactic glucocorticoids should be given while results are pending. *(Cecil, p. 1186)*

30. (B) Renal glycosuria would not be compatible with the noted threshold. Nonglucose melituria should not be associated with hyperglycemia. Insulin deficiency would generally be associated with an elevated hemoglobin A_1. The normal hemoglobin A_1 in the absence of hemolysis or hemoglobinopathy (unusual in the English) suggests a normal average blood sugar. In order for this to occur with the known frequently elevated blood sugars, there has to be substantial hypoglycemia. Patients with autonomic neuropathy, in particular, may have prolonged daily hypoglycemia that is not recognized. *(Bunn, Gabbay, and Gallop; Gale, Walford, and Tattersall)*

31. (D) The patient has advanced acromegaly. Since this condition is caused by hypersecretion of growth hormone, the appropriate diagnostic test is to determine whether growth hormone secretion can be suppressed by hyperglycemia. Exercise and insulin hypoglycemia are *provocative* tests of growth hormone secretion that assess hormone reserve, not suppressibility. Visual field determination or computed tomography may be indicated in the assessment of the patient, but will not confirm the diagnosis of acromegaly. *(Cecil, pp. 1174, 1188–1191)*

32. (B) Alpha-adrenergic stimulation leads to insulin suppression, which may contribute to the glucose intolerance of pheochromocytoma. *(Cecil, p. 1056)*

33. (A) Disordered secretion of growth hormone is the most commonly observed abnormality of pituitary function in adult hypopituitarism. Provocative studies of growth hormone secretion (e.g., insulin-induced hypoglycemia) are therefore indicated in evaluating such patients. Depressed gonadal function is the commonest symptom-causing abnormality in these patients. Impaired secretion of TSH or ACTH is much less common and normal function is often retained even in advanced pituitary disease. Elevated prolactin secretion may be seen in hypothalamic disease or with pituitary prolactinomas, but it is abnormal less often than is growth hormone response to hypoglycemia. *(Cecil, pp. 1173–1174)*

34. (D) Although all these problems may develop in ketoacidosis, a normal serum potassium at the time of presentation with moderately severe acidosis should alert one to the severe total body potassium depletion seen in a chronically untreated patient. This may be aggravated by treatment. *(Cecil, p. 1064)*

35. (C) Growth hormone induces the formation of somatomedin, which in turn is thought to promote bone and cartilage growth. These anabolic actions are accompanied by nitrogen retention. Growth hormone also antagonizes the action of insulin, leading to a high incidence of abnormal glucose tolerance or frank diabetes mellitus in patients with acromegaly. Despite the growth-promoting action of growth hormone, there is no fat accumulation. In fact, fat mobilization and ketone production occur under the influence of growth hormone. *(Cecil, p. 1173)*

36. (B) The secretion of most anterior pituitary hormones is thought to occur in response to elaboration of appropriate *releasing factors* by hypothalamic neurons. Hypothalamic damage results in loss of these releasing factors, with secondary loss of pituitary output. One exception is prolactin, whose release is *suppressed* by hypothalamic secretion of dopamine. Loss of dopamine therefore results in increased serum prolactin in states of hypothalamic disease. On the other hand, destruction of the pituitary itself causes loss of all secretory function, including that for prolactin. *(Cecil, p. 1168)*

37. (D) Chlorpropamide is excreted unchanged by the kidneys and is contraindicated in renal insufficiency for fear of prolonged hypoglycemia. *(Cecil, pp. 1066–1067)*

38. (B) All the symptoms listed can be seen with pituitary tumors. Visual symptoms are often the clues that lead to a specific diagnosis. Usually, however, endocrine disturbance (amenorrhea, impotence, loss of libido) owing to decreased gonadotropin secretion is the most common *initial* symptom. Headache is common but nonspecific, and extraocular muscle paresis is very infrequent with pituitary tumors. Diabetes insipidus is distinctly *uncommon* in pituitary neoplasms; its presence should point to hypothalamic disorder or extrapituitary parasellar tumor. *(Cecil, pp. 1179–1180)*

39. (D) Estrogens increase hepatic synthesis of TBG, thereby increasing the serum concentration of free TBG. In order to maintain free thyroxine concentration constant, thyroid hormone synthesis increases and its metabolism *decreases*. The concentration of thyroxine-bound TBG rises until the ratio of hormone-bound to free TBG is once again normal. At that point free thyroxine is once again normal, although serum concentrations of TBG-bound thyroxine (and total TBG) are increased. *(Cecil, p. 1203)*

40. (E) Diuretics and phenytoin impair insulin release. Prednisolone and oral contraceptives increase insulin resistance. Clofibrate is not associated with impaired glucose tolerance, although the hyperlipemia it is used to treat is commonly so associated. *(Cecil, p. 1065)*

41. (C) Hashimoto's thyroiditis is the most common cause of goiter in adolescents and is more common in women than in men, Nevertheless, its prevalence increases with age, so that it is more common in old women than in young women. It is thought to have an autoimmune pathogenesis, since anti-thyroid antibodies are commonly found, and it is clearly associated with other "autoimmune" states including pernicious anemia. *(Cecil, p. 1219; Hall and Evered)*

42. (A) This patient has a thyroid nodule that contains all the functioning tissue on scan. Such "hot nodules" may autonomously secrete thyroxine or triiodothyronine. In the present case, that condition is most unlikely because the free thyroxine index is low (3.7) and the TSH clearly elevated. A likely diagnosis is Hashimoto's thyroiditis (sometimes associated with normal or even elevated radioiodine uptake), which has destroyed most thyroid tissue, leaving only a single island of function — the "hot nodule." The diagnosis is made more likely by the known increased incidence of Hashimoto's thyroiditis in patients with diabetes mellitus. The only proper course of treatment at this time is a trial of thyroxine suppression. *(Cecil, p. 1219)*

43. (B) Only in pancreatitis is there absolute insulin deficiency. The other forms of diabetes are associated with varying degrees of insulin resistance. In the case of acromegaly, Cushing's syndrome, and obesity, this is entirely correctable by treating the underlying disease. *(Cecil, pp. 1064–1065)*

44. (B) Solitary thyroid nodules raise the question of malignancy. This potential is so markedly reduced in hyperfunctioning nodules ("hot nodules") that no biopsy is needed. If the patient is euthyroid, no therapy is needed; if he is hyperthyroid, surgical removal or radioiodine ablation is appropriate. Since the free thyroxine index in this patient is normal, we now need to assess serum T_3. If it is normal, only observation is indicated; if elevated, we may presume early and (as yet) mild "T_3 thyrotoxicosis," and the nodule should be removed or destroyed. *(Cecil, p. 1221)*

45. (B) The hyperthyroidism of subacute thyroiditis is transient. Indeed, it may be followed by a period of hypothyroidism until the thyroid gland regains its ability to take up iodine normally and to produce thyroid hormones. The hyperthyroidism seen during the acute phase is believed to occur because of the release of large amounts of thyroid hormone stores from a damaged gland. Consequently, definitive therapy, such as subtotal thyroidectomy or radioiodine, is contraindicated. Iodine administration likewise will be without effect on the release of thyroid hormones from the thyroid, in contrast to its effect on the thyroid in Graves' disease. The administration of blockers of thyroid hormone synthesis will not treat the fundamental cause of the hyperthyroidism. Transient symptoms of hyperthyroidism may be relieved with the beta-adrenergic antagonist propranolol. *(Cecil, pp. 1217–1218; Volpé)*

46. (D) It is unlikely that regular insulin given in the morning would contribute much in the evening without causing hypoglycemia in the interim. The morning dose of lente insulin is already limited by the normal fasting plasma glucose. Increasing exercise in the evening would tend to lower the urinary sugar, but it may also lower plasma glucose for too long; hypoglycemia after vigorous exercise may occur 12 to 24 hours after the exercise from increased insulin absorption, altered insulin distribution, and the slow rate of glycogen resynthesis. Omitting the bedtime snack would increase the risk of nocturnal hypoglycemia without having any effect on bedtime urinary sugar, which is usually tested before the snack. The safest approach would be to use a flexible regimen with short- and intermediate-acting insulin before breakfast and supper. *(Koivisto and Felig; Wahren, Felig, and Hagenfeldt)*

47. (B) Among the possible causes of goiter resulting from a congenital error in thyroid metabolism, an iodine-trapping defect can be excluded by the radioiodine uptake of 30% after two hours. The discharge of 20% of the accumulated radioiodine following the administration of potassium perchlorate strongly suggests a defect in the organification of iodide in the thyroid. Normally, iodide taken up by the thyroid is immediately organified and stored in the follicular colloid. When an enzymatic defect in iodide organification is present, iodide is "trapped" within the thyroid follicular cells by the iodide transport mechanism, but is not organified. The potassium perchlorate blocks the iodide transport process and allows the escape of the inorganic iodide back into the blood stream. An iodide-organification defect in association with nerve deafness carries the eponym of Pendred's syndrome. *(Cecil, p. 1233)*

48. (E) "Hypothyroid" connotes depressed function: low energy and strength, low metabolic rate, low serum thyroxine, slow intestinal and cardiac function. It is surprising, therefore, to realize that blood pressure, especially diastolic blood pressure, may be *high*. In this regard, hypothyroidism represents one of the most treatable forms of hypertension. Although, of course, the hypertension may be independent and persist after treatment, it is wise to defer antihypertensive therapy until the patient is euthyroid. *(Cecil, p. 1214)*

49. (D) Although the function of the eye muscles is disturbed in Graves' disease, the mechanism is *not* one of paralysis. Instead, the eye muscles, particularly the inferior rectus, become swollen and fibrotic, restricting movement of the eyeball. The commonly noted impairment of upward gaze is not due to weakness of the superior rectus, but rather to a tethering action of the inferior rectus. The other signs listed are all noted with some frequency in Graves' disease and are occasionally the presenting complaint. *(Cecil, p. 1208; Day)*

50. (C) Only non–insulin-dependent twins have a very high concordance. The risk for this patient has fallen below the maximum of 50% seen in the first year or two after onset in the other twin, but it would not be expected to fall below the population risk, which is 2 to 4%. *(Cecil, p. 1057)*

51. (A) Under normal conditions more than 99% of both thyroxine and triiodothyronine is bound to serum proteins. The percentage of free (i.e., unbound) triiodothyronine (0.3%) is tenfold greater than the free thyroxine (0.02%), but both are well under 1%. This large reservoir of protein-bound hormone explains why clinically significant changes in thyroid function can be missed (or erroneously attributed) unless the free hormone concentration is measured or estimated. *(Cecil, p. 1202)*

52. (A) Diabetes affects the nervous system in many ways, the most common being the peripheral neuropathy demonstrated in this patient's feet. In addition, the marked predilection of the diabetic to atherosclerosis predisposes to single peripheral nerve infarction with sudden loss of motor and sensory function. This frequently involves one of the oculomotor nerves, as in this patient, producing acute ophthalmoplegia. Fortunately, collateral circulation usually corrects most or all of the deficit in weeks or months. *(Cecil, pp. 1062–1063)*

53. (C) The patient has very mild symptoms of hypothyroidism, a low-normal free thyroxine index (5.1), and normal TSH. This picture is entirely compatible with the recovery of spontaneous thyroid function. The patient should return in three weeks for testing; if she remains euthyroid, further treatment is not needed. True hypothyroidism would be accompanied by more severe symptoms and more clearly abnormal thyroid function tests. *(Cecil, p. 1216; Vagenakis et al.)*

54. (A) Diabetes in all ages is associated with accelerated atherogenesis. Although many diabetics have demonstrable lipid abnormalities, the observed accelerated atherogenesis in diabetes is far out of proportion with the minimal or absent lipid abnormalities seen in most. *(Cecil, pp. 1063–1064)*

55. (B) Subacute thyroiditis may cause severe systemic symptoms; the thyroid gland is tender and exquisitely painful, with pain often being referred to the ear. Erythrocyte sedimentation rate is characteristically high. Breakdown and release of thyroglobulin is presumably responsible for elevations in thyroid hormone and hyperthyroidism. The thyroidal uptake of radioiodine is usually very *low*, and this feature clearly distinguishes subacute thyroiditis from other hyperthyroid states. *(Cecil, pp. 1217)*

56. (B) The patient has hypothyroidism both by clinical symptoms and by laboratory test (calculated free thyroxine index = 0.67 × 3.1 = 2.1, with normal ranging from 4.7 to 10.5). The most important next step is to measure serum TSH. If TSH is elevated, the diagnosis of primary hypothyroidism is secure and thyroxine replacement may begin. If TSH is normal or low, a hypothalamic-pituitary cause of the hypothyroidism should be considered. Failure to measure TSH before treatment is begun risks erroneous diagnosis and improper, even dangerous, treatment. *(Cecil, p. 1214)*

57. (A) This patient initially responded well to propylthiouracil in substantial doses. The subsequent enlargement of the goiter is likely to be due to oversuppression of thyroid function, with subsequent hypothyroidism and raised serum TSH causing goiter growth. The diagnosis can be confirmed by measurement of serum TSH in addition to the thyroid hormones already ordered. Treatment consists of lowering the dose of propylthiouracil *or* maintaining the dose and adding supplemental thyroxine by mouth to obtain euthyroidism. More propylthiouracil or methimazole would be appropriate only if the TSH were low and thyroid hormone high. *(Cecil, p. 1210)*

58. (C) A diffuse, nontender goiter in a euthyroid young woman in association with a very high antithyroglobulin antibody titer is consistent with a diagnosis of Hashimoto's thyroiditis. Although the patient is euthyroid, therapy is justified because of the size and cosmetic appearance of the goiter. The increase in goiter size may be related, at least in part, to the stimulatory effect of TSH in "driving" a thyroid gland of decreased functional reserve. There is no indication for subtotal thyroidectomy unless, despite medical therapy, the gland becomes very much larger. The administration of radioiodine would only exacerbate the situation by reducing thyroid reserve and ensuring hypothyroidism. Similarly, treatment with stable iodine is likely to make the patient hypothyroid very rapidly. The thyroid gland in Hashimoto's thyroiditis is more sensitive than the normal gland to the inhibitory effects of iodine on thyroid function. There is an excellent chance that administration of thyroid hormone to this patient will greatly reduce the size of the gland. However, the progression of the underlying disease process is unaffected. *(Cecil, p. 1219; Tunbridge et al.)*

59. (D) This patient has probably developed insulin resistance owing to circulating anti-insulin antibodies. Although all patients taking exogenous insulin develop low levels of anti-insulin antibodies (IgG), only the rare patient (less than 0.1%) develops sufficient titers to produce insulin resistance. This usually occurs in elderly patients on intermittent therapy. High doses of glucocorticoids have been effective in lowering insulin requirements in these patients, and switching from beef (found in the usual commercial insulin preparations) to the less immunogenic pure pork insulins has also been successful. Unfortunately, the newer, more purified insulin preparations (single-peak) have not been shown to have less immunogenic properties than previous preparations. High-dose insulin boluses should be avoided, as anaphylactic reactions have been reported. Amino acids in fish insulin differ considerably from those in conventional mammalian insulins. Although no neutralization of biologic activity occurs in acute situations, long-term use of fish insulin is contraindicated, owing to its high tendency to induce anti–fish-insulin antibodies. *(Cecil, p. 1069)*

60. (B) This patient is in thyroid storm. This syndrome encompasses severe hyperthyroidism, with an alteration in mental status and marked cardiovascular manifestations. The goiter with a pyramidal lobe, which is suggestive of a diffuse thyroid process, the family history of hyperthyroidism, and the history of weight loss despite a good appetite all suggest that the patient was hyperthyroid prior to the surgery, which precipitated thyroid storm. Although an infectious source for this condition cannot be excluded, the patient must be treated for thyroid storm without waiting for laboratory confirmation of the diagnosis. Propylthiouracil inhibits iodide organification in the thyroid and reduces the peripheral conversion of thyroxine to triiodothyronine. Propranolol will diminish some of the peripheral manifestations of hyperthyroidism, but will not affect the action of thyroid hormone itself. There is no strong evidence to support the use of hydrocortisone; however, it is usually administered for the theoretical consideration that its catabolism is enhanced in hyperthyroidism, and because of the possibility that there may be decreased adrenal reserve. A cooling blanket is of value for dangerous hyperpyrexia. Administration of a large dose of radioiodine is contraindicated, because the therapeutic effect does not occur soon enough and because the radioiodine may initially exacerbate the hyperthyroidism. Although antibiotics may be appropriate, they should not be the sole form of therapy. *(Cecil, p. 1212; Ingbar)*

61. (D) The patient has mild ophthalmopathy associated with Graves' disease. The disease is not severe enough to warrant therapy with glucocorticoids or surgical decompression of the orbit, but elevation of the head of the bed and the use of methylcellulose eyedrops may be of value. Since the symptoms are worse in the morning, it is possible that the palpebral fissures are not completely closed during sleep, and taping the eyelids closed at bedtime may help. Bed elevation and administration of diuretics may reduce conjunctival edema. Although the natural course of the disease is not influenced by these measures, it is generally the impression that hyperthyroidism or hypothyroidism, particularly the latter, may exacerbate ophthalmopathy. Reduction of exogenous thyroxine replacement to induce hypothyroidism is therefore contraindicated. *(Cecil, p. 1212)*

62. (B) In myxedema coma, hypothermia should be treated by covering the patient with a blanket to induce gradual, passive warming. Active warming with a heating blanket may lead to shock and death. The best method for the administration of thyroid hormone in this condition is unclear. The present consensus, however, is for the rapid intravenous injection of a large dose of L-thyroxine. Infection is often an important factor in precipitating myxedema coma, and should be carefully looked for and vigorously treated. Respiratory depression is also commonly seen in this condition, and when myxedema coma is suspected the measurement of arterial blood gas tensions is mandatory. Ventilatory assistance may be necessary. Because of diminished free-water clearance in hypothyroidism, and because of the reduced insensitive loss of water during severe hypothyroidism, these patients are at risk of developing hyponatremia and water intoxication. *(Cecil, p. 1216; Werner)*

63. (C) Cyclic 3′5′-AMP mediates most (if not all) of the effects of PTH on the kidney. These effects include the increased reabsorption of the divalent cations, magnesium and calcium, as well as the increased activation of the vitamin D metabolite 25-hydroxycholecalciferol. Bicarbonate excretion, on the other hand, is increased (as is phosphate excretion), leading to a systemic acidosis and increased serum concentrations of ionized calcium. *(Cecil, pp. 1288–1289)*

64. (E) Hyperparathyroidism results in all the symptoms listed. Nevertheless, most patients with this condition are asymptomatic and are detected because hypercalcemia is found on biochemical screening tests. *(Cecil, pp. 1290–1291)*

65. (C) A, B, and E are less likely because of the low fasting blood sugar. Hypopituitarism is usually associated with a flat glucose tolerance curve. Impaired glucose tolerance, despite fasting hypoglycemia, is not unusual in islet cell tumors, which may have sluggish release of insulin. *(Cecil, pp. 1072–1073)*

66. (B) Definitive diagnosis of hyperparathyroidism is sometimes quite difficult. In such cases, the finding of subperiosteal bone resorption (although uncommon) is considered diagnostic and points the way to definitive surgical exploration. *(Cecil, p. 1295)*

67. (D) The patient clearly has hyperparathyroidism. Even in patients who eventually prove to have large parathyroid adenomas, however, the tumor is rarely palpable in the neck. Such palpable masses usually prove to be coexisting and unrelated thyroid nodules. *(Cecil, p. 1291)*

68. (C) Surgical treatment is usually recommended in all patients with hyperparathyroidism, even when it is "mild." When observation is chosen instead of surgery, any evidence of worsening severity (using serum calcium) or the appearance of renal or osseous complications should lead to operative intervention. The serum phosphate level has not been shown to foreshadow serious complications and is not used as a criterion to change medical advice. *(Cecil, p. 1296; Neer and Potts)*

69. (B) Hypocalcemia leads to neuromuscular excitability with paresthesias, muscle spasms, tetany, and epileptiform seizures. Muscle flaccidity is not seen. The calcification of basal ganglia and lens cataracts are well described in hypocalcemia, but their pathogenesis is unknown. *(Cecil, pp. 1297–1298)*

70. (D) The calculated amended immunoreactive insulin (IRI) to glucose ratio in this patient is characteristic of fasting hyperinsulinism resulting from a functioning islet cell tumor. Pancreatic surgery will probably be required, and localization studies can improve the chances of finding the lesion. A successful preoperative trial of diazoxide is helpful in case a causative lesion is not found at surgery, since the surgeon will know that a medical therapy will be available to help manage the patient in case a tumor is left in place. The tolbutamide test, although occasionally useful, is inappropriate when the diagnosis can be made less invasively as during a fast. *(Cecil, pp. 1075–1077)*

71. (C) The hypercalcemia associated with hypophosphatemia and hyperchloremia provides strong evidence that this patient has symptomatic primary hyperparathyroidism. The intravenous urogram reveals nephrocalcinosis and urolithiasis. Multiple small calcifications are present in the pyramids of both kidneys, and there are two large laminated stones in the left ureter, overlying the psoas shadow. There is no evidence that the hypercalcemia is caused by other factors such as malignancy and sarcoidosis. Nevertheless, a normal PTH measurement in this situation may be considered disturbing and may reduce confidence in the diagnosis. A likely reason for the normal PTH value observed is that the antibody used in the assay recognized primarily the aminoterminal segment of the PTH molecule. This part of the molecule is biologically active, but is cleared relatively rapidly from the plasma, making it more difficult to detect elevations of hormone concentration. Measurement of the carboxylterminal fragments of the molecule, which are cleared more slowly from the plasma, is more likely to demonstrate such an elevation. Even in the absence of such confirmatory elevation in serum PTH, the evidence in this case is sufficient to justify neck exploration for hyperparathyroidism. *(Cecil, p. 1294)*

72. (D) The patient described has idiopathic, familial nephrogenic diabetes insipidus. In this condition pituitary secretion of vasopressin is unimpaired, but the renal tubular response to vasopressin is diminished or absent. Nephrogenic diabetes insipidus can also occur with hypercalcemia, hypokalemia, kidney parenchymal disease, and sickle cell disease, and following exposure to drugs such as lithium and dimethylchlortetracycline. Thiazide diuretics are the most effective form of therapy for this condition; they may work by lowering the glomerular filtration rate. Nicotine provokes pituitary ADH release but is not therapeutically useful. Chlorpropamide and clofibrate augment ADH action and may be useful in mild central diabetes insipidus. *(Cecil, pp. 1194, 1198)*

73. (B) Hypercalcemia and hypokalemia both induce states of relative renal refractoriness to ADH, as does excessive concentration of blood lithium. These functional disturbances are usually reversible if the ion concentration is returned to normal, although, if the situation is prolonged, the abnormal renal function may not totally regress. Sickle cell disease leads to loss of the renal papillae and, as a result, to inability to produce a hypertonic interstitial gradient. Water conservation is impaired even in the presence of ADH and there is a mild polyuria. Hypernatremia may result from polyuria and dehydration, but it is not known to impair renal response to ADH. *(Cecil, p. 1196)*

74. (A) All the modalities mentioned can be used for ADH replacement therapy. Each has certain drawbacks: posterior pituitary extract ("pituitary snuff") may cause allergic rhinitis; aqueous vasopressin and lysine vasopressin are relatively short-acting and require frequent administration; vasopressin tannate in oil requires intramuscular injection. The synthetic analogue dDAVP avoids these drawbacks. It can be used once (or twice) daily and taken by nasal inspiration. At present its use is limited only by its rather substantial expense. *(Cecil, p. 1198)*

75. (D) This patient has elevated FSH despite normal testis size, normal testosterone, and normal LH. These findings are compatible with germinal cell aplasia (Sertoli cell–only syndrome). Biopsy is unnecessary. This condition is occasionally seen after cytotoxic drugs or radiation therapy; when it occurs spontaneously, it is irreversible and the patients are infertile. The diagnosis may be confirmed by finding azoospermia in the ejaculate. There is no evidence for pituitary dysfunction or that any form of treatment will improve fertility. *(Cecil, p. 1250)*

76. (E) This girl is beyond the usual age of menarche (12.6 years), but early signs of beginning sexual maturation (early pubic hair and breast development) are present. It is reasonable to assume that menarche will occur spontaneously, and careful observation is an appropriate decision. Only if no further progression occurs or if other signs of pituitary dysfunction appear (such as growth cessation) would pituitary or gonadal investigations be appropriate. Induction of menses with gonadal steroids may be appropriate because of the patient's psychologic burden of difference from her peers. In that case, more careful laboratory definition of pituitary and gonadal function might be contemplated. *(Cecil, p. 1265)*

77. (A) The excessive and unphysiologic secretion of certain anterior pituitary hormones creates disease states termed "hyperpituitarism." Of the functioning pituitary tumors, by far the most common is the prolactinoma, distantly followed by growth hormone and ACTH-secreting neoplasms. Thus, amenorrhea-galactorrhea is a common clinical problem, whereas acromegaly and Cushing's disease are infrequent. Hypersecretion of TSH and the gonadotropins (LH and FSH) by pituitary neoplasm has been observed, but it is extraordinarily rare; TSH-mediated hyperthyroidism or hypergonadotropic gonadal dysfunction are almost never seen clinically. *(Cecil, pp. 1191–1192)*

78. (D) Intrathyroidal papillary thyroid carcinoma is associated with little, if any, increase in mortality if properly treated. The involved lobe should be removed and the patient placed on thyroxine. Use of radioiodine is controversial in the absence of known metastases. Total thyroidectomy and radical neck dissection are unnecessary. *(Cecil, p. 1222; Wang)*

79. (E) This patient has normal serum TBG concentration (resin T_3 uptake = 0.95) but elevated serum thyroxine (12.3). Calculation of the free thyroxine index (0.95 × 12.3 = 11.7) gives a value above the limits of normal (4.7–10.5), raising the question of whether the symptoms are due to hyperthyroidism. The normal serum T_3 makes this diagnosis untenable. Most likely, the patient's ingestion of contrast dye for the cholecystogram has impaired conversion of T_4 to T_3, and the symptoms are probably due to some cause other than thyroid disease. The functional block in T_3 conversion will be transient and needs no treatment. This case emphasizes the value of measuring T_3 in addition to T_4 when results of the latter are confusing or ambiguous. *(Cecil, p. 1203)*

80. (A) Detection of an elevated serum calcitonin response to provocative stimuli (calcium or pentagastrin or both) is the most sensitive indicator of medullary carcinoma of the thyroid, and can detect it at a curable stage. *All* family members should undergo testing (and total thyroidectomy if the results are abnormal) even in the absence of any other detectable abnormality. Surgery is unnecessary in normally responding individuals; biopsy is not known to be effective; thyroxine suppression is worthless since the calcitonin-producing C cells are not responsive to thyroid-stimulating hormone. *(Cecil, p. 1303)*

81. (A — True; B — True; C — True; D — False) Maternal estrogen levels represent function of the fetal and placental unit. A fall in these levels suggests placental distress, an indication for early delivery. The lecithin/sphingomyelin ratio can be used as an index of fetal pulmonary maturation so that delivery can be delayed until respiratory distress will be a minimal problem. Oxytocin challenge tests have been used to detect early signs of fetal distress. Excessive weight gain is a concern but generally does not help determine delivery date. *(Cecil, pp. 1070–1071; Gyves et al.)*

82. (A — False; B — True; C — False; D — True) Signs of isosexual precocious puberty in males include phallic enlargement and sexual hair growth. True (or complete) isosexual precocity is accompanied by testicular growth, which indicates that the syndrome is caused by gonadotropin secretion with resulting testicular response. It may result from pituitary gonadotropin secretion (sometimes caused by pituitary tumors including aberrant pinealoma) or from chorionic gonadotropin produced, for example, by a hepatoblastoma. On the other hand, incomplete precocity or precocious pseudopuberty resulting from adrenal oversecretion of androgens (as can occur with either 21- or 11-hydroxylase deficiency) can produce signs of virilization, but there is no stimulation of the testes, which remain infantile (< 1 × 1 cm). *(Cecil, p. 1247)*

83. (A — True; B — False; C — True; D — False) Replacement of glucocorticoid (with hydrocortisone, cortisone, or prednisone) and mineralocorticoid (with fludrocortisone) will restore a patient with Addison's disease to full health. Doses must be individualized to provide sufficient hormone and prevent excess. Once hormone replacement is adequate, electrolyte and carbohydrate balance will return to normal, and special diets are not needed. *(Cecil, pp. 1229–1230)*

84. (A — False; B — True; C — True; D — True) Potassium that leaves cells when displaced by hydrogen ion can re-enter very quickly after partial correction of the pH. One of the several proposed mechanisms for obtundation during recovery from ketoacidosis is a drop in spinal fluid pH, which may occur when a rising systemic pH slows respiration. Arterial P_{CO_2} rises, equilibrating quickly with the CO_2 in spinal fluid. Bicarbonate changes more slowly, leading to a fall in pH in the spinal fluid. Tissue hypoxia may result from the low red cell 2,3-diphosphoglycerate (DPG) seen in uncontrolled diabetes, which causes an increased affinity of hemoglobin for oxygen. During acidosis the Bohr effect reduces the affinity of hemoglobin for oxygen back to normal, but the effect of low DPG is unmasked when acidosis is suddenly corrected. Acidosis induces slight insulin resistance, which would be corrected by bicarbonate. (This is not a sufficient reason for using bicarbonate.) *(Cecil, p. 1068; Posner and Plum; Ditzel and Standl)*

85. (A — False; B — False; C — True; D — True; E — True) General debilitation, inability to withstand stress, and dilutional hyponatremia due to water intoxication are all signs of glucocorticoid insuffiency and *are* seen with ACTH deficiency. Similarly, adrenal androgen synthesis is ACTH-dependent and decreases in secondary adrenal insufficiency, leading to axillary hair loss in women (men preserve their axillary and pubic hair unless there is gonadal failure causing loss of testosterone). Signs of mineralocorticoid deficiency (hyperkalemia and hyponatremia due to sodium wasting) are not seen in patients with secondary hypoadrenalism, since aldosterone output is controlled by the renin-angiotensin system and is unaffected by ACTH loss. The typical mucocutaneous pigmentation of Addison's disease is not seen either, since ACTH (and MSH) secretion is decreased or absent, by definition, in *secondary* adrenal failure. *(Cecil, p. 1231)*

86. (A — False; B — True; C — False; D — True) The diagnosis of factitious hypoglycemia must be considered in a health professional whose studies give erratic results. Antibodies to insulin will develop if an antigenic preparation has been taken for a sufficient time. Lack of C-peptide immunoreactivity in the sample with the high insulin level would suggest an exogenous source. Assay for sulfonylureas might be necessary if the other studies are negative. *(Cecil, pp. 1076, 1077–1078)*

87. (A — True; B — False; C — True; D — True) The slight increase in insulin is sufficient to suppress both amino acid release from muscle and conversion to sugar in the liver. There is not sufficient insulin to increase peripheral glucose utilization, so that only the brain remains as a principal glucose utilizer. *(Cecil, p. 1055)*

88. (A — True; B — False; C — False; D — True) The patient clearly has a normal female phenotype, as judged by the external appearance. This, together with the other features described, is diagnostic of the syndrome of testicular feminization. Patients with this form of male pseudohermaphroditism have a normal male karyotype, but they are phenotypically female except for the internal genitalia. Psychologically and physically these patients are females, despite the male karyotype. The condition is caused by peripheral tissue resistance to the actions of testosterone, usually owing to the absence of cytoplasmic androgen-binding receptors. The serum testosterone concentration is usually within the normal range for adult males, but its metabolic action is not expressed because of the absence of end-organ sensitivity. The risk of developing gonadal tumors is greater in these patients than in the normal population, and surgical removal of the gonads is therefore advisable. *(Cecil, p. 1252)*

89. (A — True; B — True; C — False; D — True; E — True) Oral contraceptive steroids are the most effective known method of contraception. Nevertheless, they carry the risk of untoward side effects, the most serious of which is the increased incidence of thromboembolism. In addition to the effects noted, the estrogens in these medications may raise serum triglycerides, raise serum concentration of thyroxine-binding and cortisol-binding globulins, provoke salt and water retention, or induce serious psychologic depression. They usually cause hyperglycemia, not hypoglycemia. *(Cecil, pp. 1273–1274)*

90. (All are True) Depending on the nature of the enzyme defect, congenital adrenal hyperplasia may result in any of the conditions noted (although not all simultaneously). The most common syndrome, adrenal 21-hydroxylase deficiency, impairs mineralocorticoid production and leads to salt wasting. Adrenal 11β-hydroxylase deficiency results in increased synthesis of 11-deoxycorticosterone, a mineralocorticoid that causes hypertension in these patients. Both of these deficiencies lead to adrenal androgen excess, while certain others (e.g., 17α-hydroxylase deficiency) prevent androgen synthesis. *(Cecil, pp. 1240–1241)*

91. (A — False; B — True; C — False; D — True) A definitely elevated fasting blood sugar on repeated occasions should make the glucose tolerance test unnecessary for the diagnosis of diabetes. Strenuous avoidance of sweets can produce a curve showing glucose intolerance even when it would be normal with appropriate carbohydrate loading. Items B and D are among several appropriate precautions before glucose tolerance testing. *(Cecil, p. 1058; American Diabetes Association)*

92. (All are True) Patients with Cushing's syndrome of any cause, including iatrogenic, are susceptible to infection. The skin is easily traumatized and may provide a portal of entry; because of the excess cortisol concentrations, leukocyte function is impaired and antibody production decreased. All these effects combine to impair host defenses. Such patients may be infected with unusual organisms and may not have a typical fever response because of the antipyretic effect of cortisol. Of course, it is this very anti-inflammatory action of glucocorticoids that makes them therapeutically useful in treating pathologic inflammation such as in lupus erythematosus. *(Cecil, p. 1233)*

93. (A — True; B — False; C — False; D — True; E — True) The secretion of ACTH follows a diurnal pattern, being highest just before and at the time of arising, and falling to a nadir 12 to 14 hours later. Various forms of "stress" (including surgery, trauma, infection, pain) can increase cortisol output ten times or more. 11-Deoxycortisol, the biochemical precursor of cortisol, is unable to suppress ACTH secretion. It is this property that results in increased ACTH output when the conversion of 11-deoxycortisol to cortisol is blocked by metyrapone. Tetrahydrocortisol is a major catabolic product of cortisol, and physiologically inert. *(Cecil, p. 1227)*

94. (A — True; B — False; C — False; D — False; E — True) Clinitest tablets can provide a rough quantification of glycosuria and are therefore superior to most paper enzyme strips for evaluating insulin requirements. However, their minimal sensitivity of 0.25% is less than paper enzyme strips, which detect glycosuria as low as 0.075%. Sucrose is not a reducing substance and thus will not react with either Clinitest tablets or the paper enzyme strips. Both methods are dependent on a normal renal threshold for glucose (180 mg/dl) and can be interfered with by high-dose therapy with drugs (salicylates, L-dopa, vitamin C, Aldomet, Keflin). *(Feldman, Kelley, and Lebovitz)*

95. (A — False; B — True; C — True; D — True; E — False) Prolactin secretion is suppressed by dopamine. Dopamine precursors (L-dopa) or dopamine agonists (such as the ergot alkaloids) will inhibit prolactin secretion, therefore, whereas dopamine antagonists such as chlorpromazine will increase it. This property of the ergot alkaloids has been exploited therapeutically by using the synthetic derivative bromergocriptine to suppress prolactin hypersecretion. TRH and estrogens both promote prolactin secretion. *(Cecil, p. 1174)*

96. (A — True; B — True; C — False; D — True) Some disturbances of pituitary function are recognized as being caused by (or associated with) certain psychologic states. For example, the "functional amenorrhea" that sometimes occurs when young women leave home to attend college is considered to be due to the "stress" of separation. Such functional menstrual disturbance is second only to pregnancy as a cause of amenorrhea. Less frequent but clearly documented are the growth retardation caused by suppression of growth hormone in maternal deprivation syndrome, and the depressed growth hormone and elevated serum ACTH and cortisol concentrations that occur in some adult depressions. The secretion of TSH seems relatively unperturbable and is not known to fluctuate with psychologic input. *(Cecil, pp. 1168, 1177)*

97. (All are True) Regardless of the pathogenesis of the diabetes, there is the possibility of exhaustion of insulin reserve after continued hyperglycemia. All the treatments listed have been associated with return of endogenous insulin secretion in some patients. *(Foucar and Field; Perkins et al.; Turner et al.; Turtle)*

98. (All are True) Somogyi described the pattern of negative urines followed by an abrupt reversal to heavy glycosuria with ketonuria, suggesting unrecognized hypoglycemia. Some such patients will have had a previous history on lower doses of insulin of hypoglycemic reactions that were not recognized. When hypoglycemia becomes more severe, nightmares and morning headaches may be clues. The general trend in weight will be upward as driven by the excessive insulin. Unrecognized hypoglycemia can be detected in as many as 60% of patients with unstable diabetes, and it has been said that high fasting sugars are more likely to represent excessive than deficient insulin. Other clues include positive morning acetone without glycosuria, night sweats, and hypothermia. *(Cecil, p. 1070; Somogyi)*

99. (A — True; B — True; C — True; D — False) A history of neck irradiation, a functionless nodule ("cold nodule"), youth, and male sex are all associated with an increased likelihood that a solitary nodule is malignant. All of these make thyroidectomy, or at least biopsy of the lesion, more urgent. Hypothyroidism is *not* associated with an increased risk of cancer, even though suppression of TSH by thyroxine appears to be beneficial in patients with thyroid carcinoma. *(Cecil, pp. 1221–1222)*

100. (A — True; B — True; C — True; D — False) Hyperthyroidism in the elderly frequently is not associated with the "classic" findings seen in younger patients. Weight loss, weakness, and atrial fibrillation may be the only clues — even goiter may be absent. In this patient the slightly high free thyroxine index supports the diagnosis of hyperthyroidism, and an elevated serum T_3 and a failure of TSH response to TRH would confirm it. Since the suspicion of hyperthyroidism is high, it is appropriate to begin treatment with propylthiouracil even before the results of the diagnostic studies are known, especially if they will be slow in returning. Thyroxine suppression is clearly contraindicated since it is likely to worsen the situation. *(Cecil, p. 1224; Davis and Davis)*

101. (A — False; B — False; C — True; D — True) The acute abdomen may well be a manifestation of ketoacidosis. If it is a surgical problem, the ketoacidosis must be corrected before treatment is possible. Lipemia retinalis will be corrected only with insulin therapy. An extremely hyperglycemic patient whose blood pressure is marginal will sustain a further drop as glucose is shifted into cells. Patients with initial hypokalemia will have a further drop as insulin drives potassium into cells. In either case a few minutes could be taken to begin volume and/or potassium replacement. The delay in insulin administration should not be more than 15 to 30 minutes. *(Cecil, pp. 1067–1069)*

102. (A — True; B — True; C — False; D — True; E — True) In contrast to all other renal disorders, the proteinuria associated with diabetic nephropathy does not diminish with progressive renal failure: patients continue to excrete 10 to 11 gm of protein daily as creatinine clearance diminishes. *(Takazakura et al.)*

103. (A — True; B — False; C — True; D — True; E — True) As renal failure progresses, there is an elevation in the renal threshold at which glycosuria appears. With renal failure, many diabetics experience an increased sensitivity to insulin and a decrease in insulin requirements. This increased sensitivity is due to a decrease in renal destruction of insulin and diminished hepatic glycogen stores. As a result, serious hypoglycemic reactions can occur if insulin adjustments are not made. Hemodialysis is less satisfactory in diabetic than in nondiabetic patients, as the former tend to have more problems with clotting, fluid overload, and infection. Experience with renal transplantation has been more promising, although the mortality rate after transplantation may be twice as high as in nondiabetics. *(DeFronzo et al.; Najarian et al.)*

104. (A — False; B — False; C — False; D — True) This patient has symptomatic hyperthyroidism. A likely cause is Graves' disease, but a painless phase of subacute thyroiditis could also explain the findings. Thyroxine ingestion ("thyrotoxicosis factitia") is unlikely since there is a goiter, but this could be an independent finding. The serum T_3 measurement and TRH test would be superfluous, since the serum thyroxine measurement confirms the diagnosis. A radioiodine uptake is indicated. If increased, it favors Graves' disease; if very low, thyroiditis. A thyroid scan is not necessary with a diffuse goiter, but would be indicated if the gland were nodular. *(Cecil, pp. 1208–1209)*

105. (A — True; B — True; C — True; D — False) Glycoproteins are recognized by the liver by means of their carbohydrate component. Insulin, however, lacks this carbohydrate moiety. *(Cecil, p. 1056)*

106. (All are True) Patients treated with phenytoin (for epilepsy) or large doses of salicylates (as in rheumatoid arthritis) may be euthyroid despite a low free thyroxine index, because of displacement of thyroid hormone from its binding protein *in vivo*. Since these patients are euthyroid, TSH is normal. Similarly, individuals given triiodothyronine to "hasten" weight reduction can be euthyroid or even hyperthyroid with a low free thyroxine index, because of replacement of thyroxine by triiodothyronine. Finally, patients with low free thyroxine index may indeed be hypothyroid: a low or "normal" TSH would then point to a pituitary or hypothalamic disorder. *(Cecil, pp. 1214–1215)*

107. (A — True; B — False; C — True; D — False) Although the duration of diabetes is compatible with this degree of renal failure, the lack of proteinuria raises a question of some other causation. The predicted survival of five years between onset of significant proteinuria and severe renal failure in diabetes mellitus does not apply here. Likewise, retinopathy would be very likely only if nephropathy were the cause of the renal failure. *(Cecil, p. 1062)*

108. (A — False; B — False; C — True; D — True) Since this patient has relapsed into hyperthyroidism, some form of permanent therapy is indicated. Radioiodine treatment is appropriate, but pregnancy must be avoided during the treatment to prevent radiation damage to the fetus. The only known complication of radioiodine therapy is hypothyroidism, which occurs in 10% or more of patients in the first year after treatment, and increases at a rate of 5% per year thereafter. In general, it is wise to assume that *all* treated patients will eventually become hypothyroid and to plan appropriate surveillance. Any increased risk of malignancy to the patient or genetic damage to offspring has been so small as to be undetectable. As a result, radioiodine is the general treatment of choice for hyperthyroid adults, with surgery being reserved for special cases or circumstances. *(Cecil, p. 1211; Sofa, Schumacher, and Rodriguez-Antunez; Sarkar et al.; Holm et al.)*

109. (A — True; B — True; C — True; D — False) Parathyroid hormone maintains the serum calcium by a number of concerted mechanisms. Calcium (and phosphate) are mobilized from bone; calcium reabsorption from the renal tubule is increased; and intestinal calcium absorption is increased via an increased activation of vitamin D. Phosphate excretion in the urine is *increased* by PTH, thus eliminating excess phosphate derived from bone. *(Cecil, pp. 1288–1289)*

110. (All are True) The patient has symptoms of hypercalcemia, and the serum calcium confirms this diagnosis. Hyperparathyroidism, the use of thiazide diuretics, and the presence of hematologic (e.g., myeloma or lymphoma) and nonhematologic malignancies are common causes of hypercalcemia, whereas vitamin D or A intoxication and hyperthyroidism represent relatively uncommon causes. Careful attention to these points, together with a search for evidence of granulomatous conditions (e.g., tuberculosis and sarcoidosis) and of familial hypocalciuric hypercalcemia, will provide important clues in the differential diagnosis. *(Cecil, p. 1291; Habener and Potts)*

111. (All are False) All the techniques listed have been used, on occasion, to localize abnormal parathyroid glands. Nevertheless, they are not justified for routine use since they are relatively insensitive and expensive, and do not alter the course or outcome of surgery. These tests may well be indicated in patients whose hyperparathyroidism persists after an initial exploration. *(Cecil, p. 1295)*

112. (A — True; B — True; C — False; D — True) A history in this setting may reveal alcohol sponging at home to lower the temperature. Blood alcohol levels sufficient to impair hepatic glucose release are easy to achieve in a small child. Measuring the insulin level would detect an unrelated hyperinsulinemia. Measurement of C-peptide level should not be ordered unless the insulin level is high. *(Cecil, p. 1078)*

113. (A — True; B — True; C — False; D — True) This patient has hypocalcemia and hyperphosphatemia consistent with surgical hypoparathyroidism. Appropriate initial treatment consists of calcium replacement, both intravenous and oral, and large doses of vitamin D or dihydrotachysterol. The dihydrotachysterol dose is lowered rapidly over several days to about 1 mg daily, and the intravenous calcium is discontinued as symptomatic hypocalcemia abates. Although PTH replacement would be logical, there is as yet no suitable preparation available. *(Cecil, pp. 1299–1300; Aurbach, Marx, and Spiegel)*

114. (A — True; B — True; C — True; D — False) In sarcoidosis and vitamin D intoxication there is increased gastrointestinal absorption of calcium as a result of the action of vitamin D on the intestinal mucosal cells. Glucocorticoids reduce the absorption of calcium by diminishing the generation of active vitamin D metabolites, as well as by reducing the gastrointestinal response to 1,25-dihydroxyvitamin D. In multiple myeloma, hypercalcemia occurs because of increased bone resorption rather than increased gastrointestinal absorption. In this condition, glucocorticoids act by their effect on the neoplastic cells. Glucocorticoids do not significantly alter secretion of PTH, and therefore do not decrease the calcium-mobilizing actions of PTH on bone or its effect on increasing the renal tubular reabsorption of calcium. *(Cecil, pp. 1294–1295; Habener and Potts)*

115. (A — True; B — True; C — False; D — True; E — True) The hand film shows a short fourth metacarpal on the left and short third and fourth metacarpals on the right. This, together with the other features described, is diagnostic of pseudohypoparathyroidism. The underlying renal abnormality in this condition is tubular resistance to the action of PTH. One manifestation of this resistance is a subnormal excretory response of cyclic AMP in the urine following an injection of PTH. As is generally seen in conditions with end-organ resistance, the serum concentration of the hormone to which resistance is present, in this case PTH, is elevated. Basal ganglia calcification is a manifestation of longstanding hypoparathyroidism and pseudohypoparathyroidism. Subjects with pseudohypoparathyroidism are frequently of subnormal intelligence.

The disease is familial, but the genetics of the inheritance are unclear. *(Cecil, pp. 1300–1301)*

116. (A — True; B — False; C — True; D — False) Adrenal insufficiency and alcohol hypoglycemia are generally associated with impaired hepatic glucose release. With states of excessive insulin or insulin-like activity, glycogen storage is excellent and a response to glucagon might be expected. *(Cecil, p. 1076)*

117. (A — False; B — True; C — False; D — True) Thirst is a subjective experience that cannot be studied in animals. The behavioral correlate of thirst — drinking — is observable and has been shown to respond both to osmotic stimulation (presumably owing to "shrinkage" of the appropriate hypothalamic neurons) and to direct injection of angiotensin II. Angiotensin II is the most potent known stimulus of drinking behavior, and its presence may account for the pathologic thirst of certain overhydrated states such as congestive heart failure and hepatic cirrhosis. *(Cecil, pp. 1194–1195)*

118. (All are True) Under normal conditions release of ADH is controlled by osmotic factors. This control system can be overridden by other stimuli, resulting in ADH release even when serum osmolality is normal or low. Pain and physical stress may contribute to the antidiuretic state seen after surgery. A fall in arterial blood pressure or collapse of the left atrium (owing, for example, to increased intrathoracic pressure or to hypovolemia) will result in ADH output independent of serum osmolality. *(Cecil, p. 1194)*

119. (B); 120. (D); 121. (A); 122. (C) Islet cell tumors and insulin-like hormones cause hypoglycemia by suppressing hepatic glucose release. Cortisol deficiency reduces alanine delivery from muscle, impairing glyconeogenesis. Alcohol dehydrogenation reduces NAD, making it unavailable for glucose production. Early diabetes, with a lag in insulin release, may produce late postprandial hypoglycemia. This is also seen as decompensated diabetes improves with therapy and endogenous insulin production is partially restored. *(Cecil, pp. 1072–1073; 1077–1078)*

123. (A) The testes are slightly smaller than normal and of normal consistency. The normal serum LH concentration indicates adequate testosterone generation by the Leydig cells. Nevertheless, the elevated serum FSH concentration suggests that the germinal cells in the seminiferous tubules are absent. These data are consistent with the Sertoli cell–only syndrome, in which a phenotypically normal, well-masculinized, and potent man is nevertheless sterile. *(Cecil, p. 1250)*

124. (B) Very small and firm testes in association with elevated serum LH and FSH are typical of Klinefelter's syndrome. Elevation of both gonadotropins indicates dysfunction of both testosterone production and spermatogenesis. *(Cecil, pp. 1248–1250)*

125. (D) Lens cataract formation and frontal baldness are characteristic of the hypogonadism associated with myotonic muscular dystrophy. These patients are well androgenized but may have high serum LH concentrations. The defect in spermatogenesis leads to an elevation in the serum FSH concentration. *(Cecil, p. 1248)*

126. (C) Low, or low-normal, serum FSH and LH concentrations in association with hypogonadism and hyposmia are characteristic of Kallmann's syndrome. The hypogonadism in this condition is believed to be secondary to a hypothalamic defect, leading to decreased gonadotropin secretion by the pituitary. In none of the other conditions listed would both FSH and LH be low or low-normal. *(Cecil, p. 1251)*

127. (D) The markedly elevated serum prolactin is indicative of a prolactin-secreting pituitary tumor ("prolactinoma"), which has led to secondary suppression of gonadotropins. The clinical consequences of these changes are amenorrhea and galactorrhea, and enlargement of the tumor itself causes headache. *(Cecil, pp. 1270, 1271)*

128. (C) Atrophic vaginitis indicates loss of estrogen production (ovarian failure). As a result, serum gonadotropins, freed of feedback inhibition, are high. Amenorrhea and vasomotor instability ("hot flashes") are typical of menopausal loss of ovarian function. *(Cecil, pp. 1270, 1272)*

129. (B) This is amenorrhea traumatica, which can result from postabortal endometritis or overvigorous curettage. All hormonal functions are normal, for the amenorrhea is mechanical, owing to absence of a responsive endometrium; it would be unresponsive to administered estrogen and progesterone. *(Cecil, pp. 1270–1271)*

130. (A) The constellation of polycystic ovaries with menstrual irregularity, hirsutism, and acne is typical of the Stein-Leventhal syndrome. Hormonal findings typically show increased serum LH (greater than FSH) concentration and normal prolactin. In addition, serum testosterone concentrations may be somewhat elevated, but almost always less than 0.20 μg/dl. *(Cecil, pp. 1270–1271)*

131. (E) Undeveloped genitalia are evidence of hypogonadotropic hypogonadism. The accompanying anosmia leads to a diagnosis of Kallmann's syndrome. Consistent with this diagnosis are the markedly low levels of FSH and LH. *(Cecil, p. 1268)*

132. (D) Adrenocortical carcinoma is a likely diagnosis in this patient with signs of virilism and a palpable flank mass. These tumors can produce excess cortisol but generally are inefficient synthesizers of steroids. As a result, large amounts of 17-ketosteroids are excreted and are the hallmark of this condition. *(Cecil, pp. 1237, 1276–1277)*

133. (F) Oral contraceptives raise plasma transcortin levels. As a result, plasma cortisol levels are high but other measures of adrenal function (ACTH, urine excretion, suppressibility) are normal. *(Cecil, p. 1235)*

134. (A) Failure of urinary 17-OH corticoids to suppress when the patient is given low-dose dexamethasone establishes the diagnosis of Cushing's syndrome. The decrease in 17-OH corticoids (>50% fall from baseline) after high-dose dexamethasone makes Cushing's *disease* highly likely. Plasma cortisol levels are elevated, and diurnal variation is absent; urinary steroid excretion is high, consistent with this diagnosis. Plasma ACTH is measurable but not elevated in many cases of Cushing's disease, although it does increase markedly after adrenalectomy. *(Cecil, p. 1235)*

135. (E) This patient has ectopic ACTH syndrome owing to a lung cancer. Many tumors, especially oat cell carcinoma of the lung, have been shown to secrete ACTH. Typical body habitus of Cushing's syndrome may be lacking, but marked elevation of plasma and urinary 17-OH and ketosteroids is the rule. Plasma ACTH may be very high (in contrast to pituitary Cushing's disease). Dexamethasone does not suppress cortisol secretion. *(Cecil, pp. 1236–1237)*

136. (C) This patient has isosexual precocious pseudopuberty caused by congenital adrenal hyperplasia. The hypertension points to an adrenal 11-hydroxylase deficiency that leads to serum and urinary accumulation of 11-deoxycortisol and 11-deoxycorticosterone. Measurement of these compounds would aid diagnosis, as does the easy suppressibility of urinary 17-OH and ketosteroids. Basal 17-ketosteroids are elevated because of increased adrenal androgen synthesis; the 17-OH steroids are increased because 11-deoxycortisol, although inert metabolically, is excreted as a 17-OH corticoid. Plasma cortisol (measured by specific means) is in the low-normal range because sufficient adrenal function is present for excessive stimulation to produce cortisol (albeit at the price of causing the adrenogenital syndrome). *(Cecil, pp. 1240–1242)*

137. (B) This patient has typical Cushing's syndrome. The adrenal mass (usually not palpable, but detectable by computerized tomography or arteriography) points to an adrenal origin of the cortisol excess. Plasma cortisol shows no diurnal variation and ACTH is low. Basal 17-OH corticoid excretion is high and does not suppress with either low- or high-dose dexamethasone. These data confirm the diagnosis. The low urinary 17-ketosteroids make a carcinoma unlikely. The patient probably has an adrenal adenoma, and unilateral adrenalectomy will cure her. *(Cecil, p. 1236)*

138. (E) Surgical treatment consists of removal of the autonomous nodule. No further treatment is needed and return of function in surrounding, suppressed thyroid will restore euthyroidism. As an alternative, radioiodine treatment is appropriate and effective, although a larger dose of ^{131}I may be required than with Graves' disease. *(Cecil, p. 1221)*

139. (B) Since this tumor is multicentric, total thyroidectomy is indicated. The best chance for cure depends on total extirpation of the thyroid before any gross malignancy is detectable. *(Cecil, pp. 1221, 1303)*

140. (A) Since the tumor is already metastatic, treatment with ^{131}I must be contemplated. Thyroidectomy removes iodine concentrating cells (and tumor) from the neck, enhancing metastatic uptake. The patient is allowed to become hypothyroid, or exogenous TSH is given to stimulate metastases; ^{131}I is then administered in doses of 100 to 150 mCi every six to 12 months until metastases regress or until radiation toxicity becomes apparent. *(Cecil, pp. 1222–1223)*

141. (E) In contrast to patients with metastatic thyroid carcinoma (**140** above), those with intrathyroidal papillary carcinoma do so well that simple lobectomy with isthmectomy, followed by exogenous thyroxine treatment, is curative. The need for prophylactic ^{131}I treatment is not clear. *(Cecil, p. 1222)*

142. (C) Anaplastic carcinoma is aggressive and resistant to treatment. It is almost always unresectable by the time it is discovered, and treatment consists of palliative measures such as relief of airway obstruction. *(Cecil, p. 1221)*

143. (E) Solitary nodules have an increased risk of malignancy if they are functionless and occur in young people, especially men. In such individuals, excisional biopsy is indicated, subsequent therapy being based on presence or absence of malignant change. Needle aspiration has been used, but open biopsy is more appropriate when the risk of malignancy is high. *(Cecil, pp. 1221–1222)*

144. (B) Pregnancy is associated with an estrogen-induced rise in thyroxine-binding globulin (TBG). As a result, serum thyroxine rises, resin T_3 uptake decreases, and the free thyroxine index remains normal (unless the patient develops thyroid disease). In this example, the patient is euthyroid — a normal radioiodine uptake is expected and shown. This procedure is *contraindicated* in pregnancy and must be avoided: it provides no new information and may damage the fetus. *(Cecil, pp. 1204–1205)*

145. (C) Diseases of the hypothalmus or pituitary can result in thyroid hypofunction (almost never in hyperfunction). Typical findings in a patient who *does* have thyroid dysfunction on this basis (many patients are normal, of course) show the constellation of secondary hypothyroidism: low free thyroxine index without elevation of TSH. The TSH measurement is the crux of diagnosis and must not be omitted. *(Cecil, p. 1214)*

146. (A) Typical findings in Graves' disease include elevated thyroxine, resin T_3 uptake, and radioiodine uptake. TSH is low and unresponsive to TRH, a finding that can help establish a diagnosis in equivocal cases. *(Cecil, pp. 1208–1209)*

147. (D) Hashimoto's thyroiditis is a common cause of asymptomatic goiter, especially in young people. The absence of symptoms can be misleading, for often the free thyroxine index will be low-normal or even low. In either case, the elevated serum TSH is indicative of diminished thyroid reserve and an indication for treatment. After treatment, many patients will recognize that they are even more "asymptomatic" than they were before as vague symptoms (tiredness, weight gain, lethargy) improve. *(Cecil, p. 1219)*

148. (E) In contrast to patients with Graves' disease (**146** above), those with subacute thyroiditis may be clinically and biochemically hyperthyroid, but the radioiodine uptake is remarkably *low*. This distinguishing point is the reason for recommending radioiodine uptake in hyperthyroid patients. Subacute thyroiditis may be painless and the diagnosis unclear until a low radioiodine uptake is obtained to guide appropriate treatment. *(Cecil, p. 1218)*

149. (E) Since exogenous thyroxine can produce hyperthyroidism and low radioiodine uptake, thyroid function studies may mimic those of subacute thyroiditis, especially if the latter is painless and not accompanied by an elevated sedimentation rate. Suspicion of the diagnosis and observation (thyroiditis is self-limited) may help distinguish the two. *(Cecil, p. 1205)*

150. (B) As in pregnancy (**144** above), estrogen (diethylstilbestrol) administration raises TBG and produces the characteristic laboratory results. *(Cecil, pp. 1204–1205)*

151. (A) The new onset of atrial fibrillation raises the suspicion of hyperthyroidism. Many multinodular goiters are autonomous and unsuppressible. When modest doses of exogenous thyroxine are added to the autonomously produced hormone, the result is clinical hyperthyroidism. It is important that radioiodine uptake (and scan) be obtained *while the patient is hyperthyroid* to document autonomy. If thyroxine is discontinued and the patient becomes euthyroid, this opportunity is lost. *(Cecil, p. 1224)*

152. (C) After the discontinuation of exogenous thyroxine, there is a modest decrease in free thyroxine index to slightly abnormal levels, the nadir occurring at two to three weeks. TSH rises from initially suppressed levels but does not become elevated. By six weeks all thyroid function should be normal; if not, endogenous thyroid disease is likely. *(Cecil, p. 1216)*

153. (A) Polyendocrine failure often includes the adrenal and parathyroid glands. Mucocutaneous candidiasis is common, and an abnormal immune response has been postulated as the basis for the disorder. The parathyroid disorder is characterized by evidence of parathyroid hormone deficiency: hypocalcemia, hyperphosphatemia, low serum PTH, and brisk urinary cyclic AMP response to administered parathyroid extract. *(Cecil, pp. 1297–1298)*

154. (E) This patient has had only one abnormal parathyroid gland removed, and therefore surgical hypoparathyroidism is unlikely. A more reasonable explanation is the rapid uptake of calcium and phosphate into bone ("hungry bone syndrome") resulting in hypophosphatemia despite a low serum PTH. The time course is typical, and the syndrome will resolve with supplemental calcium and the return of normal parathyroid function. *(Cecil, p. 1296)*

155. (B) These siblings have physical stigmata of pseudohypoparathyroidism. Clinical hallmarks are hypocalcemia and hyperphosphatemia, despite elevated serum PTH. Confirmation of renal refractoriness to PTH is found in the lack of normal urinary cyclic AMP response. *(Cecil, pp. 1300–1302)*

156. (A) This patient has had a *total* thyroidectomy, making surgical hypoparathyroidism likely. The biochemical findings are identical to those in polyendocrine failure (**153** above), since the mechanism is the same — lack of PTH. Surgical technique is of the utmost importance in preventing this unhappy situation. *(Cecil, p. 1297)*

157. (D) Hypophosphatemia in the presence of *hypo*calcemia implies a primary deficiency in calcium with a resultant secondary hyperparathyroidism, leading to phosphate wasting. The elevated serum PTH is compatible with this diagnosis. *(Cecil, p. 1298)*

158. (B); 159. (D); 160. (C); 161. (A) *(Cecil, pp. 1069–1070)*

162. (D) This patient has familial hypocalciuric hypercalcemia. The findings of elevated serum calcium and low-normal serum phosphate often lead to unsuccessful neck exploration. Clues to the correct diagnosis are the family history and the distinctly low urinary calcium excretion. Since surgery is unhelpful and the course in these individuals is benign, no treatment is needed. *(Cecil, pp. 1292–1293)*

163. (B) This patient most likely has hypercalcemia of malignancy. There is marked hypercalcemia, borderline low serum phosphate, and grossly excessive hypercalciuria. The serum PTH is detectable but not truly elevated. These findings have led to speculation that such tumors elaborate an abnormal ("ectopic") PTH, although other explanations have included ectopic production of prostaglandins or other bone-resorbing substances. *(Cecil, pp. 1291–1292, 1294)*

164. (A) This patient has symptoms of hyperparathyroidism. Typical findings include moderate hypercalcemia, depressed serum phosphate, elevated serum chloride, and raised serum PTH. The urinary calcium is not markedly elevated, despite the hypercalcemia, because of the increased renal tubular reabsorption of calcium due to PTH. *(Cecil, pp. 1293–1294)*

165. (C) Thiazide diuretics cause increased renal calcium reabsorption and may result in hypercalcemia, usually of a modest degree. Since release of PTH is usually depressed, hypophosphatemia is not usual; hypokalemic alkalosis and hypochloremia may result from inhibited renal chloride reabsorption. Urinary calcium excretion tends to be increased by the hypercalcemia and decreased by the diuretic effect, leading to relatively normal excretion. *(Cecil, p. 1293)*

166. (E) Vitamin D intoxication leading to hypercalcemia can occur with daily ingestion of 10,000 to 50,000 units in adults. The clinical picture is similar to **165** above (normal serum phosphate; low serum PTH), except that serum chloride is normal, and massive hypercalciuria results from hypercalcemia and the absence of parathyroid action on the kidney (calcium reabsorption). *(Cecil, p. 1293)*

167. (B); 168. (E); 169. (C); 170. (A); 171. (D). *(Cecil, pp. 1192–1195, 1196–1197)*

167. The values are consistent with diabetes insipidus associated with a complete deficiency of antidiuretic hormone (ADH). At the end of the period of dehydration the patient's urinary osmolality is far below serum osmolality, which is dangerously high. Nevertheless, when given an injection of ADH (vasopressin), the subject is able to concentrate urine approximately threefold, to a degree that the urinary osmolality is now considerably greater than the serum osmolality. This indicates that the renal tubules are responsive to ADH, but that the endogenous production of ADH is extremely low or totally deficient. **168.** At the end of the period of dehydration, this subject is able to concentrate the urine markedly, and serum osmolality has not increased above normal. An injection of vasopressin does not further increase the urinary osmolality, indicating that it is already maximally concentrated. These data are consistent with a normal, healthy subject. **169.** These data are consistent with nephrogenic diabetes insipidus. Thus, as in complete, "central" diabetes insipidus, this patient is unable to concentrate the urine to a degree greater than the serum osmolality, despite the fact that the latter is dangerously high. In contrast to the results in patients with ADH deficiency, an injection of vasopressin still does not increase the urinary osmolality above the serum osmolality. Thus, there is renal tubular resistance to the action of vasopressin. **170.** In this subject, dehydration results in a modest increase in urinary osmolality: it does increase to above the serum osmolality, but not by a great margin. Serum osmolality increases to the high-normal range after dehydration. After injection of vasopressin, the urinary osmolality increases by 25%. This demonstrates that the renal tubules are responsive to ADH, and that secretion of endogenous ADH is suboptimal, suggesting partial ADH deficiency. **171.** Two features suggest that this subject is a compulsive water drinker. First, the maximal urinary osmolality attained after dehydration is not as great as is seen in most normal subjects. Second, the urinary osmolality does not increase significantly after an injection of vasopressin. This suggests that the tubules are already being stimulated maximally, but that their response is subnormal. Nevertheless, in contrast to the patient with congenital nephrogenic diabetes insipidus (**169** above), this patient is able to concentrate urine above serum osmolality, and he does not develop a hypertonic serum following the period of dehydration. It is believed that the chronic water ingestion decreases the osmolality in the interstitium of the kidney medulla, and thereby diminishes the ability of the kidney to concentrate the urine maximally despite an adequate ADH stimulus.

BIBLIOGRAPHY

American Diabetes Association: Standardization of the glucose tolerance test. Report of the Committee on Statistics. Diabetes *18*:299, 1969.

Aurbach, G. D., Marx, S. J., and Spiegel, A. M.: Parathyroid hormone, calcitonin, and the calciferols. *In* Williams, R. H. (ed.): Textbook of Endocrinology. 6th ed. Philadelphia, W. B. Saunders Company, 1981, p. 922.

Bunn, H. P., Gabbay, K. H., and Gallop, P. M.: The glycosylation of hemoglobin: relevance to diabetes mellitus. Science, *200*:21, 1978.

Citrin, W., Ellis, G. J., and Skyler, J. S.: Glycosylated hemoglobin: a tool in identifying psychological problems? Diabetes Care, *3*:563, 1980.

Davis, P. J., and Davis, F. B.: Hyperthyroidism in patients over the age of 60 years. Medicine, *53*:161, 1974.

Day, R. M.: Clinical manifestations. *In* Werner, S. C., and Ingbar, S. H. (eds.): The Thryoid. 4th ed. New York, Harper & Row, 1978, p. 663.

DeFronzo, R. A., Andres, R., Edgar, P., et al.: Carbohydrate metabolism in uremia: a review. Medicine, *52*:469, 1973.

DeGroot, L. J. (ed.): Endocrinology. New York, Grune & Stratton, 1979.

Ditzel, J., and Standl, E.: The oxygen transport system of red blood cells during diabetic ketoacidosis and recovery. Diabetologia, *11*:255, 1975.

Doar, J. W. H., Thompson, M. E., Wilde, C. E., and Sewell, P. F. J.: Influence of treatment with diet alone on oral glucose-tolerance test and plasma sugar and insulin levels in patients with maturity-onset diabetes mellitus. Lancet, *1*:1263, 1975.

Ehrlich, E. N.: Adrenocortical regulation of salt and water metabolism: physiology, pathophysiology, and clinical syndromes. *In* DeGroot, L. J. (ed.): Endocrinology. New York, Grune & Stratton, 1979, p. 1883.

Feldman, J. M., Kelley, W. N., and Lebovitz, H. E.: Inhibition of glucose oxidase paper tests by reducing metabolites. Diabetes, *19*:337, 1970.

Foucar, E., and Field, J. B.: Effect of control of hyperglycemia on plasma insulin responses to various stimuli in newly diagnosed ketosis-prone patients. J. Clin. Endocrinol. Metab., *35*:288, 1972.

Gale, E. A. M., Walford, S., and Tattersall, R. B.: Nocturnal hypoglycemia and haemoglobin A. Lancet, *2*:1240, 1979.

Gyves, M. T., Rodman, H. M., Little, A. B., et al.: A modern approach to management of pregnant diabetics: a two-year analysis of perinatal outcomes. Am. J. Obstet. Gynecol., *128*:606, 1977.

Habener, J. F., and Potts, J. T., Jr.: Diagnosis and differential diagnosis of primary hyperparathyroidism. *In* DeGroot, L. J. (ed.): Endocrinology. New York, Grune & Stratton, 1979, p. 703.

Hall, R., and Evered, D. C.: Autoimmune thyroid disease: thyroiditis. *In* DeGroot, L. J. (ed.): Endocrinology. New York, Grune & Stratton, 1979, p. 461.

Holm, L. E., Dahlquist, I., Israelsson, A., and Lundell, G.: Malignant thyroid tumors after iodine-131 therapy. N. Engl. J. Med., *303*:188, 1980.

Ingbar, S. H.: Thyroid storm or crisis. *In* Werner, S. C., and Ingbar, S. H. (eds.): The Thyroid. 4th ed. New York, Harper & Row, 1978, p. 800.

Jackson, R. L., and Guthrie, R. A.: The child with diabetes mellitus. Upjohn Scope Monograph, 1975.

Koivisto, V. A., and Felig, P.: Effects of leg exercise on insulin absorption in diabetic patients. N. Engl. J. Med., *298*:79, 1978.

Najarian, J. S., Kjellstrand, C. M., Simmons, R. L., et al.: Renal transplantation for diabetic glomerulosclerosis. Ann. Surg., *178*:477, 1973.

Neer, R. M., and Potts, J. T., Jr.: Medical management of hypercalcemia and hyperparathyroidism. *In* DeGroot, L. J. (ed.): Endocrinology. New York, Grune & Stratton, 1979, p. 725.

Perkins, J. R., West, T. E. T., Sonksen, P. H., et al.: The effects of energy and carbohydrate restriction in patients with chronic diabetes mellitus. Diabetologia, *13*:607, 1977.

Posner, J. B., and Plum, F.: Spinal fluid pH and neurologic symptoms in acidosis. N. Engl. J. Med., *277*:605, 1967.

Sarkar, S. D., Beierwaltes, W. H., Gill, S. F., and Cowley, B. J.: Subsequent fertility and birth histories of children and adolescents treated with ^{131}I for thyroid cancer. J. Nucl. Med., *17*:460, 1976.

Sherwood, L. M., and Gould, V. E.: Ectopic hormone syndromes and multiple endocrine neoplasia. *In* DeGroot, L. J. (ed.): Endocrinology. New York, Grune & Stratton, 1979, p. 1733.

Sofa, A. M., Schumacher, O. P., and Rodriguez-Antunez, A.: Long-term followup results in children and adolescents treated with radioactive iodine (^{131}I) for hyperthyroidism. N. Engl. J. Med., *292*:167, 1975.

Somogyi, M.: Exacerbation of diabetes by excess insulin action. Am. J. Med., *26*:169, 1959.

Takazakura, E., Nakamoto, Y., Hayakawa, H., et al.: Onset and progression of diabetic glomerulosclerosis: a prospective study based on serial renal biopsies. Diabetes, *24*:1, 1975.

Tunbridge, W. M. G., Brewis, M., French, J. M., et al.: Natural history of autoimmune thyroiditis. Br. Med. J., *282*:258, 1981.

Turner, R. C., McCarthy, S. T., Holman, R. R., and Harris, E.: Beta-cell function improved by supplementing basal insulin secretion in mild diabetes. Br. Med. J., *1*:1252, 1976.

Turtle, J. R.: Glucose and insulin secretory response patterns following diet and tolazamide therapy in diabetes. Br. Med. J., *3*:606, 1970.

Tyrrell, J. B., Brooks, R. M., Fitzgerald, P. A., et al.: Cushing's disease: selective trans-sphenoidal resection of pituitary microadenomas. N. Engl. J. Med., *298*:753, 1978.

Vagenakis, A. G., Braverman, L. E., Azizi, F., et al.: Recovery of pituitary thyrotropic function after withdrawal of prolonged thyroid-suppression therapy. N. Engl. J. Med., *293*:681, 1975.

Volpé, R.: Subacute (nonsuppurative) thyroiditis. *In* Werner, S. C., and Ingbar, S. H. (eds.): The Thyroid. 4th ed. New York, Harper & Row, 1978, p. 986.

Wahren, J., Felig, P., and Hagenfeldt, L.: Physical exercise and fuel homeostasis in diabetes mellitus. Diabetologia, *14*:213, 1978.

Wang, C.: Thyroid cancer: treatment. *In* Werner, S. C., and Ingbar, S. H. (eds.): The Thyroid. 4th ed. New York, Harper & Row, 1978, p. 558.

Werner, S. C.: Myxedema coma. *In* Werner, S. C., and Ingbar, S. H. (eds.): The Thyroid. 4th ed. New York, Harper & Row, 1978, p. 971.

Werner, S. C., and Ingbar, S. H. (eds.): The Thyroid. 4th ed. New York, Harper & Row, 1978.

Williams, R. H. (ed.): Textbook of Endocrinology. 6th ed. Philadelphia, W. B. Saunders Company, 1981.

PART 8

INFECTIOUS DISEASES

Vincent G. Pons and Richard A. Jacobs

DIRECTIONS: For questions 1 to 44, choose the ONE BEST answer to each question.

1. A 22-year-old man consults you because of a painful lesion on his penis. The lesion is not indurated and has a necrotic, dirty-appearing base. There is tender left inguinal lymphadenopathy. Gram stain of material from the base of the lesion reveals parallel arrays of small, gram-negative coccobacilli. Which of the following is the most appropriate treatment?

A. Cephalexin
B. Benzathine penicillin
C. Procaine penicillin plus probenecid
D. Sulfisoxazole
E. Chloramphenicol

2. A 22-year-old man presents with a painless, papular penile lesion. Lymph nodes above and below the inguinal ligament are swollen, tender, and fluctuant. Aspiration of one of the nodes yields viscous purulent material that on Gram stain reveals numerous polymorphonuclear leukocytes but no organisms. Which of the following is the most appropriate therapy?

A. Procaine penicillin plus probenecid
B. Dicloxacillin
C. Tetracycline
D. Chloramphenicol
E. Cephalexin

3. A 35-year-old woman with a history of recurrent urinary tract infections comes to your office with a one-day history of dysuria and frequency of urination. There is no evidence of vaginitis. Microscopic urinalysis reveals one to two polymorphonuclear leukocytes per high-power field and no bacteria. Which of the following is most appropriate for this patient?

A. Observation without therapy
B. Ampicillin
C. Tetracycline
D. Benzathine penicillin, 4.8 units intramuscularly
E. Cephalexin

4. A 16-year-old boy is brought to your office 12 hours after he was bitten on the hand by a cat while playing at a friend's house. The hand is markedly swollen. The wound is purulent and draining and surrounded by fiery-red cellulitis. There is axillary adenopathy. Gram stain of the exudate would most likely reveal

A. gram-positive cocci in chains
B. gram-positive cocci in clusters
C. gram-negative rods
D. a mixture of gram-positive cocci in pairs, chains, clusters; long, slender, gram-negative rods; and gram-positive rods

5. All the following uses of prophylactic antibiotics are appropriate EXCEPT

A. cefazolin, 1.0 gm intravenously every six hours starting one hour before planned total hip arthroplasty and continuing for 48 hours thereafter
B. cefazolin, 1.0 gm intravenously every six hours starting one hour before planned vaginal hysterectomy and continuing for 48 hours thereafter
C. cefazolin, 1.0 gm intravenously every six hours starting four hours before planned cardiac catheterization and continuing for 48 hours thereafter
D. oral nonabsorbable antibiotics starting several days before a planned colectomy
E. *no* prophylactic antibiotics given to a patient prior to elective craniotomy for removal of a meningioma

6. The pneumococcal vaccine is indicated for all the following patients EXCEPT

A. a 20-year-old black woman with sickle cell anemia
B. a 40-year-old male executive with alcoholic cirrhosis of the liver
C. a 65-year-old man with chronic obstructive pulmonary disease (COPD)
D. a 1-year-old boy with congenital heart disease
E. a 3-year-old girl who had a traumatic splenectomy

7. A 27-year-old male drug addict is admitted to the hospital with fever (temperature 102°F) and back pain in the L2–L3 area. Physical examination is unremarkable except for tenderness in the low back area. Leukocyte count is 16,500/cu mm; erythrocyte sedimentation rate is 60 mm/hour. Roentgenograms of the spine show cortical destruction of the L3 vertebral body. Blood cultures grow *Staphylococcus aureus*. Which of the following is most appropriate for this patient?

A. Tetracycline, 500 mg orally four times daily for three weeks
B. Nafcillin, 1.0 gm intravenously every four hours for four weeks
C. Chloramphenicol, 500 mg intravenously every six hours for four weeks
D. Rifampin, 600 mg orally daily plus dicloxacillin, 500 mg orally four times daily for six weeks
E. Strict immobilization with a body cast for six weeks and no antibiotic therapy

8. Filariasis due to *Wuchereria bancrofti* causes all the following EXCEPT

A. Calabar swellings
B. lymphangitis
C. chronic lymphadenopathy
D. epididymitis
E. chyluria

9. All the following were important factors in the apparent eradication of smallpox EXCEPT

A. absence of an animal reservoir
B. a high level of "herd immunity" due to vaccination
C. vaccination of contacts as soon as possible after a case was identified
D. administration of vaccinia immune globulin to household contacts as soon as possible after a case was identified
E. use of mobile public health teams to detect and contain outbreaks rapidly

10. A 23-year-old woman in the first trimester of pregnancy attends a suburban lunch party during which she picks up and comforts a fractious child who is later found to have rubella. A hemagglutination inhibition (HI) titer is performed at once on the woman's blood, and proves negative. You should now

A. offer an abortion, if the mother so wishes
B. administer cytosine arabinoside (ara-A)
C. administer rubella vaccine and gamma globulin
D. administer human immune serum globulin
E. wait two to three weeks and repeat the HI titer

11. Which of the following statements about vancomycin is correct?

A. It should be given only intramuscularly
B. It has no activity against gram-negative bacteria
C. It has no activity against anaerobic bacteria
D. It causes peripheral neuropathy
E. It should be avoided in patients with renal failure

12. All the following may produce gas in the tissues of a patient with cellulitis EXCEPT

A. *Bacteroides* species
B. *Escherichia coli*
C. *Peptostreptococcus intermedius*
D. *Pseudomonas aeruginosa*
E. *Clostridium perfringens*

13. A nurse working in the renal dialysis unit sticks her finger with a needle contaminated with the blood of a dialysis patient. This patient was found to be hepatitis B surface antigen (HB_sAg)-positive when last tested nine months ago. Which of the following should you do first?

A. Administer hepatitis B immune globulin (H-BIG) and repeat the dose in one month
B. Administer human gamma globulin and repeat the dose in one month
C. Test the patient for HB_sAg and "e" antigen
D. Test the nurse for HB_sAg and "e" antigen
E. Test both patient and nurse for both HB_sAg and antibody to HB_sAg

14. A 46-year-old habitual drunkard was knocked down in a fight six days ago and has noticed a thin discharge from one nostril ever since. He develops signs of meningitis and is admitted to the hospital. Cerebrospinal fluid findings are glucose 30 mg/dl, protein 96 mg/dl, cells 2250/cu mm, with 97% neutrophils. No organisms are seen on Gram stain. Which of the following is the best initial treatment for this patient?

A. Aqueous penicillin G, 24 million units intravenously daily
B. Aqueous penicillin G, 24 million units, plus chloramphenicol, 4 gm intravenously daily
C. Ampicillin, 12 gm, plus chloramphenicol, 4 gm intravenously daily
D. Ampicillin, 12 gm intravenously daily, plus isoniazid and ethambutol until further lab results are available
E. Nafcillin, 10 gm, plus gentamicin, 5 mg/kg, intravenously daily

15. A 10-month-old infant is brought to the emergency room because of a high fever of 12 hours' duration. On examination he appears toxic and seriously ill. There is an area of bluish-red facial cellulitis on the right cheek. The best initial antibiotic treatment would be

A. methicillin
B. aqueous penicillin G
C. ampicillin plus chloramphenicol
D. tetracycline
E. cephalothin plus clindamycin

16. A 67-year-old farmer comes to the emergency room eight hours after deeply puncturing his calf with a splintered piece of wood while working in his barnyard. He cannot recall having received any immunizations in the past and he has not served in any military units. He reports having suffered a severe urticarial reaction to penicillin nine years ago. The wound is clean, with minimal bleeding. Roentgenogram of the calf shows no foreign body. The best management is

A. careful probing of the wound, local application of peroxide, a course of tetanous toxoid, and tetracycline
B. tetanus antitoxin, careful probing of the wound, local application of peroxide, tetanus toxoid, and tetracycline
C. surgical exploration of the wound, tetanus toxoid, and desensitization to penicillin followed by treatment with penicillin
D. tetanus antitoxin, surgical exploration of the wound, tetanus toxoid, and desensitization to penicillin followed by treatment with penicillin
E. tetanus antitoxin, surgical exploration of the wound, tetanus toxoid, and chemoprophylaxis with tetracycline

17. A 28-year-old airplane pilot was treated for gonorrhea two weeks ago with aqueous procaine penicillin G, 4.8 million units intramuscularly, plus probenecid. His symptoms resolved, but over the last three days mild dysuria and urethral discharge have recurred. Gram stain of the discharge shows many polymorphonuclear leukocytes and rare gram-positive cocci. What is the best management?

A. Repeat the same regimen and send a urethral swab to the CDC for testing for penicillin resistance
B. Withhold treatment for now and send a urethral swab to the CDC for testing for penicillin resistance
C. Send a urethral culture to the routine laboratory and administer tetracycline, 0.5 gm orally four times daily for seven days
D. Send a urethral culture to the routine laboratory and administer ampicillin, 0.5 gm orally four times daily for ten days
E. Administer spectinomycin, 2 gm intramuscularly

18. A 31-year-old heroin addict with staphylococcal endocarditis of the aortic valve had been receiving methicillin, 4 gm intravenously every six hours for 19 days, when he developed recurrent fever, eosinophilia, gross hematuria, and a rise in serum creatinine from 1.6 mg/dl to 2.3 mg/dl. The best management would be to

A. stop methicillin and observe
B. stop methicillin, begin oxacillin, and observe
C. stop methicillin, begin cephalothin, and observe
D. stop methicillin, begin vancomycin, and perform a kidney biopsy
E. continue methicillin and perform a kidney biopsy

19. Hepatic disease due to *Schistosoma mansoni* is most often manifest by

A. mild jaundice
B. hematemesis
C. encephalopathy and asterixis
D. hematuria
E. spider angiomas

20. All the following are manifestations of trichinellosis (trichinosis) EXCEPT

A. periorbital edema and splinter hemorrhages
B. hypoalbuminemia and normal erythrocyte sedimentation rate
C. gastrointestinal upset
D. myocarditis, meningitis, and encephalitis
E. positive Casoni test

21. All the following side effects have been described in patients taking nitrofurantoin EXCEPT

A. acute or chronic pneumonitis
B. polyneuropathy
C. hemolytic anemia in patients with glucose-6-phosphate dehydrogenase (G6PD) deficiency
D. cholestatic hepatitis
E. aplastic anemia

22. Which of the following statements regarding tularemia is correct?

A. It occurs mainly in summer
B. It is caused by an organism that cannot be cultured *in vitro*
C. It causes granulomas in tissue
D. It infects skin, lymph nodes, and blood, but not the lungs
E. It should be treated with high doses of ampicillin

23. All the following are associated with *Candida* infections EXCEPT

A. chronic granulomatous disease
B. hypercalcemia
C. narcotic addiction
D. terminal gastric cancer
E. hyperalimentation

24. Counterimmunoelectrophoresis (CIE) is presently used as an adjunctive diagnostic test for infections due to all of the following EXCEPT

A. *Streptococcus pneumoniae*
B. *Hemophilus influenzae type B*
C. *Neisseria meningitidis*
D. *Neisseria gonorrhoeae*
E. *Escherichia coli* K1

25. The tetracyclines may cause all the following EXCEPT

A. neuromuscular blockade
B. acute fatty degeneration of the liver
C. photosensitivity dermatitis
D. increased cerebrospinal fluid pressure in infants
E. hypoplasia and discoloration of dental enamel in children

26. Enterobiasis may cause all the following complications EXCEPT

A. appendicitis
B. vulvitis
C. prostatitis
D. hepatitis
E. ischiorectal abscess

27. Trichuriasis (whipworm infection) can be complicated by all the following EXCEPT

A. bloody diarrhea
B. mild eosinophilia
C. migration of larvae through the lung
D. rectal prolapse
E. anemia

28. Mebendazole is a first-line drug for treatment of infections due to all the following nematodes EXCEPT

A. *Necator americanus*
B. *Trichuris trichiura*
C. *Strongyloides stercoralis*
D. *Enterobius vermicularis*
E. *Ascaris lumbricoides*

29. A patient from West Africa with an itching, erythematous, papular skin rash, subcutaneous nodules, punctate keratitis, and corneal scarring is most likely suffering from which one of the following?

A. Trachoma and scabies
B. Onchocerciasis
C. *Loa loa* infection
D. Dracontiasis (guinea worm infection)
E. Schistosomiasis

30. Tropical pyomyositis is usually due to infection with which one of the following?

A. *Staphylococcus aureus*
B. Mixed aerobic and anaerobic flora
C. *Dirofilaria tenuis*
D. *Pseudomonas pseudomallei*
E. None of the above

31. *Yersinia enterocolitica* is commonly associated with all the following EXCEPT

A. arthritis
B. bacteremia
C. osteomyelitis
D. bloody diarrhea
E. abdominal pain

32. Toxocariasis (visceral larva migrans) is associated with all the following EXCEPT

A. fever and tender hepatomegaly
B. endophthalmitis, sometimes simulating a retinal tumor
C. high eosinophil count (>50%)
D. exposure to dogs
E. intestinal obstruction or intussusception

33. A 38-year-old homosexual male with secondary syphilis is treated in the emergency room with benzathine penicillin, 2.4 million units intramuscularly. Six hours later he returns, complaining of severe generalized aching pains, chills, and headache. On examination he looks ill, with high fever and rigors. Which of the following is most appropriate?

A. Admit to intensive care unit and prepare to treat shock or bronchospasm
B. Admit to general ward for observation
C. Admit to general ward, give intramuscular diphenhydramine and oral aspirin, and observe
D. Immediately administer methylprednisolone, 1 gm intravenously, plus cephalothin and gentamicin, and observe
E. Prescribe aspirin and ask him to return to the emergency room if symptoms do not resolve in six hours

34. A farmer developed a painless, 1-cm papule on the dorsum of the right thumb. After two weeks, it ulcerated and drained a small amount of pus. Meanwhile, a series of six similar lesions developed in a chain extending up the forearm. There were no systemic symptoms. Biopsy of one of these papules showed a granulomatous reaction and dimorphic fungi in the skin, with branching, septate, hyphae-bearing conidia. Which one of the following would you recommend?

A. Saturated solution of potassium iodide, 2 ml orally four times daily
B. Amphotericin B intravenously, to a total of 2 gm
C. Flucytosine, 100 mg/kg orally daily for six weeks
D. Miconazole, 1 gm intravenously daily
E. Sulfadiazine, 1 gm orally four times daily

35. The best treatment of brucellosis is

A. tetracycline
B. streptomycin
C. tetracycline plus streptomycin
D. trimethoprim-sulfamethoxazole (co-trimoxazole)
E. none of the above

36. Staphylococci cause all the following EXCEPT

A. scalded skin syndrome
B. enterocolitis
C. carbuncles
D. ecthyma gangrenosum
E. parotitis

37. Major manifestations of rheumatic fever include all the following EXCEPT

A. carditis
B. polyarthritis
C. chorea
D. subcutaneous nodules
E. erythema nodosum

38. Rickettsial diseases commonly cause all the following EXCEPT

A. headache
B. hypotension
C. leukocytosis
D. disseminated focal infection of small blood vessels
E. altered mental status

39. All the following drugs are potentially useful for treatment of anaerobic infections EXCEPT

A. metronidazole
B. cefoxitin
C. amikacin
D. doxycycline
E. ticarcillin

40. Amphotericin B can cause all the following side effects EXCEPT

A. hypokalemia
B. shaking chills, headache
C. anemia
D. neuromuscular blockade
E. renal tubular acidosis

41. Ecthyma gangrenosum is a manifestation of infection with

A. *Pseudomonas aeruginosa*
B. *Bacillus anthracis* (anthrax)
C. *Erysipelothrix*
D. Group A β-hemolytic streptococci
E. *Clostridium perfringens*

42. All the following may cause retinal abnormalities EXCEPT

A. *Mycobacterium tuberculosis*
B. *Pneumocystis carinii*
C. *Candida albicans*
D. *Toxoplasma gondii*
E. *Histoplasma capsulatum*

43. Which of the following is the prophylactic regimen of choice for close household contacts of a patient with meningococcemia, before the sensitivity of the organism is known?

A. Minocycline, 250 mg orally four times daily for seven days
B. Sulfadiazine, 1.0 gm orally twice daily for two days
C. Penicillin V, 250 mg orally four times daily for seven days
D. Rifampin, 600 mg orally twice daily for two days
E. Polyvalent meningococcal vaccine

44. Which of the following is most appropriate to assess the response to therapy of a patient with neurosyphilis?

A. CSF cell count and VDRL titer
B. CSF cell count, protein, and VDRL titer
C. CSF cell count, glucose, and protein
D. CSF fluorescent treponemal antibody-absorbed (FTA-ABS) titer
E. Serum FTA-ABS titer and CSF VDRL titer

DIRECTIONS: For questions 45 to 106, you are to decide whether EACH choice is true or false. Any combination of answers, from all true to all false, may be present. Mark the answer sheet "T" or "F" in the space provided.

45. Which of the following statements about babesiosis is/are true?

A. It has not been reported in the United States
B. It is caused by a protozoan that infects red blood cells
C. Tetracycline is the preferred treatment
D. It is transmitted from animals to man by ticks
E. Fever and hemolytic anemia are part of the clinical presentation

46. Which of the following statements is/are true about the treatment of leprosy?

A. Dapsone is the drug of choice
B. Thalidomide is active against *Mycobacterium leprae,* but its teratogenic effects limit its routine use
C. The usual duration of therapy is one year
D. Clofazimine is active against *Mycobacterium leprae,* but its use is limited to prophylaxis for household contacts of active cases

47. Which of the following statements is/are true about *Klebsiella pneumoniae* pneumonia?

A. Multiple lobes are frequently involved
B. There is a predilection for upper-lobe involvement
C. It is a necrotizing pneumonia that can progress to abscess formation and empyema
D. Pleuritic chest pain is a common complaint
E. It is frequently associated with alcoholism

48. Which of the following statements is/are true about aspiration pneumonia?

A. Community-acquired aspiration pneumonia is usually caused by anaerobic bacteria
B. Hospital-acquired aspiration pneumonia is usually of mixed etiology involving both aerobic and anaerobic bacteria
C. A cephalosporin is the treatment of choice for the penicillin-allergic patient with community-acquired aspiration pneumonia
D. Bacterial pneumonia occurs in 75 to 80% of patients following aspiration of gastric contents

49. Which of the following statements is/are true about trimethoprim-sulfamethoxazole?

A. It is effective in prevention of recurrent urinary tract infections in women
B. It penetrates into the cerebral spinal fluid
C. It can be used in treatment of peptostreptococcal infections
D. It is the treatment of choice for *Pneumocystis carinii* pneumonia
E. It is active against *Hemophilus influenzae*

50. Which of the following statements is/are true about cat-scratch disease?

A. It is caused by a cell wall–deficient mycoplasma
B. It is best treated with tetracycline
C. It is the most common cause of *chronic* regional adenitis in children and adolescents in the United States
D. It is usually transmitted by a cat that appears perfectly well
E. It is associated with lymphangitis and lymphadenitis

51. Which of the following statements is/are true about rabies?

A. Bites from rodents such as wild rats, rabbits, and squirrels require rabies immunoprophylaxis
B. A wild animal that has been captured following a bite should be sacrificed only if the animal becomes ill
C. Immunofluorescent antibody stain for rabies on brain tissue provides a definitive diagnosis of animal rabies
D. Because the incubation period of rabies is long (about 60 days), rabies immunoprophylaxis can be safely deferred for seven to ten days

52. Which of the following statements is/are true about nongonococcal urethritis?

A. It is most commonly caused by *Chlamydia trachomatis*
B. It is usually associated with a spontaneous, purulent urethral discharge
C. Symptoms usually occur acutely, as with gonococcal urethritis
D. Urethral culture is best for routine diagnosis

53. Which of the following is/are commonly associated with secondary bacterial pneumonia following primary influenza A infection?

A. *Streptococcus pneumoniae*
B. *Staphylococcus aureus*
C. *Legionella pneumophila*
D. *Mycoplasma pneumoniae*
E. *Hemophilus influenzae*

54. Which of the following statements is/are true about endogenous pyrogen?

A. It is a low-molecular-weight protein synthesized by phagocytic cells
B. It is one of several substances produced by human cells that are known to cause elevation of body temperature
C. Its synthesis is inhibited by antipyretics
D. Its primary site of action is the anterior hypothalamus

55. Which of the following statements regarding syphilitic aortitis is/are true?

A. It causes characteristic calcification in the arch of the aorta
B. It is one cause of dissecting aortic aneurysm
C. It occurs as a result of congenital syphilis
D. It is associated with neurosyphilis in about 75% of cases
E. It can cause aortic stenosis

56. Which of the following statements regarding plague is/are correct?

A. In the United States it usually occurs in the Southeast
B. In severe cases it often causes neutropenia
C. It is transmitted from rats to men by lice
D. High-dose penicillin is the treatment of choice
E. It commonly causes disseminated intravascular coagulation

57. Which of the following statements regarding shigellosis is/are correct?

A. The incubation period is 36 to 72 hours
B. It has become rare in the United States over the past decade
C. Many mononuclear leukocytes appear in the stool
D. It usually causes inflammation in both the colon and the small bowel
E. Treatment with antibiotics may prolong the carrier state

58. Which of the following statements regarding varicella-zoster is/are true?

A. A susceptible child exposed to a patient with shingles (herpes zoster) has about a 50% chance of developing chickenpox
B. The secondary attack rate in susceptible children exposed to chickenpox is greater than 80%
C. Inapparent (subclinical) infections with chickenpox are common
D. Up to one third of adults with chickenpox will show evidence of pneumonia
E. Therapy with adenine arabinoside (ara-A) is effective in the immunocompromised host

59. Enteroviruses cause

A. herpangina
B. pericarditis and myocarditis
C. pleurodynia
D. hand-foot-and-mouth disease

60. Which of the following statements regarding live attenuated mumps virus vaccine is/are true?

A. It is contraindicated in children with eczema
B. It protects more than 90% of recipients
C. When combined with measles and rubella vaccines, it should be given to children 9 to 12 months old
D. It induces an inapparent infection that is noncommunicable
E. Children with leukemia should be protected with it

61. Pneumococcal capsular polysaccharide

A. can be detected in the blood, urine, and cerebrospinal fluid of patients with pneumococcal meningitis
B. confers virulence on pneumococci
C. forms the basis for distinguishing more than 80 individual pneumococcal types
D. causes fever, toxemia, and shock in severe cases of pneumococcal disease

62. Which of the following statements regarding mucormycosis (zygomycosis) is/are true?

A. It most often affects patients with serious underlying diseases like diabetes, cancer, or uremia
B. It causes thrombosis in small and medium arteries
C. It causes lung lesions that are clinically indistinguishable from *Aspergillus* bronchopneumonia
D. The rhinocerebral form of the disease often responds to therapy with amphotericin B alone

63. A 7-year-old child with meningococcal meningitis dies in the hospital despite appropriate treatment. Who should receive chemoprophylaxis?

A. The child's parents
B. The child's classmates in school
C. The child's siblings
D. The nurses and residents who cared for the child in the hospital

64. Manifestations of tetanus include

A. extreme hypertension and sudden bradycardia
B. hyperpyrexia, with major losses of salt and water through sweating
C. supraventricular tachycardia
D. vasoconstriction

65. *Mycoplasma pneumoniae* pneumonia

A. is often associated with headache
B. is often associated with pharyngitis, and sometimes with bullous myringitis
C. occurs most often in winter
D. usually causes bilateral infiltrates

66. Colorado tick fever

A. is best treated with tetracycline
B. often has a biphasic course lasting about one week
C. has an incubation period of three to seven days
D. often causes striking leukopenia

67. Which of the following statements regarding cutaneous diphtheria is/are true?

A. It occurs commonly among poor children in underdeveloped tropical countries
B. Diphtheritic myocarditis or neuropathy are occasional complications
C. It is infectious for contacts
D. It should be treated with antitoxin, intravenously

68. Pulmonary *Nocardia asteroides* infection

A. is a relatively common complication in alveolar proteinosis
B. may be associated with abscesses in skin and brain
C. is often a self-limited disease
D. should be treated with high-dose sulfadiazine

69. The prognosis for a patient with infective endocarditis is much worse if there is

A. aortic valve involvement with heart failure
B. infection on a prosthetic valve
C. a high titer of circulating immune complexes
D. gross hematuria due to renal infarction

70. *Aspergillus fumigatus* is recovered repeatedly from small specimens of mucoid sputum obtained from a patient who complains of intermittent wheezing and dyspnea. Which of the following is/are likely to be true?

A. Precipitins to *Aspergillus* are present in the serum
B. Counterimmunoelectrophoresis (CIE) will show *Aspergillus* antigen in the blood and sputum
C. Eosinophilia is present in the peripheral blood
D. The patient should receive a course of amphotericin B, intravenously

71. Meningitis due to *Escherichia coli*

A. is usually caused by strains carrying the K100 antigen
B. is frequently complicated by ventriculitis
C. is most common in children between 1 and 5 years of age
D. results in a mortality rate of approximately 50%

72. Fecal polymorphonuclear leukocytes (PMNs) are likely to be found in which of the following disorders?

A. Traveler's diarrhea
B. Staphylococcal enterocolitis
C. Ulcerative colitis
D. Shigellosis

73. Antiviral agents effective in prophylaxis or therapy of viral infections include

A. amantadine
B. thiosemicarbazone
C. adenine arabinoside (ara-A)
D. idoxuridine

74. A patient recovering from untreated secondary syphilis has approximately a

A. 25% chance of relapsing, with recurrent manifestations of secondary syphilis
B. 30% chance of developing tertiary syphilis
C. 10% chance of developing cardiovascular syphilis
D. 7% chance of developing neurosyphilis

75. Infection with *Neisseria gonorrhoeae* is asymptomatic in

A. 10 to 20% of men with urethral infection
B. most patients with pharyngeal infection
C. most patients with rectal infection
D. most women with gonococcal pelvic inflammatory disease

76. The Weil-Felix reaction

A. is specific for rickettsial disease
B. is a simple agglutination reaction
C. turns positive after three weeks of illness
D. occasionally yields false-positive results in patients with leptospirosis or *Proteus* infections

77. Acute gastroenteritis due to rotaviruses

A. usually occurs during winter months
B. is unusual in patients over 4 years of age
C. usually causes leukocytes to appear in stools
D. has an incubation period of one to four days

78. Legionnaires' disease

A. has a case-fatality rate of 5% in otherwise healthy persons
B. is more common in immunosuppressed hosts
C. commonly causes diarrhea
D. is caused by a fastidious anaerobic bacterium that will not grow on agar

79. *Cryptococcus neoformans*

A. rarely causes meningitis except in severely immunosuppressed patients
B. must be treated with antifungal agents once diagnosis of pulmonary infection is confirmed
C. is often moderately resistant to amphotericin B *in vitro*
D. usually disseminates from a primary focus in the lung

80. The Jarisch-Herxheimer reaction has been reported to occur during the early stages of treatment of

A. toxoplasmosis
B. syphilis
C. Q fever
D. leptospirosis

81. Which of the following has/have been shown to cause immune-complex nephritis?

A. *Plasmodium vivax*
B. *Treponema pallidum*
C. *Schistosoma mansoni*
D. *Streptococcus sanguis*

82. Which of the following predispose(s) a patient to tuberculosis?

A. Diabetes mellitus
B. Hodgkin's disease
C. Silicosis
D. Gastrectomy

83. BCG (bacille Calmette-Guérin) vaccine

A. is a strain of *Mycobacterium bovis* with attenuated virulence
B. provides protection against leprosy
C. is about 80% effective in preventing tuberculosis
D. reduces the incidence of tuberculous meningitis

84. Pseudomembranous colitis

A. is a complication of therapy with lincomycin or clindamycin, but does not occur with other antibiotics
B. is caused by a toxin produced by clostridia
C. often responds to treatment with vancomycin
D. should be treated with inhibitors of peristalsis, such as diphenoxylate and atropine (Lomotil)

85. Cholera

A. will infect many patients who ingest as few as 1000 vibrios
B. occurs with increased incidence in patients who have undergone total or subtotal gastrectomy
C. produces an enterotoxin that stimulates adenyl cyclase
D. damages the small-bowel mucosa, releasing leukocytes into the stool

86. Cutaneous anthrax characteristically causes

A. severe pain
B. intense, local, nonpitting edema around an ulcer
C. lymphangitis and large regional lymph nodes
D. a papule that becomes necrotic, forming an ulcer covered with a dark-colored eschar

87. Congenital toxoplasmosis causes

A. microphthalmia
B. hydrocephalus
C. retinochoroiditis
D. liver abscess

88. Giardiasis

A. affects predominantly the small, not the large, intestine
B. need not be treated if the patient is asymptomatic
C. causes malabsorption
D. occurs more commonly in patients with hypogammaglobulinemia than in normal patients

89. Leptospirosis

A. causes fewer than 100 reported cases each year in the United States
B. has an incubation period of about ten days, ranging from two to 26 days
C. is typically a biphasic illness
D. has approximately 10% mortality

90. Pulmonary infection with atypical mycobacteria

A. most often affects young children
B. causes multiple thin-walled cavities and slowly progressive fibrosis
C. usually results in death
D. seldom occurs in previously normal lungs

91. Rat-bite fever is caused by an organism that

A. induces fever, arthritis, and a morbilliform, petechial rash over the feet and hands
B. is transmitted by a bite from an ill, infected rat
C. responds to treatment with penicillin or tetracycline
D. cannot be cultured

92. Which of the following antimicrobials will appear in significant quantities in breast milk if given to a nursing mother?

A. Chloroquine
B. Sulfonamides
C. Chloramphenicol
D. Tetracyclines

93. Acute epiglottitis

A. is often associated with bacteremia
B. is usually caused by *Hemophilus parainfluenzae*
C. is uncommon in neonates and in children over 6 years old
D. should be treated with ampicillin alone

94. Which of the following organisms cause(s) food poisoning?

A. *Staphylococcus aureus*
B. *Clostridium perfringens*
C. *Bacillus cereus*
D. *Bacteroides fragilis*

95. Which of the following statements regarding typhoid fever is/are true?

A. Chloramphenicol reduces the likelihood that patients will become chronic carriers of *Salmonella typhi*
B. About 20% of patients become chronic carriers of *S. typhi*
C. It does not occur in subjects who already have antibodies to common *S. typhi* antigens
D. Relapse is more common after chloramphenicol treatment than after no treatment

96. The common cold may be caused by

A. rotavirus
B. parainfluenza 1, 2, 3
C. influenza A, B
D. respiratory syncytial virus

97. Measles vaccine

A. is a killed virus preparation
B. provides greater than 90% protection against measles
C. should be administered to children at 12 months of age
D. should be given as a booster on entering school

98. Scarlet fever

A. causes a red rash on the palms and soles
B. usually causes desquamation of the skin
C. commonly causes eosinophilia
D. does not result in glomerulonephritis

99. Strains of gonococci that cause disseminated infection are likely to show

A. a need for special nutritional supplements *in vitro*
B. extreme sensitivity to penicillin
C. relative resistance to lysis by complement
D. a tendency to cause asymptomatic infection

100. Acute suppurative otitis media is often caused by

A. *Streptococcus pyogenes*
B. *Streptococcus pneumoniae*
C. *Hemophilus influenzae*
D. *Pseudomonas aeruginosa*

101. Clostridial myonecrosis (gas gangrene) usually should be treated with

A. gentamicin
B. polyvalent antitoxin
C. penicillin
D. hyperbaric oxygen

102. Complications of *Mycoplasma pneumoniae* pneumonia include which of the following?

A. One or more relapses
B. Meningoencephalitis or Guillain-Barré syndrome
C. Stevens-Johnson syndrome
D. Pancreatitis or hepatitis

103. Which of the following statements about brucellosis is/are true?

A. It is more likely to affect women than men
B. Clinically, it may resemble rheumatic fever, with arthritis, myocarditis, and pericarditis
C. It may cause vertebral osteomyelitis
D. It is usually diagnosed by serology, rather than by blood or bone marrow culture

104. A previously asymptomatic 53-year-old man admitted for a diaphragmatic myocardial infarction was noted to have a coin lesion in the right upper lobe on a routine chest x-ray. After recovering from the myocardial infarction, he underwent thoracotomy and resection of the nodule, which grew *Cryptococcus neoformans* on culture. Which of the following would you now do?

A. Perform a bone scan
B. Perform a spinal tap
C. Administer amphotericin B intravenously over a six-month period
D. Re-evaluate the patient at regular intervals

105. False-positive, nonspecific serologic tests for syphilis are associated with which of the following?

A. Narcotic addiction
B. Old age
C. Malaria
D. Lymphoma

106. Pneumococcal infections are associated with which of the following?

A. Hypogammaglobulinemia
B. Congenital or acquired asplenia
C. Cerebrospinal fluid rhinorrhea
D. Recurrent bacterial meningitis

DIRECTIONS: Questions 107 to 202 are matching questions. For each numbered item, select the most likely associated lettered item from those provided. Each numbered item has ONLY ONE answer. Within each group, each lettered item may be the answer to one, more than one, or none of the numbered items, unless otherwise specified.

QUESTIONS 107–112

For each of the following patients, choose the most appropriate therapy.

A. Institute isoniazid therapy; check the tuberculin skin test (PPD) in three months, and if it is negative discontinue therapy
B. Institute isoniazid therapy for one year
C. Observe without therapy

107. A 1-year-old girl who lives in the same house with a parent recently diagnosed as having active tuberculosis

108. A 25-year-old man with a positive intermediate-strength tuberculin skin test (PPD); roentgenogram of the chest is normal; no previous skin tests have been performed

109. A 50-year-old man with a positive intermediate-strength PPD; roentgenogram of the chest is normal; no previous skin tests have been performed

110. A 50-year-old man with a positive intermediate-strength PPD; no previous skin tests have been performed; roentgenogram of the chest shows apical scarring, but a chest film taken five years ago also shows the same changes

111. A 50-year-old man with a positive intermediate-strength PPD; a skin test performed 18 months ago was negative; roentgenogram of the chest is normal

112. A 25-year-old man with a positive intermediate-strength PPD; the last skin test 18 months ago was negative; roentgenogram of the chest is normal

QUESTIONS 113–117

For each of the infections listed below, select the most appropriate antibiotic.

A. Trimethoprim-sulfamethoxazole
B. Ampicillin
C. Tetracycline
D. Metronidazole
E. Erythromycin

113. Lymphogranuloma venereum

114. Legionnaires' disease

115. Nonspecific vaginitis

116. *Listeria* meningitis

117. *Pneumocystis carinii* pneumonia

QUESTIONS 118–122

For each of the following statements, select the lettered item to which it applies.

A. Rheumatic fever
B. Poststreptococcal glomerulonephritis
C. Both of the above
D. Neither of the above

118. Known to follow streptococcal impetigo

119. Known to follow streptococcal pharyngitis

120. Prevented by penicillin therapy

121. Probably immunologic in origin

122. Prophylactic therapy is required to prevent recurrences

QUESTIONS 123–127

For each of the diseases listed below, select the most likely etiologic agent.

A. *Chlamydia trachomatis*
B. *Neisseria gonorrhoeae*
C. *Escherichia coli*
D. *Ureaplasma urealyticum*

123. Afebrile neonatal pneumonia

124. Acute epididymitis in men over 35

125. Urethral syndrome

126. Community-acquired urinary tract infection

127. Arthritis-dermatitis syndrome

QUESTIONS 128–133

For each of the characteristics listed below, indicate whether it is associated primarily with:

A. Tuberculoid leprosy
B. Lepromatous leprosy
C. Both

128. Positive skin test to lepromin

129. Skin biopsy that shows epithelioid cells, Langhans' giant cells, and no *Mycobacterium leprae* organisms

130. Skin biopsy that shows many *Mycobacterium leprae* organisms and foamy histiocytes

131. Few skin lesions asymmetrically distributed

132. Nasopharyngeal shedding of *Mycobacterium leprae*

133. Erythema nodosum leprosum

QUESTIONS 134–138

For each of the following patients, select the most appropriate therapeutic regimen.

A. Amphotericin B, 0.3 mg/kg intravenously daily plus flucytosine, 150 mg/kg orally daily in four divided doses, for a total of six weeks
B. Amphotericin B, 0.5 mg/kg intravenously daily to a total dose of 1 to 2 gm
C. Amphotericin B, 0.5 to 1.0 mg/kg intravenously daily to a total dose of at least 2.0 gm plus intrathecal or intraventricular amphotericin B, 0.5 mg three times per week

D. Adenine arabinoside (ara-A), 15 mg/kg intravenously daily for ten days
E. Ampicillin, 1.5 gm intravenously every four hours for at least two weeks
F. Supportive care; no chemotherapy is indicated

134. A 27-year-old man with acute leukemia has headache and fever. Lumbar puncture reveals the CSF to have a glucose of 25 mg/dl, protein of 75 mg/dl, and a positive serologic test for the antigen to *Cryptococcus neoformans*.

135. A 65-year-old man with stage IV-B lymphoma who recently completed a course of chemotherapy with cyclophosphamide (Cytoxan), vincristine, and prednisone develops signs and symptoms of meningitis. Examination of CSF reveals gram-positive rods.

136. A 40-year-old Filipino man travels to California for a visit, and after two weeks develops a febrile illness with a nonproductive cough that resolves without treatment in about ten days. Several months later he begins to have headaches and low-grade fever that gradually progress over two to three weeks. Lumbar puncture reveals abnormal CSF containing antibody for *Coccidioides immitis*.

137. A 20-year-old college student comes to the emergency room because of the sudden onset of headache, fever to 102° F, stiff neck, and nausea. Lumbar puncture reveals CSF with normal glucose, slightly elevated protein, and 65 cells/cu mm (all lymphocytes). No organisms are seen on Gram stain of the CSF.

138. A 19-year-old woman is admitted to the neurology service with photophobia, fever, agitation, and meningismus. Her condition progresses to delirium in several hours. Temporal lobe seizures are documented by the neurologist. Computerized tomography shows an enhanced area in the frontotemporal region.

QUESTIONS 139–143

For each of the infections listed below, select the cerebrospinal fluid data with which it is most likely to be associated. Each set of CSF findings should be used only once.

Leukocytes	Protein	Glucose	Culture
A. Few to 1000s; lymphocytes predominate (PMNs seen early in disease)	Elevated	Usually normal	Usually negative
B. Several to 1000s; PMNs predominate	Elevated	Usually decreased (<2/3 of serum value)	Usually diagnostic
C. Few to 100s; lymphocytes predominate	Elevated	Markedly decreased (usually <40 mg/dl)	Diagnostic in ~50% of cases
D. None to several hundred; lymphocytes predominate	Elevated	Decreased in ≈50% of cases	Usually negative
E. Few to several hundred; usually mixed PMNs and lymphocytes	Elevated	Usually normal	Usually negative

139. Fungal meningitis *(Cryptococcus, Coccidioides)*

140. Bacterial meningitis

141. Viral meningitis

142. Brain abscess

143. Tuberculous meningitis

QUESTIONS 144–147

For each of the clinical situations below, select the therapeutic or diagnostic modality most likely to be useful.

A. Antibiotics and daily leukocyte transfusions
B. Empiric use of an aminoglycoside and carbenicillin
C. Open lung biopsy
D. Amphotericin B, isoniazid, rifampin, and erythromycin
E. Trimethoprim-sulfamethoxazole
F. Bronchoscopy with bronchial lavage for culture

144. Documented *Pseudomonas aeruginosa* septicemia not responding to antibiotic therapy in a granulocytopenic patient with acute leukemia

145. Acute, rapidly progressing, diffuse pulmonary infiltrates in a 61-year-old man undergoing chemotherapy for non-Hodgkin's lymphoma

146. An afebrile 6-year-old girl about to receive therapy for just-diagnosed lymphocytic leukemia

147. An acute fever spike in a 27-year-old man with leukemia. There are fewer than 500 circulating granulocytes per cu mm, but no obvious source of infection. The granulocytopenia was documented over the last two days.

QUESTIONS 148–153

For each of the antimicrobials listed below, select its mode of action.

A. Inhibition of cell wall synthesis
B. Inhibition of enzymes requiring pyridoxal as a cofactor
C. Binding to 50S ribosomes, interfering with protein synthesis
D. Binding to 30S ribosomes, interfering with protein synthesis
E. Interaction with sterols in cell membranes of pathogenic microbes

148. Vancomycin

149. Amphotericin B

150. Cefazolin

151. Erythromycin

152. Tobramycin

153. Chloramphenicol

QUESTIONS 154–158

For each of the rickettsiae listed below, select the disease it causes and its usual arthropod vector.

A. Trench fever, body louse
B. Endemic (murine) typhus, flea
C. Epidemic typhus, body louse
D. Rocky Mountain spotted fever, tick
E. Scrub typhus, chigger (trombiculid mite)

154. *R. typhi (mooseri)*

155. *R. prowazekii*

156. *R. rickettsii*

157. *R. tsutsugamushi*

158. *R. quintana*

QUESTIONS 159–163

For each of the helminths listed below, select the drug that is most appropriate for its treatment.

A. Diethylcarbamazine
B. Niridazole
C. Thiabendazole
D. Suramin
E. Niclosamide

159. *Schistosoma haematobium*

160. *Trichinella spiralis*

161. *Onchocerca volvulus* (adult worms)

162. *Wuchereria bancrofti*

163. *Taenia saginata*

QUESTIONS 164–168

For each of the diseases due to *Aspergillus* listed below, select the most appropriate treatment.

A. Amphotericin B
B. Flucytosine
C. A surgical procedure
D. A surgical procedure plus amphotericin B
E. None of the above

164. Necrotizing *Aspergillus* bronchopneumonia

165. *Aspergillus* endocarditis

166. Allergic bronchopulmonary aspergillosis

167. Aspergilloma in a lung cavity causing repeated hemoptysis

168. *Aspergillus* brain abscess

QUESTIONS 169–173

For each of the indications for penicillin therapy listed below, select the most appropriate preparation and dosage of penicillin for initial therapy.

A. Benzathine penicillin G, 1.2 million units intramuscularly monthly
B. Benzathine penicillin G, 2.4 million units intramuscularly weekly
C. Procaine penicillin G, 4.8 million units intramuscularly, plus probenecid, 1.0 gm orally
D. Procaine penicillin G, 1.2 million units intramuscularly twice daily
E. Aqueous penicillin G, 24 million units intravenously daily

169. Late latent syphilis

170. Gonorrhea

171. Pneumococcal pneumonia

172. Pneumococcal meningitis

173. Prevention of rheumatic fever

QUESTIONS 174–179

Below are six descriptions of ulcers occurring on the genitals. For each, select the most appropriate diagnosis.

A. Syphilis
B. Herpes simplex virus type 2
C. Behçet's syndrome
D. Chancroid
E. Lymphogranuloma venereum
F. Granuloma inguinale

174. A vesicle forms on the penis, breaks down to form a small ulcer, and heals in a week; the patient then develops enlarged, matted, painful inguinal nodes, which later discharge pus through two sinus tracts

175. A single painless, clean-based, indurated ulcer with raised, firm borders at the anal margin in a male homosexual; there is no inguinal adenopathy

176. Five shallow, very painful ulcers on the shaft of the penis, 3 mm across and 2 mm apart, healing and then recurring three times in seven months

177. Two painful, exudative, nonindurated ulcers at the border of the glans penis, with regional lymphadenopathy; material from the ulcer is negative on dark-field examination; aspirate from a suppurating inguinal lymph node grows a species of *Hemophilus*

178. A single circular, painless ulcer with a sharply demarcated margin on the shaft of the penis; material from the ulcer is negative on dark-field examination, but pleomorphic coccobacilli can be found within monocytes

179. Four painless, punched-out ulcers on the scrotum in a patient with concomitant oral ulcers and superficial thrombophlebitis

QUESTIONS 180–186

For each of the protozoa listed below, select the drug that is most appropriate for its treatment.

A. Sodium stibogluconate (Pentostam, pentavalent antimony)
B. Pyrimethamine and sulfadiazine
C. Metronidazole
D. Trimethoprim-sulfamethoxazole
E. Suramin
F. Pyrimethamine, sulfadiazine, and quinine

180. *Entamoeba histolytica*

181. *Leishmania donovani*

182. *Plasmodium falciparum*

183. *Trichomonas vaginalis*

184. *Toxoplasma gondii*

185. *Pneumocystis carinii*

186. *Giardia lamblia*

QUESTIONS 187–193

For each of the patients listed below, select the group of organisms that is MOST LIKELY to cause secondary infections.

A. Herpes zoster, *Cryptococcus, Listeria, Mycobacteria*
B. *Pseudomonas, Staphylococcus aureus*
C. *Staphylococcus aureus, Pseudomonas, Klebsiella, Serratia, Enterobacter, Escherichia coli*
D. *Pneumococcus, Salmonella*
E. Cytomegalovirus, *Cryptococcus, Nocardia,* hepatitis B virus

187. Renal transplant recipient receiving steroids and azathioprine

188. Child with chronic granulomatous disease

189. Patient with Hodgkin's disease

190. Child with sickle cell anemia

191. Patient with acute myeloid leukemia who is neutropenic as a result of chemotherapy

192. Elderly patient with obstructive pulmonary disease who is recovering slowly in the intensive care unit after lobectomy for a pulmonary mass

193. Child with cystic fibrosis

QUESTIONS 194–199

For each of the antimicrobial agents listed below, select the most characteristic group of side effects.

A. Anemia, pancytopenia, "gray baby" syndrome
B. Nausea, vomiting, photosensitivity dermatitis, acute fatty liver, staining of teeth
C. Nephrotoxicity, ototoxicity, neuromuscular blockade
D. Nausea, vomiting, diarrhea, pseudomembranous colitis, leukopenia
E. Folic acid deficiency, hemolytic anemia
F. Nephrotoxicity, ototoxicity, phlebitis

194. Clindamycin

195. Trimethoprim-sulfamethoxazole

196. Doxycycline

197. Gentamicin

198. Chloramphenicol

199. Vancomycin

QUESTIONS 200–202

Match the age-range listed below with the organism most likely to cause septic arthritis in that age-group.

A. *Streptococcus pyogenes*
B. *Staphylococcus aureus*
C. *Streptococcus pneumoniae*
D. *Neisseria gonorrhoeae*
E. *Hemophilus influenzae* type b

200. 0 to 15 years of age

201. 16 to 50 years of age

202. >50 years of age

PART 8

INFECTIOUS DISEASES

ANSWERS

1. (D) This is a classic presentation of a patient with chancroid (soft chancre). The disease is caused by *Hemophilus ducreyi,* a gram-negative pleomorphic bacillus. Classically, patients present with a painful genital lesion that has a necrotic base and nonindurated edges. Lymphadenopathy occurs in about 50% of patients, usually unilaterally (two thirds of those with adenopathy). The therapy of choice is sulfisoxazole, 1 gm four times daily for 10 to 14 days. Alternatively, tetracycline, 500 mg four times daily, can be used. *(Cecil, pp. 1572–1573; Braude, pp. 1230–1232)*

2. (C) This patient has lymphogranuloma venereum, a disease caused by *Chlamydia trachomatis.* The presentation is atypical in that the primary, painless genital lesion is usually transient and is not present when adenopathy develops. The remainder of the presentation, however, is classic. Adenopathy is usually painful and bilateral. In about 10 to 20% of patients, nodes above and below the inguinal ligament are involved, giving rise to the classic "groove sign." With time, nodes may become fluctuant and drain. Chlamydiae are sensitive to tetracycline, erythromycin, and sulfonamides, but tetracycline is the drug of choice. *(Cecil, pp. 1571–1572; Braude, pp. 1227–1230)*

3. (A) Women with the urethral syndrome fall into one of three groups: (1) those with low-grade bladder bacteriuria (usually *Escherichia coli*); (2) those with infections due to *Chlamydia trachomatis;* and (3) those without an identifiable etiologic agent. Patients in the first two categories frequently have pyuria and will respond to tetracycline therapy. Those without a known etiologic agent do *not* have pyuria, and usually have a self-limited disease that does not require antibiotic therapy. *(Stamm et al.)*

4. (C) The most likely etiologic agent in this setting is *Pasteurella multocida,* an aerobic, gram-negative bacillus that is part of the oral flora of many cats and dogs. Infections with this organism occur more commonly after cat bites than after dog bites. The interval between the injury and the onset of symptoms is short (less than 24 hours). The infection progresses rapidly, and by the time the patient seeks medical attention the wound is usually purulent, with a surrounding cellulitis; local adenopathy is commonly present, and there may be associated systemic symptoms such as fever and malaise. The most rapid way of making a diagnosis is by demonstration of gram-negative rods on Gram stain of the wound, although definitive diagnosis depends upon culturing the organism. *Staphylococcus aureus* and streptococci cause most infections that become clinically evident more than 24 hours after a bite injury, and Gram stain in that setting will show gram-positive cocci in pairs, chains, and clusters. *(Braude, p. 1788).*

5. (C) Several studies have shown that prophylactic antibiotics, in order to be effective, should be started immediately before surgery. The exception to this is oral, nonabsorbable antibiotics used for bowel surgery. Too early use of antibiotics (one to two days before) only promotes resistant organisms and therefore may impair the drug's effectiveness in decreasing the postoperative infection rate. The postoperative infection rate has been shown to decrease with the use of prophylactic antibiotics in vaginal hysterectomy and in high-risk cesarean sections, as well as in clean orthopedic surgery for implanting a prosthetic hip. Antibiotics are not indicated in cardiac catheterization, and there are no convincing data on the usefulness of prophylactic antibiotics in clean neurosurgical procedures not involving a shunt. *(Cecil, p. 82; Conte; Lett et al.; Jennings)*

6. (D) Pneumococcal vaccine is contraindicated in persons less than 2 years of age. It is indicated in persons with underlying chronic diseases such as heart disease, COPD, diabetes, alcoholism with cirrhosis, and chronic renal failure. It is also recommended for anyone over 2 years of age who has had a splenectomy, and for the elderly and the immunocompromised host. *(Cecil, p. 1426; Mandell, Douglas, and Bennett, pp. 1601–1602)*

7. (B) Acute vertebral osteomyelitis is commonly seen in drug addicts. The therapy of choice in adults is at least four weeks of the appropriate parenteral antibiotic. No oral antibiotic therapy is generally recommended for adults with this disorder. Strict immobilization with a body cast is not needed; simple bed rest suffices. *(Cecil, pp. 1470–1471; Mandell, Douglas, and Bennett, pp. 946–956)*

8. (A) Filaria live and mature in lymphatics, where they cause an allergic inflammatory reaction typified by chronic lymphadenopathy and lymphangitis. Lymphatic obstruction causes chronic edema, which may progress to elephantiasis. Inflammatory reaction to the worms also occurs in the testis and epididymis. Chyluria may result from obstruction of lymphatics in the kidney or bladder. A "Calabar swelling" is a subcutaneous reaction to adult worms of another distinct filarial species, *Loa loa. (Cecil, pp. 1774–1775; Braude, pp. 1502, 1621–1622)*

9. (B) Although monkeypox is a related disease, no animal reservoir for smallpox has been found. Total eradication of the disease by elimination of human cases is therefore possible. Vaccination of contacts and travelers and early diagnosis of outbreaks by public health teams are important in smallpox control. Serious outbreaks that have occurred in populations with a high percentage of vaccinees demonstrate that the existence of "herd immunity" does not eliminate the risk of an outbreak of smallpox. *(Cecil, 1659–1660)*

10. (E) This woman is susceptible to rubella, and if she acquires it during the first trimester there is a 30 to 50% chance that the fetus will suffer significant congenital defects. However, brief exposure to a child with rubella will not always transmit infection. Therefore, she should be re-tested in two to three weeks; if the HI titer has risen significantly, infection has occurred and therapeutic abortion should be advised. Ara-A has no effect on the rubella virus, since it is an RNA virus. Human immunoglobulin may mask infection without protecting the fetus, and should not be given, except in the special case in which it is known at the outset that the mother will certainly refuse an abortion, even if infection occurs. In this circumstance, answer D would be correct, since human gamma globulin probably offers some protection against infection of the fetus. Vaccination during pregnancy is contraindicated, because it is already too late to prevent natural infection from the contact and because the live vaccine virus theoretically could infect the fetus and cause congenital anomalies. *(Cecil, p. 1641; Braude, pp. 1693–1694)*

11. (B) Vancomycin can be given orally to treat staphylococcal enterocolitis or to help eliminate normal bowel flora, in which case it is combined with other nonabsorbable antibiotics. It is an irritant substance that should never be given intramuscularly. It is active against gram-positive organisms, including some gram-positive anaerobes. It does not cause peripheral neuropathy. It should be given in reduced dosage in cases of renal failure, but has proved very useful for treatment of shunt infections in patients on dialysis. *(Cecil, pp. 78, 1472)*

12. (D) All these organisms are capable of playing an etiologic role in gas-forming cellulitis except *P. aeruginosa*, which does not produce gas. *C. perfringens* causes cellulitis with gas in the tissues, or classic clostridial myonecrosis (gas gangrene). Two or more of the species listed are often present together in the tissues in a case of cellulitis with gas formation. *(Cecil, p. 1494)*

13. (E) The patient should be tested for HB_sAg, since he may not be a chronic carrier. If he is antigen-negative, no further action is required. The nurse should be tested for antibody to hepatitis B; if she is antibody-positive, no further action is required, since she already has humoral immunity of the same type that could be given by passive immunization with human serum globulin. The nurse should also be tested for HB_sAg, since she herself may have had a recent inapparent infection or be a chronic carrier. *If* the patient is HB_sAg-positive and the nurse is antibody-negative, the nurse should be given H-BIG, as in answer A. *(Cecil, pp. 784–785; Morbidity and Mortality Weekly Report, 1977)*

14. (A) Pneumococcal meningitis is most likely in a 46-year-old with probable CSF rhinorrhea. *Hemophilus influenzae* type b is unlikely in this setting, so ampicillin plus chloramphenicol is not required initially. Staphylococcal infection is possible, as are a host of other bacterial pathogens that occasionally cause meningitis in adults. The best approach is to treat with high-dose penicillin, observe the early course closely, and be ready to re-tap without hesitation as early as six to 12 hours later if progress is not satisfactory. Counterimmunoelectrophoresis of CSF is sometimes helpful by detecting species-specific bacterial antigen before culture results are available. Tuberculous meningitis is very unlikely in view of the acute onset and high neutrophil count in CSF. *(Cecil, pp. 1473, 1477–1478; Braude, pp. 1234–1238)*

15. (C) *Hemophilus influenzae* type b is a common cause of facial cellulitis in young children. Pending culture of the organism from the blood or skin lesion, it is best to use both ampicillin and chloramphenicol, since these children are often seriously ill with bacteremia, and up to 15% of stains of *H. influenzae* are resistant to ampicillin in some cities. High-dose ampicillin should be adequate as initial therapy if the pathogen later proves to be *Streptococcus pyogenes*. Staphylococcal infection is possible but less likely. Anaerobic organisms are unlikely to cause facial cellulitis in young children. *(Cecil, pp. 1484–1486)*

16. (E) A deep puncture wound sustained in a barnyard is a classic example of a "tetanus-prone" wound. Surgical exploration is indicated to remove any devitalized tissue and possible foreign bodies, which may be radiolucent. *Clostridium tetani* is fully susceptible to a variety of antibiotics, including penicillin, tetracycline, and erythromycin, so an alternative antibiotic such as tetracycline can be given if the patient has a history of penicillin allergy. Because chemoprophylaxis with antibiotic may not be effective if delayed more than four to six hours after injury, this patient should receive human tetanus antitoxin prior to surgery. Since his immunization status is uncertain, he should also receive a full course of three doses of tetanus toxoid. *(Cecil, pp. 1502–1503)*

17. (C) This man probably has postgonococcal urethritis (PGU). A routine urethral culture should be obtained to exclude relapse or reinfection with gonococcus; meanwhile, he can be treated for PGU with tetracycline. Gonococcal isolates from cases of penicillin treatment failure should be tested for β-lactamase production in a local laboratory, and if positive should be reported to the CDC. PGU is frequently due to infection with *Chlamydia trachomatis (Cecil, pp. 1563–1564; Braude, pp. 1201–1203, 1209)*

18. (C) This sequence of events is typical for methicillin-induced interstitial nephritis. With eosinophilia, fever, and hematuria, the diagnosis is so likely that kidney biopsy is unnecessary in most cases. Antibiotic treatment must be continued, since 19 days of therapy is inadequate for staphylococcal endocarditis. Oxacillin and nafcillin are contraindicated, since there is a strong chance that these agents would perpetuate the nephritis. Cephalothin is a potent antistaphylococcal drug that is much less likely than methicillin to cause nephritis. Vancomycin should be kept in reserve for patients in whom semisynthetic penicillins or cephalosporins cannot be used. *(Cecil, pp. 77–78, 554; Ditlove et al.)*

19. (B) *S. mansoni* causes fibrosis of hepatic portal radicles (pipestem fibrosis). This causes portal hypertension, which in turn results in splenomegaly and esophageal varices. Hepatocellular failure, with its typical associations such as encephalopathy and spider angiomas, seldom occurs. Infections by *S. haematobium* (not *S. mansoni*) commonly cause hematuria. *(Cecil, pp. 1758–*1759; Braude, pp. 1098, 1099—1100)

20. (E) Transient upper gastrointestinal upset (cramping epigastric pains and vomiting) is common in trichinosis during the first one to two weeks, during the stage of maturation of larvae to adult worms in the upper small intestine. When the stage of muscle penetration begins, periorbital edema and splinter hemorrhages are commonly seen, along with fever, eosinophilia, and painful tender muscles. The widespread foci of inflammation cause leakage from capillaries and hypoalbuminemia. The sedimentation rate usually is normal or only slightly elevated, which is a surprising finding in a febrile, toxic patient. The larvae do not form mature cysts in myocardium, meninges, or brain, but may cause inflammation in these organs during the stage of muscle invasion. This can be fatal in very heavy infestations. The Casoni test is a skin test to detect echinococcal infection; it has no relevance to trichinosis. *(Cecil, pp. 1771–1772; Braude, pp. 1834–1835)*

21. (E) Nitrofurantoin occasionally causes a syndrome of fever, rash, eosinophilia, and pulmonary infiltrates, which may be either acute or chronic. It may also cause polyneuropathy, cholestatic hepatitis, and hemolytic anemia in patients with G6PD deficiency. Aplasia of the marrow has not been described. *(Cecil, p. 81)*

22. (C) Tularemia occurs in all seasons, being transmitted by ticks, deer flies, and mosquitoes in spring and summer and by contact with infected small game in autumn and winter. *Francisella tularensis* can be cultured (on blood-glucose-cystine agar) from ulcers and draining regional lymph nodes in ulceroglandular disease, and occasionally from bronchial secretions in those patients (about 30%) with tularemia pneumonia. The disease causes caseating granulomas and small abscesses in lymph nodes, liver, and spleen. Patients respond rapidly to treatment with tetracycline, streptomycin, or chloramphenicol. *(Cecil, 1524–1526; Braude, pp. 1791–1793, 1795)*

23. (B) Patients with chronic granulomatous disease commonly suffer *Candida* infections in addition to bacterial infections (especially those due to *Staph. aureus* and enteric bacilli). Intravenous heroin abusers are prone to endocarditis due to *Candida parapsilosis* and other *Candida* species. Debilitated and cachectic patients with a terminal malignancy (such as gastric cancer) often become infected with *Candida.* Hyperalimentation lines may become infected, causing *Candida* septicemia. Chronic cutaneous candidiasis occurs in some patients who have hypocalcemia, not hypercalcemia. *(Cecil, pp. 1706–1707)*

24. (D) CIE is an improved version of gel precipitation in which the application of an electrical gradient enhances both the speed and sensitivity of the test. It is presently being used for detection of bacterial antigens in body fluids such as CSF, pleural fluid, serum, and urine, and can be of value in rapid diagnosis of bacterial meningitis when the Gram stain is negative. It is not yet used for routine detection of gonococcal antigens, but it can detect soluble antigen derived from all the other organisms listed. *(Hoeprich, p. 123)*

25. (A) Tetracyclines should be avoided whenever possible in pregnant women and patients with renal failure, since their use in these patients sometimes causes acute fatty degeneration of the liver. Dermatitis may appear in sun-exposed areas in patients taking long-acting tetracyclines such as demethylchlortetracycline. In infants, tetracyclines can cause pseudotumor cerebri, with bulging fontanelles. In children, these drugs cause a characteristic yellowish-brown staining and hypoplasia of dental enamel. Neuromuscular blockade is a rare complication of therapy with aminoglycosides, not tetracyclines. *(Cecil, p. 80)*

26. (D) Enterobiasis (infestation with pinworms, *Enterobius vermicularis*) is often asymptomatic and is usually harmless. Migrating worms occasionally cause appendicitis, vulvitis, and prostatitis. Ischiorectal abscesses sometimes occur as a complication of perianal excoriation from itching and scratching. Major organ involvement such as in hepatitis does not occur. *(Cecil, pp. 1770–1771)*

27. (C) *Trichuris* does not have a tissue phase, and unlike *Ascaris* the larvae do not migrate through the lung. *Trichuris* eggs ingested by man hatch in the small intestine; larvae pass down into the large bowel after three to ten days. The anterior part of the worm buries deep into the colonic submucosa, from which each worm abstracts 0.005 ml blood per day. Light infections are asymptomatic; with high worm loads, colic, bloody diarrhea, prolapse of the rectum, and anemia may occur. Eosinophilia can occur, but is usually mild, since *Trichuris* is primarily an intraluminal parasite and does not cause inflammation in tissues. Eosinophilia occurs most typically in those metazoan parasitic infections in which tissue invasion occurs, such as strongyloidiasis. *(Cecil, p. 1770)*

28. (C) The advent of mebendazole, a broad-spectrum nematocide, has simplified the treatment of nematode infections in man. It may be used to treat infections caused by all the organisms listed except *Strongyloides,* which is treated with thiabendazole, 25 mg/kg twice daily for two days. *(Cecil, pp. 1764–1765; Blumenthal)*

29. (B) Trachoma causes conjunctivitis and secondary corneal scarring, but not punctate keratitis. Scabies is a common cause of an itchy, papular rash (often with secondary bacterial infection) in the tropics as well as in temperate zones, but it does not cause true subcutaneous nodules. *Loa loa* causes subcutaneous nodules ("Calabar swellings") and may migrate across the eye, but does not cause an itchy skin rash or blindness. The female guinea worm, which is up to 1 meter long, lives in the subcutaneous tissues. The anterior end emerges at the center of a chronic ulcer and discharges eggs on contact with water. Schistosomiasis does not typically affect the eye. All the findings listed in this question are typical of onchocerciasis: subcutaneous nodules are due to an inflammatory reaction to adult worms, and migrating microfilariae can produce punctate keratitis, corneal scarring, and blindness. *(Cecil, pp. 1777–1778)*

30. (A) Tropical pyomyositis is characterized by one or more large, deep-seated abscesses in voluntary muscles. The organism isolated is usually *S. aureus;* why it commonly causes pyomyositis in the tropics and not elsewhere is unknown. *Dirofilaria* is a rare cause of granulomatous nodules in skin or lung. Melioidosis (*P. pseudomallei*) usually causes abscesses in skin or lung rather than muscle. *(Cecil, p. 1472; Braude, p. 1563)*

31. (C) Infection with *Y. enterocolitica* is often misdiagnosed as appendicitis or regional enteritis, since patients have abdominal pain and diarrhea. Bacteremia is common, as is arthritis, but osteomyelitis is very rare. *(Braude, pp. 1065–1066; Jacobs)*

32. (E) Toxocariasis is due to larvae of *Toxocara cati* or *T. canis.* After a patient ingests eggs from the feces of household cats or dogs, larvae penetrate the abdominal wall and pass to liver, brain, or eye. A systemic illness characterized by mild fever, tender hepatomegaly, and eosinophilia occurs. Granulomas forming around larvae in the eye may simulate retinoblastoma. Underprivileged children living in rural areas are more prone to infection with *Toxocara.* Adult worms are rarely present in the bowel. Intestinal obstruction or intussusception is a complication of heavy *Ascaris lumbricoides* infection, not toxocariasis. *(Cecil, p. 1769; Braude, pp. 1837–1839)*

33. (C) These symptoms probably represent a Jarisch-Herxheimer reaction, which commonly occurs soon after penicillin is first given for treatment of secondary syphilis. If the symptoms are severe, as in this case, the patient should be admitted to the hospital for supportive treatment and exclusion of more serious diseases. However, the Jarisch-Herxheimer reaction is usually self-limited and not life-threatening, so intensive care units, high-dose intravenous steroids, and broad-spectrum antibiotics are not indicated. Antihistamine and aspirin may relieve the symptoms. *(Cecil, p. 1583)*

34. (A) This is a standard description of the cutaneous lymphatic form of sporotrichosis, which is an occupational disease of florists, nurserymen, and farmers that is caused by the fungus *Sporothrix schenckii.* This form of the infection usually responds slowly to iodide therapy, which may have to be continued for months. The disseminated form of the disease, which causes lesions in lungs, bones, and skin by hematogenous spread, is best treated with amphotericin B. *(Cecil, pp. 1705–1706; Braude, pp. 1573–1577)*

35. (C) Both tetracycline and streptomycin are active against *Brucella*. The best results have been obtained by using a combination of the two antibiotics, as follows: tetracycline, 2 gm/day orally in four divided doses for six weeks, plus streptomycin, 1 gm/day intramuscularly for the first two weeks. Relapses will occur in less than 5% of patients receiving this regimen. Co-trimoxazole may be active against *Brucella*, but is not a first-line drug at present. *(Cecil, pp. 1535–1537)*

36. (D) Scalded skin syndrome is caused by an epidermolytic exotoxin released by staphylococci of bacteriophage group II. Staphylococcal enterocolitis is a serious condition that occasionally occurs in patients on antibiotic therapy, or after surgery. A carbuncle is a staphylococcal skin infection consisting of a cluster of furuncles in an area of thick skin (such as the back of the neck). Acute suppurative parotitis in dehydrated, cachectic, or uremic patients is often caused by staphylococci. Ecthyma gangrenosum is a distinctive necrotic skin lesion caused by *Pseudomonas aeruginosa*, not staphylococci. *(Cecil, p. 1468–1469, 1516)*

37. (E) All the conditions listed are major manifestations of rheumatic fever (according to the revised Duckett-Jones criteria) except erythema nodosum, which is nonspecific and uncommon in rheumatic fever. Erythema marginatum is the fifth major criterion, appearing occasionally in childhood cases. This is a circinate, multiform erythema that appears on the extremities or trunk and spreads centrifugally, often coalescing to form combined lesions with serpiginous borders. This lesion is easily distinguished from erythema nodosum by its appearance. *(Cecil, p. 1453)*

38. (C) The single most important pathophysiologic feature of rickettsial disease is disseminated focal infection of capillaries, arteries, and venules. Headache, altered mental status, and hypotension are common features of rickettsial disease as well as of many other acute illnesses. The leukocyte count is usually normal or low in acute rickettsial infection. *(Cecil, pp. 1604–1605)*

39. (C) The aminoglycosides, including amikacin, bind to the 30S ribosome of bacteria in an energy-requiring reaction; these antibiotics have no significant activity against anaerobes. The other drugs listed all possess broad-spectrum antianaerobic activity, but no single drug can be relied on to inhibit all strains of anaerobes. Cefoxitin is a cephamycin compound (related to cephalosporins) that is more active than other cephalosporins against *Bacteroides* species. *(Cecil, pp. 1506–1507; Washington et al.)*

40. (D) Treatment with amphotericin B results in a wide range of side effects. Fever, rigors, headache, nausea, vomiting, and phlebitis are all common. Anaphylaxis, arrhythmias, hepatic toxicity, and thrombocytopenia occur much less often. Nephrotoxicity frequently occurs during therapy, and renal tubular acidosis may develop. Hypokalemia often requires replacement therapy with potassium. Anemia occurs owing to reversible bone-marrow suppression. Neuromuscular blockade is a complication of aminoglycoside therapy, and does not occur with amphotericin. *(Cecil, p. 81; Hoeprich, pp. 182–184)*

41. (A) Ecthyma gangrenosum is a striking skin lesion produced by *P. aeruginosa*. In immunocompromised patients, these bacilli can invade the walls of cutaneous arterioles and multiply rapidly, causing thrombosis of the vessel and infarction of overlying skin. The lesion has a dark black center surrounded by an erythematous margin, which is painful. Blood cultures are positive and the patients are seriously ill, often with bacteremic shock. *(Cecil, p. 1516; Braude, pp. 1391–1392; Dorff et al.)*

42. (B) Retinal involvement may occur as a manifestation of disseminated candidiasis and miliary tuberculosis. Uveitis is a classic complication of histoplasmosis, and choroidoretinitis is a characteristic late result of congenital infection with *T. gondii*. Infection with *Pneumocystis*, on the other hand, is limited to the lungs. *(Cecil, pp. 1553, 1699, 1707, 1741, 1743)*

43. (D) Rifampin is effective in eradicating the carrier state and is the drug of choice here. Minocycline is also effective but causes vestibular dysfunction in many patients, especially women. Sulfas are recommended as drugs of choice for prophylaxis, but *only* if the infecting strain has already been shown to be sensitive to sulfas in the laboratory. Penicillin V is not recommended. Meningococcal vaccines are given to large susceptible populations such as military recruits entering training camps, and usually are not administered to household contacts of sporadic cases. *(Cecil, p. 1483)*

44. (B) Pleocytosis and elevated CSF protein should resolve slowly after successful treatment of neurosyphilis, and VDRL titer in the CSF should fall in most patients. The *serum* VDRL titer is not a reliable indicator of disease activity in the CNS. The FTA-ABS test result is reported only as positive, negative, or equivocal; it is not titered out. FTA-ABS in CSF is of less value than the VDRL titer in assessment of neurosyphilis. CSF glucose is usually normal in neurosyphilis. *(Cecil, p. 1583)*

45. (A — False; B — True; C — False; D — True; E — True) Babesiosis is an acute, febrile illness with hemolytic anemia, caused by intraerythrocyte protozoa *(Babesia bovis, B. microti,* and so forth) that are transmitted from infected animals to man by ticks. Several cases occur yearly in the United States, mostly from Nantucket or Martha's Vineyard. Tetracycline is not effective in therapy. In the past, chloroquine has been recommended for treatment; however, studies show that parasitemia persists following treatment with chloroquine, and it is now believed that the beneficial effects of this drug are attributable to its anti-inflammatory properties. Experimental babesiosis in animals responds well to aromatic diamidines such as pentamidine. Most human cases of babesiosis are mild and require symptomatic therapy only. In splenectomized patients or those whose condition deteriorates with symptomatic treatment, pentamidine should be given. *(Cecil, pp. 1744–1746; Miller, Neva, and Gill; Ruebush and Spielman)*

46. (A — True; B — False; C — False; D — False) A number of drugs are active against *Mycobacterium leprae* including dapsone, rifampin, clofazimine, ethionamide, and prothionamide. The number of drugs used and duration of therapy depend on the form of leprosy being treated. For tuberculoid (TT) and borderline tuberculoid (BT) leprosy, the bacterial load is small and single-drug therapy is sufficient. Dapsone is the drug of choice. The duration of therapy is three years for TT and five years for BT. Forms of the disease associated with a higher tubercle burden (borderline, borderline lepromatous, and lepromatous) are treated initially with a combination of drugs — either dapsone and rifampin or dapsone and clofazimine. Both drugs are generally used for six months, and therapy then continues with dapsone alone for at least ten years.

Clofazimine not only has antibacterial activity but also has anti-inflammatory properties, and thus may be advantageous in treating erythema nodosum leprosum and lepra reactions. Thalidomide is not active against *M. leprae*, but is very useful in treating erythema nodosum leprosum. Its use is limited to postmenopausal women and to men because of its teratogenic effects. The question of who should receive prophylatic therapy is controversial, but the only drug with proved efficacy in this setting is dapsone. *(Cecil, pp. 1560–1561; Braude, pp. 1378–1385)*

47. (All are True) Pneumonia caused by *K. pneumoniae* is usually a very severe disease and characteristically is associated with tissue destruction. Multilobe involvement is common (two thirds of patients) and there is predilection for upper-lobe involvement, although any lobe can be affected. Because of the associated tissue destruction, abscess formation and the development of empyema are common. The pleural surface is covered by a fibrinous exudate, accounting for the pleuritic pain that is a complaint in 80% of patients. *K. pneumoniae* pneumonia is associated with alcoholism in 66% of cases. It is also seen in patients with chronic bronchopulmonary disease and diabetes mellitus, but its association with these diseases is not as striking as that with alcoholism. *(Cecil, pp. 1430–1432; Braude, pp. 918–921)*

48. (A — True; B — True; C — False; D — False) The bacterial etiology of aspiration pneumonia varies depending on the clinical setting. Most community-acquired aspiration pneumonia is caused by anaerobic bacteria (about two thirds) or mixtures of aerobic and anaerobic bacteria (about one fourth). In contrast, aspiration that occurs in the hospital is most commonly caused by a mixture of aerobic and anaerobic bacteria (about 60%), with aerobic bacteria alone causing about 19% of cases. In community-acquired infections, both the aerobic and anaerobic bacteria originate from the mouth and are sensitive to penicillin. In the penicillin-allergic patient, clindamycin is the most reliable antibiotic and is the most used in clinical experience. Although most patients will demonstrate pulmonary infiltrates following aspiration of acid material, this is a chemical pneumonitis, and only about 25% of patients actually develop bacterial pneumonia. *(Cecil, pp. 1435–1438)*

49. (A — True; B — True; C — False; D — True; E — True) Trimethoprim-sulfamethoxazole blocks sequential steps in folic acid biosynthesis. It affects bacterial and protozoan folate synthesis much more than it does the mammalian enzyme systems. It has a broad range of clinical uses, is often bactericidal, and is the most effective antimicrobial agent in prevention of recurrent urinary tract infections in women. It can be given as infrequently as three times per week for this purpose. Trimethoprim-sulfamethoxazole penetrates into most body tissues, including the central nervous system, and has been used to treat gram-negative meningitis in certain select situations. It is the treatment of choice for *P. carinii* pneumonia in both children and adults. In addition it is active against *H. influenzae*, including β-lactamase–producing strains. It is *inactive* against anaerobic bacteria, such as *Peptostreptococcus*, and should not be used to treat diseases caused by these organisms. *(Cecil, p. 81)*

50. (A — False; B — False; C — True; D — True; E — False) Cat-scratch disease is the most common cause of chronic regional lymphadenitis in children and adolescents in the United States. The causative agent is as yet unknown and is presumed to be a virus. Extensive studies have excluded bacteria and fungi as etiologic agents. The disease is characterized by a papule or pustule at the site of the scratch (53% of patients), followed in several weeks by regional lymphadenitis. Lymphangitis does not occur in this disease. Cats that transmit the disease should not be destroyed, since they usually appear perfectly well and transmit the unidentified causative agent for no longer than two to three weeks. The prognosis of the disease is excellent, with lymphadenopathy usually regressing spontaneously in two to three months. Antimicrobial therapy offers no benefit. *(Cecil, pp. 1695–1697)*

51. (A — False; B — False; C — True; D — False) Some animals are much more likely to be infected with rabies virus than others. Carnivores such as skunks, raccoons, coyotes, and foxes as well as bats are most commonly infected. These animals should be considered to be rabid unless they are tested and specifically shown not to be. In contrast, rodents rarely are found to have rabies and have not been known to cause human rabies in the United States. Thus, bites from these animals do not require rabies immunoprophylaxis. Since signs of rabies in wild animals cannot be interpreted reliably, any wild animal that bites or scratches a person should be killed at once and the brain then submitted for examination. The brains of animals suspected of having rabies should be examined by the fluorescent antibody technique. If this test is positive, it is assumed that rabies virus is excreted in the saliva of the animal, and immunoprophylaxis should be instituted. If the test is negative, no therapy is needed. Although the incubation period of rabies is usually long (about 20 to 60 days), one should not delay in starting immunoprophylaxis; the sooner therapy is started, the more likely it is to be effective. *(Cecil, pp. 2097–2100; Morbidity and Mortality Weekly Report, 1980)*

52. (A — True; B — False; C — False; D — False) Nongonococcal urethritis affects males and is characterized by dysuria or urethral discharge, or both. Most cases are caused by *C. trachomatis*, although *Ureaplasma urealyticum* has been identified as a causative agent in about 20% of cases. There are several ways to distinguish gonococcal from nongonococcal urethritis. Gonococcal urethritis is usually of acute onset and is associated with a spontaneous, purulent urethral discharge. Patients with nongonococcal urethritis have a less dramatic onset and usually have symptoms for several days before seeking medical attention. The discharge is more commonly mucoid than purulent and almost always requires stripping of the urethra for demonstration. Although one could culture *C. trachomatis* from the discharge, this is time-consuming and expensive. A Gram stain of the urethral exudate that demonstrates numerous polymorphonuclear leukocytes *without* gram-negative diplococci is strong presumptive evidence for the presence of nongonococcal urethritis. *(Cecil, pp. 1563–1564; Jacobs and Krauss)*

53. (A — True; B — True; C — False; D — False; E — True) Pneumococci, staphylococci, and *H. influenzae* are the most common bacterial pathogens associated with influenza A infections of the lung. Helpful clues to the presence of the bacterial infections include Gram stain and culture of sputum, a localized area of consolidation on roentgenogram, and the classic clinical story of the initial influenzal illness followed by a period of improvement and subsequent relapse owing to the superimposed bacterial infection. *(Mandell, Douglas, and Bennett, p. 1151)*

54. (A — True; B — False; C — False; D — True) Endogenous pyrogen is a low-molecular-weight protein produced by phagocytic cells including peripheral circulating leukocytes and monocytes as well as fixed tissue phagocytes such as Kupffer cells, alveolar macrophages, and splenic sinusoidal cells. A number of different *exogenous* pyrogens (endotoxin of gram-negative bacteria, androgen breakdown products, synthetic polynucleotides) can stimulate *endogenous* pyrogen synthesis. Endogenous pyrogen, however, seems to be the "final common pathway" of fever production in humans and is the only known fever-causing substance produced by the host. It acts on the preoptic area of the anterior hypothalamus and is associated with an increase in monoamines and prostaglandins in the vicinity of the thermoregulatory center. Antipyretics have no direct effect on endogenous pyrogen synthesis, but instead reduce fever indirectly by inhibiting pyrogen-induced prostaglandin synthesis. *(Cecil, pp. 1393–1394)*

55. (All are False) Congenital syphilis does not cause syphilitic aortitis — this is an unexplained phenomenon. Calcification in the arch of the aorta suggests arteriosclerosis; syphilis causes linear calcifications in the *ascending* aorta. Syphilitic aortitis does not cause dissection, and is associated with neurosyphilis in only 10 to 25% of cases. Dilatation of the ascending aorta stretches the aortic valve ring, causing aortic incompetence, not stenosis. *(Cecil, p. 1578)*

56. (A — False; B — False; C — False; D — False; E — True) Only about seven cases of plague occur in the United States each year, usually originating in southwestern or western states. Plague is transmitted from rats to man by the rat flea *(Xenopsylla cheopis)*, not by lice. Neutrophilia is typical, often reaching 30,000/cu mm or more in severe cases; such patients often also develop disseminated intravascular coagulation (DIC). (Purpura and peripheral gangrene due to DIC probably led to the term "black death.") Patients with plague should be treated with streptomycin, tetracycline, or chloramphenicol. *(Cecil, pp. 1521–1523; Braude, pp. 1796–1803)*

57. (A — True; B — False; C — False; D — False; E — False) Shigellosis has a brief incubation period of 1½ to three days. It remains a fairly common disease, especially in nursery schools and homes for the retarded; over 16,000 cases were reported in 1976 in the United States. Most cases are now caused by *Shigella sonnei*. In shigellosis, erythrocytes and polymorphonuclear leukocytes (blood and pus) are usually found in the stool, in contrast to salmonellosis, which is associated with predominantly mononuclear cells in the stool. Inflammation is usually confined to the large bowel. Both duration of symptoms and duration of fecal carriage of *Shigella* are significantly reduced by treatment with ampicillin, tetracycline, or trimethoprim-sulfamethoxazole. *(Cecil, pp. 1517–1519)*

58. (A — False; B — True; C — False; D — True; E — True) The secondary attack rate is much higher in susceptible children exposed to a case of chickenpox (87%) than after exposure to a patient with shingles (15%). Subclinical varicella infections are rare. Clinical and radiologic evidence of pneumonitis occurs in 16 to 33% of adults. In the immunocompromised host, especially patients with lymphoma, ara-A has been shown to ameliorate symptoms and prevent dissemination. *(Cecil, pp. 1654–1658; Braude, pp. 1652–1653; Whitley et al., 1976)*

59. (All are True) Enteroviruses (poliovirus, coxsackie A and B, and echovirus) cause all the syndromes listed, as well as aseptic meningitis, encephalitis, paralysis, orchitis, hepatitis, pharyngitis, and generalized disease of the newborn. *(Cecil, pp. 1663–1665)*.

60. (A — False; B — True; C — False; D — True; E — False) The vaccine is extremely safe, and there are no contraindications except allergy to egg proteins or neomycin. (All live virus vaccines should be avoided in pregnant and immunocompromised patients.) It produces a protective antibody response in more than 90% of recipients, but the duration of protection is not established, since it has been in use for only 12 years. It may be given to persons of any age above 12 months, but when combined with measles and rubella vaccines ("MMR") should not be given before age 15 months, since the immune response to measles vaccine is unreliable in younger infants. *(Cecil, p. 1644, Braude, p. 894)*

61. (A — True; B — True; C — True; D — False) Pneumococcal polysaccharide forms the capsule of smooth strains of pneumococci. This substance is associated with virulence by conferring resistance to phagocytosis. More than 80 types of pneumococci can be distinguished on the basis of antibody reactions with capsular polysaccharides. The capsular material is very stable and can be detected in body fluids during pneumococcal infection, sometimes persisting for days or weeks after recovery has occurred. Unlike endotoxin, it does not cause fever, toxemia, or shock. *(Cecil, pp. 1420–1422)*

62. (A — True; B — True; C — True; D — False) Mucormycosis is an acute, often fatal fungus infection caused by species of *Rhizopus* or *Mucor*. It has a strong tendency to affect patients with uncontrolled diabetes, especially during episodes of ketoacidosis. The characteristic infarctions of nasal turbinates or brain are due to invasion of vessels by the fungus, with subsequent thrombosis. These fungi can also cause a rapidly progressive bronchopneumonia (sometimes with infarction, necrosis, and cavity formation) that is clinically indistinguishable from *Aspergillus* bronchopneumonia. The disease has high mortality even when correctly diagnosed and treated. Rhinocerebral mucormycosis can sometimes be cured, but surgical debridement is necessary; there is little chance of curing the infection with amphotericin B alone. *(Cecil, pp. 1710–1711; Braude, pp. 850–852)*

63. (A — True; B — False; C — True; D — False) Close household contacts of a child with meningococcal disease should receive chemoprophylaxis. It is not indicated for playmates and classmates, nor for hospital staff providing routine care of the patient. However, it may be prudent to advise contacts to report immediately for evaluation if any symptoms develop. *(Cecil, p. 1483)*

64. (All are True) All these manifestations may occur in a patient with tetanus, owing to the uncoordinated overactivity of the sympathetic nervous system that is typical of the action of tetanospasmin on neural tissue. *(Cecil, pp. 1499–1501)*

65. (A — True; B — True; C — False; D — False) Headache is common in patients with mycoplasma pneumonia, as is pharyngitis. Bullous myringitis occurs in about 15% of cases. There is no seasonal clustering of cases. Although bilateral infiltrates may occur, roentgenogram of the chest usually shows a unilateral lower lobe infiltrate, more prominent near the hilum. *(Cecil, pp. 1427–1428)*

66. (A — False; B — True; C — True; D — True) Colorado tick fever is caused by an arbovirus, not rickettsiae, so antibiotic treatment is futile. The typical biphasic course, seen in 50% or more of cases, helps to differentiate this disease from Rocky Mountain spotted fever on clinical grounds. Onset of illness is three to seven days after a bite by an infected tick *(Dermacentor andersoni)*. Leukopenia is usual. *(Cecil, pp. 1676–1678; Braude, pp. 1856–1860)*

67. (A — True; B — True; C — True; D — False) Cutaneous diphtheria is common among poor children in tropical areas, and among "skid row" inhabitants in certain U.S. cities. Although strains of *Corynebacterium diphtheriae* recovered from the skin are often nontoxigenic, cutaneous diphtheria occasionally causes myocarditis or neuropathy. It is infectious for contacts, especially under crowded, dirty conditions. Poor children in underdeveloped areas may acquire immunity to pharyngeal infection from cutaneous diphtheria. This infection responds to erythromycin or penicillin. Antitoxin is not routinely indicated, because the incidence of disease due to toxin absorption is low. *(Cecil, pp. 1490–1493; Braude, pp. 817–823)*

68. (A — True; B — True; C — False; D — True) There is a strong association between alveolar proteinosis and *Nocardia* infection. Nocardiosis also occurs in patients with neoplasia or immune defects, and in renal transplant recipients. The tissues most often affected are lung, brain, and skin; in immunosuppressed patients the organism may disseminate to all these sites. The disease is usually fatal unless appropriate treatment is given; this usually consists of high-dose sulfonamide therapy. Alternatives are erythromycin or trimethoprim-sulfamethoxazole. *(Cecil, pp. 1533–1535; Hoeprich, pp. 356–364)*

69. (A — True; B — True; C — False; D — False) Heart failure is the single most important indicator of poor prognosis in infective endocarditis. The outlook is also worse in elderly patients and in patients with aortic valve involvement. Cure of prosthetic valve endocarditis often requires valve replacement, with associated increased mortality. Circulating immune complexes are present in more than 95% of patients with infective endocarditis. Their presence does not alter prognosis, therefore, but mortality is higher if immune-complex glomerulonephritis occurs and causes renal failure. Renal infarction due to emboli may cause gross hematuria and severe flank pain, but usually does not cause renal failure or affect the overall survival rate adversely. *(Cecil, p. 1465; Bayer et al.; Karchmer et al.)*

70. (A — True; B — False; C — True; D — False) This patient probably has allergic bronchopulmonary aspergillosis. Such patients usually have eosinophilia, and precipitins to *Aspergillus* are present in serum. CIE has not yet been proved useful for routine detection of *Aspergillus* antigens. Endobronchial colonization with *Aspergillus* does not respond to systemic administration of amphotericin B. *(Cecil, pp. 1708–1710)*

71. (A — False; B — True; C — False; D — True) Strains with the Kl (not K100) polysaccharide antigen are most likely to cause meningitis. Ventriculitis occurs commonly and may be a major factor in treatment failure. *E. coli* meningitis is most common before two months of age and carries approximately 50% mortality. *(Sarff et al.; Bortolussi et al.)*

72. (A — False; B — True; C — True; D — True) Shigellosis, staphylococcal enterocolitis, and ulcerative colitis are all inflammatory diseases involving the colonic mucosa, from which PMNs are shed into the lumen. Cholera, staphylococcal food poisoning, and diarrhea due to enterotoxigenic *E. coli* are not inflammatory diseases, and PMNs are not found in the stool. A few cases of traveler's diarrhea are due to shigellosis, but most are due to *E. coli;* PMNs therefore are not a frequent finding in the stools of patients suffering from "Montezuma's revenge." *(Cecil, pp. 676, 703, 1472, 1517)*

73. (All are True) Amantadine has been shown to be effective in preventing influenza during epidemics in highly susceptible groups such as elderly inpatients. Thiosemicarbazone may be effective as a prophylactic agent after exposure to smallpox. Ara-A can reduce mortality and sequelae in *Herpes simplex* encephalitis if used early, before coma supervenes. Idoxuridine is useful in topical therapy of herpes keratitis (dendritic ulcer). *(Cecil, pp. 83–86; Hoeprich, pp. 726, 735; Whitley et al., 1977)*

74. (All are True) In the well-known Oslo Study, 2000 untreated patients with syphilis were followed over a period of 60 years (1891-1951). One or more relapses of secondary syphilis occurred in about 25% of these cases. One third of all patients developed tertiary syphilis. The majority with tertiary disease had gummas involving skin, mucous membrane, or skeleton; about 10% had cardiovascular syphilis; and about 7% developed neurosyphilis. *(Cecil, p. 1575; Gjestland)*

75. (A — True; B — True; C — True; D — False) *N. gonorrhoeae* often causes asymptomatic infections. It is well known that most women with gonorrhea have few or no symptoms, but less well known that 10 to 20% of males with gonococcal urethritis are also asymptomatic. These men are particularly important in spreading infection, since they often remain untreated. Gonococci can cause sore throat and severe proctitis, but most patients with throat and rectal infections are asymptomatic. Pelvic inflammatory disease, however, usually causes acute or subacute pain in the lower abdomen or low back, and striking tenderness on pelvic examination. *(Cecil, pp. 1567, 1568)*

76. (A — False; B — True; C — False; D — True) The Weil-Felix reaction is a simple agglutination test based on polysaccharide antigens shared between *Proteus* OX-2, OX-19, and OX-K, and certain rickettsiae. By its nature, therefore, it is a nonspecific test. False-positive results may occur during leptospirosis, relapsing fever, and *Proteus* infections. One reason why this nonspecific test has remained useful is that it turns positive early, at the end of the first week of illness. *(Cecil, p. 1606)*

77. (A — True; B — True; C — False; D — True) Rotaviruses are probably the commonest cause of acute gastroenteritis in small children. Rotavirus may affect neonates, is most common between 6 and 24 months of age, and is unusual after 4 years of age. The disease is most common in winter (it is sometimes called "winter vomiting disease"), and may occur sporadically or in epidemics. Incubation period during epidemics is one to four days. Fecal leukocytes are usually absent; this helps to differentiate acute viral gastroenteritis from shigellosis. *(Cecil, pp. 1670–1671; Braude, pp. 1106–1107)*

78. (A — True; B — True; C — True; D — False) The case-fatality ratio for Legionnaires' disease is quite low (about 5%) in otherwise healthy people, but may be as high as 30% in the presence of underlying chronic conditions such as cardiorespiratory disease. The disease occurs with increased incidence in immunosuppressed hosts, especially patients with renal transplants taking immunosuppressive drugs. About 50% of patients have diarrhea. The organism is an aerobic bacterium that forms colonies slowly (three to five days) on supplemented Mueller-Hinton agar. *(Cecil, pp. 1439–1440; Kirby et al.)*

79. (A — False; B — False; C — False; D — True) Cryptococcal meningitis commonly occurs in patients who have Hodgkin's disease or are taking corticosteroids, but about

50% of cases occur in those who have no recognizable form of immunosuppression. "Cryptococcomas" in the lungs of otherwise healthy persons may resolve spontaneously and do not always require drug treatment, provided that the patient is kept under observation. Disseminated disease and meningitis are usually fatal unless adequate treatment is given. *C. neoformans* is usually sensitive to amphotericin B, but combined therapy with amphotericin B and 5-fluorocytosine may give better results for treatment of cryptococcal meningitis. The organisms usually disseminate to skin, bone, and CNS by blood-borne spread from a primary focus in the lung. *(Cecil, pp. 1703–1705)*

80. (A — False; B — True; C — False; D — True) The Jarisch-Herxheimer reaction consists of malaise, fever, rigors, headache, and myalgias occurring a few hours after the first dose of an antibiotic (usually penicillin) given for treatment of certain spirochetal infections: syphilis, leptospirosis, and relapsing fever. The reaction is presumed to be due to rapid release of "endotoxins" or antigens from the cell walls of spirochetes as they are destroyed by antibiotic. The reaction does not occur during treatment of protozoan and rickettsial infections. *(Cecil, p. 1583)*

81. (All are True) All the organisms listed may cause subacute or chronic infections, during which immune complexes may be formed between antigen released by the organism and host antibody. These complexes may deposit in glomerular basement membrane, causing nephritis and sometimes the nephrotic syndrome. *(Cecil, pp. 1460, 1577, 1719, 1755–1756)*

82. (All are True) Diabetes is associated with a somewhat increased frequency and severity of tuberculosis. Silicosis predisposes to both typical and atypical tuberculous infections. Gastric resection may cause reactivation of old pulmonary foci by an unknown mechanism in 4 to 6% of cases. In years past it was said that "tuberculosis follows Hodgkin's disease like a shadow," presumably because of depressed cellular immune function. *(Cecil, p. 1541)*

83. (All are True) Vaccination with BCG (an attenuated strain of *M. bovis*) will prevent development of approximately four of every five cases of tuberculosis that would have occurred in the absence of vaccination. In those who develop tuberculosis despite vaccination, miliary disease and tuberculous meningitis are notably rare. BCG may also provide significant protection against infection with *M. leprae*. *(Cecil, p. 1541)*

84. (A — False; B — True; C — True; D — False) Pseudomembranous colitis was originally described *before* the introduction of antibiotics, as a rare complication of surgery. More recently, most cases have occurred after use of antibiotics. Although a wide range of different antibiotics have been implicated, the most frequent association has been with lincomycin or clindamycin therapy (hence the term "clindamycin colitis"). It is probably due to disturbance of normal bowel flora by the antibiotics, allowing proliferation of *Clostridium difficile*, which elaborates an exotoxin affecting the gut. These organisms are sensitive to vancomycin, which may be given orally for treatment. Inhibitors of intestinal motility are probably contraindicated, since they may lead to retention of toxin in the bowel. *(Cecil, pp. 1497–1498; Tedesco, Barton, and Alpers)*

85. (A — False; B — True; C — True; D — False) *Vibrio cholerae* is highly susceptible to gastric acid; therefore, a very high inoculum (10 billion organisms or more) is necessary to infect most normal subjects. After gastrectomy, patients are susceptible to a lower inoculum. The cholera enterotoxin binds to the small-bowel epithelial cells and stimulates adenyl cyclase. A resultant increase in 3′,5′-cyclic adenosine monophosphate leads to massive excretion of isotonic fluid into the small bowel lumen. The small bowel mucosa appears normal morphologically, and the stool does not contain leukocytes or red cells unless another disease is also present. *(Cecil, pp. 1519–1521)*

86. (A — False; B — True; C — False; D — True) Cutaneous anthrax is a rare disease in the United States. In contrast to common skin infections such as furunculosis and cellulitis, there is usually little pain, no lymphangitis, and only minor involvement of regional nodes. The characteristic features are intense, nonpitting edema surrounding an ulcer covered by dark-colored eschar. The area is more often pruritic than painful. Occasionally, anthrax disseminates via the blood stream to cause hemorrhagic mediastinitis or meningitis. *(Cecil, pp. 1526–1528; Braude, pp. 1806–1810)*

87. (A — True; B — True; C — True; D — False) Congenital toxoplasmosis is manifest by fever, hepatosplenomegaly, pneumonitis, rash, microphthalmia, microcephaly, seizures, and retardation. If the aqueduct of Sylvius is obstructed, hydrocephalus occurs. Retinochoroiditis is a late result of congenital toxoplasmosis. Toxoplasmosis causes hepatitis, not hepatic abscesses. *(Cecil, p. 1741)*

88. (A — True; B — False; C — True; D — True) *Giardia lamblia* is a protozoan that inhabits the upper small bowel. Once diagnosed, even asymptomatic patients should be treated with quinacrine or metronidazole to prevent possible future complications. Cysts appear in the stool, but trophozoites will be found there only in patients with rapid bowel transit times. Heavy infections result in steatorrhea. Giardiasis is particularly common in patients with hypogammaglobulinemia. *(Cecil, pp. 1746–1747; Braude, pp. 1075–1078)*

89. (All are True) Leptospirosis is an uncommon disease in the United States. It is typically biphasic, with the first ("leptospiremic") phase lasting four to nine days, followed by a brief remission for one to three days, and then relapse into the second ("immune") phase. Mortality is closely related to age, being about 10% overall, but up to 50% in patients over 50 years of age. *(Cecil, pp. 1595–1597; Braude, pp. 1841–1847)*

90. (A — False; B — True; C — False; D — True) Atypical tuberculosis of the lungs is most common in older, white males. It is much less common in blacks and females, and is rare in children. It tends to be slowly progressive over years, forming multiple thin-walled cavities and causing secondary fibrosis. Pre-existing chronic lung disease such as emphysema or pneumoconiosis usually must be present before atypical mycobacteria can gain a foothold. The patient usually dies of other causes; only 15% or fewer die as a result of the infection, even though antimicrobial therapy often fails to eradicate the organisms. *(Cecil, p. 1555)*

91. (A — True; B — False; C — True; D — False) Rat-bite fever is caused by a pleomorphic gram-negative bacillus, *Streptobacillus moniliformis*. It is most likely to affect children living in poverty and crowded conditions, which set the stage for nocturnal rat bites. The organism is found in the mouths of *healthy* rats; therefore, biomedical laboratory workers are also at risk. Diagnosis is made by culturing the bacillus from blood or joint fluid, not by serology. For treatment, low-dose penicillin, or tetracycline, 500 mg orally q.i.d., are the drugs of choice. *(Cecil, pp. 1594–1595; Braude, pp. 1789–1790)*

92. (A — False; B — True; C — True; D — True) In three studies, chloroquine concentration in breast milk was less than the lower limit detectable by the assay employed. Sulfonamides pass into breast milk in sufficient quantities to cause hemolytic anemia in G6PD-deficient infants, or neonatal jaundice due to displacement of bilirubin from plasma proteins. Chloramphenicol reaches about 50% of blood levels in milk — this is not sufficient to cause the "gray baby syndrome," but it can cause marrow suppression. Tetracyclines also appear in breast milk at concentrations about 40% of serum levels, which theoretically could result in mottling of the infant's teeth. Since the calcium in milk retards tetracycline absorption, this may not be a real danger. *(Anderson)*

93. (A — True; B — False; C — True; D — False) Acute epiglottitis is a serious disease caused by *Hemophilus influenzae* type b. This is an invasive pathogen, and bacteremia is commonly present. The infection is unusual in neonates (who possess maternal antibody) and in children over 6 years of age (who usually possess bactericidal antibody to *H. influenzae* type b). The first aim of management is to secure the airway, usually by intubation. Antibiotic therapy with *both* ampicillin and chloramphenicol should then be given, since 5 to 15% of strains of *H. influenzae* type b are now resistant to ampicillin. *(Braude, pp. 841–843)*

94. (A — True; B — True; C — True; D — False) Certain phage groups (III and IV) of *S. aureus* cause food poisoning by elaborating a heat-stable exotoxin, which is absorbed and then acts on the central nervous system to cause symptoms. *C. perfringens* type A and *B. cereus* also cause a significant number of cases of food poisoning each year in the United States. *B. fragilis* forms a major proportion of the normal flora of the bowel and does not cause food poisoning. *(Cecil, pp. 742–744)*

95. (A — False; B — False; C — False; D — True) Relapse occurs in 8 to 10% of untreated cases of typhoid fever, and is *more* common (15 to 20%) in patients treated with chloramphenicol. Only about 3% of patients become chronic carriers; in undeveloped countries, those with schistosomiasis are more likely to become chronic urinary carriers of *S. typhi*. Immunity is not related to presence of antibodies to the common *S. typhi* antigens O, H, or Vi, since volunteers with such antibodies can still be infected with *S. typhi*. Cellular immunity is probably more important in conferring resistance to typhoid fever. Treatment with chloramphenicol does not reduce the likelihood that patients will become chronic carriers and will not eradicate the carrier state. Long-term, high-dose ampicillin with probenecid will eradicate the carrier state in some patients, but if gallbladder disease is present, cholecystectomy is usually necessary to terminate carriage of *S. typhi*. *(Cecil, pp. 1507–1510; Braude, pp. 1399–1407)*

96. (A — False; B — True; C — True; D — True) The largest single etiologic group of viruses causing the common cold is the rhinoviruses. Rotavirus is the commonest cause of infantile diarrhea, but does not cause coryza. Parainfluenza 1, 2, and 3; influenza A and B; and respiratory syncytial virus can all cause common colds. Infection with two distinct viruses at once is not rare. *(Cecil, p. 1624)*

97. (A — False; B — True; C — False; D — False) Measles vaccine is a live attenuated strain originally derived from Dr. John Enders' Edmonston strain. Vaccination causes seroversion in 90 to 97% of children; the cases that still occur are mainly due to failure of vaccination programs to reach all children, rather than to failure of the vaccine itself. Failure of immunization can occur if the vaccine is given to infants 12 months of age or less, possibly owing to persisting maternal antibody. Therefore, the vaccine should not be given before children reach 15 months of age. Since the live vaccine induces a subclinical infection, immunity is solid and "booster" injections are not required. *(Cecil, p. 1639)*

98. (A — False; B — True; C — True; D — False) Scarlet fever occurs when Group A streptococci causing streptococcal pharyngitis happen to be themselves infected by a bacteriophage that causes them to elaborate erythrogenic toxin. The rash of scarlet fever is found most typically on the face, trunk, inner aspects of the arms and thighs, and especially in the axillae and groins. The palms and soles usually are not red. Desquamation of the skin occurs during the recovery phase, and can help to make a retrospective diagnosis after a case of pharyngitis has resolved. Eosinophilia (up to 20% of the total leukocytes) is common during the recovery phase; it often passes unnoticed because blood smears are seldom examined after the child begins to recover. Scarlet fever is a classic cause of both acute rheumatic fever and acute glomerulonephritis, but rarely in the same patient. *(Cecil, pp. 1445–1446)*

99. (All are True) There is a fairly strong association between all the characteristics listed and the tendency of strains of gonococci to cause disseminated infection. These organisms require arginine, hypoxanthine, and uracil for growth *in vitro*, are sensitive to $<0.125\ \mu g$ penicillin G/ml, and are relatively resistant to complement-mediated lysis. In the study cited, these strains were recovered from 42% of whites and 9% of blacks with gonorrhea. *(Knapp et al.)*

100. (A — True; B — True; C — True; D — False) *Strep. pneumoniae* is the commonest cause of acute bacterial otitis media, accounting for over 50% of cases at all ages. *Strep. pyogenes* (about 10% of cases) is now less common than formerly. *H. influenzae* (most often untypable strains) also causes a significant proportion of cases. *P. aeruginosa* is often recovered from cases of otitis externa and chronic otitis media with perforated drum, but does not cause acute otitis media. *(Braude, pp. 834–835, 839)*

101. (A — False; B — False; C — True; D — True) Gentamicin is inactive against anaerobes and has no place in treatment of gas gangrene. Polyvalent antitoxin should not be used because it is ineffective; *Clostridia* spp. elaborate a number of different toxins, and commercially available antitoxin neutralizes only a few of them. Adequate surgical debridement, excision, or amputation is the key to successful management of gas gangrene. Next in importance is antibiotic therapy, consisting of aqueous penicillin G, 300,000 to 400,000 units/kg intravenously daily. Finally, hyperbaric oxygen is probably of value in selected cases, but it is important that surgery, penicillin, and supportive therapy not be delayed by the logistics of arranging for hyperbaric oxygen treatment. *(Cecil, pp. 1494–1495; Braude, pp. 1780–1781)*

102. (All are True) Pulmonary mycoplasma infection is occasionally accompanied by one or more of a wide range of complications, including all those listed. Others are intravascular hemolysis, neuropathy, cerebellar ataxia, bullous myringitis, urticaria, erythema nodosum, pericarditis, myocarditis, arthritis, bronchiectasis, and thrombocytopenic pupura. *(Cecil, pp. 1428–1429)*

103. (A—False; B—True; C—True; D—True) Brucellosis most often affects meat packers, veterinarians, and farmers; hence, men are affected six times more frequently than women. The organisms, disseminating via the blood stream, can infect almost any tissue, including bone and heart valves; the differential diagnosis is therefore wide, including rheumatic fever, connective tissue diseases, many viral infections, tuberculosis, sarcoidosis, Hodgkin's disease, and other disorders. Although blood cultures are positive in 50 to 75% of untreated cases early in the disease, most cases (80–85%) in the United States are diagnosed by serology, not culture. *(Cecil, pp. 1535–1537)*

104. (A — True; B — True; C — False; D — True) Cryptococcosis limited to the lung in normal hosts usually has a good prognosis; pulmonary lesions often will resolve spontaneously without amphotericin B therapy. Nevertheless, it is mandatory to exclude extrapulmonary lesions (especially in CNS and bone) in patients with a cryptococcoma in the lung before deciding whether treatment is required. In this patient, all further tests were negative and no therapy was given; he remained well when seen for follow-up at regular intervals over two years and no new lesions appeared on roentgenogram of the chest. *(Cecil, pp. 1703–1705; Braude, pp. 986–988; Hammerman et al.)*

105. (All are True) A large number of heterogeneous conditions may be associated with biologic false-positive serologic tests for syphilis (STS). For example, false-positives occur in 8 to 20% of patients with systemic lupus erythematosus, up to 30% of narcotic addicts, and 10% of patients over 80 years of age. Acute false-positive STS (lasting less than six months) are found occasionally in patients with malaria or mycoplasma infections, or after vaccinations. Chronic false-positive STS (lasting more than six months) may occur in narcotic addicts and patients with autoimmune diseases or leprosy. Most false-positive tests are in low titer (<1:8), but high-titer false-positives have occasionally been recorded in patients with lymphoma. *(Cecil, p. 1581)*

106. (All are True) Alcoholism predisposes to pneumococcal pneumonia, bacteremia, endocarditis, and meningitis, as does congenital or acquired hypogammaglobulinemia. Asplenia is associated with fulminant pneumococcal septicemia. About 80% of cases of meningitis occurring in patients with CSF rhinorrhea are due to pneumococci. When a patient suffers *recurrent* bacterial meningitis, pneumococci are involved about *ten times* as frequently as any other bacterial species. *(Cecil, pp. 1420–1427, 1473–1478)*

107–112 *(Cecil, pp. 1541–1542; Mandell, Douglas, and Bennett, pp. 1920–1923)*
107. (A) Any person living in the same household as a person with active tuberculosis has a high risk of developing infection (2.5% in the first year, and 5% for patients already skin-test–positive at the time of examination). The rate may be even higher in infants, and infection can be very severe. It is recommended that children, regardless of PPD status, be treated with isoniazid for three months and the PPD then rechecked. If it is positive at that time, therapy should be continued; if negative, therapy can be discontinued. **108. (B)** In patients 20 to 34 years of age the risk of isoniazid-induced hepatitis is up to 0.3%. The risk of developing active tuberculosis exceeds this if the skin test is positive and the chest x-ray normal. Thus, patients under 35 who have a positive skin test and no evidence of active disease should receive one year of isoniazid prophylaxis. **109. (C)** The risk of isoniazid hepatitis is as high as 1.2% in persons 35 to 49 years of age, and the risk in persons of 50 and older is 2.3%. The risk of developing hepatitis is felt to outweigh the benefits of isoniazid prophylaxis. Thus, isoniazid would not be routinely recommended in the patient described. **110. (C)** Persons with a positive skin test who have a history of untreated tuberculosis or roentgenographic evidence of nonprogressive disease should be treated if they are 35 years of age or younger. The risk of hepatitis is such that older patients should be carefully followed without isoniazid prophylaxis. **111. (B)**; **112. (B)** Newly infected persons are defined as those who have converted from skin-test–negative to skin-test–positive in the last two years. The risk of active disease in this group is high, approximately 5% in the first year. Thus, recent converters of any age should receive one year of isoniazid prophylaxis.

113. (C) L. venereum is a sexually transmitted disease caused by certain serotypes (L1, L2, L3) of *Chlamydia trachomatis*. All strains of *Chlamydia* are sensitive to tetracycline, which is the drug of choice. *(Cecil, p. 1572; Braude, pp. 1229–1230)*

114. (E) Legionnaires' disease is caused by *Legionella pneumophila*, an organism that produces β-lactamase, and penicillins and cephalosporins are not indicated. Erythromycin has been used most commonly for treatment and is associated with a low case-fatality rate. Tetracycline has also been used, but both *in vitro* and *in vivo* data suggest that it is less effective than erythromycin. *(Cecil, pp. 1440–1441)*

115. (D) Nonspecific vaginitis is associated with infections caused by *Gardnerella vaginalis* (formerly *Hemophilus vaginalis*). Metronidazole has been shown to be more effective than other commonly used regimens. *(Cecil, pp. 1565-1566)*

116. (B) *Listeria monocytogenes* is a gram-positive bacillus that frequently causes meningitis in neonates. The organism is sensitive to penicillin and ampicillin, *in vitro* sensitivity being superior for ampicillin. Ampicillin penetrates into the central nervous system and is the drug of choice. *(Cecil, p. 1478; Braude, pp. 1237–1238)*

117. (A) *P. carinii* causes pneumonia in immunosuppressed patients. Pentamidine and trimethoprim-sulfamethoxazole are of about equal efficacy in treatment of this disease, but pentamidine is much more toxic. Trimethoprim-sulfamethoxazole is the drug of choice in both children and adults. *(Cecil, pp. 81, 1395–1402)*

118–122 *(Cecil, pp. 1444–1445)*
118. (B); **119. (C)** Nephritogenic strains of group A streptococcus cause impetigo and pharyngitis; in contrast, rheumatogenic strains cause only pharyngitis. Thus, glomerulonephritis can follow either pharyngitis or skin infection, but acute rheumatic fever follows pharyngitis only. **120. (A)** Treatment of streptococcal pharyngitis with penicillin is effective in preventing rheumatic fever, and this protective effect lasts for several weeks after the acute pharyngitis. Penicillin does not prevent glomerulonephritis. **121. (C)** Both acute rheumatic fever and poststreptococcal glomerulonephritis are thought to be immune-mediated diseases, although the responsible streptococcal antigen has not been identified. **122. (A)** Patients who have had rheumatic fever are at high risk of developing recurrent disease following significant streptococcal upper respiratory tract disease. Thus, patients with acute rheu-

matic fever require continuous prophylaxis to prevent recurrences. Because recurrent episodes of glomerulonephritis are extremely rare, prophylaxis is not needed.

123. (A) *C. trachomatis* has a complex developmental cycle and causes a number of diseases. The two most common chlamydial diseases that affect neonates are inclusion conjunctivitis and interstitial pneumonia. The pneumonia is distinctive. It is gradual in onset, with a peak incidence at 13 months of age. Infants are afebrile, with a characteristic cough (a series of closely spaced staccato coughs, separated by a brief inspiration) and slight eosinophilia. The illness can last several weeks. *(Cecil, p. 1598; Beem and Saxon; Mandell, Douglas, and Bennett, pp. 1464–1476)*

124. (C) The etiologic agent of acute epididymitis appears to depend on the age of the patient. Men with epididymitis who are 35 or younger tend to be infected with either *C. trachomatis* or *N. gonorrhoeae*. In men over 35, the most common etiologic agent is *E. coli*, with *Proteus* species and *Pseudomonas aeruginosa* playing a lesser role. *(Berger et al.)*

125. (C) The urethral syndrome is a disease of women that is characterized by dysuria, frequency of urination, and the isolation of *fewer than* 10^5 organisms per milliliter of a sterile urine specimen. Forty-six per cent of women with these symptoms actually have low-grade bladder bacteriuria as confirmed by suprapubic aspiration, despite the fact that their urine has fewer than 10^5 organisms per milliliter. The most common etiologic agent in this group is *E. coli*. Only 19% of these patients have evidence of a recent infection with *C. trachomatis*. The remainder (35%) have no known etiologic agent to explain their symptoms. *(Cecil, pp. 1564–1565; Stamm et al.)*

126. (C) Community-acquired urinary tract infections are most commonly caused by *E. coli* (80 to 90%), most of the remainder being caused by *Proteus mirabilis* and *Klebsiella pneumoniae*. *(Cecil, p. 566)*

127. (B) *N. gonorrhoeae* can cause localized disease such as urethritis, cervicitis, proctitis, pharyngitis, and so forth, as well as disseminated disease, known as disseminated gonococcal infection (DGI) or the arthritis-dermatitis syndrome. It is most common in women and has an onset around the time of menses. The characteristic rash is manifest as five to 40 tender, discrete, pustular lesions on an erythematous base. The lesions most commonly occur on the extremities; the trunk and face are spared. Tenosynovitis frequently occurs, as does septic arthritis that usually involves one or two large joints. *(Cecil, p. 1569; Braude, pp. 1407–1410)*

128. (A); 129. (A); 130. (B); 131. (A); 132. (B); 133. (B) Leprosy is a chronic granulomatous disease caused by *Mycobacterium leprae*, with a wide spectrum of clinical manifestations. At one end of the spectrum is tuberculoid leprosy in which disease is limited to a few areas of the skin and associated nerve supply. Patients with this form of leprosy have a low burden of organisms and intact cellular immunity. As a result, skin biopsy usually reveals no acid-fast organisms, although well-developed granulomas are seen and the lepromin skin test is positive. At the other end of the spectrum is lepromatous leprosy, a disease characterized by diffuse infiltration of the skin with *M. leprae*, with multiple cutaneous lesions. Patients with this form of leprosy have a generalized impairment of cell-mediated immunity. Skin biopsies reveal numerous acid-fast bacilli (without granuloma formation), but the skin test to lepromin is negative. Because of the overwhelming infection, nasal secretions contain enormous numbers of organisms (up to 2×10^8 in a single nose-blow). Erythema nodosum leprosum is a reactional state usually seen in patients with high bacterial loads after initiation of therapy; it is characterized by the appearance of painful red papules or nodules. *(Cecil, pp. 1556–1560; Braude, pp. 1378–1387)*

134. (A) The therapy for cryptococcal meningitis is combination amphotericin B plus flucytosine. Excellent results were obtained in a recent controlled clinical trial. *(Cecil, p. 1705; Bennett et al.)*

135. (E) *Listeria* meningitis is an infection of the immunocompromised host, especially renal transplant and lymphoma patients. Therapy usually consists of high doses of ampicillin for at least two weeks; some would recommend three to four weeks. *(Cecil, p. 1531; Mandell, Douglas, and Bennett, pp. 1630–1632; Braude, pp. 1234–1235)*

136. (C) The therapy for coccidioidal meningitis is amphotericin B, both intravenously and intrathecally. The duration of therapy is variable and depends on host defense mechanisms and response to therapy. Usually 2.0 to 3.0 gm of intravenously administered amphotericin B are needed. Intrathecal amphotericin B is also necessary, but intracisternal or intraventricular administration achieves the same purpose; i.e., direct placement of the drug into the CSF. Frequently an Ommaya reservoir is needed. *(Cecil, p. 1701; Drutz and Catanzaro; Braude, pp. 1251–1253)*

137. (F) Aseptic viral meningitis is frequently caused by the enteroviruses, especially echovirus, but also coxsackievirus B. It is usually a benign, self-limited infection that requires no special therapy. *(Cecil, pp. 1664–1665; Braude, pp. 1365–1373)*

138. (D) This is a typical case of herpes simplex I meningoencephalitis. Several publications have argued for brain biopsy as the means of making the diagnosis, since CSF culture and serologic tests are not usually useful. Therapy with ara-A has been shown to improve the outcome if initiated early in the course of the meningoencephalitis. *(Braude, pp. 1309–1328; Whitley et al., 1977; Whitley et al., 1981)*

139. (D) The most common causes of fungal meningitis include *Cryptococcus, Coccidioides*, and *Candida*. *Candida* will be cultured; however, cryptococcal and coccidioidal meningitis are usually diagnosed with serologic testing of the CSF for the antigen of *Cryptococcus* and the antibody for *Coccidioides*, present in more than 90% of cases. *(Pons and Hoff)*

140. (B) Bacterial meningitis is almost always diagnosed by CSF culture (exceptions include *Listeria monocytogenes* meningitis in which blood cultures are positive but CSF is negative, and partially treated bacterial meningitis). The CSF pleocytosis is predominantly PMNs, and the CSF glucose is decreased. Early diagnosis of pneumococcal, meningococcal, and *Hemophilus influenzae* meningitis can be made rapidly with counterimmunoelectrophoresis. *(Cecil, pp. 1475–1476)*

141. (A) Aseptic viral meningitis is usually caused by the enteroviruses, which are rarely cultured from CSF. CSF pleocytosis shows lymphocytes predominantly, although early in the course of a viral meningitis some PMNs can be seen. *(Cecil, pp. 1664–1665)*

142. (E) Brain abscess can cause irritation of the meninges and produce the CSF findings described in E. Spinal tap carries a risk in brain abscess, and deaths associated with brain herniation have been described. Unless the abscess ruptures into the CSF, information obtained from the CSF (culture, cell count, and chemical tests) is generally of little help *(Cecil, pp. 2075–2076)*

143. (C) Tuberculous meningitis may be difficult to diagnose since acid-fast stains are usually negative and culture of the CSF is positive in only about 50% of cases. Since several weeks are needed for the culture data, the acute illness is often misdiagnosed. The diagnosis should be suspected with CSF data as described in C. *(Cecil, p. 1475)*

144. (A) Patients with granulocytopenic leukemia and documented *Pseudomonas* septicemia are best treated with a synergistic combination of antibiotics (an aminoglycoside plus carbenicillin) as well as leukocyte transfusions, especially if there is a poor response to antibiotics alone. The therapy should be continued until either the patient recovers or the peripheral granulocyte count returns to normal. *(Cecil, pp. 1395–1405; Grieco, pp. 886–888)*

145. (C) The differential diagnosis of rapidly progressing pulmonary infiltrates in this patient includes viral (cytomegalovirus), parasitic *(Pneumocystis)*, fungal, and other diseases caused by opportunistic organisms (tuberculosis, Legionnaires' disease). Open lung biopsy has been useful in rapidly securing the diagnosis and directing specific therapy with little morbidity. Bronchoscopy is a grossly contaminated procedure and is not appropriate for obtaining specimens for culture. *(Leight and Michaelis)*

146. (E) The use of trimethoprim-sulfamethoxazole has been shown to be effective in preventing infections with *Pneumocystis carinii* in children with lymphocytic leukemia. The use of this antibiotic for prevention of *Pneumocystis* and bacterial infections in adults with leukemia has yet to be conclusively established. *(Hughes et al.)*

147. (B) Broad-spectrum antibiotics are warranted since most of these episodes of fever in patients such as this are associated with enteric gram-negative bacteria; gram-positive organisms are less likely. The EORTC (European Organization for the Research and Treatment of Cancer) study indicated the usefulness of initial empiric therapy with an aminoglycoside plus carbenicillin in this clinical situation. *(EORTC Antimicrobial Therapy Project Group)*

148. (A); 149. (E); 150. (A); 151. (C); 152. (D); 153. (C) Cefazolin, like all cephalosporins and penicillins, inhibits cell wall synthesis. Vancomycin also inhibits cell wall synthesis, but at another site in the synthetic pathway. Amphotericin B damages the membrane of eukaryotic cells (for example, cells of fungi and man) by interacting with sterols in the membrane. Erythromycin, clindamycin, and chloramphenicol all bind to 50S ribosomes, where they interfere with protein synthesis. Tobramycin, like all aminoglycosides, binds to 30S ribosomes and inhibits protein synthesis. *(Cecil, pp. 71–83; Braude, pp. 234–246)*

154. (B) *R. typhi* (previously *R. mooseri*) is the cause of endemic (murine) typhus. This disease is spread from rodents to man by fleas. Man can be infected when flea feces containing rickettsiae contact broken skin, or when an infected aerosol is inhaled. *(Cecil, p. 1603; Braude, p. 1446)*

155. (C) *R. prowazekii* is the cause of epidemic typhus. This organism and *R. quintana* (the cause of trench fever) are the only major rickettsiae for which man rather than rodents, small mammals, or arthropods is the reservoir. Infection is spread by contact between the crushed lice or their feces and broken skin, or by inhalation of infected aerosols. *(Cecil, p. 1603; Braude, pp. 1441–1442)*

156. (D) *R. rickettsii* is the cause of Rocky Mountain spotted fever. Ixodid ticks and small mammals form the reservoir for *R. rickettsii*, which is transmitted to man by the bites of infected ticks. *(Cecil, p. 1603; Braude, pp. 1448–1450)*

157. (E) *R. tsutsugamushi* causes scrub typhus. This rickettsia is transferred to man by the bites of chiggers (trombiculid mites). These small arthropods live in scrub and grassland in Asia, Australia, and New Guinea, and on islands in the Pacific. *(Cecil, p. 1603; Braude, pp. 1448–1450)*

158. (A) See also answer to question 155. *R. quintana* is the causative agent of trench fever. It is spread by contact between the crushed lice or their feces and broken skin, or by inhalation of infected aerosols. This organism has recently been reclassified into the genus *Rochalimaea*. *(Cecil, p. 1603; Braude, pp. 1472–1473)*

159. (B) Schistosomiasis should not be treated unless living eggs are present in feces or tissue. The aim of treatment is to reduce the worm burden, not to achieve complete cure. Niridazole, 25 mg/kg/day, is administered in two divided doses for five to seven days. Side effects include vomiting, diarrhea, cramps, and dizziness. *(Cecil, pp. 1757–1758)*

160. (C) The prognosis of trichinosis is usually good, even if no specific treatment is given. Symptomatic treatment includes analgesics and steroids. In severe infection, the drug of choice is thiabendazole, 25 mg/kg/day for five to seven days *(Cecil, p 1772)*

161. (D) Accessible nodules containing adult *O. volvulus* worms should be excised if possible, to reduce the worm load. Remaining adult worms may be killed by suramin, 1 gm intravenously weekly for five weeks. Microfilariae are killed by diethylcarbamazine, 6 to 9 mg/kg/day in three divided doses. *(Cecil, p. 1778)*

162. (A) All patients with *W. bancrofti* microfilaremia should be treated with diethylcarbamazine, which kills both microfilariae and adult worms. A low dose should be given at first, and increased to 6 to 9 mg/kg/day in three divided doses for 14 days. Microfilaremia is usually absent in established elephantiasis; chemotherapy will not relieve this late complication of *W. bancrofti* infection. *(Cecil, p. 1775)*

163. (E) All the major tapeworms that infect humans (beef, pork, and fish tapeworms) may be treated with niclosamide. Two 0.5-gm tablets are chewed and swallowed with a little water on an empty stomach, and the same dose is repeated one hour later. Since the worm disintegrates and the head of the worm cannot be found in feces, follow-up stool examination should be done after six months to ensure that the worm was killed *(Cecil, pp. 1753–1754)*

164. (A) Necrotizing bronchopneumonia due to *Aspergillus* species occurs almost exclusively in immunocompromised patients, especially those with neutropenia. Recovery from invasive aspergillosis is unusual unless restoration of the host's defense mechanisms occurs during treatment. Unfortunately, *Aspergillus* species are often resistant or partially resistant to amphotericin B, which is the only antimicrobial agent presently available for therapy. This drug should be given in an attempt to suppress the infection while the return of host defenses toward normal is awaited. Use of flucytosine is ineffective. *(Cecil, pp. 1709–1710)*

165. (D) *Aspergillus* is second in frequency only to *Candida* species as a cause of fungal endocarditis on prosthetic heart valves. Primary treatment consists of surgical replacement of the infected prosthesis, but amphotericin B is usually administered also in the hope of eradicating any remaining foci of infection or preventing reinfection of the new prosthesis. Without surgery, the prognosis is virtually hopeless. *(Cecil, p. 1710; Kammer and Utz)*

166. (E) Allergic bronchopulmonary aspergillosis is an allergic reaction to *Aspergillus* or its spores, not an invasive infection. Precipitins to *Aspergillus* antigens are usually present in the patient's serum. Treatment includes corticosteroids and bronchodilators; antifungal agents are not effective. *(Cecil, p. 1709; Braude, pp. 1008–1013)*

167. (C) An aspergilloma (fungus ball) in a lung cavity or cyst may be asymptomatic or may cause hemoptysis of varying severity. Fungus balls will sometimes break up and disappear spontaneously. Cure can be achieved by surgical excision, which is indicated if the patient experiences repeated or severe hemoptysis. Antifungal drugs are ineffective. *(Cecil, p. 1709; Braude, p. 1013)*

168. (D) *Aspergillus* species can cause a wide variety of CNS lesions, including meningitis, meningoencephalitis, granulomas, isolated brain abscess, and multiple brain abscesses. Treatment of an isolated brain abscess consists of surgical drainage and/or excision of the abscess, plus a course of amphotericin B. *(Cecil, pp. 1709–1710; Young et al.)*

169. (B) The regimen recommended by the CDC for treatment of late latent syphilis is benzathine penicillin G, 2.4 million units intramuscularly once weekly for three weeks. (Some authorities now feel that asymptomatic neurosyphilis should be treated with higher doses of penicillin, e.g., aqueous penicillin G, 12 to 24 million units intravenously daily for ten days.) *(Cecil, p. 1582)*

170. (C) The CDC has recommended procaine penicillin G, 4.8 million units intramuscularly plus probenecid, 1 gm orally as the regimen of first choice for treatment of uncomplicated gonorrhea in both males and females. This regimen has two major advantages: (1) the entire dose is given under supervision, in one session; and (2) it cures incubating syphilis, thus avoiding the need for follow-up serology. *(Cecil, p. 1568)*

171. (D) Pneumococcal pneumonia will respond equally favorably to many penicillin regimens, since most pneumococci are highly sensitive (MIC <0.1 μg/ml). Procaine penicillin G is often chosen for treatment of pneumococcal pneumonia for reasons of convenience to patient and staff, since fewer injections are needed than with the shorter-acting aqueous penicillin G. The dose of penicillin listed under regimen E is unnecessarily high for pneumococcal pneumonia. Penicillin-resistant pneumococci have appeared in South Africa, but have not yet become a significant problem in the United States. *(Cecil, p. 1425)*

172. (E) Aqueous penicillin G is used for treatment of meningitis whenever possible. It should be given intravenously at frequent intervals (every two to four hours) in high doses (18 to 24 million units per day). Penetration into CSF is adequate in the presence of meningeal inflammation; the dose should not be reduced when the patient begins to improve. *(Cecil, p. 1477)*

173. (A) The most effective regimen for prevention of rheumatic fever is benzathine penicillin, 1.2 million units intramuscularly monthly. Since it is given under supervision, patient compliance is better than for alternative oral regimens such as penicillin V, 250 mg orally twice daily. *(Cecil, p. 1450)*

174. (E) Lymphogranuloma venereum typically causes marked inguinal adenopathy with suppuration, discharging sinuses, and associated systemic symptoms. Late complications include chronic fibrosis, rectal strictures, and lymphatic obstruction. The LGV chlamydiae may be treated with sulfonamide or tetracycline. *(Cecil, pp. 1571–1572)*

175. (A) This is a classic description of a primary syphilitic chancre. Syphilis, which is now relatively common among promiscuous male homosexuals, should be suspected in all cases of genital or perianal ulceration. Even when the lesions are not typical, dark-field examination and serology are usually advisable to exclude this diagnosis. Inguinal adenopathy is often absent in the presence of a rectal chancre. *(Cecil, p. 1575)*

176. (B) Multiple shallow, painful ulcers with a strong tendency to recurrence are typical of genital herpes, caused by herpes simplex virus type 2. This distressing disease has increased greatly in frequency in the past ten years. *(Cecil, pp. 1564, 1647; Braude, pp. 1218–1227)*

177. (D) Chancroid is caused by *Hemophilus ducreyi*. It is characterized by painful, nonindurated ulcers with associated enlarged inguinal nodes, which frequently suppurate. Coexisting syphilis should always be carefully excluded, after which chancroid may be treated with sulfisoxazole. *(Cecil, pp. 1572–1573; Braude, pp. 1230–1232)*

178. (F) Granuloma inguinale is an indolent granulomatous and ulcerative disease caused by a pleomorphic coccobacillus, *Calymmatobacterium granulomatis*, which is related to *Klebsiella*. These bacilli may be seen within monocytes in scrapings from the genital lesion. After coexisting syphilis has been excluded, this infection may be treated with tetracycline. *(Cecil, p. 1572)*

179. (C) Scrotal ulcers, often associated with oral ulcerations, venous thromboses, and inflammation of the eye, suggest Behçet's syndrome. This is a vasculitis of unknown etiology that may be associated with a wide spectrum of additional manifestations, including arthritis and gastrointestinal symptoms. *(Cecil, pp. 1899–1900; Dowling; Kansu et al.)*

180. (C) Metronidazole, 800 mg orally three times daily for eight days, is effective against both intraluminal and tissue amebas. Alternatives are emetine (which is more toxic) and chloroquine. Intraluminal amebas can be treated with diiodohydroxyquin. *(Cecil, p. 1738; Braude, pp. 1074–1075)*

181. (A) Visceral leishmaniasis (kala-azar) is best treated with pentavalent antimony compounds. The dose of sodium stibogluconate is 20 mg/kg/day intravenously or intramuscularly for six to 30 days; side effects are rare. *(Cecil, p. 1733; Braude, p. 1140)*

182. (F) Many strains of *P. falciparum* are now resistant to chloroquine. A standard regimen for falciparum malaria is quinine sulfate, 650 mg orally three times daily for ten to 14 days, *plus* pyrimethamine, 50 mg orally daily for one to three days, *plus* sulfadiazine, 0.5 gm orally four times daily for five to ten days. *(Cecil, pp. 1720–1721)*

183. (C) Trichomonas vaginitis responds well to metronidazole, either 200 mg orally three times daily for eight days, or a single oral dose of 2.0 gm. Reinfection is likely to occur if the sexual partner is not treated simultaneously. *(Cecil, p. 1565)*

184. (B) Toxoplasmosis may be treated with pyrimethamine plus sulfadiazine. Folinic acid, 6 mg orally daily, should be given to prevent folate deficiency during treatment. *(Cecil, p. 1742)*

185. (D) Pneumocystosis responds to treatment with pentamidine isethionate, but sulfamethoxazole, 100 mg/kg/day, plus trimethoprim, 20 mg/kg/day orally or intravenously, has recently proved equally effective and less toxic. It has therefore become the drug of choice, but a trial of pentamidine, 4 mg/kg/day intramuscularly for 14 days, should still be considered if the patient does not respond. *(Cecil, p. 1744; Braude, pp. 1031–1032)*

186. (C) Giardiasis can be cured in about 80% of cases by metronidazole, 200 mg orally three times daily for ten days. Treatment failures may be given quinacrine hydrochloride (Atabrine), 100 mg orally three times daily after food for seven days, which yields a similar success rate. *(Cecil, p. 1747; Braude, p. 1078)*

187. (E) Renal transplant recipients have severely depressed cell-mediated immunity owing to treatment with steroids and azathioprine. They may suffer from a wide variety of secondary infections, ranging from a gram-negative bacteria in the urinary tract and at the site of the transplant to *Pneumocystis* in the lungs. Cytomegalovirus and hepatitis B infections are so common among dialysis and renal transplant patients that answer E, which includes these two viruses, is correct here. *(Cecil, pp. 1395–1402)*

188. (C) Children with CGD suffer severe, recurrent infections with *Staph. aureus*, gram-negative bacilli, *Candida*, and other pathogens. They are not more susceptible than normal subjects to streptococci and pneumococci, because these organisms produce hydrogen peroxide and thus remedy the inherited metabolic defect in CGD neutrophils. *(Cecil, pp. 1395–1402)*

189. (A) Hodgkin's disease is associated with an abnormality of cell-mediated immunity that predisposes to such diverse infections as varicella-zoster, cryptococcosis, and listeriosis. About 20% of these patients developed tuberculosis in the past. The present incidence is lower, about 1 to 2%. *(Cecil, pp. 1395–1402)*

190. (D) Sickle cell disease predisposes the patient to infection with pneumococci and salmonellae. The mechanisms involved include repeated splenic infarctions leading to "autosplenectomy," and a subtle defect in opsonization of bacteria. Patients with sickle cell anemia should be vaccinated with the 14-valent pneumococcal polysaccharide vaccine (Pneumovax). *(Cecil, pp. 1395–1402; Amman et al.)*

191. (C) Neutropenia of 500/cu mm or less predisposes to frequent severe bacterial and fungal infections, often caused by one or more of the organisms listed in answer C. *Pneumocystis* pneumonitis also may occur. *(Cecil, pp. 1395–1402)*

192. (C) Older patients with pre-existing diseases are at high risk to develp nosocomial pneumonia after major surgery. Gram-negative bacilli and/or *Staph. aureus* usually colonize the pharynx in such patients; since nosocomial pneumonias often arise from aspiration of pharyngeal material, these organisms are the predominant etiologic agents. Fungi are less commonly responsible. *(Cecil, pp. 1432–1435)*

193. (B) The lungs of children with cystic fibrosis are almost always colonized with *Pseudomonas* and *Staph. aureus*. If one sputum sample is negative for these two species, culture of further specimens usually reveals one or both of them. It is usually impossible to eradicate these organisms for more than brief periods by using antibiotics. *(Cecil, pp. 387–388)*

194. (D) The best-known complication of clindamycin therapy is diarrhea, which occasionally progresses to fully developed pseudomembranous colitis. This serious condition is due to an exotoxin produced by *Clostridia* species that proliferate during treatment. Other side effects of clindamycin are uncommon. *(Cecil, pp. 78–79)*

195. (E) Trimethoprim is a folic acid antagonist that can deprive the patient as well as the bacteria of folate, sometimes causing anemia. This is not a problem during short courses of the drug. Sulfamethoxazole, like all sulfas, can cause hemolysis in patients with G6PD deficiency. *(Cecil, p. 81)*

196. (B) Like all the tetracyclines, doxycycline can cause nonspecific gastrointestinal upset and unsightly staining of the teeth if given to pregnant women or children less than 8 years old. Pregnant women also suffer acute fatty degeneration of the liver as a result of taking tetracyclines. Doxycycline and the other long-acting tetracyclines sometimes cause photosensitivity dermatitis. *(Cecil, p. 80)*

197. (C) Gentamicin, like all the aminoglycosides, is nephrotoxic and neurotoxic. If absorbed or injected too rapidly, it can cause respiratory paralysis owing to neuromuscular blockade. *(Cecil, pp. 79–80)*

198. (A) Chloramphenicol commonly induces reversible, dose-related bone marrow depression causing anemia. Once in 40,000 courses of therapy it produces irreversible pancytopenia, which is often fatal. This form of marrow toxicity is not dose-related. In neonates, chloramphenicol can produce fatal circulatory collapse — the "gray baby syndrome." The drug should be avoided in neonates unless serum levels can be monitored. *(Cecil, p. 80)*

199. (F) Vancomycin is an irritant antibiotic that cannot be given intramuscularly because of pain. Phlebitis often occurs at injection sites. Nephrotoxicity and ototoxicity occur occasionally. *(Cecil, p. 78)*

200. (B) *Staph. aureus* is the leading cause of septic arthritis in children less than 15 years of age. Streptococci are second in frequency in this age-group. *H. influenzae* accounts for 30% of cases in children less than 2 years old, but is much less common thereafter. *(Hoeprich, pp. 1125–1132)*

201. (D) *N. gonorrhoeae* is by far the most common cause of septic arthritis in young adults (75% of cases). *Staph. aureus* is next in frequency (15%), and a small number of cases are caused by *Strep. pneumoniae* and the gram-negative bacilli. Meningococci, *Brucella*, salmonellae, tuberculosis, and fungi all may cause interesting forms of septic arthritis, but together make up only a small proportion of cases. *(Hoeprich, pp. 1125–1132)*

202. (B) In the elderly, *Staph. aureus* once again becomes the leading cause of septic arthritis, accounting for 75% of cases. The remaining 25% are due chiefly to streptococci and gram-negative bacilli. Septic arthritis in the aged often is superimposed upon rheumatoid arthritis or other chronic joint disease. *(Hoeprich, pp. 1125–1132)*

BIBLIOGRAPHY

Amman, A. J., Addiego, J., Wara, D. W., et al.: Polyvalent pneumococcal-polysaccharide immunization of patients with sickle-cell anemia and patients with splenectomy. N. Engl. J. Med., *297*:897, 1977.

Anderson, P. O.: Drugs and breast feeding — review. Drug Intelligence and Clinical Pharmacy, *11*:208, 1977.

Bayer, A. S., Theofilopoulos, A. N., Eisenberg, R., et al.: Circulating immune complexes in infective endocarditis. N. Engl. J. Med., *295*:1500, 1976.

Beem, M. O., and Saxon, E. M.: Respiratory tract colonization and a distinctive pneumonia syndrome in infants infected with *Chlamydia trachomatis.* N. Engl. J. Med., *296*:306, 1977.

Bennett, J. E., Dismukes, W. E., Duma, R. J., et al.: A comparison of amphotericin B alone and combined with flucytosine in the treatment of cryptococcal meningitis. N. Engl. J. Med., *301*:126, 1979.

Berger, R. E., Alexander, R., Monda, G. D., et al.: *Chlamydia trachomatis* as a cause of acute "idiopathic" epididymitis. N. Engl. J. Med., *298*:301, 1978.

Blumenthal, D. S.: Current concepts — intestinal nematodes in United States. N. Engl. J. Med., *297*:1437, 1977.

Bortolussi, R., Krishnan, C., Armstrong, D., and Tovichayathamrong, P.: Prognosis for survival in neonatal meningitis — clinical and pathologic review of 52 cases. Can. Med. Assoc. J., *118*:165, 1978.

Braude, A. I. (ed.): Medical Microbiology and Infectious Diseases. Philadelphia, W. B. Saunders Company, 1981.

Conte, J. E.: Manual of Antibiotics and Infectious Disease. Philadelphia, Lea & Febiger, 1981.

Ditlove, J., Weidmann, P., Bernstein, M., and Massry, S. G.: Methicillin nephritis. Medicine, *56*:483, 1977.

Dorff, G. J., Geimer, N. F., Rosenthal, D. R., et al.: Pseudomonas septicemia. Illustrated evolution of its skin lesion. Arch. Intern. Med., *128*:591, 1977.

Dowling, G. B.: Behçet's disease. Proc. R. Soc. Med., *54*:101, 1961.

Drutz, D. J., and Catanzaro, A.: Coccidioidomycosis: state of the art. Parts 1 and 2. Am. Rev. Respir. Dis., *117*:559, 727, 1978.

EORTC Antimicrobial Therapy Project Group: Three antibiotic regimens in the treatment of infection in febrile granulocytopenia patients with cancer. J. Infect. Dis., *137*:14, 1978.

Gjestland, T.: Oslo study of untreated syphilis; epidemiologic investigation of natural course of syphilitic infection based upon re-study of Boeck-Bruusgaard material. Acta Derm. Venereol., *35* (Suppl. 34):1, 1955.

Grieco, M. H. (ed.): Infection in the Abnormal Host. New York, Yorke Medical Books, 1980.

Hammerman, K. J. Powell, K. E., Christianson, C. S., et al.: Pulmonary cryptococcosis; clinical forms and treatment. A Center for Disease Control cooperative mycoses study. Am. Rev. Respir. Dis., *108*:1116, 1973.

Hoeprich, P. D. (ed.): Infectious Diseases. 2nd ed. New York, Harper & Row, 1977.

Hughes, W. T., Kuhn, S., Chaudhary, S., et al.: Successful chemoprophylaxis for *Pneumocystis carinii* pneumonitis. N. Engl. J. Med., *297*:1419, 1977.

Jacobs, J. C.: *Yersinia enterocolitica* arthritis. Pediatrics, *55*:236, 1975.

Jacobs, N. F., and Krauss, S. J.: Gonococcal and nongonococcal urethritis in men — clinical and laboratory differentiation. Ann. Intern. Med., *82*:7, 1975.

Jennings, R. H.: Prophylactic antibiotics in vaginal and abdominal hysterectomy. South. Med. J., *71*:251, 1978.

Kammer, R. B., and Utz, J. P.: Aspergillus species endocarditis: the new face of a not so rare disease. Am. J. Med., *56*:506, 1974.

Kansu, E., Ozer, F. L., Akalin, E., et al.: Behçet's syndrome with obstruction of the venae cavae. A report of seven cases. Q. J. Med., *41*:151, 1972.

Karchmer, A. W., Dismukes, W. E., Buckley, M. J., et al.: Prosthetic valve endocarditis — clinical features influencing therapy. Am. J. Med., *64*:199, 1978.

Kirby, B. D., Snyder, K. M., Meyer, R. D., et al.: Legionnaires' disease: clinical features of 24 cases. Ann. Intern. Med., *89*:297, 1978.

Knapp, J. S., Thornsberry, C., Schoolnik, G. A., et al.: Phenotypic and epidemiologic correlates of auxotype in *Neisseria gonorrhoeae*. J. Infect. Dis., *138*:160, 1978.

Leight, G. S., and Michaelis, L. L.: Open lung biopsy for the diagnosis of acute, diffuse pulmonary infiltrates in the immunosuppressed patient. Chest, *73*:4, 1978.

Lett, W. J., Ansbacher, R., Davison, B. L., et al.: Prophylactic antibiotics for women undergoing vaginal hysterectomy. J. Reprod. Med., *19*:51, 1977.

Mandell, G. L., Douglas, R. G., and Bennett, J. E. (eds.): Principles and Practice of Infectious Diseases. New York, John Wiley & Sons, 1979.

Miller, L. H., Neva, F. A., and Gill, F.: Failure of chloroquine in human babesiosis *(Babesia microti)* — case report and chemotherapeutic trials in hamsters. Ann. Intern. Med., *88*:200, 1978.

Morbidity and Mortality Weekly Report, *26*:425, 441, 1977.

Morbidity and Mortality Weekly Report, *29*:265, 1980.

Pons, V. G., and Hoff, J. T.: Infections of the CNS. *In* Wilson, C. B. (ed.): Current Surgical Management of Neurological Diseases. New York, Churchill-Livingstone, 1980, pp. 268–269.

Ruebush, T. K., and Spielman, A.: Human babesiosis in the United States (editorial). Ann. Intern. Med., *88*:263, 1978.

Sarff, L. D., McCracken, G. H., Schiffer, M. S., et al.: Epidemiology of *Escherichia coli* K1 in healthy and diseased newborns. Lancet, *1*:1099, 1975.

Stamm, W. E., Wagner, K. F., Amsel, R., et al.: Causes of the acute urethral syndrome in women. N. Engl. J. Med., *303*:409, 1980.

Tedesco, F. J., Barton, R. W., and Alpers, D. H.: Clindamycin-associated colitis. A prospective study. Ann. Intern. Med., *81*:429, 1974.

Washington, J. A., 2d, Snyder, R. J., Kohner, P. C., et al.: Effect of cation content of agar on the activity of gentamicin, tobramycin, and amikacin against *Pseudomonas aeruginosa*. J. Infect. Dis., *137*:103, 1978.

Whitley, R. J., Ch'ien, L. T., Dolin, R., et al.: Adenine arabinoside therapy of herpes zoster in the immunosuppressed: the NIAID collaborative antiviral study. N. Engl. J. Med., *294*:1193, 1976.

Whitley, R. J., Soong, S., Dolin, R., et al.: Adenine arabinoside therapy of biopsy-proved herpes simplex encephalitis. National Institute of Allergy and Infectious Diseases collaborative antiviral study. N. Engl. J. Med., *297*:289, 1977.

Whitley, R. J., Soong, S., Hirsch, H. S., et al.: Herpes simplex encephalitis: vitarabine therapy and diagnostic problems. N. Engl. J. Med., *304*:313, 1981.

Young, R. C., Bennett, J. E., Vogel, C. L., et al.: Aspergillosis: the spectrum of the disease in 98 patients. Medicine, *49*:147, 1970.

PART 9
CLINICAL IMMUNOLOGY AND RHEUMATOLOGY

David S. Pisetsky and John R. Rice

DIRECTIONS: For questions 1 to 39, choose the ONE BEST answer to each question.

1. The organism most likely to cause septic arthritis in an adult patient with longstanding rheumatoid arthritis is

A. *Staphylococcus aureus*
B. *Pseudomonas aeruginosa*
C. *Streptococcus pyogenes*
D. *Streptococcus (Diplococcus) pneumoniae*
E. *Hemophilus influenzae*

QUESTIONS 2–3

2. A 2-year-old boy who was bitten by a wild bat is to be treated with horse antirabies serum. Which of the following should be done first?

A. Administer full doses of horse antiserum
B. Administer corticosteroids
C. Administer epinephrine and diphenhydramine (Benadryl)
D. Measure serum complement levels
E. Obtain a careful history concerning possible sensitivity to horse products

3. Two weeks after the initiation of horse serum therapy, the patient develops fever, urticaria, arthritis, and edema. The erythrocyte sedimentation rate and leukocyte count are elevated. Urinalysis shows trace proteinuria and 2 to 5 RBCs/hpf. Which of the following should be done now?

A. Discontinue horse antirabies serum
B. Reduce the concentration of antirabies serum
C. Administer epinephrine intravenously with diphenhydramine (Benadryl) intramuscularly
D. Administer antibiotics and local care to the injection sites
E. Begin a short course of prednisone and attempt to obtain human antirabies serum

---

4. Markers for T lymphocytes include

A. E rosettes
B. EAC rosettes
C. C3 receptors
D. monomeric IgM
E. Ia antigens

5. A 47-year-old woman with rheumatoid arthritis develops pain and swelling in the left calf after an afternoon of gardening. Which of the following would be the most useful diagnostic test?

A. Doppler flow studies of the lower extremities
B. Venography of the lower left extremity
C. Arthrography of the left knee
D. Examination of synovial fluid from the left knee
E. Bilateral plain knee films with standing views

6. Dr antigens are

A. found on T cells
B. associated with β_2-microglobulin
C. found on macrophages
D. identified by immune response genes
E. capable of eliciting strong cell-mediated cytotoxicity

7. Uveitis is a common or characteristic manifestation of each of the following disorders EXCEPT

A. ankylosing spondylitis
B. adult-onset rheumatoid arthritis
C. Behçet's disease
D. sarcoidosis
E. juvenile rheumatoid arthritis

8. Of the following studies, the most sensitive screening test for systemic lupus erythematosus is

A. anti-ribonucleoprotein antibody titer
B. anti–double-stranded DNA antibody titer
C. anti-Sm antibody titer
D. LE cell preparation
E. IgG antinuclear antibody titer

9. The use of aspirin in the treatment of inflammatory disease has been associated with all the following EXCEPT

A. hepatitis
B. renal insufficiency
C. irreversible deafness
D. asthma
E. bleeding disorders

10. In evaluation of the patient whose hands are illustrated, all the following tests might be useful EXCEPT

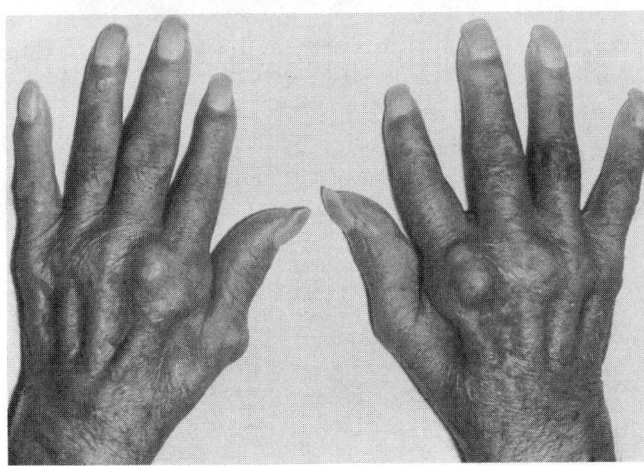

A. serum iron and total iron-binding capacity
B. plain films of the hands

C. serum uric acid level
D. muscle biopsy
E. latex test for rheumatoid factor

11. All the following are useful in the treatment of psoriatic arthritis EXCEPT

A. aspirin
B. hydroxychloroquine (Plaquenil)
C. methotrexate
D. 6-mercaptopurine
E. indomethacin

12. Muscular weakness in association with an elevation in serum muscle enzymes is characteristic of each of the following disorders EXCEPT

A. childhood dermatomyositis
B. myxedema
C. muscular dystrophy
D. Cushing's syndrome
E. alcoholic rhabdomyolysis

13. All the following statements regarding renal disease resulting from immune-complex deposition are true EXCEPT

A. DNA–anti-DNA complexes cause renal disease in patients with systemic lupus erythematosus
B. Penicillamine induces drug–anti-drug complexes
C. The presence of circulating immune complexes correlates strongly with the occurrence of glomerulonephritis
D. Immunofluorescent studies of glomeruli involved in immune-complex disease reveal granular or lumpy patterns of deposition
E. Immune complex–mediated tissue damage involves an interaction of the complement system and neutrophils at the local site

14. A 20-year-old man complains that after running in warm weather he develops hives, abdominal pain, diaphoresis, and headache. The wheals that occur on the face are small and are surrounded by large "axon" flares. The patient has light hair and freckles; stroking the freckles does not cause a wheal. Intradermal injection of methacholine induces a large wheal. The most likely diagnosis is

A. hereditary angioedema
B. cholinergic urticaria
C. cold urticaria
D. solar urticaria
E. urticaria pigmentosa

15. A patient with systemic lupus erythematosus has fever, maculopapular skin rash, and arthralgias. There is no evidence of other organ involvement. Initial management should include all the following EXCEPT

A. topical sun screens
B. topical corticosteroids
C. systemic corticosteroids
D. acetylsalicylic acid
E. antimalarial drugs

16. Major and minor criteria for the diagnosis of Behçet's disease include all the following EXCEPT

A. photosensitivity
B. uveitis
C. oral and genital ulceration
D. thrombophlebitis
E. colitis

17. A 55-year-old woman has had deforming rheumatoid arthritis for 20 years for which she has been receiving 10 mg of prednisone daily. She reports the gradual onset of weakness in both lower extremities and she has had one episode of urinary incontinence. The most useful diagnostic procedure in the evaluation of this patient's complaint is

A. nerve conduction studies
B. muscle biopsy
C. cervical spine films
D. computerized tomography of the brain
E. lumbar discography

18. Hypocalcemic tetany is a presenting sign of which immunodeficiency disease?

A. Severe combined immunodeficiency disease
B. Nezelof's syndrome
C. Wiskott-Aldrich syndrome
D. X-linked agammaglobulinemia
E. DiGeorge's syndrome

19. A 42-year-old man has a ten-day history of fever, pain in the right knee, and painful, nodular lesions over the pretibial areas bilaterally. The lesions are raised, diffusely marginated, erythematous, and tender, and involve subcutaneous tissue as well as the overlying skin. The differential diagnosis includes all the following EXCEPT

A. sarcoidosis
B. Takayasu's syndrome
C. tuberculosis
D. inflammatory bowel disease
E. drug hypersensitivity

20. Renal involvement is NOT a feature of which one of the following disorders?

A. Hypersensitivity angiitis
B. Midline granuloma
C. Churg-Strauss allergic granulomatosis
D. Wegener's granulomatosis
E. Lymphomatoid granulomatosis

21. A 26-year-old man is stung by a bee, and shortly thereafter a wheal develops at the site of the sting. He soon feels flushed and develops hives, rhinorrhea, and tightness in the chest. He is brought to your office. Immediate therapy should be

A. transfer to a local hospital emergency room
B. cold compress to site of the sting
C. epinephrine, subcutaneously
D. isoproterenol, sublingually
E. parenteral administration of antihistamines and steroids

22. A 57-year-old woman with rheumatoid arthritis is taking 12 aspirin tablets daily with mild tinnitus and poor control of symptoms. You should

A. increase the aspirin dose to 16 tablets per day
B. add low doses of corticosteroids
C. discontinue aspirin and begin gold therapy
D. discontinue aspirin and begin an alternative anti-inflammatory drug
E. measure the serum salicylate level

23. A 23-year-old woman presents with findings suggestive of systemic lupus erythematosus (SLE). Laboratory studies reveal a low total serum complement (CH_{50}) with undetectable C4 and normal C3. What is the most likely diagnosis?

A. SLE with hereditary C4 deficiency
B. SLE with immune-complex nephritis
C. SLE with hereditary angioneurotic edema
D. SLE with alternate complement pathway activation
E. SLE with minimal immune-complex deposition

24. Which of the following side effects is NOT matched properly with a drug?

A. Proteinuria — hydroxychloroquine
B. Rash — gold
C. Stomatitis — penicillamine
D. Hepatitis — aspirin
E. Renal dysfunction — indomethacin

25. The most common pattern of joint involvement in psoriatic arthritis is

A. psoriatic spondylosis
B. asymmetric large and small joint arthritis
C. arthritis mutilans
D. symmetric distal interphalangeal arthritis
E. symmetric polyarthritis

26. The biopsy illustrated opposite is from small bowel and contains numerous macrophages laden with PAS-positive material. The patient complains of weight loss, joint pain, and diarrhea. The most probable diagnosis is

A. ulcerative colitis
B. intestinal lymphoma
C. nontropical sprue
D. Whipple's disease
E. lymphomatoid granulomatosis

27. Clinical and laboratory features of polymyalgia rheumatica include all the following EXCEPT

A. lymphadenopathy
B. morning stiffness
C. limitation of shoulder motion
D. inguinal discomfort
E. erythrocyte sedimentation rate of 50 mm/hour or greater (Westergren)

28. The following statements about gold are true EXCEPT

A. It is ineffective in laboratory models of inflammation
B. Proteinuria is a serious side effect
C. It can be restarted at lower doses after resolution of a drug-related rash
D. It is a first-line remittive therapy for erosive arthritis
E. It should be given to a total dose of 1 gm and then stopped

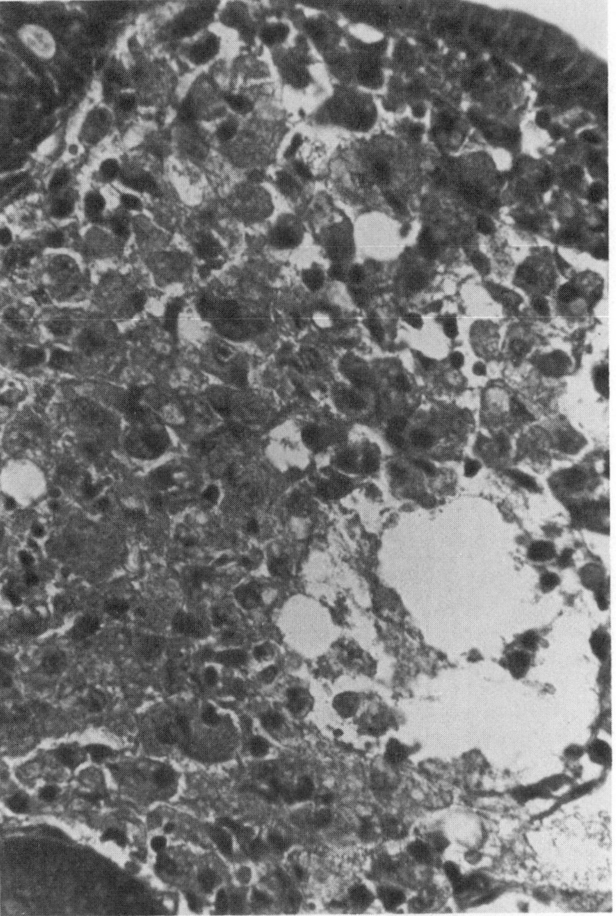

29. The treatment of choice for midline granuloma is

A. wide surgical excision with skin grafts
B. systemic corticosteroids
C. cyclophosphamide (Cytoxan)
D. local radiation therapy with 1000 rads
E. local radiation therapy with 5000 rads

30. Which one of the following synovial fluid findings would be consistent with Reiter's syndrome but not with rheumatoid arthritis?

A. Total leukocyte count greater than 40,000/cu mm
B. Total protein levels greater than twice serum levels
C. Increased viscosity in unclotted fluid
D. Elevated levels of total hemolytic complement
E. Inclusion bodies in leukocytes

31. Laboratory features of hydralazine-induced systemic lupus erythematosus include each of the following EXCEPT

A. leukopenia
B. elevated erythrocyte sedimentation rate
C. positive antinuclear antibody titer
D. positive anti–double-stranded DNA titer
E. positive lupus erythematosus cell preparation

32. Which of the following factors is associated with the skin lesions depicted in the illustrations on p. 244?

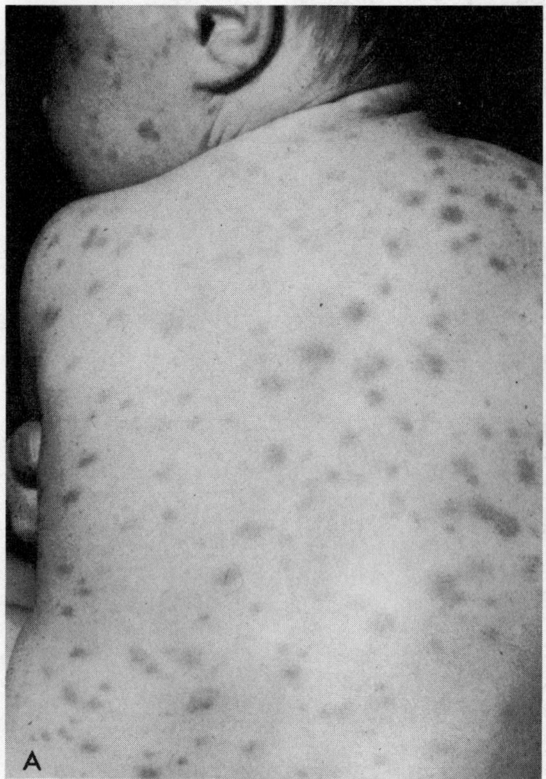

A, Widespread distribution of lesions over the body.

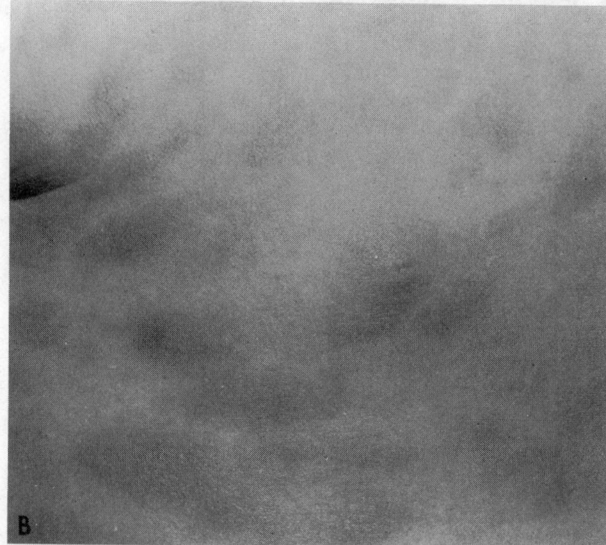

B, Wheal and flares are seen after stroking affected areas. (From Bellanti, J.: Immunology II. Philadelphia, W.B. Saunders Co., 1978, p. 487.)

A. Food allergy
B. Excessive sun exposure
C. Exposure to the resins of the plants of *Rhus* genus
D. Mast cell infiltration of the skin
E. Eruptions following subcutaneous administration of methacholine

33. A patient with polymyositis presents with marked proximal muscle weakness and an elevation in serum creatine phosphokinase (CPK) levels. After three months of therapy with prednisone, 60 mg daily, muscle strength and CPK values are normal. Prednisone is continued at a dosage of 40 mg daily; however, proximal weakness recurs in spite of continued normal CPK levels. You should

A. search for an occult malignancy
B. order a muscle biopsy
C. add methotrexate to the program
D. gradually reduce the prednisone dosage
E. increase prednisone back to 60 mg daily

34. Common sites of involvement by primary degenerative joint disease (osteoarthritis) include all the following EXCEPT

A. distal interphalangeal joints
B. proximal interphalangeal joints
C. wrists
D. knees
E. hips

35. The combination of roentgenograms most likely to demonstrate chondrocalcinosis in pseudogout is

A. wrists, knees, pelvis
B. shoulders, elbows, ankles
C. ankles, hips, elbows
D. knees, elbows, shoulders
E. hips, elbows, thoracic spine

36. Disseminated neisserial infection is associated with deficiency of which component of complement?

A. C1r
B. C1s
C. C4
D. C6
E. C9

QUESTIONS 37–38

A 25-year-old woman complains of fatigue and a six-week history of right knee pain. She has had some back pain and stiffness over the past two years. There is pitting of several fingernails, and an erythematous, scaly plaque involving the umbilicus and surrounding skin is noted. The right knee is warm and effused. The patient is unable to fully flex the lumbar spine, and there is synovitis involving the proximal interphalangeal joint on the left ring finger and the distal interphalangeal joint on the right index finger.

37. The most likely diagnosis is

A. gout
B. Reiter's syndrome
C. rheumatoid arthritis
D. psoriatic arthritis
E. arthropathy of inflammatory bowel disease

38. The LEAST useful diagnostic study from the list below would be

A. examination of knee fluid
B. HLA-B27 antigen screen
C. latex test for rheumatoid factor
D. plain films of the hands
E. plain films of the back and sacroiliac joints

---

39. Which of the following immunoglobulin classes is found on the surface of B lymphocytes?

A. IgD
B. IgE
C. IgG1
D. IgG3
E. IgA

DIRECTIONS: For questions 40 to 60, you are to decide whether EACH choice is true or false. Any combination of answers, from all true to all false, may be present. Mark the answer sheet "T" or "F" in the space provided.

40. Which of the following statements regarding rheumatoid lung disease is/are true?

A. Pneumoconiosis protects against development of lung nodules
B. Women are affected more often than men
C. Pleural fluid glucose may be 10 to 20% of serum levels
D. The pulmonary nodules do not cavitate
E. Most patients with rheumatoid lung have negative tests for rheumatoid factor

41. Appropriate management of nongonococcal septic arthritis would include which of the following?

A. Splinting of the affected joint to minimize pain
B. Infusion of the joint space with antibiotics
C. Non–weight-bearing during the period of acute inflammation
D. Drainage of the involved joint
E. Withholding antibiotics 48 to 72 hours pending results of culture and sensitivity testing

42. Which of the following statements regarding Felty's syndrome is/are correct?

A. Splenectomy should be carried out once the total leukocyte count is consistently less than 2000/cu mm
B. Chronic leg ulceration will usually respond to the addition of lithium to the therapeutic program
C. Early therapy with corticosteroids will often increase the leukocyte count and prevent subsequent infectious complications
D. Development of bacterial pneumonia with no improvement after 48 to 72 hours of antibiotic therapy is an indication for emergency splenectomy
E. Gold therapy may afford improvement in active joint disease and in depressed leukocyte counts

43. Which of the following radiographic findings is/are compatible with the diagnosis of rheumatoid arthritis?

A. Soft tissue swellings
B. New bone formation
C. Periosteal elevation
D. Juxta-articular osteoporosis
E. Erosions

44. Which of the following statements about rheumatic manifestations of inflammatory bowel disease is/are true?

A. Persistent arthritis is an indication for colectomy in patients with ulcerative colitis
B. Peripheral joint involvement is associated with the HLA-B27 haplotype
C. Clinical activity of the bowel disease and associated spondylitis are closely correlated
D. Erythema nodosum and uveitis are common findings in patients with rheumatic manifestations of inflammatory bowel disease

45. In which of the following diseases is the administration of gamma globulin indicated for the prevention of infections?

A. Severe combined immunodeficiency disease
B. IgA deficiency
C. Transient hypogammaglobulinemia of infancy
D. Immunodeficiency with elevated IgM
E. Common variable agammaglobulinemia

46. Clinical features consistent with a diagnosis of polymyositis or dermatomyositis include

A. muscle wasting (atrophy)
B. postexertional cramping
C. muscle fasciculations
D. dysphagia
E. weakness of facial musculature

47. Which of the following statements about juvenile rheumatoid arthritis (JRA) is/are true?

A. Tests for rheumatoid factor are positive in most patients
B. Boys with pauciarticular disease have a high incidence of HLA-B27
C. Gold should be used in patients with chronic progressive synovitis and deformity.
D. Iridocyclitis is associated with a positive antinuclear antibody titer
E. Monoarticular disease occurs less frequently in JRA than in adult disease

48. Depression of total serum complement levels (CH_{50}) occurs in which of the following?

A. Hereditary C4 deficiency
B. Active systemic lupus erythematosus with nephritis
C. Rheumatoid vasculitis
D. Acute attacks of hereditary angioneurotic edema

49. Which of the following statements concerning insect sting allergy is/are true?

A. The RAST (radioallergosorbent test) is the most sensitive diagnostic test
B. Most patients with this allergy are sensitive to both bee and vespid venom
C. IgG antibodies are protective
D. Whole body extract is effective in desensitization immunotherapy
E. Desensitization immunotherapy should be administered over a prolonged period to reduce the incidence of side effects

50. Which of the following statements regarding the management of reflex sympathetic dystrophy is/are true?

A. The finding of severe osteopenia on plain films is an indication for splinting or non–weight-bearing of the affected part
B. A three-week tapering course of systemic corticosteroids often accelerates resolution of pain and promotes early mobilization of the symptomatic area
C. Coolness and diaphoresis of the involved extremity often indicate proximal vascular obstruction
D. Pain medications or anti-inflammatory agents should be used sparingly in order to avoid obscuring the clinical response to therapy
E. Rheumatoid factor titers often afford a useful tool in following disease activity to therapy

51. As a diagnostic tool, synovial biopsy is often indicated in patients suspected of having

A. hemochromatosis
B. rheumatoid arthritis
C. tuberculous arthritis
D. amyloid joint disease
E. psoriatic arthritis

52. HLA-A and HLA-B antigens elicit

A. organ graft rejection
B. mixed lymphocyte reactivity
C. cell-mediated cytotoxicity
D. graft-versus-host disease
E. immune suppression

53. Clinical and laboratory findings consistent with a diagnosis of Sjögren's syndrome include

A. recurrent epistaxis
B. interstitial pneumonitis
C. renal tubular acidosis
D. generalized lymphadenopathy
E. absent salivary β_2-microglobulin

54. Which of the following statements regarding systemic lupus erythematosus is/are true?

A. Corticosteroids should not be used during pregnancy because of potential teratogenic effects on the fetus
B. A patient should be advised to consider pregnancy only when all clinical and laboratory evidence of major system disease has been controlled
C. Oral contraceptives should be avoided as a method of birth control
D. Exacerbations of disease activity often occur during the last trimester of pregnancy or immediately post partum
E. A newborn infant may exhibit transient serologic and clinical evidence of lupus as a result of transplacental transfer of maternal antibody

55. A 10-year-old boy has a history consistent with allergy to grass and ragweed pollen. Which of the following statements about his condition is/are true?

A. A high dose of ragweed antigen is required for release of leukocyte histamine
B. Successful immunotherapy will result in decreased leukocyte sensitivity to ragweed and grass challenge
C. The RAST (radioallergosorbent test) is the most sensitive diagnostic test
D. Radioallergosorbent testing of the serum will probably show a high degree of binding to ragweed antigen E
E. The symptoms will have a seasonal pattern

56. A renal arteriogram such as the one shown is characteristic of which of the following?

A. Henoch-Schönlein purpura
B. Giant cell arteritis
C. Systemic lupus erythematosus
D. Polyarteritis nodosa
E. Fabry's disease

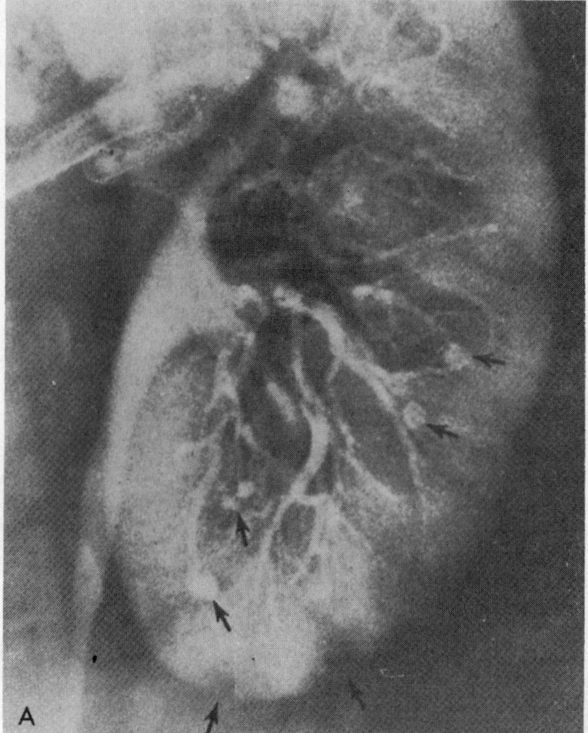

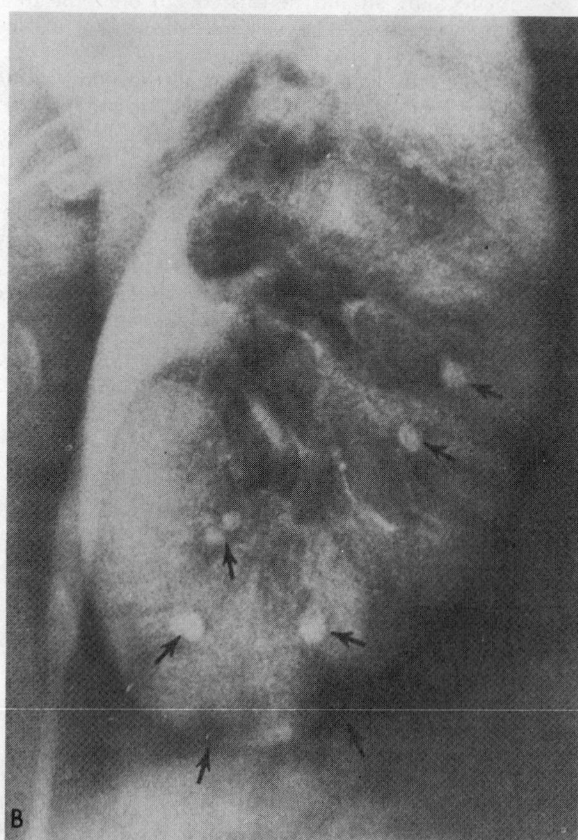

Renal arteriogram in *(A)* arterial and *(B)* capillary phases. (From Fauci, A., et al.: Am. J. Med., *64*:890, 1978. Yorke Medical Group)

57. Which of the following statements about cold urticaria is/are true?

A. It is transferable by serum
B. It occurs in a familial pattern with low levels of functionally normal C1 esterase inhibitor
C. Cold challenge increases plasma histamine
D. Complement consumption follows cold exposure
E. Hypotension results from severe cold exposure

58. Causes of neuropathic joint disease include which of the following conditions?

A. Cerebrovascular accidents
B. Diabetes mellitus
C. Intrapulmonary lesions
D. Syringomyelia
E. Amyotrophic lateral sclerosis

59. Which of the following statements about hereditary angioedema is/are true?

A. Inheritance is sex-linked
B. Serum C3 levels are low
C. Serum C4 levels are low
D. There is decreased activity of C1 esterase inhibitor
E. Danazol is effective preventive therapy

60. Which of the following statements regarding Wegener's granulomatosis is/are true

A. Prominent hilar adenopathy is a characteristic radiographic finding
B. Renal disease should be treated with cyclophosphamide if there is no response to a trial of high-dose corticosteroids
C. Laboratory findings usually do not include eosinophilia
D. Biopsy of skin lesions shows necrotizing arteritis without evidence of granulomatous inflammation
E. Renal disease is characterized by the presence of antibodies to glomerular basement membrane

DIRECTIONS: Questions 61 to 105 are matching questions. For each numbered item, choose the most likely associated lettered item from those provided. Each numbered item has ONLY ONE answer. Within each group, each lettered item may be the answer to one, more than one, or none of the numbered items, unless otherwise specified.

QUESTIONS 61–64

For each of the following, choose the most likely associated immunoglobulin.

A. IgG3
B. IgD
C. IgE
D. IgA

61. Antigen receptor on B cells

62. Complement activation via the alternate pathway

63. Major immunoglobulin in secretions

64. Reaginic antibody

QUESTIONS 65–69

For each histopathologic description, select the most likely form of vasculitis.

A. Lymphomatoid granulomatosis
B. Churg-Strauss disease
C. Takayasu's syndrome
D. Henoch-Schönlein purpura
E. Kawasaki disease

65. Infiltration of large muscular arteries with giant cells

66. Leukocytoclasis involving small venules

67. Infiltration of both arteries and veins by atypical lymphocytes

68. Inflammation of medium-sized arteries, eosinophilia, and pulmonary granulomas

69. Coronary arteritis with aneurysms

QUESTIONS 70–72

For each disease, select the HLA locus with which it is most closely associated.

A. HLA-A
B. HLA-B
C. HLA-D

70. Sjögren's syndrome

71. Juvenile-onset diabetes mellitus

72. Hemochromatosis

QUESTIONS 73–76

For each of the following clinical manifestations, select the most likely infectious agent.

A. *Trichinella spiralis*
B. β-Hemolytic streptococcus
C. Hepatitis B virus
D. *Mycobacterium tuberculosis*

73. Myalgias, periorbital edema, and eosinophilia

74. Hip destruction

75. Subcutaneous nodules

76. Polyarthralgias, hypocomplementemia, and urticaria

QUESTIONS 77–81

For each of the following patients, select the most suitable diagnosis. Use each lettered item ONLY ONCE.

A. Reiter's syndrome
B. Gonococcal arthritis
C. Staphylococcal arthritis
D. Gout
E. Pseudogout

77. A 52-year-old obese woman with discomfort and swelling in the right knee for three weeks; there is no previous history of joint complaints

78. A 27-year-old man with persistent pain, swelling, and erythema involving the right subtalar joint for the past six weeks; five days ago he began to have pain in the plantar area of the left heel

79. A 48-year-old male alcoholic with an acutely painful and swollen left tibiotalar joint; a similar episode occurred in the left great toe six months ago but resolved spontaneously in seven days

80. A 22-year-old female college student with acute pain and soft tissue swelling over the right wrist and extensor tendons of the right hand; she also had transient discomfort in the left wrist and knee three days ago

81. A 61-year-old man with longstanding rheumatoid arthritis and acute, severe pain and swelling in the left knee — other joints are minimally symptomatic; the patient is being treated with aspirin and gold

QUESTIONS 82–86

For each disease, select the characteristic findings or underlying metabolic disturbance.

A. Thrombocytopenia and eczema
B. Deficiency of purine nucleoside phosphorylase
C. Deficiency of adenosine deaminase
D. Low levels of IgA and high levels of α-fetoprotein
E. Glutathione peroxidase deficiency

82. Severe combined immunodeficiency disease (SCID)

83. Nezelof's syndrome

84. Chronic granulomatous disease

85. Ataxia telangiectasia

86. Wiskott-Aldrich syndrome

QUESTIONS 87–91

For each of the following heritable disorders, select the most likely physical findings.

A. Cartilage pigmentation in the external ear
B. Joint hypermobility
C. Blue sclerae
D. Angiokeratoma
E. Lenticular subluxation

87. Ehlers-Danlos syndrome

88. Osteogenesis imperfecta

89. Homocystinuria

90. Ochronosis (alcaptonuria)

91. Fabry's disease

QUESTIONS 92–95

For each of the following disorders, select the most likely finding.

A. Aseptic necrosis of the femoral head
B. Erythema chronicum migrans
C. Weakly positive birefringent crystals in joint fluid
D. Reddish-brown cutaneous nodules

92. Pseudogout

93. Hemoglobin SC disease

94. Lyme arthritis

95. Multicentric reticulohistiocytosis

QUESTIONS 96–100

For each of the following disorders, select the most likely clinical feature.

A. Nail pitting
B. Thrombophlebitis
C. Photosensitivity
D. Lupus pernio
E. Urethritis

96. Reiter's syndrome

97. Systemic lupus erythematosus

98. Psoriatic arthritis

99. Behçet's disease

100. Sarcoidosis

QUESTIONS 101–105

For each manifestation of drug hypersensitivity listed below, select the drug that is the most likely offender.

A. Aspirin
B. Sulfonamides
C. Penicillin
D. Isoniazid
E. Quinidine

101. Systemic lupus erythematosus–like disease

102. Asthma

103. Thrombocytopenic purpura

104. Erythema nodosum

105. Hemolytic anemia

PART 9

CLINICAL IMMUNOLOGY AND RHEUMATOLOGY

ANSWERS

1. (A) *Staph. aureus* is the most common organism involved in nongonococcal septic arthritis in both adults and children. The bulk of septic arthritis in rheumatoid disease is caused by this agent. Gram-negative organisms play an important role in pyarthrosis in the immunocompromised host. *H. influenzae* and streptococcal infections may occur, but they are seen most frequently in children from 6 months to 2 years of age. *(Cecil, p. 1876)*

2. (E) Because of the danger of allergic reactions to horse serum products, patients to be treated with such preparations should be evaluated carefully for possible sensitivity. Detailed questioning should determine previous exposure and sensitivity to such products, and skin testing with diluted test serum should be performed. If the history suggests an allergy, there should be precautions for anaphylaxis. If skin testing fails to induce wheal and flare reaction after 30 minutes, there is little likelihood that the patient will experience an immediate hypersensitivity reaction to horse serum therapy. *(Cecil, p. 1816)*

3. (E) Serum sickness is an immunologically mediated reaction that may follow antigenic exposure to foreign proteins. This reaction is usually self-limited, although prednisone may be of considerable symptomatic benefit. Because of the short duration of treatment, steroid-related side effects generally are not a significant clinical problem. *(Cecil, p. 1816)*

4. (A) In the evaluation of immunologic function, enumeration of the different immune cell populations found in the peripheral blood provides useful information. Such cells differ in their activities, as well as in cell surface antigens that represent differentiation markers. T cells, which are involved in cellular immunity and immunologic regulation; B cells, which are the important effector element in humoral immunity; and monocytes can all be identified on this basis. The formation of E rosettes (the adherence of sheep red blood cells to the cell surface) is a unique feature of T cells and reflects poorly understood properties of their cell surfaces. The E rosette test, although nonspecific, allows ready identification and enumeration of T cells. Formation of EAC rosettes and the presence of receptors for the third component of complement (C3) are properties of B lymphocytes. Monomeric IgM is the form of IgM that occurs on the surface of B lymphocytes along with IgD; the usual assays for B cells involve measurement of surface immunoglobulin rather than the specific subclass. Finally, Ia antigens (or Dr antigens in the human) are found on B cells and monocytes, not on resting T cells. *(Cecil, pp. 1782–1783, 1812)*

5. (C) Definitive diagnosis of a ruptured popliteal cyst is made by arthrography. Ultrasound examination of the popliteal area and calf may also be useful. Extrinsic compression of venous return may cause difficulty in the interpretation of venograms or flow studies. Concomitant thrombophlebitis in association with a ruptured popliteal cyst has been reported, but is uncommon. *(Cecil, p. 1847)*

6. (C) Ia antigens (Dr antigens in the human) are cell surface antigens encoded by genes within the major histocompatibility complex. They are considered class II antigens and are related to the determinants that are responsible for inducing a mixed lymphocyte reaction (MLR). Unlike class I antigens, they are not present on all cells or associated with β_2-microglobulin. They are predominantly found on B cells and represent a major means of distinguishing B and T cells. These antigens are also present on monocytes, where they may play a role in "antigen presentation." Immune response genes have not been definitely identified in humans although it would be expected that they would be associated with Ia-like antigens by analogy to other species. These antigens do not elicit strong cell-mediated cytotoxicity, although they are associated with a strong mixed lymphocyte reaction. *Cecil, pp. 1782, 1812–1813)*

7. (B) Acute anterior segment uveitis occurs with increased frequency in ankylosing spondylitis, in Behçet's disease, and in sarcoidosis. Chronic, often asymptomatic uveitis occurs in juvenile rheumatoid arthritis and may cause visual loss if not detected and treated; girls with ANA-positive disease are the most commonly affected. Adult rheumatoid arthritis is not associated with uveitis in spite of the frequency of other eye problems. *(Cecil, pp. 1878–1879, 1899–1900, 2298–2299, 2301–2311)*

8. (E) IgG antinuclear antibodies are found in over 95 per cent of patients with active SLE. Anti–double-stranded DNA and anti-Sm antibodies are relatively specific for SLE, but are found in roughly 70 per cent and 30 per cent of patients respectively. A positive LE prep is neither sensitive nor specific. *(Cecil, p. 1856)*

9. (C) A variety of side effects has been associated with the use of aspirin in the treatment of inflammatory disease. Some are related to the inhibition of prostaglandin synthesis by aspirin, and others result from its other pharmacologic actions. Awareness of these side effects is important, as cessation or modification of dose can lessen morbidity and, in some instances, avert the need for costly diagnostic studies.

Ototoxicity is a frequent problem with aspirin and is usually manifest as tinnitus at high serum levels of the drug. In some patients, particularly older individuals, there is hearing loss that is dose-related. Nevertheless, these problems are reversible with cessation of the medication. Hepatitis, manifest by liver function abnormalities, occurs in the setting of active inflammatory disease. Renal insufficiency may be related to interference with prostaglandin metabolism. In patients with SLE, in which renal disease can be a prominent feature, the influence of aspirin as well as other anti-inflammatory agents on the kidney must be considered when renal function deteriorates. Cessation of aspirin can lead to improved function, thus avoiding invasive diagnostic procedures or the need to change to more aggressive therapy. Hypersensitivity to aspirin can be accompanied by severe asthmatic reactions. It is important to note that salicylates other than aspirin can induce these reactions, and that these compounds are found in a very large number of proprietary preparations. Finally, bleeding problems secondary to aspirin action on platelet function can lead to chronic blood loss. In some situations it can be associated with more serious hemorrhage. *(Cecil, pp. 632, 787, 981, 1849)*

10. (D) The differential diagnosis of a symmetric polyarthritis with involvement of the wrist and metacarpophalangeal and proximal interphalangeal joints includes rheumatoid arthritis, gout, and hemochromatosis. Arthritis of this extent and distribution would not be associated with polymyositis. *(Cecil, pp. 1848–1849)*

11. (B) Several forms of psoriatic arthritis can be distinguished on the basis of clinical features such as distribution of affected joints, presence of sacroiliitis, and extent of joint destruction. Although the approach to therapy varies with the clinical pattern as well as the severity of the accompanying skin disease, several agents with general utility have been identified. Both aspirin and indomethacin are effective anti-inflammatory agents in patients with psoriatic arthritis; patients with the spondylitis pattern may benefit from indomethacin particularly. Methotrexate and 6-mercaptopurine are effective in the treatment of psoriatic skin disease and can be used in patients with more serious skin involvement, as well as in those with more destructive joint disease. Plaquenil is not recommended in these patients because of the danger of exfoliative skin reactions. *(Cecil, pp. 1880–1881)*

12. (D) Although proximal muscle weakness may be quite pronounced in Cushing's syndrome, creatine phosphokinase and other muscle enzymes are not increased. Extreme but rapidly reversible muscle weakness and enzyme elevations are often seen in alcoholic rhabdomyolysis. Some forms of muscular dystrophy may mimic polymyositis in presentation, and a careful family history must be taken when evaluating this group of disorders. *(Cecil, pp. 1873–1875)*

13. (C) Immune complexes in serum are detected by techniques based on their physical and chemical properties or their ability to bind to complement. In several conditions in which circulating complexes can be demonstrated (e.g., rheumatoid arthritis, pregnancy) renal disease is not a significant problem. Presumably the complexes occurring in these situations, because of their size, specificity, or other immunochemical properties, do not lead to significant glomerular deposition. *(Cecil, pp. 1807–1809)*

14. (B) A variety of physical and chemical stimuli can precipitate urticarial reactions in sensitive individuals. In this patient the diagnosis of cholinergic urticaria is supported by its relationship to exercise and the development of hives following administration of methacholine. *(Cecil, p. 1798)*

15. (C) Not all patients with SLE require therapy with systemic corticosteroids. Skin disease will often respond to sun avoidance and to topical corticosteroids. Nondeforming arthritis may be helped by salicylates or alternate anti-inflammatory drugs. Antimalarial drugs are useful in the treatment of both skin and joint manifestations. *(Cecil, pp. 1856–1857)*

16. (A) Skin lesions in Behçet's disease are common and include various forms of pyoderma, erythema nodosum, and vasculitis. Photosensitivity is not a feature of this disorder. *(Cecil, pp. 1899–1900)*

17. (C) Weakness in a patient with rheumatoid arthritis can result from a variety of pathologic processes. With joint pain and immobility, muscle strength can decline with disuse; in some patients there can be "overlap" with other inflammatory diseases such as coexistent polymyositis; neuropathy, perhaps the result of vasculitis, can present with sensorimotor deficits. Although these causes of muscle weakness are related to significant morbidity, they are not likely to cause the immediate catastrophic problem that results from compression on the cord by subluxation of the cervical spine. Instability of the joints of the cervical spine occurs commonly in longstanding erosive rheumatoid disease, and results from the same type of inflammatory damage that occurs elsewhere. The diagnosis can be made by flexion-extension views of the cervical spine with the demonstration of a separation between C1 and C2 of greater than 2.5 to 3 mm. Occasionally, subluxation of other cervical articulations is detected. Fortunately, most patients with subluxation are without neurologic findings. Nevertheless, in some patients there is impingement of the cord, and the findings of symmetric lower extremity weakness with bowel and bladder dysfunction should lead to prompt evaluation of the joints of this area. *(Cecil, p. 1848)*

18. (E) Diagnosis and classification of the immunodeficiency states are based primarily on the assessment of cellular and humoral components of the immune system. Characteristic abnormalities of B- and/or T-cell function usually dominate the clinical picture by causing increased susceptibility to various types of infection. In some instances, however, symptoms related to another organ system are clinically prominent and may even be the first sign of disease. In DiGeorge's syndrome there is dysgenesis of the third and fourth pharyngeal pouches, leading to aplasia or hypoplasia of the thymus and parathyroid glands as well as a variety of other related structural anomalies. Tetany or hypocalcemia secondary to involvement of the parathyroids can occur in the neonatal period. This feature of DiGeorge's syndrome can lead to its early recognition, unlike other immunodeficiency states in which diagnosis may not be made until infectious complications supervene. *(Cecil, pp. 1793–1794)*

19. (B) Erythema nodosum occurs in association with a wide variety of infectious diseases, as a manifestation of drug sensitivity, and in some patients with inflammatory bowel disease, sarcoidosis, or Behçet's disease. Panniculitis is not a manifestation of giant cell arteritis or Takayasu's syndrome. *(Cecil, pp. 1899, 2280)*

20. (B) Midline granuloma is a destructive granulomatous disorder of unknown etiology; involvement is limited to the upper airways and surrounding structures. Renal involvement in lymphomatoid granulomatosis consists of characteristic nodular cellular aggregates. In the remaining disorders, renal involvement is predominantly a glomerulopathy. *(Cecil, pp. 1865, 1867, 1870, 1896)*

21. (C) Systemic hypersensitivity reactions can result from stings of insects of the order Hymenoptera. Immediate therapy for systemic reactions is epinephrine given subcutaneously if there is no evidence of shock, or intravenously if vascular collapse has occurred. Antihistamines and steroids may be beneficial in the treatment of some urticarial reactions, but the possibility of a severe anaphylactic reaction demands prompt administration of epinephrine. *(Cecil, pp. 1806–1807)*

22. (E) To achieve maximal anti-inflammatory effects from salicylates, a minimum serum level of 20 to 25 mg/dl must be maintained. Documentation of an adequate salicylate level at maximal tolerated doses avoids continued ineffective use of the drug in patients unable to achieve therapeutic levels, suggests a need for use of a remittive drug such as gold or penicillamine if symptoms persist in spite of adequate aspirin therapy, and checks for compliance with the therapeutic regimen. *(Cecil, p. 1849)*

23. (A) Hereditary deficiency of several different complement components has been associated with SLE. In this patient, the presence of low C4 with normal C3 suggests a deficiency state rather than activation by immune complexes, in which case C3 levels would also be low. In hereditary angioneurotic edema, C4 levels are only moderately decreased, and the CH_{50} is normal in quiescent periods. With activation of the alternate pathway, depression of the C3 level would result. In early stages of immune-complex disease, there can be decreases in C4 levels with normal CH_{50}. *(Cecil, pp. 1788–1789)*

24. (A) The treatment of arthritic disorders is frequently limited by the occurrence of side effects of anti-inflammatory and remittive agents. It is necessary to be aware of these medication-related problems and to perform appropriate surveillance to detect early toxicity. Of the drugs listed, hydroxychloroquine (Plaquenil) is not properly matched with its side effect. The most serious complication from the use of this antimalarial agent is retinopathy. Although uncommon, the irreversible nature of the retinopathy and severe consequence of blindness demand close monitoring with frequent ophthalmoscopic examinations. *(Cecil, p. 1850)*

25. (B) Approximately 70% of patients with psoriatic arthritis present with asymmetric involvement of both large and small joints. Oligo- or polyarthritis may occur in this pattern. A "sausage toe" or inflammatory distal interphalangeal joint arthritis may suggest a diagnosis of psoriatic arthritis in patients in whom joint disease precedes the onset of skin lesions. Seronegative rheumatoid-like disease occurs in approximately 15 per cent of patients with psoriatic arthritis; other patterns of joint disease are less common. *(Cecil, pp. 1880–1881)*

26. (D) The biopsy is characteristic of Whipple's disease. Joint complaints in the disorder often precede other symptoms by several years and may mimic those of seronegative rheumatoid arthritis. *(Cecil, pp. 689, 1887)*

27. (A) Lymphadenopathy is not a feature of polymyalgia rheumatica or of giant cell arteritis. Morning stiffness and evidence of mild articular involvement, including both adhesive shoulder capsulitis and small knee effusions, are not uncommon. In some patients the distinction between polymyalgia rheumatica and early seronegative rheumatoid arthritis may be difficult or impossible without a period of clinical observation. *(Cecil, p. 1871)*

28. (E) Gold salts have been shown to be effective agents in the treatment of rheumatoid arthritis. They are not anti-inflammatory and have actions that have been termed "anti-rheumatoid" or "remittive." They can be used in patients who have progressive disease despite an adequate anti-inflammatory program, in patients with poor prognosis, or in patients with erosive disease as demonstrated by roentgenogram. An initial course consists of weekly intramuscular injections to a total dose of approximately 1 gm. If a response is demonstrated, the frequency of injections should be reduced, but the drug should be continued indefinitely. A variety of serious side effects, including proteinuria and rash, limit the use of gold and demand careful selection of patients for treatment. Since there are only a limited number of therapeutic options in patients with severe progressive rheumatoid arthritis, it is important to recognize that not all side effects are absolute contraindications to further therapy. Thus, following a skin reaction, gold can be restarted at a lower dose without recurrence in many patients. *(Cecil, p. 1850)*

29. (E) Midline granuloma is a progressive inflammatory disease that results in severe local tissue destruction of the nose, sinuses, and other structures of the face. Local radiation therapy has been of benefit, with high doses (5000 rads) resulting in a higher percentage of long-term remissions than lower doses. Other approaches to therapy have not been successful, as reflected in the previous designation of this disease as "lethal" midline granuloma. *(Cecil, p. 1897)*

30. (D) In both Reiter's syndrome and psoriatic arthritis, synovial fluid hemolytic complement levels may be elevated. Complement levels in rheumatoid joint fluid are normal or depressed. *(Cecil, p. 1880)*

31. (D) Drug-induced SLE resembles the naturally occurring disease in many respects, but antibodies to double-stranded DNA are not found. *(Cecil, p. 1856)*

32. (D) Urticaria pigmentosa, or systemic mastocytosis, results from the infiltration of skin by mast cells in a neoplastic proliferation of very slow growth. These cells can release mediators of hypersensitivity that provoke a variety of painful and distressing symptoms. The involved areas have freckle-like lesions that will produce a wheal and flare when stroked (Darier's sign). In some patients, stroking uninvolved skin produces a wheal of dermatographia. Food allergy is unrelated to urticaria pigmentosa, and the other listed conditions and agents are not associated with the skin infiltrate. *(Cecil, p. 1819)*

33. (D) Proximal weakness in spite of continued normal enzyme levels suggests emergence of steroid-induced myopathy. The only reliable "test" for this complication of therapy is a reduction in corticosteroid dosage coupled with sequential muscle testing. *(Cecil, p. 1875)*

34. (C) Although osteoarthritis is thought to be related to a degenerative noninflammatory process, certain joints are curiously spared. For example, the wrist and ankles are infrequently involved, although both are subject to considerable use or weight-bearing. The presence of wrist involvement in patients thought to have osteoarthritis should lead to other diagnostic considerations such as rheumatoid arthritis, crystal deposition disease, infection, or trauma. *(Cecil, pp. 1882–1883)*

35. (A) Pseudogout may present in a variety of patterns ranging from an acute monarthritis to a polyarticular form resembling rheumatoid arthritis. Since chondrocalcinosis is not always seen radiographically in symptomatic joints, a survey of other joints is often useful. It appears in the knees, wrists, and symphysis pubis. *(Cecil, p. 1881)*

36. (D) Disseminated or recurrent neisserial infections have been associated with deficiencies of several of the later components of the complement system including C5,

C6, C7, and C8. C1r, C1s, and C4 deficiencies have been associated with SLE; no clinical condition as yet has been ascribed to C9 deficiency. *(Cecil, p. 1788)*

37. (D) Psoriatic arthritis is suggested by the nail pitting and umbilical lesion in association with an asymmetric pattern of joint involvement including a DIP joint. Back complaints raise a question of associated spondyloarthropathy. *(Cecil, pp. 1880–1881)*

38. (B) The HLA-B27 antigen occurs in increased frequency in psoriatic arthritis, especially if there is associated spondylitis. The test, however, has little value in the evaluation of an individual patient since the antigen is found in 7% or so of normal controls (Caucasian) and is not invariably present even in the setting of florid spondyloarthropathy. The same logic applies in considering the HLA-B27 screen as a diagnostic tool in patients with other forms of suspected spondyloarthropathy. *(Cecil, pp. 1880–1881)*

39. (A) B lymphocytes bear immunoglobulin molecules that function as antigen-specific receptors and targets of regulatory interactions. In the role of surface receptors, the predominant immunoglobulin classes are IgD and IgM, which occur in a monomeric form that may serve distinct functions in terms of cell maturation and activation. It is interesting that, despite its abundance on the surface of cells, IgD is not well represented in the serum. The other immunoglobulin classes are not found to an appreciable extent as intrinsic cell surface proteins. *(Cecil, p. 1782)*

40. (A — False; B — False; C — True; D — False; E — False) Although not invariably low, pleural fluid glucose levels in rheumatoid pleurisy may reach levels of 10 mg/dl or less as a result of impaired transport mechanisms. Rheumatoid lung involvement tends to occur in men more than in women. It is usually associated with high titers of rheumatoid factor. Rheumatoid nodules may cavitate, and they have no radiographic features that allow sure differentiation from other nodular lung lesions. *(Cecil, pp. 1846, 1847)*

41. (A — True; B — False; C — True; D — True; E — False) Non–weight-bearing and splinting minimize pain and subsequent contracture in patients with septic arthritis. Infusion of antibiotics directly into the joint space is not required since parenteral administration of antibiotics provides adequate drug levels in the synovium and articular space. Two of the major factors contributing to a favorable outcome in septic arthritis are a lack of delay in treatment and adequate drainage of the affected joint. Antibiotics should be started without delay after cultures are taken. Choice of antibiotic should be based on the Gram stain and other special stains, as well as on the clinical setting. Any joint not amenable to thorough drainage by repeat needle aspiration should be opened surgically. *(Cecil, p. 1877)*

42. (A — False; B — False; C — False; D — False; E — True) There are no absolute criteria in Felty's syndrome for splenectomy based solely on the leukocyte count. Recurrent infections and persistent leg ulceration may improve after removal of the spleen. Corticosteroids or lithium may increase the leukocyte count, but have no proved benefit in the management of infectious complications. Any major surgery, including splenectomy, carried out in a patient with active, significant infection carries a high risk of perioperative mortality, and should be avoided. Gold therapy may be used cautiously in patients with leukopenia, and may ameliorate both the hematologic and clinical problems associated with Felty's syndrome. *(Cecil, p. 1851)*

43. (A — True; B — False; C — False; D — True; E — True) Roentgenographic studies of the joints can be very useful in distinguishing the various forms of arthritis. Although the findings in rheumatoid arthritis (RA) may vary depending on the duration and severity of disease, certain patterns of soft tissue and joint involvement signify a characteristic inflammatory process. Hand films are particularly useful because this area is commonly involved at all stages of the disease. Symmetric fusiform soft tissue swelling and juxta-articular osteoporosis are frequent findings. Erosions at characteristic locations and without surrounding reaction occur in some patients with RA and distinguish a more aggressive form of the disease with a tendency to deformity. Bony reaction and new bone formation are not usual features of RA and occur more frequently in osteoarthritis. Similarly, periosteal elevation is not a finding indicative of RA. *(Cecil, p. 1844)*

44. (A — False; B — False; C — False; D — True) Patients with inflammatory bowel disease can suffer from two forms of arthritis. In the spondylitic pattern, there is involvement of the spine similar to that in ankylosing spondylitis. HLA-B27 occurs frequently in these patients, whose clinical course is not dissimilar from that of those with ankylosing spondylitis without the bowel problem. The severity of the spine disease is not related to the activity of the bowel inflammation. In the second pattern there is involvement of peripheral joints, especially the knees, elbows, and ankles. These patients do *not* have an increased incidence of HLA-B27, although they frequently have other inflammatory conditions such as erythema nodosum and uveitis. The clinical activity of this form of arthritis is more closely correlated with the bowel disease, but the decision concerning surgery should be based on the status of the gastrointestinal disease, not the arthropathy. *(Cecil, p. 1841)*

45. (A — True; B — False; C — False; D — True; E — True) Gamma globulin preparations can be very valuable in preventing infection in patients with immunodeficiency disease. Nevertheless, such therapy can be complicated by serious side effects or undesired biologic actions. For example, an IgA-deficient individual can respond to administered IgA as if it were foreign. As a consequence of this sensitization, later exposure to IgA (particularly in the form of blood product transfusions) can lead to fatal anaphylaxis. Therefore, globulin preparations are contraindicated in these patients. Even if gamma globulin could be administered safely, it would not correct the lack of IgA in secretions, which is where IgA exerts its most important protective activity. In transient hypogammaglobulinemia of infancy, the immunologic disturbance is self-limited. Exogenously provided globulins can suppress the development of immunologic capabilities of affected children and may prolong the deficiency state. *(Cecil, pp. 1791–1792, 1794–1795)*

46. (A — True; B — False; C — False; D — True; E — False) In the course of severe or untreated polymyositis or dermatomyositis, atrophy of involved muscles may occur. Postexertional cramping is characteristic of metabolic muscle defects as in McArdle's disease or carnitine palmityltransferase deficiency. Muscle fasciculations suggest denervation rather than myopathic disease. Weakness of the facial musculature is rare in these disorders, and suggests myasthenia gravis. *(Cecil, p. 1873)*

47. (A — False; B — True; C — True; D — True; E — False) JRA most likely represents a series of diseases that are linked by the occurrence of joint inflammation. There is considerable heterogeneity in the clinical presentation of patients with this diagnosis, prompting some to use other terminologies to reflect the differences from adult rheumatoid disease. It is important, therefore, to identify features that distinguish adult and juvenile rheumatoid disease, as well as similarities that can be encountered in patients with JRA. Most patients with the diagnosis of JRA do not have positive serologic tests for rheumatoid factor, and monoarticular disease is more frequent than in adult RA. There are, however, children with the diagnosis of JRA who appear genuinely to have an early onset of rheumatoid disease; for these individuals with chronic disease and deformity, gold is appropriate as remittive therapy (as in the adult). Different subsets of patients with JRA have been distinguished by clinical and serologic features that provide prognostic information and guidelines for follow-up. For example, boys with pauciarticular disease show a high incidence of HLA-B27 and may represent an early onset of ankylosing spondylitis. The presence of positive ANA titers is associated with iridocyclitis, and directs attention to the need for frequent ophthalmologic evaluation. *(Cecil, pp. 1851–1852)*

48. (A — True; B — True; C — True; D — False) Depression in the total hemolytic complement can occur via at least two different mechanisms: (1) isolated deficiency of a single component of the system, as in hereditary C4 deficiency disease; and (2) consumption of various components through activation by immune complexes, as in SLE, rheumatoid vasculitis, and other vasculitic disorders. In hereditary angioneurotic edema, C2 and C4 are decreased during acute attacks, but not to levels at which the CH_{50} is affected. *(Cecil, pp. 1788–1789, 1853, 1864–1865; Samter, pp. 244–280)*

49. (A — False; B — False; C — True; D — False; E — False) Because of the severe and sometimes fatal results of allergic reactions to insect stings, physicians must be aware of the proper approach to diagnosis, treatment, and prevention. There are multiple antigens borne by insects of the order Hymenoptera, and use of improved antigen preparations and immunologic testing have allowed patterns of susceptibility to these materials to be investigated. The skin test is the most sensitive and specific technique for documenting allergy. This and the RAST show that only about 10% of patients with such allergies are sensitive to both bee and vespid venom. After the nature of the antigen to which a sensitive patient is allergic has been documented, immunotherapy can be undertaken. This treatment presumably leads to the production of IgG antibodies, which are protective, unlike IgE antibodies, which lead to anaphylactic reactions. Venom therapy should be employed, as whole body extract has been shown to be ineffective. Desensitization therapy should be performed rapidly over a six- to eight-week period, as this schedule is associated with both improved responsiveness and a lower incidence of adverse reactions. *(Cecil, pp. 1805–1807)*

50. (A — False; B — True; C — False; D — False; E — False) Marked regional osteopenia is characteristic of reflex sympathetic dystrophy. Protecting the affected part may actually prolong the clinical course. Use of the involved extremity in spite of pain should be encouraged, and pain medications, anti-inflammatory drugs, and corticosteroids all may be useful in reducing symptoms. Coolness and diaphoresis of an involved limb result from regional redistribution of blood flow, not from proximal obstruction. There are no serologic abnormalities with reflex dystrophy. *(Cecil, p. 1947)*

51. (A — False; B — False; C — True; D — True; E — False) Synovial biopsy has limited application as a diagnostic tool. In most forms of inflammatory joint disease, such as rheumatoid disease and psoriatic arthritis, the histologic appearance of the synovium is nonspecific. Increased synovial iron deposition is nonspecific and is not diagnostic of hemochromatosis. Indications for biopsy include a suspicion of amyloid joint disease; chronic, "culture-negative" arthritis suspected of being tuberculous or fungal in nature; and the evaluation of suspected pigmented villonodular synovitis. *(Cecil, p. 1842)*

52. (A — True; B — False; C — True; D — False; E — False) In all mammalian species studied there is a genetic region, termed the "major histocompatibility complex" (MHC), which is associated with a variety of immunologic functions, most prominently rejection of foreign tissue grafts and control of immune responses. Within this region various subloci have been identified, each determining specific cell surface antigens as well as functional activities. These antigens differ in structure and cell distribution. HLA-A and HLA-B locus antigens, also called class I, are found on the surface of all cells. They are responsible for strong organ graft rejection and, perhaps as a correlate *in vitro*, they can induce cytotoxic T cells with specificity for that antigen. Mixed lymphocyte reactivity is a proliferative reaction resulting from antigenic differences at the HLA-D locus, the analog of the I region in humans. Graft-versus-host reactions, most commonly encountered in bone marrow transplants in immunologically compromised individuals, are also associated with the I region. Suppression of specific immune response has not yet been clearly identified in humans, but in animals the linkage has also been to the I region. *(Cecil, p. 1812)*

53. (A — True; B — True; C — True; D — True; E — False) Sjögren's syndrome is a chronic inflammatory disease marked by inflammation and destruction of the salivary and lacrimal glands. It occurs in both a primary and secondary form, with distinguishing features including the association with another rheumatic disease, as well as certain immunogenetic and serologic findings. Elements of the sicca complex usually dominate the clinical picture with dryness of the eyes, mouth, and other mucous membranes producing a variety of distressing symptoms; nasal mucosal involvement can lead to recurrent epistaxis. Lymphocytic infiltrates can lead to both renal and pulmonary dysfunction. An important feature of Sjögren's syndrome is disturbance of immune function. Abnormalities of cells of the B-cell lineage may culminate in monoclonal gammopathies, macroglobulinemia, pseudolymphoma, and malignant lymphomas. Elevation of the β_2-microglobulin level in the saliva of patients with this condition may provide a clue to the course of the disease. *(Cecil, pp. 1861–1862)*

54. (A — False; B — True; C — True; D — True; E — True) Patients with SLE should consider pregnancy only when all major system involvement is stable and well controlled. Because oral contraceptives may exacerbate lupus, alternate methods of birth control are preferable. During pregnancy systemic corticosteroid requirements will continue; there are no known teratogenic effects related to corticosteroid therapy. Disease activity may increase in the last trimester of pregnancy or immediately post partum. Newborn infants may have serologic evidence or limited clinical manifestations of lupus at birth and for a limited time thereafter as a result of passive transfer of maternal antibodies *in utero*. *(Zurier)*

55. (A — False; B — True; C — False; D — True; E — True) Allergy to pollens results from the release of mediators by sensitized cells when they are exposed to very low doses of antigens. This condition involves specific IgE antibodies, although the diagnosis is best made by careful history regarding seasonal allergy as well as the judicious use of skin tests. Immunotherapy with pollen extracts can reduce sensitivity, possibly through the induction of IgG antibodies to the allergens. *(Cecil, pp. 1800–1802)*

56. (A — False; B — False; C — False; D — True; E — False) Renal microaneurysms are rarely seen in vasculitic syndromes other than polyarteritis nodosa. Renal artery involvement occurs occasionally in giant cell arteritis, but it does not affect smaller intrarenal vasculature. Renal dysfunction in Fabry's disease results from glycosphingolipid accumulation in glomerular, tubular, and endothelial cells. *(Cecil, pp. 1867, 1871; Baker and Robinson)*

57. (A — True; B — False; C — True; D — False; E — True) Cold urticaria exists in inherited and acquired forms, but does not involve complement components. Although skin reactions are the usual result of exposure to cold objects, attacks may involve angioedema or vascular collapse when bodily exposure to cold occurs. The mechanisms responsible for this condition are suggested by the facts that it is transferred by serum and that histamine is released following cold exposure. *(Cecil, p. 1798)*

58. (A — False; B — True; C — False; D — True; E — False) Neuropathic joint disease (Charcot joints) is a progressive degenerative arthritis resulting from a variety of neurologic disorders. Proprioceptive and pain sensations are impaired in the affected joints, resulting in loss of normal protective reactions and joint deterioration from weight-bearing and motion. Diseases that affect sensation are the usual causes of this disorder, with syphilis and diabetes the most common associated conditions. Syringomyelia and myelomeningocele are other causes. Cerebrovascular accidents are associated with the syndrome of reflex sympathetic dystrophy; intrapulmonary lesions may be accompanied by hypertrophic pulmonary osteoarthropathy. *(Cecil, p. 1888)*

59. (A — False; B — False; C — True; D — True; E — True) Hereditary angioneurotic edema results from the absence of function of the inhibitor of the activated form of the first complement protein of the classical pathway. Acute attacks may be marked by angioedema or acute abdominal pain that sometimes mimics a surgical abdominal condition. Low levels of C4 result from spontaneous activation of the complement cascade. Specific therapy for termination of acute attacks is not well established, but anabolic steroids such as danazol are effective in preventing them. The inheritance of this condition is autosomal dominant; however, the absence of a family history should not exclude the diagnosis. *(Cecil, pp. 1788, 1798)*

60. (A — False; B — False; C — True; D — True; E — False) Pulmonary disease in Wegener's granulomatosis is characterized by nodular and infiltrative lesions without enlargement of hilar nodes. Cyclophosphamide is the drug of choice and should be instituted immediately if renal disease is present. The role of corticosteroids given in combination with immunosuppressive therapy is controversial; given as a single agent they are of no documented benefit. Laboratory findings in Wegener's disease are nonspecific and include leukocytosis and diffuse hypergammaglobulinemia. Eosinophilia is rare. Biopsy of vasculitic skin lesions may or may not demonstrate evidence of granulomatous inflammation in conjunction with necrotizing vascular disease. Antibodies to glomerular basement membrane are seen in Goodpasture's syndrome, not Wegener's. *(Cecil, pp. 1869–1871)*

61. (B); 62. (D); 63. (D); 64. (C) Several different classes of antibody molecules have been distinguished on the basis of their immunochemical and functional properties. Immunoglobulins D and M are found on the surface of B cells, where they function as antigen specific receptors. IgM and IgG can fix complement, with the IgG1 and IgG3 subclasses activating complement via the classical pathway. IgA antibody molecules can initiate complement activation via the alternate pathway. IgA antibodies are the predominant immunoglobulin in secretions, where they play a critical role in establishing local immunity. IgE antibodies mediate allergic reactions by binding to mast cells causing mediator release; they have been termed "reaginic antibodies" because of this role in immediate hypersensitivity reactions. *(Cecil, pp. 1779–1780)*

65. (C); 66. (D); 67. (A); 68. (B); 69. (E) A significant advance in the treatment of patients with vasculitic disorders has resulted from improved diagnosis and classification of patients on the basis of histopathologic findings such as the size and location of involved vessels and the nature of the inflammatory cells in the infiltrate. Takayasu's disease, like temporal or giant cell arteritis, involves large arteries with the presence of giant cells as a distinguishing feature. The two diseases differ in the age of the patients, with Takayasu's affecting younger women. Takayasu's disease also shows a predilection for the aorta and its branches, in contrast to temporal arteritis, which affects primarily the cranial circulation. In Henoch-Schönlein purpura, as well as in hypersensitivity vasculitis, there is skin involvement frequently manifested as palpable purpura; small vessels are affected, and there is leukocytoclasis or nuclear debris in the infiltrate. Lymphomatoid granulomatosis resembles Wegener's granulomatosis in some clinical features but can be differentiated on the basis of invasion of blood vessels by atypical lymphocytes; culmination in lymphoma or lymphoproliferative disease is not uncommon. Pulmonary involvement and eosinophilia distinguish Churg-Strauss disease from periarteritis nodosa. Kawasaki's disease, which is more commonly encountered in Japan, is characterized by vasculitis with coronary artery involvement as an important clinical finding; angiography is useful for detecting the aneurysms. *(Cecil, pp. 1863–1866)*

70. (C); 71. (C); 72. (A) Since the antigens of the major histocompatibility complex (MHC) were described in humans, there have been many studies seeking to associate the occurrence of disease with specific HLA haplotypes. Because of the role of the MHC in the control of immune responses, immunologic or inflammatory diseases have been important targets for these investigations, and a variety of conditions have been shown to occur with greater frequency in certain HLA haplotypes. Diseases not usually considered to be immunologic in origin have also been associated with this gene region. Different diseases are related to the different loci of the HLA complex, suggesting mechanistic differences in the nature of these associations. Ankylosing spondylitis is associated with the B locus antigen, HLA-B27; rheumatoid arthritis, SLE, and Sjögren's syndrome are associated with the D locus. Juvenile-onset diabetes mellitus is also associated with a D locus antigen. Hemochromatosis, not usually grouped with inflammatory diseases, is associated with the A2 antigen. These associations have important implications in studies of the pathogenesis of various diseases, but the precise role for HLA typing in clinical practice is still uncertain. *(Cecil, pp. 1813–1814)*

73. (A) *Trichinella* larvae are produced in the intestine by developing adult nematodes; they invade the circulation and encyst in muscle. Myalgia occurs if the number of parasites is large. Fever, periorbital edema, eosinophilia, and subconjunctival hemorrhage may also occur. *(Cecil, pp. 1771–1772)*

74. (D) Tuberculous infection of the hip may lead to advanced joint destruction because symptoms are relatively mild at onset in comparison with those caused by the more common offending agents in septic hip disease. *(Cecil, p. 1877)*

75. (B) β-Hemolytic streptococcal pharyngitis, untreated, may induce acute rheumatic fever with characteristic subcutaneous nodules. *(Cecil, pp. 1445, 1450–1456)*

76. (C) Hepatitis B infection may result in systemic disease with urticaria and arthralgias as a prodrome; it occasionally progresses to a full-blown vasculitic syndrome resembling polyarteritis nodosa. Accompanying hypocomplementemia suggests an immune complex–mediated process. *(Cecil, pp. 1877–1878)*

77. (E) Pseudogout, unlike gout, occurs commonly in both men and women; it usually presents as a monarthritis of the knee rather than the toe or ankle, as in gout. Rarely, both gout and pseudogout may occur simultaneously in the same joint. *(Cecil, p. 1881)*

78. (A) Subtalar involvement can occur in any of the disorders listed, but the associated plantar heel pain suggests enthesopathy as commonly seen in Reiter's syndrome. *(Cecil, pp. 1879–1880)*

79. (D) Alcohol ingestion results in increased serum uric acid levels and may be associated with gout. Reiter's syndrome might also present with a self-limited monarthritis, but Reiter's usually occurs in younger patients, and an episode of joint inflammation often takes weeks or months to resolve as opposed to the seven- to ten-day course of initial gouty episodes. *(Cecil, pp. 1113, 1879)*

80. (B) Gonococcal arthritis is seen most commonly in sexually active women. Tenosynovitis is a frequent element of the pattern of joint involvement. *(Cecil, p. 1877)*

81. (C) A disproportionately painful joint in a patient with otherwise controlled joint disease should arouse suspicion of septic arthritis. *Staphylococcus aureus* is the most common offending organism. *(Cecil, pp. 1878–1879)*

82. (C) Some patients with SCID lack the enzyme adenosine deaminase (ADA) and show disorders in several products of purine metabolism. *(Cecil, pp. 1794–1795)*

83. (B) Nezelof's syndrome, although differing in the nature of the immune deficiency found, also has disturbances in purine metabolism; the enzyme involved in this disorder is purine nucleoside phosphorylase (PNP). ADA and PNP act sequentially in the purine salvage pathway; their relationship to immunodeficiency suggests that lymphocyte populations may be especially sensitive to the products of these enzymatic reactions. *(Cecil, p. 1794)*

84. (E) In chronic granulomatous disease neutrophil disturbances lead to sensitivity to infection. Impaired generation of peroxide, attributable in some patients to glutathione peroxidase deficiency, appears to underlie the inability of the leukocytes to handle infection. Other conditions in this group are marked by certain clinical and laboratory findings, but their relationship to disease pathogenesis remains to be fully defined. *(Cecil, pp. 910–912)*

85. (D) In ataxia telangiectasia, which is marked by complex multisystem abnormalities and an increased incidence of malignancy, low levels of IgA and high levels of the α-fetoprotein have been demonstrated. *(Cecil, p. 1795)*

86. (A) Eczema, thrombocytopenia, and susceptibility to infection represent a diagnostic triad in the Wiskott-Aldrich syndrome. *(Cecil, p. 1795)*

87. (B) The Ehlers-Danlos syndromes are a group of genetic disorders sharing a variety of clinical features including joint hypermobility, hyperextensible skin, and connective tissue friability. *(Cecil, pp. 1138–1139)*

88. (C) Osteogenesis imperfecta is characterized by abnormal bone composition and structure resulting in multiple pathologic fractures; blue sclerae are seen in the more severe congenita variant. *(Cecil, p. 1335)*

89. (E) Homocystinuria may also be associated with bone abnormalities and fractures, but the characteristic ocular lesion is ectopia lentis. *(Cecil, p. 1106)*

90. (A) Ochronosis results from the absence of homogentisic acid oxidase and is characterized by pigmentation in the sclerae, ears, and other tissues. Late clinical manifestations include axial and large joint degenerative arthritis. Degenerative, heavily calcified intervertebral discs seen throughout the spine are virtually pathognomonic of the disorder. *(Cecil, p. 1102)*

91. (D) Fabry's disease is an X-linked lysosomal storage disease resulting from deficiency of α-galactosidase A. Gradual cellular dysfunction is caused by intracellular accumulation of glycosphingolipid in a variety of cells including endothelium. Angiokeratomas are characteristic superficial vascular lesions, especially in the pelvic girdle area. Diagnosis is confirmed by slit-lamp examination of the cornea and by biochemical determination of trihexosyl ceramide in blood or urine. *(Cecil, p. 1092)*

92. (C) A diagnosis of pseudogout is confirmed by the finding of synovial fluid PMNs containing positively birefringent crystals of calcium pyrophosphate. Monosodium urate crystals of gout are negatively birefringent, needle-shaped, and easily distinguished from those seen in pseudogout. *(Cecil, p. 1881)*

93. (A) Aseptic necrosis of the femoral head may develop spontaneously in a variety of disorders, including sickle cell disease and hemoglobin SC disease. It occurs most frequently as a complication of corticosteroid therapy. *(Cecil, pp. 889, 1851)*

94. (B) Lyme arthritis is a recently characterized disorder in which the skin lesions of erythema chronicum migrans commonly precede the onset of asymmetric large joint arthritis by four to six weeks. *(Cecil, p. 1878)*

95. (D) Multicentric reticulohistiocytosis is a rare disease in which deforming arthritis is accompanied by reddish-brown skin nodules. Biopsy of a skin nodule will show infiltration of the skin and subcutaneous tissues with numerous macrophages and histiocytes containing PAS-positive material. *(Cecil, p. 1888)*

96. (E) Nongonococcal urethritis or other forms of inflammatory genitourinary disease in association with arthritis should suggest a diagnosis of Reiter's syndrome. *(Cecil, pp. 1879–1880)*

97. (C) Both skin and joint symptoms in SLE may be exacerbated by exposure to ultraviolet irradiation in the form of sunlight or intense fluorescent lighting. *(Cecil, pp. 1852–1854)*

98. (A) Nail pitting and dystrophy may occur in Reiter's syndrome but are more characteristic of psoriasis and psoriatic arthritis. *(Cecil, pp. 1880–1881)*

99. (B) Recurrent thrombophlebitis is a major clinical problem in Behçet's disease and may contribute to considerable morbidity. *(Cecil, pp. 1899–1900)*

100. (D) Lupus pernio in sarcoidosis may resemble a discoid malar eruption in SLE, but is easily distinguished by biopsy. *(Cecil, pp. 1893–1894)*

101. (D); 102. (A); 103. (E); 104. (B); 105. (C) 101. Isoniazid, along with hydralazine, phenytoin, and procainamide, has been implicated in the induction of an illness with features of SLE. **102.** Aspirin hypersensitivity can be manifest as asthmatic attacks, especially in individuals with nasal polyps. **103.** Quinidine has been associated with thrombocytopenia. **104.** Sulfa drugs are associated with a wide variety of side effects including inflammatory disturbances; they are a leading cause of drug-associated erythema nodosum. **105.** Penicillin can participate in several forms of immune reaction, including allergy and the induction of hemolytic anemia. In the latter a determinant formed by penicillin with a component of the red cell membrane is the target of the antibody reaction. *(Cecil, pp. 1816–1818)*

BIBLIOGRAPHY

Baker, S. B., and Robinson, D. R.: Unusual renal manifestations of Wegener's granulomatosis. Report of two cases. Am. J. Med., *64*:883, 1978.

Samter, M. (ed.): Immunological Diseases. 3rd ed. Boston, Little, Brown & Company, 1978.

Zurier: R. B.: Systemic lupus erythematosus and pregnancy. Clin. Rheumat. Dis., *1*:613, 1975.

PART 10
NEUROLOGIC DISEASE

Barrie J. Hurwitz and J. Scott Luther

DIRECTIONS: For questions 1 to 77, choose the ONE BEST answer to each question.

1. A 48-year-old man has had progressive tingling and numbness of the feet for the last six months. On examination he is alert and oriented but a little vague. Cranial nerves and muscle strength are normal; tone is slightly increased in the legs. Vibration and position sense are decreased in the distal legs and to a lesser degree in the hands. Pain and temperature senses are slightly decreased in the feet. Patellar reflexes are hyperactive, Achilles reflexes are absent, and bilateral extensor plantar responses are present. Hematocrit is 40%; leukocyte count is 6800/cu mm; blood urea nitrogen is 16 mg/dl; serum glucose is 85 mg/dl; and serum electrolytes are normal. Results of which one of the following studies would most likely be abnormal?

A. Roentgenograms of the cervical spine
B. Computerized tomography (CT scan) of the brain
C. Schilling test
D. Glucose tolerance test
E. Hepatic function tests

2. A 30-year-old man has a one-week history of low back pain that intermittently radiates into the left leg and is associated with numbness of the left foot. Which one of the following signs would most reliably indicate a herniated low lumbar intervertebral disc in this patient?

A. Low back pain exacerbated by forward flexion of the trunk and relieved by lying down
B. Point tenderness on firm percussion over the lumbar spine
C. Pain radiating from the back into the left leg when the nonpainful extended right leg is raised
D. Pain radiating from the back into the extended left leg when it is raised
E. Pain in the lumbar area produced by neck flexion

3. All the following statements regarding amyotrophic lateral sclerosis are true EXCEPT

A. Neuronal loss occurs in the cerebral cortex
B. Neuronal loss occurs in motor cranial nerve nuclei
C. Neuronal loss occurs in the anterior horns of the spinal cord
D. Visible multiple fasciculations are common
E. Motor nerve conduction velocities are abnormally slow

4. A somnolent and confused 36-year-old man is brought to the emergency room, having been found in this condition by neighbors. No other history is available. He is tremulous and moves all four extremities semipurposefully. There are brisk oculocephalic responses with generalized hyperreflexia. The remainder of the neurologic examination is normal. Respiratory rate is 36 per minute. Arterial blood studies show a pH of 7.51, a Pa_{CO_2} of 25 mm Hg, and a Pa_{O_2} of 80 mm Hg; serum bicarbonate is 21 mEq/L. What is the most likely diagnosis?

A. Diabetic ketoacidosis
B. Uremic encephalopathy
C. Salicylate intoxication
D. Hepatic encephalopathy
E. Depressant drug poisoning

5. Which of the following conditions is the most likely cause of sudden recurrent syncope in a middle-aged man?

A. Multifocal premature ventricular contractions
B. Vertebrobasilar transient ischemic attacks (TIAs)
C. Hyperventilation attacks
D. Aortic stenosis
E. Left carotid artery TIAs

6. The vegetative state is characterized by all the following EXCEPT

A. sleep-wake cycles
B. spontaneous swallowing, chewing, and eye opening
C. retained mental content with inability to express mentation
D. spontaneous respirations not usually requiring ventilatory support
E. retained spontaneous circulatory control

7. All the following neurologic disorders are transmitted by autosomal dominant inheritance EXCEPT

A. tuberous sclerosis
B. Huntington's disease
C. myotonic muscular dystrophy
D. Duchenne muscular dystrophy
E. von Recklinghausen's disease (neurofibromatosis)

8. Peripheral neuropathy may be caused by any of the following drugs EXCEPT

A. nitrofurantoin
B. isoniazid
C. vincristine
D. phenytoin
E. gentamicin

9. The abrupt onset of diplopia may be caused by any of the following conditions EXCEPT

A. multiple sclerosis
B. myasthenic syndrome
C. Wernicke's encephalopathy
D. cavernous sinus thrombosis
E. lateral pontine infarction

10. Accepted criteria for the diagnosis of brain death include all the following EXCEPT

A. absent deep tendon reflexes
B. absent oculovestibular reflexes

C. isoelectric electrocardiogram for 30 minutes at maximal gain
D. negative drug screen
E. absent brain-stem function for 12 to 24 hours

11. A 61-year-old woman is being evaluated for episodic right upper quadrant pain, which you think may represent recurrent bouts of cholecystitis with cholelithiasis. She has no neurologic complaints. During the physical examination you detect a left carotid bruit, which is maximal in intensity near the angle of the jaw. The patient is probably going to require cholecystectomy. With regard to the left carotid bruit, the most appropriate approach would be

A. carotid arteriography
B. anticoagulation
C. noninvasive studies (Doppler)
D. papaverine hydrochloride
E. observation with no further studies

12. A 30-year-old alcoholic is admitted to the hospital for evaluation of suspected withdrawal seizures. After two days he becomes confused, disoriented, and hyperpyretic, and has visual hallucinations. Which of the following is the most appropriate therapy?

A. Vitamin B complex
B. Phenytoin
C. Chlordiazepoxide
D. Alcohol
E. Corticosteroids

13. Which of the following is the most reliable diagnostic feature of carpal tunnel syndrome?

A. Presence of Tinel's sign
B. Thenar atrophy
C. Nocturnal paresthesia of the hand
D. Numbness of the hand
E. Hypothenar atrophy

14. You are asked to confirm the diagnosis of amyotrophic lateral sclerosis in a 45-year-old man with recent onset of bulbar signs and symptoms. The differential diagnosis must include all the following EXCEPT

A. inflammatory polyradiculoneuropathy (Guillain-Barré syndrome)
B. myasthenia gravis
C. botulism
D. avitaminosis B_{12}
E. poliomyelitis

15. A 38-year-old woman is brought to the emergency room after suffering a seizure. There is a two-day history of headache and lethargy, but no previous seizures. On examination, she has poor attention span and memory function. Plantar response on the left is extensor. Computerized tomography of the brain is normal. Which of the following is the most likely diagnosis?

A. Herpes simplex encephalitis
B. Glioblastoma multiforme
C. Intracerebral hemorrhage
D. Embolic occlusion at the trifurcation of the right middle cerebral artery
E. Todd's paralysis

16. Which of the following is the most common idiopathic seizure type occurring in the adult population?

A. Generalized tonic-clonic (grand mal)
B. Absence (petit mal)
C. Akinetic
D. Partial (focal)
E. Myoclonic

17. A 19-year-old man with a chronic seizure disorder comes to the emergency room stating he has had two seizures in the past four hours. While waiting to be seen, he has a 90-second generalized major motor seizure. He is now postictal. Which one of the following should be administered?

A. Diazepam, 10-mg intravenous bolus
B. Diazepam, 10 mg intramuscularly
C. Phenytoin, 250 mg intramuscularly
D. Phenytoin, 250-mg intravenous bolus
E. Phenytoin 250 mg intravenously over five minutes

18. A 26-year-old woman is brought to hospital at midnight screaming hysterically and complaining of headache. The patient speaks little English and translation is difficult, but her family says she suddenly collapsed while seeing her mother onto a plane in an emotional departure. When the patient awoke from her faint she reported a headache. She has a history of headaches for many years, and the current one is different only in intensity. Her visits to the medical clinic for headaches have been frequent, but the absence of signs during these visits has provoked a psychiatric referral to be effected next month. Your detailed neurologic and general medical examination is normal. Which of the following is most appropriate?

A. Immediate psychiatric consultation
B. Referral to psychiatric clinic in the morning
C. Immediate computerized tomography of the brain
D. Lumbar puncture
E. Diazepam, 5 mg orally, and observation overnight in the emergency room

19. All the following statements regarding the management of parkinsonism are true EXCEPT

A. Early treatment will halt progression
B. Psychotherapy is important in its management
C. Regular physical therapy is a useful adjunct
D. The introduction of levodopa has significantly lowered the mortality rate
E. The "on-off" phenomenon is a disabling complication of chronic levodopa therapy

20. All the following drugs are useful in the prophylactic treatment of migraine EXCEPT

A. propranolol
B. amitriptyline
C. methysergide
D. cyproheptadine
E. oxycodone

21. Symptoms and signs of marijuana abuse include all the following EXCEPT

A. impaired memory and driving performance
B. enhanced perception of sounds and colors
C. conjunctival vascular congestion
D. depression and acute panic reactions
E. withdrawal seizures in chronic abusers

22. Characteristics of multiple sclerosis include all the following EXCEPT

A. ataxia
B. aphasia

C. facial pain
D. internuclear ophthalmoplegia
E. nystagmus

23. Which one of the following lesions would NOT be expected to cause coma?

A. Hemorrhage in the pons
B. Cerebellar hemorrhage with secondary compression of the brain stem
C. Right hemisphere glioblastoma causing uncal herniation
D. An infarct in the dominant cerebral hemisphere
E. Metabolic depression of both hemispheres due to barbiturate intoxication

24. Parkinsonism may occur as a predominant manifestation of all the following EXCEPT

A. generalized anoxia-ischemia
B. manganese intoxication
C. brain tumor
D. cerebral atherosclerosis
E. phenothiazine ingestion

25. In a patient with disordered thinking and behavior, which of the following suggests an organic delirium rather than a psychiatric disease?

A. Auditory hallucinations
B. A normal awake electroencephalogram
C. Asterixis and myoclonus
D. Confusion as to personal identity, place, and time
E. Normal cognitive function (e.g., abstractions, calculations)

26. A 65-year-old housewife is brought to the emergency room because of the sudden onset of disordered speech and behavior. On examination there is a rapid, irregularly irregular pulse. Speech is fluent with frequent nonsense words; the rest of the neurologic examination is only "probably" normal because the patient does not understand or does not cooperate with any verbal commands. The most likely diagnosis is

A. embolic stroke involving Broca's area
B. embolic stroke involving the superior temporal gyrus
C. left putamenal hemorrhage
D. acute schizophrenic word-salad
E. hysteria

27. Korsakoff's syndrome is characterized by all the following EXCEPT

A. loss of remote memories
B. failure to lay down new memories
C. severe impairment of intellectual functions other than memory
D. confabulation
E. lack of insight into disability

28. You are called to the emergency room to see a young man in coma. No history is available. Examination reveals that the pupils are 3 mm, equal, and reactive. Doll's eyes and oculovestibular responses are absent. The limbs are flaccid, and respirations are slow and irregular. The most likely diagnosis is

A. pontine infarction or hemorrhage
B. metabolic encephalopathy
C. late diencephalic stage of central herniation
D. psychogenic unresponsiveness
E. uncal herniation

29. You are called to the emergency room to see an intoxicated middle-aged man suffering from lethargy and confusion. When you arrive 15 minutes later, he is unresponsive to voice; noxious supraorbital stimulation produces extension of the right arm and leg (decerebrate), and flexion of the left arm and leg (decorticate). The left pupil is 8 mm and unreactive; the right is 5 mm and minimally reactive. The eyes are dysconjugate without doll's eyes. Which of the following would you do first?

A. Check the oculovestibular reflex with ice water
B. Obtain a roentgenogram of the skull to look for a fracture
C. Perform lumbar puncture to rule out subarachnoid hemorrhage
D. Hyperventilate the patient and administer mannitol intravenously
E. Draw blood for alcohol level

30. Coma resulting from sedative drug overdose is commonly associated with all the following EXCEPT

A. prolonged coma with absence of any sign of brain function
B. concomitant use of alcohol
C. hypothermia unless aspiration pneumonia is present
D. reactive pupils
E. asymmetric neurologic signs

31. When a patient is admitted in coma or slips into unconsciousness while in the hospital, which of the following would you do first?

A. Establish a clear airway
B. Treat infection and convulsions
C. Administer glucose, 25 gm intravenously
D. Perform a lumbar puncture
E. Administer naloxone

32. You are called to the emergency room to see a previously healthy 65-year-old woman complaining of vertigo of sudden onset. On examination she is pale, diaphoretic, and lying on her right side with her eyes closed. When she opens her eyes there is nystagmus to the right on forward gaze that increases on right gaze; she becomes nauseated and vomits. Blood pressure is normal; extraocular movements and hearing are intact. The patient falls to the left and past points to the left; neurologic examination is otherwise normal. The most likely diagnosis is

A. Meniere's disease
B. left lateral medullary infarct
C. syndrome of internal auditory artery occlusion
D. multiple sclerosis
E. vestibular neuronitis

33. The INITIAL procedure of choice to assess occlusion of the superior sagittal sinus is

A. electroencephalography
B. cerebral angiography
C. pneumoencephalography
D. dynamic radionuclide brain scanning
E. computerized tomography of the brain

34. A 45-year-old man has a two-year history of impotence, and describes the recent onset of faintness on arising to an erect position and after a few minutes of standing. Examination reveals a normal blood pressure in the supine position, but when the patient stands systolic and diastolic pressures drop 40 and 20 mm Hg respectively without an increase in heart rate. There is lack of facial expression, diffuse muscle rigidity, and a resting tremor of both hands. The remainder of the examination is normal. The most likely diagnosis is

A. chronic hyperventilation syndrome
B. idiopathic autonomic insufficiency
C. cerebral artery occlusive disease
D. postencephalitic parkinsonism
E. drug-induced parkinsonism

35. A 65-year-old man complains of several episodes of blindness in the left eye lasting up to five minutes, and he now has persisting headache, difficulty with expression, and weakness of the right hand and of the face. The most likely diagnosis is

A. occlusion of the left middle cerebral artery
B. focal seizures involving the left motor cortex
C. left internal carotid artery occlusion
D. chronic subdural hematoma
E. hemiplegic migraine

36. You are called to the emergency room to see a 65-year-old woman who is experiencing sudden nausea, vomiting, headache, and inability to walk. The patient is alert; blood pressure is 240/150 mm Hg. On neurologic examination there is paralysis of upward gaze and of left lateral gaze; pupils are 3 mm, equal, and reactive; there is a left lower motor neuron facial palsy; and ataxia of the left arm and leg is noted. All four extremities move with good strength, and the plantar response is flexor bilaterally. There are no sensory abnormalities. The most likely diagnosis is

A. left vertebral occlusion
B. left internal auditory artery occlusion
C. pontine hemorrhage
D. thalamic hemorrhage
E. cerebellar hemorrhage

37. A 45-year-old hypertensive man is brought to the hospital by his family because of drowsiness and confusion of more than 24 hours' duration. The patient is nauseated, and complains of a headache and difficulty with vision. On examination blood pressure is 225/140 mm Hg. There is bilateral papilledema, and the patient cannot count fingers held before his eyes. Both pupils react. The neck is supple. There are no motor or sensory deficits, but both plantar reflexes are extensor. Which of the following is the most likely diagnosis?

A. Progressive subcortical encephalopathy
B. Ruptured anterior communicating aneurysm
C. Hypertensive encephalopathy
D. Thalamic hemorrhage
E. Pseudotumor cerebri

38. All the following occur frequently in Reye's syndrome EXCEPT

A. antecedent influenza B infection
B. persistent vomiting
C. seizures
D. jaundice
E. increased intracranial pressure

39. You are asked to see a 39-year-old woman because of the sudden onset of paralysis of the right side. Physical examination reveals an alert, mute woman who does not understand verbal commands. Blood pressure is normal. Pulse is irregular and there is midsystolic cardiac murmur. There is a flaccid right hemiplegia involving the face, arm, and leg equally, with an associated sensory deficit and homonymous hemianopia. There is right hyperreflexia, and plantar response on the right is extensor. Strength is normal on the left side. Which of the following is the most likely diagnosis?

A. Embolic occlusion of a branch of the middle cerebral artery to the motor cortex
B. Embolic occlusion of the anterior cerebral artery
C. Embolic occlusion at the origin of the middle cerebral artery
D. Putamenal hemorrhage
E. Rupture of a mycotic aneurysm

40. A 60-year-old alcoholic man is brought to the emergency room by the police. He is afebrile, drowsy, poorly oriented, and uncooperative. His breath smells of alcohol. The right pupil is 4 mm, and the left 3 mm; both react to light, and eye movements are full without hemianopia. Facial movements are symmetric. The left arm and leg are weak, and the left plantar response is extensor. Roentgenograms of the skull are negative for fracture, and the calcified pineal is midline. Which of the following is correct?

A. The findings accord best with Wernicke-Korsakoff syndrome
B. The normal skull film rules out a subdural hematoma
C. Early uncal herniation is unlikely
D. A lumbar puncture should be performed to look for xanthochromia
E. Computerized tomography of the brain or cerebral angiography is indicated

41. All the following statements regarding brain abscesses are true EXCEPT

A. They commonly occur in patients with cyanotic heart disease
B. They commonly stem from ear and sinus infections
C. They are more common in acute than in subacute bacterial endocarditis
D. The clinical course is often that of an expanding brain tumor
E. They usually present as acute meningitis

42. Which of the following is the most common viral agent associated with encephalitis?

A. Mumps
B. Influenza
C. Herpes simplex
D. Herpes zoster
E. Lymphocytic choriomeningitis (LCM) virus

43. A 32-year-old woman, previously in good health, developed severe midback pain 24 hours before both legs became weak and the left leg numb. Over the subsequent seven days sensory loss and numbness ascended to the nipples; there was flaccid paraplegia with urinary retention, and she lost vision in the right eye. The most likely diagnosis is

A. Guillain-Barré syndrome
B. Brown-Séquard syndrome
C. neuromyelitis optica
D. poliomyelitis
E. metastatic carcinoma

44. Hearing loss in Meniere's disease has all the following clinical features EXCEPT

A. tone decay
B. good speech discrimination
C. low-tone hearing loss early
D. recruitment
E. short increment sensitivity index test 78%

45. Clinical manifestations of hyperkalemic periodic paralysis (PP) include all the following EXCEPT

A. myotonia
B. lid-lag
C. Chvostek's sign
D. attacks of weakness lasting days or more
E. dominant pattern of inheritance

46. Characteristics of narcolepsy include all the following EXCEPT

A. somnambulism
B. sleep paralysis
C. hypnagogic hallucinations
D. cataplexy
E. positive family history

47. Typical findings in Wernicke-Korsakoff syndrome include all the following EXCEPT

A. optic atrophy
B. cerebellar ataxia
C. bilateral lateral rectus weakness
D. nystagmus
E. polyneuropathy

48. Which of the following sets of symptoms is most characteristic of alcoholic cerebellar degeneration?

A. Nystagmus, gait ataxia, and dysarthria
B. Upper extremity dysmetria and gait ataxia
C. Lower extremity dysmetria and gait ataxia
D. Upper extremity dysmetria, gait ataxia, and nystagmus
E. Lower extremity dysmetria, gait ataxia, and nystagmus

49. Typical characteristics of nontraumatic brachial plexus neuropathy (brachial plexitis) include all the following EXCEPT

A. distal muscles more involved than proximal muscles
B. pain in the affected extremity
C. prominent wasting of the involved muscles
D. motor impairment much greater than sensory impairment
E. complete recovery is the rule

50. Characteristics of Duchenne muscular dystrophy include all the following EXCEPT

A. childhood onset
B. normal serum creatine phosphokinase
C. shortened life expectancy
D. motor impairment much greater than sensory impairment
E. well-formed calf muscles

51. Accepted therapies for myasthenia gravis include all the following EXCEPT

A. sodium valproate
B. thymectomy
C. pyridostigmine
D. corticosteroids
E. plasmapheresis

52. Idiopathic trigeminal neuralgia (tic douloureux) is characterized by all the following EXCEPT

A. There is a constant burning pain in the distribution of the trigeminal nerve unilaterally
B. There are normal neurologic examination results
C. Carbamazepine (Tegretol) is the treatment of choice
D. It most commonly affects the second and third division of the trigeminal nerve
E. It frequently is precipitated by touching the lips or mouth

53. Common characteristics of essential tremor (familial tremor) include all the following EXCEPT

A. Upper and lower extremities are equally affected
B. It commonly begins before age 30
C. Tremor is suppressed by alcohol
D. It is an inherited disorder
E. Propranolol reduces the tremor in more than 50% of patients

54. The clinical presentation of subarachnoid hemorrhage from ruptured berry aneurysm usually includes all the following EXCEPT

A. bruit heard on auscultation over orbit
B. headache
C. stiff neck
D. subhyaloid hemorrhage on funduscopic examination
E. Brudzinski's sign

55. Cerebrospinal gamma globulin is commonly elevated in which one of the following disorders?

A. Brain abscess
B. Multiple sclerosis
C. Thrombotic cerebral infarction
D. Subarachnoid hemorrhage
E. Guillain-Barré syndrome

56. Typical findings in tabes dorsalis include all the following EXCEPT

A. hyperreflexia
B. small pupils that accommodate better than they react to light
C. history of "lightning pains"
D. ataxic gait
E. loss of proprioception

57. Periodic paralysis may be associated with any of the following EXCEPT

A. hyperthyroidism
B. hypothyroidism
C. hyperkalemia
D. hypokalemia
E. normokalemia

58. Manifestations of neurosyphilis include all the following EXCEPT

A. meningitis
B. dementia
C. optic atrophy
D. pupils that react to light but do not accommodate
E. cerebral infarction

59. Metabolic causes of seizures include all the following EXCEPT

A. hypoglycemia
B. hyperglycemia
C. short-acting barbiturate withdrawal
D. hypercalcemia
E. hyponatremia

60. Neurologic complications of corticosteroids include all the following EXCEPT

A. myopathy
B. psychosis
C. pseudotumor cerebri (benign intracranial hypertension)
D. neuropathy
E. compression fractures with radiculoneuropathy

61. Paraneoplastic syndromes may present with any of the following EXCEPT

A. aphasia
B. myositis
C. cerebellar degeneration
D. peripheral neuropathy
E. opsoclonus

62. Toxic neuropathies may be caused by any of the following EXCEPT

A. arsenic
B. lead
C. vincristine
D. botulism
E. thallium

63. Autonomic insufficiency is associated with all the following EXCEPT

A. diabetes mellitus
B. Wilson's disease
C. amyloidosis
D. Guillain-Barré syndrome
E. Riley-Day syndrome

64. Characteristics of amyotrophic lateral sclerosis include all the following EXCEPT

A. decreased vibration and position sense
B. hyperreflexia
C. extensor plantar response
D. muscle wasting
E. muscle fasciculations

65. In a comatose patient, which of the following is most compatible with a metabolic etiology?

A. Pupillary constriction to light
B. Intact deep tendon reflexes
C. Decerebrate posturing
D. Extensor plantar responses
E. Internuclear ophthalmoplegia

66. Which of the following is most characteristic of nondominant hemisphere lesions?

A. Contralateral hemiparesis
B. Aphasia
C. Gerstmann's syndrome
D. Anosognosia (denial or neglect of neurologic disability)
E. Alexia

67. A 35-year-old man has a one-week history of severe, episodic, unilateral headaches occurring most frequently at night. The headaches are often induced by drinking alcohol and are associated with ipsilateral rhinorrhea, tearing, and Horner's syndrome. What is the most likely diagnosis?

A. Common migraine
B. Classic migraine
C. Tic douloureux
D. Cluster headache
E. Temporomandibular joint dysfunction

68. Benign intracranial hypertension (pseudotumor cerebri) has been associated with all the following EXCEPT

A. pregnancy
B. withdrawal of corticosteroids
C. hypervitaminosis A
D. hypervitaminosis C
E. chronic hypercapnia

69. A unilateral nonpulsatile ocular bruit suggests the diagnosis of

A. traumatic internal jugular vein occlusion
B. acute traumatic glaucoma
C. sagittal sinus thrombosis
D. intracavernous carotid stenosis
E. subdural hematoma

70. All the following are typical of Parkinson's disease EXCEPT

A. resting tremor accentuated with active movement of limb
B. muscular rigidity on passive movement of joint
C. tremor that disappears during sleep
D. diminished facial expression
E. bradykinesia with festination of gait

71. A 26-year-old man has a ten-year history of multifocal tics, echolalia, and compulsive utterances of profanity. What is the most likely diagnosis?

A. Torsion dystonia
B. Paranoid schizophrenia
C. Gilles de la Tourette's syndrome
D. Sydenham's chorea
E. Huntington's chorea

72. In a comatose patient not exposed to cold, hypothermia suggests any of the following EXCEPT

A. pontine hemorrhage
B. barbiturate intoxication
C. hypoglycemia
D. Wernicke's encephalopathy
E. myxedema

73. Which of the following is diagnostic of multiple sclerosis?

A. Unilateral optic atrophy
B. Paraplegia
C. Intranuclear ophthalmoplegia
D. Nystagmus on vertical gaze with unilateral lower extremity spasticity
E. Hemianesthesia with contralateral hemiparesis

74. Which of the following movement disorders has been associated with a discrete anatomic central nervous system lesion?

A. Athetosis
B. Myoclonus
C. Dystonia
D. Ballismus
E. Chorea

75. The Kayser-Fleischer ring about the cornea is found in which one of the following?

A. Torsion dystonia
B. Wegener's granulomatosis
C. Wilson's disease (hepatolenticular degeneration)
D. Devic's disease (neuromyelitis optica)
E. Sydenham's chorea

76. Adrenocorticosteroids are effective in all the following disorders EXCEPT

A. polymyalgia rheumatica
B. increased intracranial pressure secondary to metastatic tumor
C. temporal arteritis
D. thrombotic cerebral infarction
E. myasthenia gravis

77. Each of the following is found in myotonic muscular dystrophy EXCEPT

A. greater weakness in proximal than in distal muscles
B. frontal baldness
C. testicular atrophy
D. difficulty in relaxation of grip
E. cataracts

DIRECTIONS: For questions 78 to 118, you are to decide whether EACH choice is true or false. Any combination of answers, from all true to all false, may be present. Mark the answer sheet "T" or "F" in the space provided.

78. Which of the following statements regarding peripheral neuropathy is/are true?

A. Both primary and secondary amyloidosis cause peripheral neuropathy
B. Uremic neuropathy usually worsens following renal transplantation
C. Diabetic amyotrophy is characterized by the sudden onset of severe pain and weakness of both thighs
D. Hypothyroidism is associated with both a mononeuropathy and a diffuse peripheral neuropathy
E. Sarcoidosis causes a facial paralysis indistinguishable from Bell's palsy

79. Which of the following statements regarding the Guillain-Barré syndrome (idiopathic inflammatory polyradiculoneuropathy) is/are true?

A. A subacute initial presentation is the rule
B. Corticosteroids produce significant improvement in more than 50% of patients
C. An ascending paralysis occurs in more than 70% of cases
D. Inappropriate antidiuretic hormone secretion frequently complicates severe cases
E. Approximately 90% of patients make a good recovery
F. Tachyarrhythmias frequently occur

80. Which of the following statements concerning cerebrovascular disease is/are correct?

A. As life expectancy of the general population is increasing, so the incidence of stroke appears to be rising significantly
B. Chronic atrial fibrillation alone, without valvular heart disease, results in a fivefold increased risk of stroke
C. Atherosclerosis of the middle and anterior cerebral arteries is the cause of most strokes
D. Complete occlusion of an internal carotid artery at its origin usually produces a dense contralateral hemiparesis
E. Palpation and auscultation of the internal carotid arteries is a valuable bedside test

81. Which of the following statements about sleep apnea syndrome is/are true?

A. The patient complains of excessive daytime sleepiness
B. The patient complains of difficulty in breathing
C. Snoring is a prominent sign
D. Men are more commonly affected than women
E. Tracheostomy is the treatment of choice in the peripheral type

82. Which of the following statements concerning the management of chronic pain is/are true?

A. Analgesic doses should be spaced as far apart as possible to prevent drug abuse
B. Drug combinations are to be avoided
C. Antidepressants should be reserved for patients with concomitant depression
D. Tolerance develops to all narcotic analgesics
E. Minor analgesics are of little benefit and should be avoided

83. Which of the following statements about the benzodiazepines is/are true?

A. Drug dependence is common
B. They are central nervous system depressants
C. Seizures may occur as part of an acute abstinence syndrome
D. Intoxication produces nystagmus, dysarthria, and ataxia
E. Specific receptor sites have been found in the central nervous system

84. Which of the following statements regarding alcohol withdrawal seizures is/are true?

A. They usually occur 12 to 24 hours after cessation of drinking
B. They are usually focal
C. They are multiple in about 40% of cases
D. They respond to phenytoin sodium
E. They recur when delirium tremens supervenes

85. Which of the following statements regarding myasthenia gravis is/are true?

A. There is an increased incidence of thymoma
B. The cranial nerve–innervated muscles are spared
C. Sensory impairment never occurs
D. Alteration in intellectual function frequently occurs
E. Fatigue occurs with repetitive muscle activity or exercise

86. Which of the following statements regarding petit mal seizures is/are true?

A. Onset is in childhood
B. They occur as often as 100 times a day
C. Hyperventilation may transiently increase the frequency or duration of spells
D. There are three-per-second spike and wave complexes on electroencephalogram
E. They readily respond to phenytoin therapy

87. Which of the following is/are consistent with a diagnosis of benign intracranial hypertension (pseudotumor cerebri)?

A. Computerized tomography that shows moderate enlargement of the ventricular system
B. Lumbar puncture: opening pressure greater than 300 mm, acellular, protein 76 mg/dl, glucose 30 mg/dl
C. An electroencephalogram that shows generalized slowing
D. Lumbar-peritoneal shunt required
E. Visual loss as a presenting complaint

88. Which of the following statements regarding cutaneous herpes is/are true?

A. Thoracic dermatomes are most often affected
B. The rash precedes the pain by four to five days

C. Cutaneous dissemination is most common in patients with underlying malignancies
D. Pain may persist for months to years following regression of the cutaneous lesions
E. Herpes simplex is the agent most commonly isolated

89. Which of the following statements regarding tuberous sclerosis is/are true?

A. Seizures are common
B. Most patients are mentally retarded
C. Café au lait spots typically occur
D. Unilateral port wine facial nevi typically occur
E. Hypertelorism typically occurs

90. Which of the following drug doses is/are equivalent to morphine, 10 mg intramuscularly every four hours?

A. Codeine, 130 mg intramuscularly every four hours
B. Levorphanol, 4 mg orally every four hours
C. Meperidine, 75 mg intramuscularly every three hours
D. Pentazocine, 60 mg intramuscularly every four hours
E. Methadone, 20 mg orally every four hours

91. Which of the following studies is/are frequently of value in establishing a diagnosis of multiple sclerosis?

A. Somatosensory and visual evoked potentials
B. Computerized tomography
C. Cerebral arteriography
D. Lumbar puncture
E. Electromyography and nerve conduction studies

92. Which of the following statements regarding chronic subdural hematomas is/are true?

A. Seizures are common presenting symptoms
B. Headache and lethargy are common presenting symptoms
C. The syndrome is common in chronic alcoholics
D. They almost never occur in the absence of antecedent head injury
E. A negative CT scan excludes the diagnosis

93. Which of the following statements is/are true regarding heroin addiction?

A. The incidence has been declining significantly in the United States since the late 1970s
B. It is a leading cause of death in young men
C. Cross-tolerance to all narcotics occurs
D. Withdrawal symptoms peak within 36 to 48 hours
E. Addicts are generally initiated by a nonaddicted drug dealer

94. Neurologic complications of street heroin include which of the following?

A. Transverse myelitis
B. Acute inflammatory polyradiculoneuropathy
C. Amblyopia
D. Rhabdomyolysis
E. Chronic fibrosing myopathy

95. Which of the following tumors frequently show(s) areas of calcification on roentgenogram or computerized tomography?

A. Glioblastoma multiforme
B. Oligodendroglioma
C. Ependymoma
D. Craniopharyngioma
E. Chromophobe adenoma

96. Which of the following statements regarding lumbar puncture is/are true?

A. A platelet count below 30,000 cu mm is an absolute contraindication
B. It is always indicated if meningitis is suspected
C. Infection in tissues overlying the lumbar spine is an absolute contraindication
D. It is indicated before anticoagulant therapy for cerebrovascular disease if computerized tomography is not available
E. It is best deferred in a comatose patient with persisting asymmetric neurologic signs of increased intracranial pressure

97. Which of the following statements regarding mania and depression is/are true?

A. Lithium carbonate is useful in controlling attacks of depression
B. Repetitive attacks of depression are the most common manifestation
C. In the manic phase the patient is characteristically self-confident, jocular, and cooperative
D. The possibility of homicide should always be considered in depressed patients
E. Delusional beliefs are commonly part of manic-depressive psychosis

98. Which of the following statements regarding a depressive response is/are true?

A. Anxiety is a typical example that illustrates common features of the depressive response
B. The best treatment is electroconvulsive therapy (ECT)
C. It is the same as depression in a manic-depressive psychosis
D. It is common in patients who have had a stroke
E. It often complicates hysterical personality disorders

99. If the Wechsler Adult Intelligence Scale (WAIS) indicates that a subject has a performance IQ well below verbal IQ, possible explanations include which of the following?

A. Alzheimer's disease
B. Anxiety
C. Depression
D. Poor education
E. Korsakoff's syndrome

100. Immediate management of severe sedative drug overdose includes which of the following?

A. Intravenous access
B. Analeptic drugs to stimulate respirations
C. Tracheal intubation
D. Gastric lavage
E. Hemodialysis

101. Acute destruction or metabolic derangement of the posterior hypothalamus is associated with which of the following?

A. Gastrointestinal hemorrhage and acute ulceration
B. Poikilothermia

C. Hypersomnolence
D. Impaired recent memory
E. Diabetes insipidus

102. Headache occurs from distortion of which of the following structures?

A. Arteries of the scalp
B. Superior sagittal sinus
C. Tentorium cerebelli
D. Parenchyma of the brain
E. Second cervical root

103. Which of the following statements regarding rigidity is/are true?

A. It occurs most commonly in Parkinson's disease
B. It follows large lesions of area 4 or its subcortical connections
C. It frequently responds to baclofen or dantrolene
D. It follows a discrete lesion in the subthalamic nucleus
E. There is continuous activity in the involved muscles

104. Parkinson's disease is characterized by which of the following?

A. A deficiency of striatal dopamine
B. A tremor at rest with suppression during sleep
C. Postural instability
D. Cholinergic hypoactivity in the basal ganglia
E. Dopamine hyperactivity in the basal ganglia

105. The prognosis in completed cerebral infarction may be favorably affected by which of the following?

A. Surgical treatment (thromboendarterectomy)
B. Use of corticosteroids
C. Effective treatment of hypertension
D. Programs of rehabilitation
E. Anticoagulation

106. Which of the following statements regarding herpes zoster (shingles) is/are true?

A. It is due to the same virus that causes chickenpox
B. It frequently occurs in adults exposed to children with chickenpox
C. It is associated with activation of varicella virus latent in sensory ganglia
D. It frequently occurs in adults exposed to zoster
E. Oral corticosteroids, if used early, diminish the incidence of postherpetic neuralgia

107. Dissociated sensory loss (impairment in pain and temperature sensation with preservation of the sense of touch) is associated with which of the following?

A. Syringomyelia
B. Lepromatous neuropathy
C. Intramedullary neoplasm of the spinal cord
D. Syphilitic aortitis
E. Avitaminosis B_{12}

108. Characteristics of the neuropathy associated with diabetes mellitus include which of the following?

A. Proximal weakness of a lower limb
B. Cranial neuropathy
C. Charcot joint
D. Elevation of cerebrospinal fluid protein
E. Lower extremity hyperpathia

109. Which of the following statements regarding compression of the spinal cord in the thoracic region is/are true?

A. It is associated with spastic legs and flaccid arms
B. It is often caused by a herniated intervertebral disc
C. It is associated with weakness of the intercostal muscles
D. It often produces Beevor's sign
E. Localized pain often precedes objective neurologic signs

110. Which of the following produce(s) a parkinsonian state?

A. Carbon monoxide poisoning
B. Phenothiazines
C. Encephalitis
D. Manganese poisoning
E. Thallium intoxication

111. Spinal arachnoiditis is a complication of which of the following?

A. Spinal epidural hemorrhage
B. Tuberculous meningitis
C. Subarachnoid hemorrhage
D. Spinal anesthesia
E. Myelography

112. Which of the following neurologic diseases is/are associated with respiratory failure?

A. Guillain-Barré syndrome
B. Botulism
C. Poliomyelitis
D. High cervical spinal cord trauma
E. Myasthenia gravis

113. Which of the following tumors is/are found in neurofibromatosis?

A. Oligodendroglioma
B. Acoustic neuroma
C. Pheochromocytoma
D. Optic gliomas
E. Meningiomas

114. Which of the following disorders is/are characterized by involvement of the skin and the central nervous system?

A. Ataxia telangiectasia
B. Sturge-Weber syndrome
C. Neurofibromatosis
D. Tuberous sclerosis
E. Pellagra

115. Which of the following is/are true of anosmia?

A. It is a result of basilar skull fracture
B. It is usually reported as an alteration or decrease in taste
C. It is most commonly caused by rhinitis
D. It is an important finding in a demented patient
E. It may result from brain tumor

116. Which of the following statements regarding acoustic neuroma is/are true?

A. It is associated with reduced cerebrospinal fluid glucose
B. The vestibular portion of the eighth cranial nerve is commonly spared

C. Episodic vertigo is common
D. Cerebrospinal fluid protein is markedly elevated (100 to 500 mg/dl)
E. The fifth cranial nerve is commonly involved

117. Which of the following is/are true of radiation myelopathy?

A. Lhermitte's sign occurs
B. Symptoms begin 12 months or more after radiation exposure
C. The peripheral nerves are relatively resistant to radiation injury
D. The spinal cord is more susceptible to injury than the brain
E. Lesions are usually restricted to white matter

118. Characteristics of cerebral cysticercosis include which of the following?

A. Hydrocephalus
B. Intestinal infection with *Taenia solium*
C. Cerebral calcification
D. Eosinophilia and increased protein in the cerebrospinal fluid
E. Seizures

DIRECTIONS: Questions 119 to 192 are matching questions. For each numbered item, choose the most likely associated lettered item from those provided. Each numbered item has ONLY ONE answer. Within each group, each lettered item may be the answer to one, more than one, or none of the numbered items.

QUESTIONS 119–123

For each of the following anticonvulsants, select the most likely associated side effect that occurs shortly after the institution of therapy.

A. Leukopenia
B. Drowsiness
C. Anorexia, nausea
D. Nystagmus, ataxia
E. Hepatotoxicity

119. Phenytoin

120. Carbamazepine

121. Phenobarbital

122. Ethosuximide

123. Valproic acid

QUESTIONS 124–128

For each of the following patients, select the most likely diagnosis.

A. Subacute sclerosing panencephalitis
B. Creutzfeldt-Jakob disease
C. Progressive multifocal leukoencephalopathy
D. Alzheimer's disease
E. Huntington's chorea
F. Multiple sclerosis

124. A 55-year-old man with myoclonus, cerebral ataxia, a slow electroencephalogram with bursts of sharp waves, and spongiform cerebral cortex at biopsy

125. A 40-year-old man with a family history of dementia and caudate atrophy seen on computerized tomography

126. An 18-year-old woman with myoclonus, very high measles antibody titers, and perivascular infiltrates and intranuclear inclusions on brain biopsy

127. A 60-year-old woman with seizures, dementia, and neurofibrillar tangles on brain biopsy

128. A 30-year-old woman with hemiparesis and dysarthria, previously treated lymphoma with intranuclear inclusions, foci of demyelination, and JC virus identified at brain biopsy

QUESTIONS 129–134

For each of the following abnormal eye movements, select the most likely diagnosis.

A. Vestibular neuronitis
B. Neuroblastoma
C. Phenytoin intoxication
D. Multiple sclerosis
E. Cerebral infarction of the right frontal lobe
F. Arnold-Chiari malformation

129. Left conjugate gaze-induced jerk nystagmus of the left eye with loss of adduction of the right eye

130. Bidirectional gaze-evoked nystagmus

131. Left gaze-evoked jerk nystagmus with vertigo

132. Left conjugate gaze preference without nystagmus

133. Down-beat nystagmus

134. Opsoclonus

QUESTIONS 135–140

For each of the following clinical syndromes, select the most likely site of lesion.

A. Peroneal nerve
B. Radial nerve
C. Femoral nerve
D. C7 root
E. L4 root
F. S1 root
G. L5 root

135. Decreased sensation of dorsum of foot; weakness of ankle dorsiflexion, inversion, and eversion of foot; intact reflexes

136. Decreased sensation behind lateral malleolus; weak plantar flexion and eversion of foot; absent Achilles reflex

137. Decreased sensation of medial leg; weakness of foot inversion; diminished knee reflex

138. Pain in anterior thigh; weak knee extension; absent knee reflex

139. Decreased sensation of dorsum of thumb; weakness of triceps, wrist and finger extensors, brachioradials, and supinator of forearm; absent triceps and supinator reflexes

140. Decreased sensation of middle finger; weakness of latissimus dorsi, pectoralis major, triceps, and wrist extensors and flexors; decreased triceps reflex

QUESTIONS 141–145

For each of the following sets of cerebrospinal fluid profiles, select the most likely diagnosis.

A. Pneumococcal meningitis
B. Meningeal carcinomatosis
C. Multiple sclerosis
D. Herpes simplex encephalitis
E. Guillain-Barré syndrome

	WBCs (per cu mm)	RBCs (per cu mm)	Glucose (mg/dl)	Protein (mg/dl)
141.	300 (80% lymphs)	100	70	65
142.	300 (80% PMNs)	0	15	150
143.	4 (100% lymphs)	0	70	150
144.	20 (80% lymphs)	0	70	65
145.	20 (80% lymphs)	0	15	150

QUESTIONS 146–150

For each of the following visual abnormalities, select the most likely diagnosis.

A. Carotid artery stenosis
B. Craniopharyngioma
C. Multiple sclerosis
D. Sphenoid wing meningioma
E. Glioblastoma
F. Retinal detachment

146. Unilateral papilledema with decreased visual acuity

147. Unilateral optic atrophy with decreased visual acuity

148. Bitemporal hemianopia

149. Homonymous hemianopia

150. Transient unilateral visual loss

QUESTIONS 151–155

For each of the following unilateral pupillary abnormalities, select the most likely diagnosis.

A. Diabetes mellitus
B. Syphilis
C. Horner's syndrome
D. Adie's syndrome
E. Berry aneurysm

151. 2 mm, irregular; fixed to light; constricts to accommodation

152. 6 mm, regular; fixed to light; accommodates slowly

153. 2 mm; reacts to light; ptosis

154. 6 mm; reacts to light; ptosis

155. 6 mm; fixed to light; ptosis

QUESTIONS 156–160

For each of the following drugs, select the most appropriate treatment for an overdose.

A. Chlorpromazine
B. Naloxone
C. Diazepam
D. Hemodialysis
E. Physostigmine

156. Meperidine

157. Lithium

158. Methylphenidate (amphetamine)

159. LSD

160. Amitriptyline

QUESTIONS 161–164

For each of the following descriptions, select the most likely associated pain syndrome.

A. Postherpetic neuralgia
B. Trigeminal neuralgia
C. Phantom limb pain
D. Causalgia

161. Chronic severe pain with trigger spots; surgery directed against the central nervous system is often unhelpful

162. Hyperpathic and burning pain; cutaneous densitization is often helpful

163. Brief stabbing pain with trigger spots; surgery directed against the peripheral nervous system is often helpful

164. Continuous hyperpathic pain; sympathectomy is often helpful

QUESTIONS 165–168

For each of the following sets of clinical findings, select the most likely congenital infection.

A. Cytomegalovirus infection
B. Toxoplasmosis
C. Rubella
D. Herpes simplex

165. Hepatosplenomegaly, jaundice, microcephaly, periventricular calcifications

166. Cataracts, glaucoma, cardiac malformations

167. Chorioretinitis, seizures, scattered intracranial calcifications

168. Encephalitis, pneumonitis

QUESTIONS 169–173

For each of the following descriptions, select the most likely tumor.

A. Glioblastoma multiforme
B. Astrocytoma
C. Medulloblastoma
D. Meningioma
E. Hemangioblastoma

169. The most common primary cerebellar tumor in adults

170. A cerebellar hemisphere tumor in children

171. A benign tumor

172. Metastasizes throughout the subarachnoid space

173. The most malignant primary brain tumor

QUESTIONS 174–178

For each of the following descriptions, select the most likely disorder.

A. Cerebral concussion
B. Subdural hematoma
C. Epidural hematoma
D. Basilar skull fracture
E. Penetrating brain injury

174. Prompt, complete recovery is the rule

175. Lucid interval precedes deterioration

176. May follow a trivial injury to head

177. Epilepsy occurs in approximately 40% of patients

178. The presence of cerebrospinal fluid rhinorrhea is diagnostic

QUESTIONS 179–182

For each of the following clinical descriptions, select the most likely associated type of epilepsy.

A. Petit mal
B. Akinetic seizures
C. Temporal lobe seizures
D. Myoclonus
E. Supplementary motor area seizures
F. Jacksonian seizures

179. May be mistaken for daydreaming or inattention in children

180. Arrest of activity, lip smacking, chewing or aimless movements

181. Involuntary jerks precipitated by sensory stimulation or movement

182. Focal motor seizures that spread up the extremity toward the trunk

QUESTIONS 183–187

For each of the following types of epilepsy, select the most appropriate anticonvulsant drug; each drug may be used only once.

A. Phenytoin
B. Phenobarbital
C. Carbamazepine
D. Ethosuximide
E. None of the above

183. Petit mal

184. Generalized and focal motor seizures in adults

185. Temporal lobe seizures

186. Febrile seizures

187. Alcohol withdrawal seizures

QUESTIONS 188–192

For each of the following roentgenographic features, select the most appropriate diagnosis.

A. Von Recklinghausen's disease
B. Sturge-Weber syndrome
C. Arnold-Chiari malformation
D. Platybasia
E. Klippel-Feil syndrome

188. Downward displacement of the cerebellum through the foramen magnum

189. Fusion of one or more cervical vertebrae

190. Flattening of the base of the skull

191. Scoliosis, lordosis, kyphosis, and pseudarthrosis

192. "Railroad track" intracranial calcifications

PART 10

NEUROLOGIC DISEASE

ANSWERS

1. (C) The clinical picture is that of a predominantly large fiber sensory neuropathy affecting both lower and upper extremities. Bilateral Babinski signs and hyperreflexia at the knees suggest pyramidal tract dysfunction. The mental vagueness suggests a mild encephalopathy. These signs are characteristic of vitamin B_{12} deficiency. The normal hematocrit does not militate against this. Cervical spine disease should not produce a dissociated sensory neuropathy with absent Achilles reflexes. Cerebral symptoms are not features of cervical cord disease. Diabetic peripheral neuropathy is rarely dissociated, and bilateral pyramidal tract signs are not part of the illness. Hepatic failure produces encephalopathy, but pyramidal tract signs are rare in mild cases, as is a dissociated sensory peripheral neuropathy. *(Cecil, pp. 2049–2050, 2156–2157; Rundles)*

2. (C) Pain referred to the contralateral back or leg when the nonpainful leg is raised (crossed straight leg raising) implies root compression within the spinal canal, and is the most accurate sign of a significant herniated intervertebral disc. The straight leg raising sign (i.e., pain radiating into an extended lower extremity when it is raised) occurs in most patients with severe low back pain, but does not indicate the underlying cause. Point tenderness over a spinous process raises the suspicion of vertebral tumor or infection. Point tenderness over muscles may indicate severe muscle spasm, which again is nondiagnostic of the underlying etiology. Low back pain exacerbated by forward flexion and relieved by lying down occurs with any cause of spasm of the paravertebral back muscles. Pain in the lumbar area produced by neck flexion suggests cervical spinal cord disease or compression. *(Cecil, pp. 2148–2150)*

3. (E) Amyotrophic lateral sclerosis is a degenerative disease of motor nerve cells arising from layers 3 and 5 of the precentral cerebral cortex and of motor cranial and spinal nerve nuclei. The clinical picture invariably reveals visible muscle fasciculations. Spasticity and hyperreflexia are common, as are muscular atrophy and weakness. Motor nerve conduction velocities are usually normal until the disease is virtually terminal. A dropout of motor nerve cells with loss of axons may lead to alterations of the amplitude of the evoked potentials in muscle, but the nerve conduction velocities are frequently normal: this separates this entity from peripheral motor neuropathies. Acute denervation is often present on electromyography. *(Cecil, pp. 2037–2038)*

4. (D) The clinical picture of encephalopathy with brisk oculocephalic responses, hyperreflexia, and no focal neurologic signs suggests a metabolic encephalopathy. Hyperventilation, an elevated pH, adequate oxygenation, low $Paco_2$, and raised serum bicarbonate level all indicate a respiratory alkalosis. Depressant drug poisoning produces hypoventilation and respiratory acidosis. The other conditions result in hyperventilation and metabolic acidosis. Salicylate intoxication may produce a mixed respiratory alkalosis and metabolic acidosis, but the bicarbonate level is rarely above 15. Brisk oculocephalic responses are characteristic of hepatic encephalopathy. *(Cecil, pp. 1915–1922)*

5. (D) Aortic stenosis, by producing global transient reduction in cerebral blood supply, and thus global transient cerebral ischemia, is a common cause of sudden syncope. Multifocal premature ventricular contractions are unlikely to produce syncope, as are any arrhythmias except for tachyarrhythmias above 160 to 180 per minute or bradyarrhythmias below 30 to 40 per minute. Vertebrobasilar TIAs rarely produce sudden syncope, but drop attacks without loss of consciousness may occur, as may focal transient neurologic deficits. Carotid TIAs usually produce focal neurologic deficits; if they are of the dominant hemisphere, speech arrest may occur, but not syncope. Hyperventilation attacks are closely related to syncope in that cerebral blood flow may be globally reduced and may lead to giddiness, faintness, and anxiety. If severe enough, syncope may occur with a superimposed Valsalva, but isolated syncope without these other symptoms is very unusual. *(Cecil, pp. 1927–1929)*

6. (C) The vegetative state reflects loss of cerebral function with intact brain-stem function. This usually follows significant hypoxic or traumatic brain damage, and consists of a profound dementia with no apparent mental activity. This is in contrast to the locked-in state, which is characterized by retained mental content but the inability to express onself, and is usually due to lower pontine or midbrain lesions involving efferent motor pathways. In the persistent vegetative state, spontaneous eye opening, swallowing, and chewing; sleep-wake cycles; spontaneous respiration not requiring ventilatory support; and circulatory control all occur. *(Cecil, pp. 1913–1914, 1926; Plum and Posner, Chapt. 1)*

7. (D) Duchenne muscular dystrophy is inherited as a sex-linked recessive condition. *(Cecil, pp. 2030, 2043, 2044, 2170)*

8. (E) Nitrofurantoin produces neuropathy when high blood levels occur with impaired renal function. Isoniazid interferes with pyridoxine metabolism; this can be prevented by pyridoxine supplementation. The vinca alkaloids, especially vincristine, produce a predominantly sensory polyneuropathy. Phenytoin, particularly in high doses, can induce a peripheral neuropathy as well as cerebellar ataxia. Gentamicin may produce ototoxicity with dysfunction of both vestibular and auditory components of the vestibular cochlear nerve. This is most severe in patients with repeated trough concentrations of gentamicin in plasma that exceed 2 mg/ml. Diffuse polyneuropathy, however, has not been described with gentamicin. *(Cecil, p. 2163; Gilman et al., pp. 1169–1175)*

9. (B) Myasthenic (Eaton-Lambert) syndrome, in contrast to myasthenia gravis, does not cause weakness of extraocular muscles. The syndrome produces mild diffuse muscular weakness of skeletal muscles. It characteristically occurs as a nonmetastatic manifestation of malignancy. Multiple sclerosis, Wernicke's encephalopathy, and lateral pontine infarction all may disrupt cranial nerve nuclei and tracts in the brain stem, leading to diplopia. Cavernous sinus thrombosis may cause diplopia by producing unilateral proptosis or compression of cranial nerves 3, 4, or 6. *(Cecil, pp. 2181, 2184)*

10. (A) The Cornell criteria for brain death include an isoelectric EEG for 30 minutes at 5-10 μV/mm. Total absence of brain-stem function, including absent oculovestibular reflexes, is mandatory. A negative drug screen and an observation period of at least 12 hours is mandatory when the cause of brain death is not immediately apparent. If a drug screen is not available, at least a 24-hour period of observation is required. Deep tendon reflexes are purely spinal reflexes and may be preserved in spite of brain death. *(Cecil, p. 1926)*

11. (E) Patients with an asymptomatic carotid bruit should be followed conservatively; although they are at a higher risk for stroke than an age-matched population without bruits, the strokes that occur in this population often are not in the distribution of the artery with the bruit. Papaverine hydrochloride is ineffective in the treatment of peripheral or cerebrovascular disease. *(Cecil, pp. 2063–2064; Heyman et al.)*

12. (C) Delirium tremens is characterized by confusion, disorientation, delusions, hallucinations, psychomotor agitation, and autonomic dysfunction. Symptoms usually begin 48 to 72 hours following the cessation of drinking, with a peak incidence at 72 to 96 hours. Chlordiazepoxide used judiciously is very effective in reducing psychomotor agitation in these patients. The routine use of corticosteroids is contraindicated; phenytoin has no effect on delirium tremens and is of questionable efficacy in controlling withdrawal seizures. *(Cecil, pp. 2021–2022)*

13. (B) Although not an early sign, thenar atrophy in the setting of the other clinical symptoms listed should establish the diagnosis of carpal tunnel syndrome. The sensation of prickly numbness and pain in the hand and fingers with a nocturnal exacerbation and presence of Tinel's sign should suggest the diagnosis prior to the onset of atrophy of the median-innervated muscles, but the diagnosis can be confirmed only by nerve conduction velocities at that time. The hypothenar muscles are ulnar-innervated and are not part of the syndrome. *(Cecil, p. 2155)*

14. (D) Bulbar symptoms may be prominent in all the disorders listed except vitamin B_{12} deficiency, and may be the presenting clinical features in any of them. Myasthenia gravis, botulism, and (less frequently) poliomyelitis may involve the oculomotor nerves or ocular muscles; amyotrophic lateral sclerosis and Guillain-Barré syndrome do not characteristically have ocular involvement. Vitamin B_{12} deficiency can produce dementia, long-tract signs, and sensory abnormalities, but it does not involve the bulbar musculature. *(Cecil, pp. 2049, 2095, 2159–2160, 2180–2181, 2184)*

15. (A) Herpes simplex encephalitis is a sporadic disease with a highly variable clinical course. Neurologic dysfunction can range from a mild encephalitis with confusion to widespread neurologic devastation. The onset is often abrupt and is frequently associated with seizures and focal neurologic findings on examination. The CT scan is often normal in the first four to five days of the disease, when cerebral biopsy is often indicated for confirmation. The EEG may be more reliable in indicating focal temporal lobe slowing. Intracerebral blood and large invasive tumors rarely escape detection by CT scan. *(Cecil, pp. 2089–2091, 2116)*

16. (D) Partial seizures, whether simple or complex, are the most common seizure type in adults and outnumber generalized seizures 2 to 1. Absence seizures usually begin in childhood between the ages of 3 and 10 years, and rarely persist beyond the age of 30. Akinetic and myoclonic seizures occur rarely in infancy and childhood and even less often in adults. *(Cecil, pp. 2114–2118; Hauser and Kurland)*

17. (E) Frequent recurrent seizures in which the patient has an intervening lucid interval or returns to normal, although disturbing, do not constitute status epilepticus and do not require intravenous diazepam. Intramuscular diazepam and phenytoin are poorly and erratically absorbed. Intravenous diazepam is used in status epilepticus, but brain and blood levels fall rapidly within 30 minutes after intravenous administration because of redistribution, and therefore must be followed by another medication. Phenytoin should not be administered at a rate greater than 50 mg per minute because of potential side effects of hypotension and cardiac arrhythmias. It is also incompatible with most intravenous solutions, and should be administered directly into the vein at the rate indicated. *(Cecil, pp. 2121–2123; Penry and Newmark)*

18. (D) Subarachnoid hemorrhage, usually from a leaking berry aneurysm, may present with only severe headache without signs of meningeal irritation or focal neurologic abnormalities. With a normal examination, in the emergency situation, and with the patient complaining of a severe headache, a lumbar puncture should be performed. It is a safe procedure that should establish or effectively rule out this diagnosis. *(Cecil, pp. 1951, 2067, 2069)*

19. (A) Psychotherapy and physical therapy are valuable adjunct treatments. Levodopa has halved the mortality rate in parkinsonism, but the disease invariably progresses in spite of any form of treatment. Levodopa increases functional capacity and delays disabling symptoms, but because of the relentless progress of the disease it is advised that this drug be used only when the patient is significantly disabled. The "on-off" phenomenon occurs with levodopa usage in approximately 40% of patients, possibly owing to desensitization of dopamine receptors. *(Cecil, pp. 2027–2029)*

20. (E) Beta-blockers, tricyclic antidepressants, cyproheptadine, and methysergide have all been shown to be more effective than placebo in the prophylactic treatment of migraine. Oxycodone is a narcotic analgesic that is most useful in the relief of acute pain; it is not indicated in the prophylactic treatment of migraine, since this would lead to tolerance and addiction. *(Cecil, pp. 1949–1950)*

21. (E) Short-term memory and coordinated tasks such as driving performance may be impaired with marijuana usage. Enhanced perception of sounds and colors classically occur. Conjunctival vascular congestion with peripheral vasodilatation are frequently found. Depression and acute panic reactions are common adverse effects. A mild withdrawal syndrome of irritability, sleep disturbance, and tremulousness may occur, but withdrawal seizures have not been described. *(Cecil, pp. 2014–2015)*

22. (B) Multiple sclerosis most commonly affects the spinal cord, brain stem, and cerebellar and visual pathways.

Atypical facial pain occurs in 2 to 10% of cases. The cerebral form of multiple sclerosis is rare, and the cerebral cortex is spared; aphasia, therefore, is very rare. *(Cecil, pp. 2109–2111)*

23. (D) The present physiologic concept of consciousness depends on the functional integrity of an arousal system in the central core of the upper brain stem (thalamus, midbrain, and rostral pons) that must interact effectively with one or both cerebral hemispheres. To produce an alteration of consciousness, a disease or dysfunction must damage or depress both hemispheres, the brain stem core, or both. The mechanisms by which neurologic diseases cause coma fall into three categories: (1) supratentorial masses that shift and compress the arousal system in the diencephalon and midbrain (e.g., uncal herniation); (2) subtentorial masses or destructive lesions that destroy or compress the centrally located activating system anywhere above the midpons; and (3) metabolic depression of the brain stem reticular formation or cerebral cortex, or both. *(Cecil, pp. 1913–1915; Adams and Victor, pp. 231–236)*

24. (D) Parkinsonism may follow carbon monoxide poisoning (anoxia-ischemia), manganese poisoning, brain tumors of the basal ganglia and other areas, cerebral trauma, intoxication with phenothiazines, and encephalitis. It is very doubtful whether parkinsonism occurs as a result of diffuse atherosclerosis. Multiple lacunar infarctions (lacunar state) in hypertensive patients are associated with pseudobulbar palsy, not parkinsonism. *(Cecil, p. 2026)*

25. (C) Psychiatric disease can be distinguished in the awake patient by examination of the mental status and motor function. Psychotic patients are oriented and have normal cognitive functions. Delirious patients are disoriented and confused but never forget their personal identities. Hallucinations in psychiatric illness are usually auditory; in metabolic illness they are usually visual. Asterixis and myoclonus are never found in purely psychiatric disease. *(Cecil, pp. 1921–1922; Adams and Victor, pp. 280–284; Morse and Litin)*

26. (B) The diagnosis is most likely an embolic occlusion of the inferior division of the left middle cerebral artery. Such a lesion will produce fluent aphasia because of infarction of Wernicke's area. There is no hemiplegia, and other neurologic signs, except for a right homonymous hemianopia, are usually absent. Broca's aphasia is characterized by impaired expression with intact comprehension. There is nearly always a right hemiparesis. Schizophrenic word-salad usually occurs in chronic schizophrenics. Aphasia is not a part of delirium. New-onset hysteria at age 65 is rare, as is lack of some cooperation. *(Cecil, pp. 2054, 2057; Adams and Victor, pp. 327–334, 534–540)*

27. (C) In Korsakoff's syndrome there is relatively little impairment of cognitive functions, so that immediate recall and ability to do calculations and make abstractions are intact. Patients with Korsakoff's syndrome may have difficulty retrieving old memories, but they never forget their personal identities and names. *(Cecil, pp. 1980, 2046–2047; Victor)*

28. (B) Metabolic brain disease is most likely because it commonly presents with preserved pupillary reactivity to light despite severe depression of the lower brain-stem mechanisms controlling respiration, circulation, and motor responses. *(Cecil, pp. 1918–1920)*

29. (D) The clinical picture is that of a supratentorial mass lesion, in this case probably a subdural hematoma, causing left-sided uncal herniation. Displacement of the hemisphere by an expanding mass causes the uncus of the temporal lobe to squeeze into the tentorial notch and against the midbrain. As the uncus slides over the tentorial edge it often compresses the third nerve, so that the pupil on the side of the herniation begins to dilate. Eventually the pupil dilates widely and becomes light-fixed, and the patient becomes stuporous. Shortly afterward the involved eye turns outward owing to paralysis of the oculomotor functions of the third nerve, while sixth nerve function (lateral rectus muscle) remains intact. Compression of the ipsilateral peduncle produces contralateral signs (hemiplegia and decerebration). *(Cecil, pp. 1914–1915, 2137–2138)*

30. (E) Stupor or coma caused by sedative drug poisoning represents severe metabolic brain disease. The depression of the central nervous system tends to be bilateral and symmetric. Respiratory and circulatory mechanisms in the lower brain stem are affected by high doses, but pupillary light reflexes are usually preserved. Prognosis is excellent for patients who reach the hospital alive. The concomitant abuse of alcohol is common. Hypothermia is the rule, and elevations of body temperature imply an infection. *(Cecil, pp. 1919–1920, 1923–1925)*

31. (A) The physician must ensure that the brain receives no further injury in the process of examining the patient in coma. Before anything else the physician must provide a free and open airway and determine that the patient is breathing. Next, the heart and blood pressure must be examined and circulation supported if necessary. Whenever the cause of coma is doubtful, 25 gm of glucose solution should be given after the blood sugar has been drawn. Naloxone should be administered if opiate intoxication is even a remote possibility. *(Cecil, pp. 1922–1923)*

32. (E) Acute labyrinthitis or vestibular neuronitis is defined as a single bout of spontaneous vertigo lasting for hours to days. Hearing is normal and there are no other neurologic signs. Nausea and vomiting in the presence of nystagmus and vertigo should not be construed as evidence of vagal nucleus or brain-stem dysfunction. Meniere's disease consists of bouts of vertigo associated with hearing loss and tinnitus. Vertigo due to cerebrovascular disease is accompanied by signs of dysfunction of the cranial nerves and the cerebellar, corticospinal, and sensory pathways. The onset of multiple sclerosis would not be expected at this patient's age. *(Cecil, pp. 1963–1964)*

33. (D) Dynamic radionuclide brain scanning is the initial procedure of choice. Cerebral blood flow can be estimated rapidly by this low-risk technique, which can be performed on an ambulatory basis. CT scanning, since it does not well visualize the cerebral blood vessels, is not the first procedure of choice but can be useful to evaluate ventricular size and to diagnose infarction or mass lesion. Pneumoencephalography has been replaced by CT scanning but may be needed to verify the presence of intrasellar arachnoid tissue if "empty sella syndrome" is suspected. Cerebral angiography may be needed to clarify the findings of radionuclide scanning. Electroencephalography provides nonspecific, limited diagnostic information except in certain types of epilepsy. *(Cecil, p. 1977; Barnes, Parker, and Anger)*

34. (B) Idiopathic autonomic insufficiency (Shy-Drager syndrome) is a progressive, usually fatal disease of the central nervous system. Symptoms of autonomic insufficiency predominate initially; as the disease progresses, a parkinson-like illness or a cerebellar type of incoordination may develop. *(Cecil, pp. 2034–2035)* Severe orthostatic hypotension is not a feature of either postencephalitic parkinsonism or drug-induced extrapyramidal syndromes. *(Cecil, pp. 2025–2026)* Patients with generalized atherosclerosis may have frequent episodes of syncope, in most instances accompanied by signs of focal neurologic deficits such as motor weakness, sensory loss, and cranial nerve disorders. These cases of "blind staggers" are thought to be due to a postural decline in cerebral blood flow superimposed upon severe stenosis or occlusion of multiple cerebral vessels. *(Cecil, p. 2060)*

35. (C) Symptoms and signs specific for occlusion or partial obstruction of the internal carotid artery consist of intermittent blindness in the eye on the side of the lesion combined with contralateral hemiparesis and sensory loss. This clinical picture often begins with a series of transient ischemic attacks of amaurosis fugax (transient monocular blindness), and only later causes permanent weakness and sensory loss. Acute occlusion of the internal carotid artery may be associated with headache, probably as a result of dilatation of branches of the external carotid artery supplying collateral blood flow. *(Cecil, p. 2057; Adams and Victor, pp. 529–533)*

36. (E) The patient has a hypertensive cerebellar hemorrhage. The onset is sudden without loss of consciousness; within minutes patients are unable to stand or walk, and most vomit repeatedly. Headache and dizziness occur in about half the patients. There is often a paresis of gaze to the side of the lesion. The pupils remain small and reactive. In half the cases there is ipsilateral facial weakness of the lower motor neuron type. Strength is normal and sensory abnormalities are absent. Loss of voluntary or reflex upward gaze is a sign of compression of the pretectum, resulting from obstructive hydrocephalus or from direct compression by the hemorrhage. Rapid diagnosis is crucial because early surgical decompression can lead to complete reversal of the neurologic deficit. *(Cecil, pp. 2071–2072; Ott et al.)*

37. (C) Hypertensive encephalopathy presents with severe generalized headache, vomiting, and drowsiness or stupor. The full syndrome may require up to 48 hours to develop and may include seizures, focal neurologic deficits, blindness of cortical or retinal origin, and coma. The cerebrospinal fluid is usually clear, but pressure and protein content are elevated. The syndrome is precipitated by an abrupt sustained rise in blood pressure that exceeds the limits of cerebrovascular autoregulation. The definitive criterion for the diagnosis of hypertensive encephalopathy is the prompt reversal of the syndrome, often within one hour, by treatment to lower the blood pressure. The syndrome must be distinguished from metabolic encephalopathy, seizures, meningitis, encephalitis, and subarachnoid hemorrhage. Hypertensive intracerebral hemorrhage can always be recognized by the sudden onset of a unifocal neurologic deficit accompanied by bloody spinal fluid. Pseudotumor cerebri is not associated with clouding of consciousness. Progressive subcortical encephalopathy is insidious in onset and follows a chronic course. *(Cecil, pp. 2065–2066; Chester)*

38. (D) Reye's syndrome is an acute and often fatal encephalopathy of childhood, characterized by acute brain swelling associated with liver dysfunction. The syndrome may follow a variety of common viral infections, including influenza B. Persistent vomiting, coma, seizures, and increased intracranial pressure are common. Bilirubin levels rise in a minority of patients; jaundice, therefore, is not characteristic of Reye's syndrome. *(Cecil, p. 2105)*

39. (C) The most likely diagnosis is occlusion of the middle cerebral artery proximal to the origin of the lenticulostriate arteries that supply the motor fibers in the internal capsule to the face, arm, and leg. Infarction of the internal capsule produces profound contralateral hemiplegia. Extensive infarction of the areas of cortex supplied by the left middle cerebral artery accounts for the total aphasia and blindness in the contralateral, homonymous visual field. Occlusions in branches of the middle cerebral artery produce a variable clinical picture; at times paresis is evident only in the arm and face. In some patients sensory impairment is the dominant, and occasionally the only, neurologic abnormality. Occlusion of the anterior cerebral artery causes infarction in the cortical areas that control motor and sensory function of the contralateral lower extremity. The etiology of the stroke in this case was a prolapsing mitral valve. Mycotic aneurysms are produced by septic emboli associated with bacterial endocarditis. They tend to be multiple and are found distally in the smaller branches of the middle cerebral artery. Intracerebral bleeding into the region of the internal capsule causes a clinical picture similar to the one described, but such a large hemorrhage would be expected to cause an alteration in consciousness and elevated intracranial pressure reflected by an elevated systemic blood pressure. *(Cecil, pp. 2057, 2066–2073; Adams and Victor, pp. 534–540; Barnett et al.)*

40. (E) Chronic subdural hematoma occurs after the age of 50, and often in alcoholics because of their frequent falls. Headache is present in 80 to 90% of cases; a change in level of consciousness in more than 50%. Hemianopia, hemiparesis, or pupillary abnormality occurs in less than half the cases. Anisocoria by itself can be the earliest sign of uncal herniation. Lumbar puncture is usually clear, but xanthochromia may be present in 25 to 50% of patients. A fractured skull is identified in one third of cases, and the pineal is displaced in only one fifth. Sudden decompensation and unexpected death may occur — therefore, the

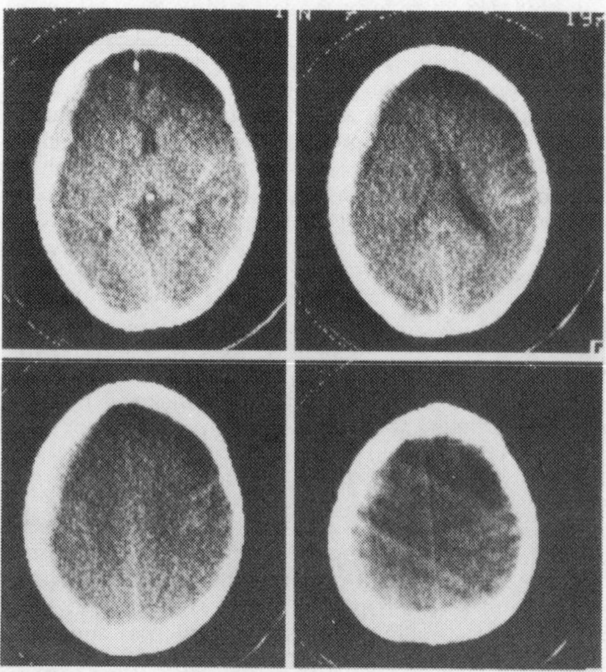

diagnosis, when suspected, should be confirmed by CT scan (illustrated on p. 276), angiography, or trephination. *(Cecil, pp. 2141–2142; McKissock, Richardson, and Bloom)*

41. (E) Brain abscess may be a consequence of an adjacent primary focus of infection (ear, mastoid, sinuses, scalp, or skull) or of infection of the lung or heart. Brain abscesses occur in acute bacterial endocarditis. Various streptococci (anaerobic or non–group A) and *Staphylococcus aureus* are the most frequently isolated organisms. Occasionally, patients with brain abscess present signs of meningitis. This syndrome is due to leaking of the abscess into the ventricular cerebrospinal fluid. The usual history of brain abscess consists of headache and a tumor-like development of focal signs. *(Cecil, pp. 2073–2075)*

42. (A) In only one third of cases of encephalitis can a specific viral agent be identified. The mumps virus accounts for more reported cases of encephalitis than any other agent. Arboviruses are common; enteroviruses are frequently recovered. Herpes simplex is a signficant cause; influenza, LCM, and herpes zoster are uncommon or rare. *(Cecil, pp. 2085–2086)*

43. (C) The history is compatible with Devic's neuromyelitis optica: necrotic myelopathy and optic nerve demyelination. It may be considered a variant of multiple sclerosis, and may occur as the initial illness or later in the course of the disease. Days or weeks may elapse between the onsets of the two symptom complexes. *(Cecil, pp. 2108–2113)* In Guillain-Barré syndrome motor paralysis is flaccid and tends to ascend the body, but demonstrable sensory deficits are absent or modest. Urinary retention develops in only 5% of patients. *(Cecil, pp. 2159–2160)* The Brown-Séquard syndrome refers to an injury to one half of the cord, in which there is spastic weakness, ipsilateral loss of position and vibration sense, and contralateral loss of pain and temperature sensation. *(Cecil, p. 2143)* Paralytic poliomyelitis causes flaccid paralysis; sensory loss does occur in acute poliomyelitis, but is extremely rare. *(Cecil, pp. 2093–2095)*

44. (A) The hearing loss of Meniere's disease is a fluctuating, low-tone "cochlear" type, although other frequencies are involved eventually. Choices B, C, D, and E describe a typical cochlear lesion; choice A, tone decay, is present in retrocochlear lesions involving the eighth nerve or the pons. *(Cecil, pp. 1958–1960)*

45. (D) Hyperkalemic PP is characterized by attacks of weakness ranging from only minutes to hours. Severe attacks lasting more than a day are seen in *hypokalemic* PP. Patients with hyperkalemic PP usually have evidence of myotonia, often limited to percussion myotonia of the tongue. Lid-lag and Chvostek's sign also may be identified in hyperkalemic PP. *(Cecil, pp. 2176–2177)*

46. (A) Narcolepsy is characterized by irresistible episodes of sleep occurring from a few to many times a day. Often, patients with narcolepsy also note cataplexy (episodic generalized weakness, precipitated by emotion and often causing the patient to fall to the ground), sleep paralysis (brief periods of sensation of total body paralysis while falling asleep or on awakening), and hypnagogic hallucinations (visual illusions while falling asleep). Somnambulism (sleepwalking) is independent of the narcolepsy symptom complex. Twenty-five percent of narcoleptic patients have sleep attacks only; 70% have both narcolepsy and cataplexy. The disease begins in young adulthood. A family history is present in half the patients. The presence of cataplexy rules out daytime sleepiness caused by withdrawal of stimulants or sleep apnea syndrome. *(Cecil, p. 1933; Zarcone; Adams and Victor, pp. 269–271)*

47. (A) The characteristic lesions in Wernicke's encephalopathy involve the periaqueductal gray matter and produce extraocular movement impairment, including nystagmus and ocular muscle palsies. Alcohol produces a toxic optic atrophy, but this is distinct from Wernicke's syndrome. Korsakoff's psychosis describes a characteristic impairment of recent memory. Polyneuropathy occurs in 50 to 80% of cases. *(Cecil, pp. 2046–2047; Adams and Victor, pp. 705–710)*

48. (C) Cerebellar degeneration from alcohol affects mainly midline cerebellar structures, producing a wide-based ataxic gait and cerebellar dysmetria (ataxia), usually confined to the lower extremities. Upper extremity dysmetria, nystagmus, and dysarthria are rare. *(Cecil, p. 1967; Adams and Victor, pp. 64, 719–720)*

49. (A) This disorder typically begins with pain in the involved extremity, most often proximal, progressing to weakness with minimal sensory loss of proximal muscles. Wasting follows, but complete recovery usually occurs over many months. *(Cecil, p. 2156; Adams and Victor, pp. 917–919; Tsairis, Dyck, and Mulder)*

50. (B) Duchenne muscular dystrophy is a genetically transmitted recessive disorder that affects males only (i.e., X-linked). First symptoms are pelvic weakness, usually noted before the age of 5 years. The disorder progresses relatively rapidly, producing incapacitation in adolescence and death from pulmonary infection in early adulthood. The serum CPK is markedly elevated. Muscular atrophy can occur, but calf muscles are frequently hypertrophic although markedly weak. In most other muscular dystrophies, significant atrophy is commonplace. *(Cecil, pp. 2170–2173; Adams and Victor, pp. 961–962)*

51. (A) Medical treatment of myasthenia gravis revolves around the anticholinesterases, i.e., neostigmine and pyridostigmine. Corticosteroids have been shown to be effective in refractory cases. Plasmapheresis produces prompt but often unsustained improvement. Early thymectomy in some cases is beneficial. Sodium valproate is an anticonvulsant and plays no role in the treatment of this disorder. *(Cecil, pp. 2182–2184; Drachman)*

52. (A) Trigeminal neuralgia is a syndrome of severe paroxysmal jabbing pain precipitated by contact with oral or facial trigger zones and affecting the second and third divisions of the trigeminal nerve. In idiopathic or typical trigeminal neuralgia, the neurologic examination is entirely normal. Atypical face pain with sensory changes in the distribution of the trigeminal nerve may be a symptom of a gasserian ganglion tumor, multiple sclerosis, or brainstem infarct. Tic pain rarely occurs at night. Carbamazepine is the drug treatment of choice. *(Cecil, p. 2154; Adams and Victor, pp. 131–132, 929–930; Lance, pp. 52–54)*

53. (A) Essential or familial tremor is an inherited movement disorder, possibly autosomal dominant in transmission. The onset of symptoms often occurs before the third decade. Tremors involve the upper extremities and head, but rarely the legs. Patients commonly report the suppression of the tremor by alcohol or propranolol. *(Cecil, p. 2029)*

54. (A) Subarachnoid hemorrhage from a ruptured aneurysm usually presents with the sudden onset of severe headache as arterial blood is released into the subarachnoid space. The resulting increase in intracranial pressure and the meningeal irritation from the blood produce subhyaloid retinal hemorrhages and neck stiffness, respectively. Bruits, however, are heard about the skull in patients with intracranial arteriovenous malformations, whether or not bleeding has occurred. *(Cecil, p. 2069; Adams and Victor, pp. 573–579)*

55. (B) Increase in the gamma globulin fraction of CSF protein is commonly found in patients with multiple sclerosis. It is also elevated in CNS syphilis, CNS sarcoid, and subacute sclerosing panencephalitis. In Guillain-Barré syndrome the total protein is elevated; however, the increase is predominantly albumin, and the gamma globulin concentration is not typically disproportionately elevated. *(Cecil, pp. 2109–2112)*

56. (A) Tabes dorsalis affects the posterior spinal nerve roots, and therefore causes retrograde degeneration of the posterior columns of the spinal cord. This involvement of the nervous system results in interruption of the spinal reflex arc and disordered proprioception, producing areflexia and gait ataxia, respectively. Lightning pains are typical of this disease (approximately 75% of cases), as are pupillary abnormalities, the most common of which is the Argyll Robertson pupil, which reacts weakly to light but accommodates normally. *(Cecil, pp. 2081–2084)*

57. (B) Periodic paralysis is characterized by episodic spells of flaccid muscle weakness most often associated with elevated or depressed levels of serum potassium during the attack. In some cases no alteration of serum potassium is noted at all. There is often a family history of similar spells. Thyrotoxic periodic paralysis mimics the urinary and serum electrolyte picture of the hypokalemic disorder, but is most frequent in Oriental patients and is rarely familial; treatment involves appropriate antithyroid therapy. *(Cecil, pp. 2176–2178; Baker and Baker, Vol. 3, Ch. 37, pp. 32–37)*

58. (D) Central nervous system involvement by syphilis may be that of acute syphilitic meningitis, general paresis (dementia), or tabes dorsalis with optic atrophy and Argyll Robertson pupils, which accommodate but fail to react to light. Cerebral infarction, now uncommon, was a frequent finding in untreated cases. *(Cecil, pp. 2081–2083; Adams and Victor, pp. 493–500)*

59. (D) Seizures may result from low levels of serum glucose and sodium, from withdrawal of daily doses of short-acting barbiturates (equivalent to 600 mg/day or more of Seconal), or in hyperosmolar states of marked hyperglycemia (330 to 350 milliosmoles/L). Hypocalcemia may be associated with seizures, but hypercalcemia produces impaired mentation, weakness, ataxia, and progressive obtundation. *(Cecil, p. 2116)*

60. (D) Steroid administration may cause alterations in mental status ranging from depression to psychosis, as well as increased intracranial pressure (pseudotumor cerebri) and weakness from muscle wasting (especially proximal). A neuropathy does not occur; reflexes are preserved. *(Cecil, p. 2132)*

61. (A) Remote effects of cancer on the nervous system include sensorimotor peripheral neuropathy, subacute cerebellar degeneration, polymyositis-dermatomyositis, dementia (limbic encephalitis), and others. Aphasia and any other evidence of a single, focal nervous system lesion are incompatible with a paraneoplastic etiology. *(Cecil, pp. 1026–1028)*

62. (D) Many drugs and the heavy metals are toxic to nerves. Botulism toxin affects the neuromuscular junction rather than the peripheral nerve. The symptoms therefore are reminiscent of myasthenia gravis, with prominent involvement of the extraocular and bulbar muscles. Alopecia one to two weeks after the development of neuropathy is characteristic of thallium exposure. *(Cecil, pp. 2163, 2184, 2218–2226; Adams and Victor, pp. 897–901)*

63. (B) Neuropathies that commonly affect the peripheral autonomic nervous system, and therefore produce symptoms of autonomic insufficiency, include diabetes mellitus, amyloidosis, and Guillain-Barré syndrome. Riley-Day syndrome is a condition of familial dysautonomia, and autonomic aberrations are a hallmark of this syndrome. *(Cecil, pp. 2159–2160, 2161, 2162, 2164)*

64. (A) Amyotrophic lateral sclerosis is a disease affecting the anterior horn cells and the lateral columns (corticospinal tracts). Patients have weakness, wasting, and fasciculations characteristic of anterior horn cell disease, and hyperreflexia and extensor plantar response characteristic of a corticospinal tract lesion. There is, however, no involvement of the sensory system; this is purely a motor disease. *(Cecil, p. 2037)*

65. (A) The pupillary light reflex is preserved in metabolic coma with only rare exceptions (glutethimide or anticholinergic drug intoxication, profound hypothermia, or anoxia). Decerebrate posturing can be seen in some metabolic encephalopathies (hepatic and anoxic encephalopathies, and early in barbiturate overdose), but this finding is most compatible with structural brain disease. The deep tendon reflexes may be present or absent in metabolic brain disease. The Babinski sign is found in structural corticospinal tract lesions and also is a manifestation of metabolic coma. Internuclear ophthalmoplegia results from a focal lesion in the medial longitudinal fasciculus, most commonly multiple sclerosis or stroke. *(Cecil, pp. 1919–1920)*

66. (D) Anosognosia is found in nondominant hemisphere disease, especially in the acute stage. Such patients may have a left hemiparesis precluding movement from bed, and yet may deny that anything is wrong. When shown their paretic left arm, patients are often unaware of whose limb they are observing. Language function or loss of same (aphasia) defines hemispheric dominance; Gerstmann's syndrome (agraphia, right-left disorientation, acalculia, and finger agnosia) is found with dominant parietal lesions. Alexia usually accompanies aphasia. *(Cecil, pp. 1936–1937, 1939)*

67. (D) The symptoms described are characteristic of cluster headache. The spells occur daily for weeks and then subside for varying periods. Each symptomatic period is termed a "cluster." During a susceptible period, even modest amounts of alcohol may precipitate a headache. Cluster headaches occur most frequently in men. They begin later in life than migraine, and have a characteristic nocturnal predominance. *(Cecil, p. 1951; Lance, pp. 208–226)*

68. (D) Although the etiology is obscure, increased intracranial pressure occurs in patients ingesting large doses of vitamin A (but not vitamin C). Various hormonal alterations also produce the syndrome, including those resulting from corticosteroid administration or withdrawal, pregnancy, the postpartum state, and oral progesterone.

Other drugs that have been associated with this syndrome are tetracycline, nalidixic acid, and acetazolamide. *(Cecil, pp. 2131–2132; Weisberg)*

69. (D) A unilateral orbital bruit indicates intracavernous stenosis of the carotid artery. *(Cecil, p. 2057)*

70. (A) Parkinsonian tremor is present at rest, diminished with active movement, and absent during sleep. The lack of facial expression is typical of the disease and has been termed a "masklike" face. Resistance to passive movement of a joint on both flexion and extension is termed "rigidity" and is characteristic of extrapyramidal disorders. Bradykinesia, with a shuffling gait in which the patient has difficulty initiating and stopping a movement, is also typical of parkinsonism. *(Cecil, pp. 2025–2026; Adams and Victor, pp. 807–812)*

71. (C) Gilles de la Tourette's syndrome is one of multifocal tics and coprolalia beginning in childhood and following a waxing-waning course. The tics are mostly facial at onset, but their location varies over the years. Haloperidol is effective treatment. *(Cecil, p. 2033; Adams and Victor, p. 77)*

72. (A) Barbiturate poisoning and hypoglycemia are common causes of hypothermia in the comatose patient. This symptom complex may be seen also with Wernicke's encephalopathy, but coma is uncommon. Pontine hemorrhage produces hyperthermia in patients surviving for more than a few days. *(Cecil, pp. 1921, 1925)*

73. (D) All the signs listed are common findings in multiple sclerosis, but only choice D requires more than a single lesion in the central nervous system. This multiplicity of lesions is essential for the diagnosis. *(Cecil, pp. 2109–2112; Adams and Victor, pp. 648–658)*

74. (D) Ballismus is the result of a lesion in the subthalamic nucleus. The anatomic lesion in the other movement disorders is unknown. *(Cecil, pp. 2024, 2031)*

75. (C) Copper accumulation in Descemet's membrane produces the characteristic Kayser-Fleischer ring of Wilson's disease. *(Cecil, pp. 1126–1128)*

76. (D) The brain edema surrounding a tumor metastatic to the central nervous system is remarkably sensitive to steroid treatment. Polymyalgia rheumatica and temporal arteritis are also steroid-responsive, and myasthenia gravis responds to steroids in certain instances. There is no role for steroids in the treatment of cerebral infarction. *(Cecil, pp. 1869, 2065, 2129, 2183)*

77. (A) Myotonic muscular dystrophy is an autosomal dominant disorder that affects distal muscles before proximal ones (as opposed to the typical pattern in muscular dystrophy). Difficulty in muscle relaxation (termed "myotonia") is characteristic. Involvement of other systems results in cataracts, frontal baldness, testicular atrophy, and diabetes mellitus. *(Cecil, p. 2172; Baker and Baker, Vol. 3, Ch. 37, pp. 25–28)*

78. (A — True; B — False; C — True; D — True; E — True) Uremic polyneuropathy is most common in patients with end-stage uremia receiving chronic hemodialysis; it usually disappears after renal transplantation. The cause of uremic neuropathy is poorly understood, but its incidence appears to be decreasing as the techniques of hemodialysis improve. Diabetic amyotrophy is thought to be a lumbosacral plexus or root lesion, perhaps vascular in origin, affecting one or both legs proximally with sudden pain and weakness followed by atrophy. This is in contrast to diabetic polyneuropathy, which is a distal, predominantly sensory, polyneuropathy. Polyneuropathy of amyloidosis is seen in both primary and secondary types such as multiple myeloma, in which amyloid deposits have been found in peripheral nerves. Hypothyroidism is associated with both mononeuropathy and polyneuropathy, which frequently improve with thyroid replacement therapy. The most common neurologic manifestation of sarcoidosis is isolated or multiple cranial neuropathy; an isolated lower motor neuron facial palsy is the most common initial presentation. *(Cecil, pp. 2161–2163)*

79. (A — True; B — False; C — False; D — True; E — True; F — True) The Guillain-Barré syndrome typically has a subacute initial presentation, although some cases may be quite acute and others fairly chronic. Controlled trials have shown that steroids prolong the disease and are of no benefit in most cases. Progression of paralysis may be ascending, descending, or patchy or diffuse. Ascending paralysis occurs in about 40% of cases. Autonomic dysfunction characterized by tachyarrhythmias and unstable blood pressure commonly occurs in severe cases. The prognosis is generally excellent. *(Cecil, pp. 2159–2160; Goodall; Announcement/NINCDS Ad Hoc Committee)*

80. (A — False; B — True; C — False; D — True; E — False) Prospective studies have shown chronic atrial fibrillation alone to be associated with a fivefold increased incidence of stroke. With valvular heart disease the increased rate is significantly higher. The incidence of strokes appears to be decreasing, perhaps as a consequence of decreased deaths due to hypertension and the sequelae of rheumatic heart disease. The cause of most strokes appears to be atherosclerosis in the major extracranial arteries to the brain, often producing artery-to-artery emboli. Complete occlusion of the internal carotid artery often produces a dense contralateral hemiparesis; however, it may also be completely asymptomatic and be an incidental finding at arteriography or autopsy. Palpation of the internal carotid artery is a difficult and unreliable bedside test. The presence of a carotid bruit may indicate underlying atherosclerosis, but not necessarily so. *(Cecil, pp. 2050–2057)*

81. (A — True; B — False; C — True; D — True; E — True) The patient is usually unaware of any difficulty with breathing, particularly while awake; the apnea occurs during sleep, when it is usually noticed by the patient's spouse. Snoring is also a disturbing feature to the spouse. Tiredness and excessive daytime sleepiness are common symptoms. Although some cases respond to weight loss, tracheostomy is the treatment of choice in severe peripheral cases. This disorder is more common in men than in women. *(Cecil, pp. 1934–1935)*

82. (A — False; B — False; C — False; D — True; E — False) Clinical and experimental evidence suggests that early prompt treatment is the most effective means of controlling chronic pain. Combination treatment is often better than a single agent alone, and the effects of minor analgesics and/or tricyclic antidepressants are often additive to the pain relief obtained from narcotics, to which tolerance will always develop. *(Cecil, p. 1943)*

83. (All are True) Depressants of the central nervous system include benzodiazepines, and specific CNS receptor sites for these drugs have been isolated. Intoxication resembles alcohol intoxication with nystagmus, dysarthria, and ataxia. Seizures may occur as part of an acute abstinence syndrome, but death is very infrequent from self-poisoning provided respiration is maintained. Drug dependence is common with this group of agents, particularly in women. *(Cecil, pp. 2010–2012)*

84. (A — True; B — False; C — True; D — False; E — False) Seizures usually occur 12 to 24 hours after cessation or reduction of drinking. Victor reported that in 40% of patients more than one seizure occurred, usually within six hours of the first; status epilepticus occurred in 3% of his patients. Phenytoin therapy is not indicated for control of alcoholic epilepsy. Alcoholic epilepsy is usually made manifest by generalized seizures; focal seizures are an indication to search for underlying disease. Delirium tremens follows seizures in a small percentage of patients but is no longer frequent, probably because of the current widespread use of diazepam for sedation; once the DTs have begun, seizures do not recur. *(Cecil, pp. 2021–2022; Victor, 1968)*

85. (A — True; B — False; C — True; D — False; E — True) Myasthenia gravis affects the myoneural junctions, and therefore produces motor weakness without impairment of sensory function or intelligence. Fatigue with repetitive exercise is typical. Involvement of muscles innervated by the cranial nerves is prominent and frequently produces the first signs or symptoms (diplopia, ptosis, dysphagia, and dysarthria). All patients with this disorder require radiologic evaluation (tomograms of anterior mediastinum, etc.) to exclude thymomas, which occur in 10 to 15%. *(Cecil, pp. 2180–2184; Baker and Baker, Vol. 3, Ch. 37, pp. 62–71)*

86. (A — True; B — True; C — True; D — True; E — False) Petit mal is a genetically transmitted disorder beginning exclusively in childhood and characterized by brief absence attacks that may occur as often as 100 or more times daily. The EEG during spells shows a characteristic 3/second spike and wave discharge (see illustration). These absence spells are often easily induced by hyperventilation. Phenytoin is of no benefit in the treatment of this seizure type, which readily responds to ethosuximide, valproic acid, or clonazepam. *(Cecil, pp. 2117, 2122)*

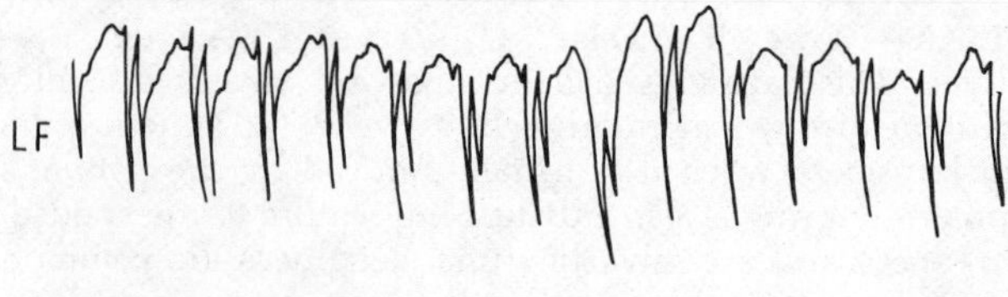

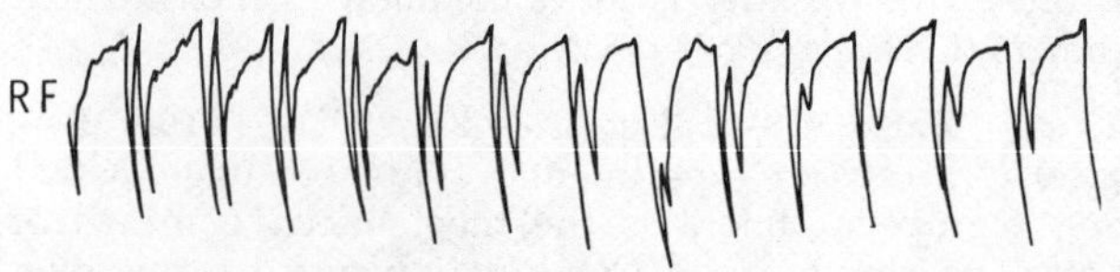

87. (A — False; B — False; C — False; D — False; E — True) Benign intracranial hypertension most commonly presents with headache and visual disturbances. Lumbar puncture reveals an elevated cerebrospinal fluid pressure, but otherwise is normal. The protein is normal and in many cases is below 15 mg/dl. The EEG is characteristically normal. The syndrome is usually self-limiting with spontaneous remission after a period of weeks to months. A few patients will require lumbar-peritoneal shunt to relieve persistent symptoms. *(Cecil, pp. 2132–2133)*

88. (A — True; B — False; C — True; D — True; E — False) Segmental herpes zoster most often presents with pain limited to one or several adjacent dermatomes upon which the vesicular lesions appear after several days. Persistence of pain following resolution of the vesicles is termed "postherpetic neuralgia." Dissemination is most common in patients with lymphoreticular malignancies. *(Cecil, pp. 2091–2093; Adams and Victor, pp. 512–515)*

89. (A — True; B — True; C — True; D — False; E — True) Tuberous sclerosis is a congenital, probably dominantly transmitted disorder with central nervous system and cutaneous manifestations. The skin has characteristic acneiform lesions about the nose and cheeks (adenoma sebaceum), which may not develop until the second decade. Hypertelorism is frequently seen in this illness. In addition, café au lait spots similar to those in von Recklinghausen's disease are found. The most prominent features of CNS involvement are mental retardation and epilepsy. The brain is studded with small, firm nodules or tubers for which the disease is named. The unilateral port wine nevus is found in another of the neurocutaneous disorders, Sturge-Weber syndrome. *(Cecil, p. 2044; Adams and Victor, pp. 845–851, 944)*

90. (All are True) *(Cecil, pp. 1944–1945)*

91. (A — True; B — True; C — False; D — True; E — False) Abnormalities of latency and wave form in visual and somatosensory evoked potentials may reveal abnormalities in different parts of the neuraxis, some of which may not be clinically evident. Computerized tomography with large-contrast bolus may reveal enhancing demyelinating plaques. An elevated gamma globulin concentration in the spinal fluid is frequently present. Electromyography and nerve conduction studies are of value in diagnosing peripheral nerve lesions, but are usually normal in multiple sclerosis. Cerebral arteriography is of no benefit except to exclude other lesions. *(Cecil, p. 2110)*

92. (A — True; B — True; C — True; D — False; E — False) Seizures, headaches, and lethargy are common presenting symptoms. Chronic subdural hematomas are more frequent among alcoholics than among nonalcoholics. Antecedent head injury is common, but the syndrome may occur spontaneously or be associated with anticoagulant usage. The CT scan, although a useful diagnostic tool, may not detect all chronic subdurals, as subtle shifts in the ventricular system may be missed. When the diagnosis is strongly suspected, a radionuclide brain scan or cerebral arteriography may be more definitive. *(Cecil, pp. 2142–2143)*

93. (A — False; B — True; C — True; D — True; E — False) Heroin use declined in the mid-1970s but has increased again since then. It is a leading cause of death in males aged 15 to 35 years, and cross-tolerance to all narcotics does occur. Withdrawal symptoms peak by 48 hours and gradually subside over five to ten days. Initiation is usually by a friend or acquaintance, and the role of the nonaddicted dealer is minimal in exposing new users. *(Cecil, pp. 2006–2010)*

94. (All are True) Toxic amblyopia may be secondary to quinine. Street heroin is adulterated with quinine, lactulose, mannitol, and numerous other substances. The sterility is questionable. *(Cecil, pp. 2006–2010)*

95. (A—False; B—True; C—False; D—True; E—False) Astrocytic tumors consist of astrocytes that proliferate and infiltrate the brain; occasionally, if benign, they calcify. Glioblastoma multiforme is the most malignant form of astrocytoma and usually is not associated with calcification. The oligodendroglioma is a cellular, globular mass that frequently calcifies; seizures are common, and these tumors rarely become malignant. Ependymomas usually are well demarcated and may be seen in the cerebrospinal fluid, but do not frequently calcify. Craniopharyngiomas frequently present as calcific sellar or suprasellar masses and may grow to a large size before detection. The chromophobe adenomas do not calcify. *(Cecil, pp. 2125–2126)*

96. (A—False; B—True; C—True; D—True; E—True) The question of when to do a lumbar puncture is always a serious one. In patients with increased intracranial pressure, the procedure sometimes induces fatal herniation of the brain through the tentorium of the foramen magnum. A patient suspected of having an expanding intracranial mass as indicated by depressed consciousness, hemiparesis, or papilledema should have other diagnostic studies (CT scan or angiography) in place of lumbar puncture. The main indications for lumbar puncture are: (1) when CNS infection is suspected, to confirm infection and identify the organism; and (2) before using anticoagulants to treat ischemic cerebrovascular disease, to be certain that cerebral hemorrhage is not present. The CT scan, if available, can replace lumbar puncture in the latter case. If lumbar epidural abscess is suspected, cervical or cisternal puncture must be used in place of the lumbar route, as attempted puncture in the latter may carry infected material into the spinal fluid. Thrombocytopenia may lead to localized bleeding, but is not an absolute contraindication. *(Cecil, pp. 1920, 1944)*

97. (A—False; B—True; C—False; D—True; E—True) Homicide is a possibility in depressed patients who harbor delusional beliefs that their family shares in their guilt and accursed characteristics. Manic patients are often overbearing, easy to anger, and suspicious that the efforts being made to control them are unjust. The prognosis for a single attack of mania or depression is excellent; the long-range prognosis is not so favorable. Lithium is effective in controlling mania; treatment of depression requires other agents. Repeated attacks of depression without intervening manic episodes are common. *(Cecil, pp. 1987–1989)*

98. (A—False; B—False; C—False; D—True; E—True) Depression as a response to illness, physiologic abnormalities, or troubled circumstances is not the same as depression as a symptom of manic-depressive disorder. Treatment of the former is based on a supportive relationship between doctor and patient. ECT is not indicated. Patients with a hysterical personality causing them to be emotionally unstable and to amplify emotional reactions are prone to depressive responses. Stroke may precipitate a mood of depression; disorders of the right hemisphere, however, may be accompanied by a state of unconcern and jocularity. The grief reaction, not anxiety, illustrates most of the common features. *(Cecil, pp. 1993–1995)*

99. (A—True; B—True; C—True; D—False; E—True) The WAIS consists of verbal and performance tests. In the verbal tests the subject is asked to define words, recognize similarities between words, interpret proverbs, and so on. In the performance tests the subject is asked to put together puzzles, work with symbols, and construct patterns with blocks. The verbal and performance scores of normal individuals are usually comparable. In brain disease, performance disturbances appear before verbal ones do. This may indicate that verbal tests measure more what an individual has learned, whereas performance tests measure his capacity to meet new problems. Emotional unrest also interferes with WAIS scores. *(Cecil, pp. 1979–1981)*

100. (A—True; B—False; C—True; D—True; E—False) The basic management of sedative drug-induced coma consists of physiologic support with attention to the airway, prevention of hypoventilation and aspiration, and maintenance of an adequate systemic circulation. Hemodialysis usually is not necessary except to shorten the duration of coma for patients who have ingested large amounts of long-acting barbiturates or glutethimide. Analeptics are contraindicated and carry the risk of producing seizures in lightly poisoned patients. Naloxone is not specifically indicated to treat sedative drug overdose; however, it should be given to any patient with coma of uncertain origin so that an unsuspected opiate overdose does not go untreated. *(Cecil, pp. 1923–1925)*

101. (A—True; B—True; C—True; D—False; E—False) Damage to the posterior hypothalamus has been associated with lethargy, hypersomnolence, and coma. Large posterior hypothalamic lesions destroy both heat loss and heat production mechanisms and result in poikilothermia; hypothermia therefore commonly results at ordinary ambient temperatures. Posterior hypothalamic lesions can produce gastrointestinal ulceration. Impaired recent memory can follow damage to the ventromedian hypothalamus, thalamus, and mamillary bodies. Hyperthermia and diabetes insipidus can follow trauma to or hemorrhage into the region of the anterior hypothalamus. *(Cecil, p. 2127)*

102. (A—True; B—True; C—True; D—False; E—True) Among intracranial structures, only a limited group of tissues can cause pain. These include the great venous sinuses; parts of the dura at the base; the dural and cerebral arteries at the base of the brain; cranial nerves V, VII, IX, and X; and nerves C1 to C3. The cranium, parenchyma of the brain, pia-arachnoid, ependyma, and choroid plexuses are not sensitive to pain. *(Cecil, p. 1949; Lance, pp. 1–2)*

103. (A—True; B—False; C—False; D—False; E—True) Heightened muscle tonus is associated with extrapyramidal disorders, especially parkinsonism. The mechanism underlying rigidity is impairment of reciprocal inhibition of agonist and antagonist muscles. Electromyography shows continuing muscle activity. Passive movements may be cogwheel or jerky. Rigidity is not associated with lesions either of the subthalamic nucleus or the pyramidal tract (area 4), which produce ballismus and flaccid paralysis, respectively. Baclofen and dantrolene are of questionable benefit in disorders resulting in spasticity, not rigidity. *(Cecil, p. 2024; Lance and McLeod, pp. 163–202)*

104. (A—True; B—True; C—True; D—False; E—False) In parkinsonism the substantia nigra degenerates. Dopamine deficiency allows for cholinergic hyperactivity in parkinsonism — hence the often favorable response of such patients to anticholinergic agents. Dopamine hyperactivity and/or cholinergic hypoactivity results in the hyperkinetic phenomena of Huntington's chorea. The tremor of extrapyramidal origin characteristically is augmented when the part is at rest, and is diminished or abolished during sleep. Patients often exhibit difficulties in positioning themselves for the simplest tasks, such as rising from a chair and getting dressed. *(Cecil, pp. 2025–2026)*

105. (A — False; B — False; C — True; D — True; E — False) The treatment of completed stroke has four aims: to preserve life, to limit the amount of brain damage, to lessen disability and deformity, and to prevent recurrence. Survival is increased by efforts directed toward maintaining respiratory function and adequate fluid, electrolyte, and caloric intake. Corticosteroids have not been effective in reducing cerebral edema after infarction. Rehabilitation programs often lessen disability after stroke by training patients in developing new skills with their remaining functions. Anticoagulation and thromboendarterectomy in patients with severe neurologic deficits or evidence of extensive atherosclerotic disease do not reduce future mortality or morbidity. Control of hypertension, especially in patients under 65, is related to a reduced risk of reinfarction. *(Cecil, pp. 2064–2065; Report from the Joint Committee for Stroke Resources XIV)*

106. (A — True; B — False; C — True; D — False; E — True) Herpes zoster is due to varicella, the same virus that causes chickenpox. Zoster rarely develops after exposure to chickenpox or other cases of zoster. The precise pathogenesis of herpes zoster is unknown, but the most widely accepted hypothesis is that varicella viruses in ganglia are activated owing to decline of immunity with age, or as a result of the development of malignancy, trauma, local x-irradiation, immunosuppressive therapy, or other factors. High-dose steroids administered early in the course of herpes zoster are thought to reduce the severity of neuralgia. *(Cecil, pp. 2091–2093; Hope-Simpson)*

107. (A — True; B — True; C — True; D — True; E — False) Lesions that destroy the pain and temperature fibers in the anterior spinal commissure, but spare the posterior columns of the spinal cord, cause a dissociated sensory loss; therefore, syringomyelia and intramedullary neoplasms of the cord are correct answers. Syphilitic vasculitis was a common cause of spinal cord ischemia before antibiotic treatment became available. Leprosy, the most common treatable neuropathy in the world, is associated with intracutaneous nerve damage; pain and temperature sense are most affected; touch and pressure sensation often remain nearly normal. Vitamin B_{12} deficiency usually affects the posterior columns, causing impairment of position and vibration much more than of pain and temperature sense. *(Cecil, pp. 2146–2147)*

108. (All are True) Diabetic neuropathies fall into two types: (1) mononeuropathy involving single large peripheral nerves such as the femoral; and (2) a distal symmetric sensorimotor polyneuropathy. In the latter, touch-pressure, vibration, and joint position sensations are affected. Charcot joints may occur. Damage to autonomic nerves leads to disturbances of intestinal motility. The protein concentration of the CSF is often elevated from 50 to 400 mg/dl. Hyperalgesic neuropathy with a burning quality occurs frequently. *(Cecil, pp. 2161–2162)*

109. (A — False; B — False; C — True; D — True; E — True) Compression of the spinal cord in the thoracic area is suggested by the finding of normal arms and spastic legs. The intercostal, abdominal, and paraspinal muscles can be wasted. When the patient raises his head, the umbilicus may elevate or may be pulled laterally (Beevor's sign), owing to asymmetric weakness of opposing muscles. Tumors are common in the thoracic spine, but herniated discs are rare. Well-localized pain of recent onset is a common presentation with minimal neurologic findings. *(Cecil, pp. 1969–1972, 2146, 2148, 2150–2152)*

110. (A — True; B — True; C — True; D — True; E — False) Postencephalitic Parkinson's disease followed the epidemic of encephalitis lethargica in the 1920s. Parkinsonism is an important sequela of the phenothiazine drugs, and an uncommon but well-recognized feature of poisoning by carbon monoxide and manganese. Cerebral vascular disease has not been shown to produce such a picture. Thallium produces a toxic peripheral neuropathy with alopecia, but not extrapyramidal symptoms. *(Cecil, p. 2026)*

111. (A — False; B — True; C — True; D — True; E — True) Spinal arachnoiditis may result from any inflammatory meningeal process, but is most commonly seen after spinal surgery or spinal anesthesia. Blood in the epidural space does not come into contact with the arachnoid. The introduction of blood, lipoidal contrast media, or antibiotics into the subarachnoid space may precipitate arachnoiditis. Although the incidence is low, arachnoiditis does follow myelography. *(Cecil, p. 2152; Adams and Victor, pp. 628–629)*

112. (All are True) Respiratory failure is caused by an acute peripheral neuropathy affecting respiratory muscles in Guillain-Barré syndrome; a myoneural junction blockage in botulism; anterior horn cell disease in poliomyelitis; a lesion of pathways between the brain-stem regulatory centers and the spinal cord in cervical cord injury; and defective myoneural junction transmission in myasthenia gravis. *(Cecil, pp. 2096, 2109–2112, 2144, 2161–2163, 2180–2182, 2184)*

113. (A — False; B — True; C — True; D — True; E — True) Neurofibromatosis is an autosomal dominant disorder characterized by café au lait spots, freckling, and neurofibromas. There is an increased incidence of benign and malignant tumors of the central nervous system, tumors of the cranial nerves, and pheochromocytomas. *(Cecil, pp. 2043–2044; Adams and Victor, pp. 847–849)*

114. (All are True) All the conditions listed are neurocutaneous syndromes, i.e., disorders characterized by involvement of the skin and the central nervous system. Ataxia telangiectasia is notable for ocular and cutaneous telangiectasia as well as cerebellar ataxia. A port wine facial nevus associated with a capillary hemangioma of the ipsilateral cerebellar cortex is termed "Sturge-Weber syndrome." Neurofibromatosis denotes cutaneous café au lait spots, with benign and sometimes malignant tumors of peripheral nerves and brain. Patients with tuberous sclerosis also have café au lait spots as a cutaneous sign as well as the characteristic facial acneiform adenoma sebaceum. These skin lesions are associated with mental retardation and seizures, together with intracranial tumors or "tubers." Niacin deficiency produces a dermatitis characterized by pigmentation and hyperkeratinization. Mental abnormalities in the form of dementia also occur. *(Cecil, pp. 2043–2045)*

115. (All are True) Patients with anosmia commonly report the disorder as a deficit in taste. Lesions producing this phenomenon may involve the olfactory system from the nasal passage to the intracranial cavity. Basilar skull fracture involving the area of the olfactory bulb and olfactory groove meningiomas are frequent causes of anosmia. These tumors may also result in dementia. Local disease in the nose accounts for anosmia in most patients. *(Cecil, pp. 2153–2154)*

116. (A — False; B — False; C — False; D — True; E — True) Neurofibromas of the eighth cranial nerve (acoustic neuroma) involve the vestibular portion initially. The presentation, however, rarely includes prominent vertigo; rather, a mild unsteadiness is noted. The CSF is remarkable for a very high protein and, unless infection is superimposed, a normal glucose. Cranial nerves 5 and 7 are often affected owing to their close proximity in the cerebellopontine angle. *(Cecil, p. 2128; Adams and Victor, pp. 462–464)*

117. (A — True; B — True; C — True; D — True; E — False) Radiation injury to the spinal cord is delayed for months to years following exposure. The susceptibility varies with the dose, length of exposure, and tissue type. The spinal cord is more susceptible than the brain, and nerves are relatively resistant. An early manifestation of radiation myelopathy is Lhermitte's sign, which is usually transient. Destruction of both gray and white matter may be extensive. *(Cecil, pp. 2130–2131)*

118. (All are True) Cysticercosis is usually produced by the pork tapeworm, *T. solium.* Human infection occurs when man ingests eggs or larvae by eating feces-contaminated food or insufficiently cooked pork containing encysted larvae. Once ingested, the eggs become larvae that penetrate the intestine and are blood-borne to muscle, liver, eye, and brain. Cerebral cysticercosis has myriad manifestations, including seizures (if the cyst is located in the cortex), hydrocephalus, and basal (eosinophilic) meningitis. Widespread infection can present with signs of increased intracranial pressure. No specific treatment is available. Hydrocephalus may require shunting of CSF, and intracranial hypertension may respond to corticosteroids. In 20 to 30% of patients, *T. solium* infects the intestines. *(Cecil, pp. 1751–1752)*

119. (D); 120. (A); 121. (B); 122. (C); 123. (E) Nystagmus is common following the institution of phenytoin therapy and may even be present with the patient's blood levels in the therapeutic range; ataxia tends to occur at higher doses. Blood dyscrasias have been reported with carbamazepine; the incidence is low, the major danger period being the first three months of therapy. Sedation and loss of concentration often follows initiation of phenobarbital therapy; these symptoms improve over time. Ethosuximide is frequently associated with anorexia and nausea, as well as headache and hiccups. Valproic acid is extensively protein-bound and interacts with other protein-bound substances such as phenytoin and phenobarbital; it usually causes an increase in serum phenobarbital levels when used in combination with that drug. Hepatic failure shortly after the beginning of therapy is a known effect of valproic acid and necessitates the monitoring of liver enzymes for several months. *(Cecil, p. 2122; Penry and Newmark; Browne)*

124. (B); 125. (E); 126. (A); 127. (D); 128. (C) Creutzfeldt-Jakob disease, usually seen in patients over 40, is transmissible from human to human/primate via inoculated brain and is presumed to be viral in origin, although virus has never been isolated. The cortex has a spongiform appearance, myoclonus is characteristic, and pyramidal as well as cerebellar signs often occur. Huntington's chorea is dominantly inherited, and chorea may or may not be seen early in the disease. Subacute sclerosing panencephalitis is a disease of children and young adults with myoclonus and a characteristic burst suppression pattern on EEG, presumably paramyxovirus-related. Alzheimer's dementia is frequently accompanied by seizures and is unusual below age 50; an abundance of neurofibrillary tangles and senile plaques is characteristic. Progressive multifocal leukoencephalopathy frequently occurs in immunosuppressed hosts, and recently a human papovavirus (JC virus) has been isolated. The pathology is characteristically multifocal demyelination, and various clinical signs can occur. Multiple sclerosis is a disease of young adults; seizures and dementia are uncommon symptoms. Demyelination occurs but viral particles and bodies have not been identified. *(Cecil, pp. 1981–1982, 2030, 2101–2102, 2110–2111)*

129. (D); 130. (C); 131. (A); 132. (E); 133. (F); 134. (B) Internuclear ophthalmoplegia indicating a lesion of the medial longitudinal fasciculus is characteristic of multiple sclerosis or midbrain stroke. Phenytoin intoxication produces gaze-evoked nystagmus. Unilateral gaze-evoked nystagmus with subjective vertigo indicates end-organ vestibular disease. A supranuclear lesion of frontal eye fields leads to lateral conjugate gaze without nystagmus. Lower basilar lesions characteristically produce down-beat nystagmus. Opsoclonus is pathognomonic of a nonmetastatic effect of malignancy and is especially seen in neuroblastoma. *(Cecil, pp. 1957–1958)*

135. (A); 136. (F); 137. (E); 138. (C); 139. (B); 140. (D) *(Cecil, pp. 1970–1971)*

141. (D); 142. (A); 143. (E); 144. (C); 145. (B) Herpes simplex encephalitis is often hemorrhagic initially, and a predominant lymphocytosis occurs in most viral infections. Bacterial meningitis is marked by a predominant PMN response, low sugar, and high protein. This may also be seen in carcinomatous meningitis, although the cell count is predominantly lymphocytes rather than PMNs. Guillain-Barré syndrome is marked by an increase in the CSF protein without an increase in lymphocytes (albuminocytologic dissociation). Acute multiple sclerosis may show some lymphocytic response and mild elevation of protein; sugar is usually normal. *(Cecil, pp. 2110, 2129, 2159)*

146. (C); 147. (D); 148. (B); 149. (E); 150. (A) Visual acuity remains normal in papilledema but is decreased in optic neuritis, commonly caused by multiple sclerosis. Sphenoid wing meningioma can compress the optic nerve, leading to unilateral optic atrophy and decreased acuity. Tumors arising out of the sella, such as craniopharyngioma, may compress the optic chiasm and produce bitemporal hemianopia. Homonymous hemianopia is commonly due to unilateral optic radiation disease; an infiltrating glioblastoma of the parietal lobe may be a likely cause. Amaurosis fugax (transient monocular blindness) is commonly due to carotid artery atherosclerotic emboli, as the ophthalmic artery is the first branch of the internal carotid artery. *(Cecil, pp. 1954–1956)*

151. (B); 152. (D); 153. (C); 154. (A); 155. (E) The Argyll Robertson pupils of syphilis are usually bilateral but may be unilateral. Myotonic pupil (Adie's) is of no pathologic significance. Horner's is a unilateral sympathetic paralysis of the eye. Diabetes frequently produces a partial third nerve palsy with retention of pupillary response. Berry aneurysm, by direct compression of the third nerve, may produce total complete third nerve palsy. *(Cecil, p. 1956)*

156. (B); 157. (D); 158. (A); 159. (C); 160. (E) Naloxone, given intravenously or intramuscularly, is a specific opiate antagonist. Lithium is dialyzable. Phenothiazines will control the acute paranoia of amphetamine intoxication, but may aggravate LSD-induced panic. Diazepam will quiet the latter. Physostigmine will block the tachyarrhythmias induced by tricyclic antidepressants. *(Cecil, p. 1924)*

161. (C); 162. (A); 163. (B); 164. (D) Phantom limb pain may be chronic with trigger points; surgical procedures are not helpful. Early cutaneous desensitization frequently helps postherpetic neuralgia, often in combination with amitriptyline or analgesics. In trigeminal neuralgia that is persistent and refractory to phenytoin or carbamazepine, destructive surgical procedures directed against the trigeminal nerve frequently help; mobilization of arteries crossing the trigeminal nerve root intracranially has been said to be helpful to some. Causalgia frequently responds to sympathectomy. *(Cecil, pp. 1946–1948)*

165. (A); 166. (C); 167. (B); 168. (D) The most frequently encountered signs of cytomegalovirus infection in symptomatic newborns are hepatosplenomegaly, jaundice, purpura, microcephaly, cerebral calcifications, and chorioretinitis. The clinical picture of congenital toxoplasmosis may be identical to that seen in CMV disease; however, chorioretinitis, anemia, and seizures are common. Cerebral calcifications in toxoplasmosis are scattered irregularly throughout the brain. Cytomegalovirus has an affinity for the subependymal cells, and deposition of calcium in this area results in characteristic periventricular calcifications. Rubella may be difficult to distinguish from CMV in the neonatal period, but the presence of central cataracts is a strong presumptive evidence of rubella. Herpes simplex infection may present as a fulminant meningoencephalitis or pneumonitis. *(Cecil, pp. 1649–1651, 2089–2091)*

169. (E); 170. (B); 171. (D); 172. (C); 173. (A) Glioblastoma multiforme is characterized by a very rapid growth rate, much tissue necrosis, and brain edema. Astrocytomas occur in the cerebellar hemispheres in children and are often cystic. Medulloblastomas are midline cerebellar tumors of children but can occur in older patients; they are malignant and frequently metastasize throughout the neuraxis. Meningiomas arise in the meninges and are usually benign, so that complete removal is often possible. Hemangioblastomas are the most frequent adult primary tumor of the cerebellum, but they also occur in the cerebrum; they may be associated with angiomatosis of the retina and cysts of the kidney and pancreas (von Hippel-Lindau syndrome). *(Cecil, pp. 2044, 2124–2128)*

174. (A); 175. (C); 176. (B); 177. (E); 178. (D) Concussion is defined as loss of consciousness after head injury without macroscopic damage to nervous tissue. A subdural hematoma (chronic) may follow a relatively minor head injury owing to tearing of a cortical or bridging vein. Epidural hematomas frequently occur as a result of a skull fracture with tearing of a meningeal artery; after a lucid interval the expanding clot caused by arterial bleeding causes brain shift, and death may result. Basilar skull fractures are usually diagnosed by drainage of blood and/or CSF from the nose or ears. Penetrating injuries have a high risk of epilepsy. *(Cecil, pp. 2136–2142)*

179. (A); 180. (C); 181. (D); 182. (F) Petit mal is marked by brief attacks of altered consciousness (absences) lasting five to 30 seconds, accompanied by a fixed stare and by blinking. Temporal lobe seizures are associated with a dreamy state and ictal automatisms; they last longer than petit mal attacks and often are followed by a major motor seizure and/or postictal confusion. Myoclonic seizures are sensitive to sensory stimulation, and may exist as an isolated phenomenon or may precede a grand mal convulsion. Jacksonian seizures are caused by a lesion in the motor cortex; they begin as a repetitive movement of a distal portion of an extremity, and then spread. *(Cecil, pp. 2116–2118; Solomon and Plum)*

183. (D); 184. (A); 185. (C); 186. (B); 187. (E) Ethosuximide is the drug of choice in the treatment of petit mal. Phenytoin is the drug of choice for treating major motor seizures in adults, and also for focal seizures and psychomotor seizures; it is ineffective for petit mal, febrile seizures, and alcohol withdrawal seizures. Carbamazepine is effective in psychomotor seizures. Phenobarbital is the drug of choice in treating the preschool child with grand mal seizures, e.g., febrile seizures. Alcohol withdrawal seizures are usually self-limited and do not respond to chronic anticonvulsant therapy. *(Cecil, pp. 2121–2123)*

188. (C); 189. (E); 190. (D); 191. (A); 192. (B) The most common neurologic syndromes associated with anomalies in the region of the foramen magnum and distortion of the cerebellum, cervical cord, and brain stem are choices C, E, and D, respectively. Von Recklinghausen's disease, or neurofibromatosis, is associated with abnormalities of the bones of the skull as well as deformities in the spine caused by the effects of enlarging neurofibromas. Calcification of a leptomeningeal hemangioma in the cortex of a patient with Sturge-Weber syndrome gives the "railroad track" pattern on a skull film (see illustration). *(Cecil, pp. 2043–2044, 2135)*

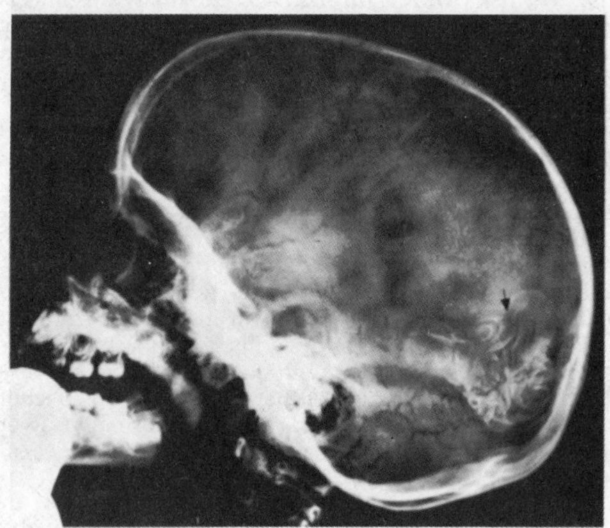

BIBLIOGRAPHY

Adams, R. D., and Victor, M.: Principles of Neurology. 2nd ed. New York, McGraw-Hill Book Company, 1981.

Announcement/NINCDS Ad Hoc Committee. Criteria for diagnosis of Guillain-Barré Syndrome. Ann. Neurol. *3*:565, 1978.

Baker, A. B., and Baker, L. H.: Clinical Neurology. New York, Harper & Row, 1975.

Barnes, B. D., Parker, H., and Anger, H. O.: Neurologic diagnosis using the 80-lens optical camera. Neurology, *27*:26, 1977.

Barnett, H. J. M., Jones, M. W., Boughner, D. R., et al.: Cerebral ischemic events associated with prolapsing mitral valve. Arch. Neurol., *33*:777, 1976.

Browne, T. R.: Valproic acid. N. Engl. J. Med., *302*:661, 1980.

Chester, E. M.: Hypertensive encephalopathy: a clinicopathologic study of 20 cases. Neurology, *28*:928, 1978.

Drachman, D. B.: Myasthenia gravis. N. Engl. J. Med., *298*:136, 1978.

Gilman, A. G., Goodman, L. S., and Gilman, A. (eds.): Goodman and Gilman's The Pharmacologic Basis of Therapeutics. 6th ed. New York, Macmillan, 1980.

Goodall, J. D. A., Kosmidis, J. C., and Geddes, A. M.: Effect of corticosteroids on course of Guillain-Barré syndrome. Lancet, *1*:524, 1974.

Hauser, W. A., and Kurland, L. T.: The epidemiology of epilepsy in Rochester, Minnesota, 1935 through 1967: Epilepsia, *16*:1, 1975.

Heyman, A., Wilkinson, W. E., Heyden, S., et al.: Risk of stroke in asymptomatic persons with cervical arterial bruits: a population study in Evans County, Georgia. N. Engl. J. Med., *302*:838, 1980.

Hope-Simpson, R. E.: Nature of herpes zoster: a long-term study and a new hypothesis. Proc. R. Soc. Med., *58*:9, 1965.

Lance, J. W.: Mechanism and Management of Headache. 3rd ed. London, Butterworths, 1975.

Lance, J. W., and McLeod, J. G.: A Physiologic Approach to Clinical Neurology. 2nd ed. London, Butterworths, 1975.

McKissock, W., Richardson, A., and Bloom, W. H.: Subdural haematoma: a review of 389 cases. Lancet, *1*:1365, 1960.

Morse, R. M., and Litin, E. M.: Postoperative delirium: a study of etiologic factors. Am. J. Psychiatry, *126*:388, 1969.

Ott, K. H., Kase, C. S., Ojemann, R. G., et al.: Cerebellar hemorrhage: diagnosis and treatment. Arch. Neurol., *31*:160, 1974.

Penry, J. K., and Newmark, M. E.: The use of antiepileptic drugs. Ann. Intern. Med., *90*:207, 1979.

Plum, F., and Posner, J. B.: The Diagnosis of Stupor and Coma. 3rd ed. Philadelphia, F. A. Davis Company, 1980.

Report from the Joint Committee for Stroke Resources XIV: Cerebral ischemia: the role of thrombosis and of antithrombotic therapy. Stroke, *8*:150, 1977.

Rundles, R. W.: Prognosis in the neurologic manifestations of pernicious anemia. Blood, *1*:209–219, 1946.

Solomon, G. E., and Plum, F.: Clinical Management of Seizures. Philadelphia, W. B. Saunders Company, 1976.

Tsairis, P., Dyck, P. J., and Mulder, D. W.: Natural history of brachial plexus neuropathy. Arch. Neurol., *27*:109, 1972.

Victor, M.: The pathophysiology of alcoholic epilepsy. Res. Publ. Assoc. Res. Nerv. Ment. Dis., *46*:431, 1968.

Victor, M.: The amnesic syndrome and its anatomical basis. Can. Med. Assoc. J., *100*:1115, 1969.

Weisberg, L. A.: Benign intracranial hypertension. Medicine, *54*:197, 1975.

Zarcone, V.: Narcolepsy. N. Engl. J. Med., *288*:1156, 1973.

PART 11
DERMATOLOGY

Peter M. Elias

DIRECTIONS: For questions 1 to 28, choose the ONE BEST answer to each question.

QUESTIONS 1–2

A 27-year-old man has a blistering eruption of three days' duration. He tells you that he has had recurrent "fever blisters" for the past two years. Physical examination reveals erythematous, hive-like plaques; tense blisters on the skin; and superficial, painful erosions in the mouth. The palms and soles have red iris lesions with dark, purpuric centers.

1. The most likely diagnosis is

A. pemphigus vulgaris
B. bullous pemphigoid
C. erythema multiforme
D. lupus erythematosus
E. leukocytoclastic vasculitis

2. All the following have been shown to trigger episodes of this disease EXCEPT

A. herpes simplex
B. *Mycoplasma pneumoniae* pneumonia
C. sulfonamides
D. deep x-ray therapy
E. ulcerative colitis

QUESTIONS 3–4

A 48-year-old man has a nonsymptomatic scaling eruption involving the scalp, eyebrows, eyelashes, molar eminences, and nasolabial folds. Examination reveals a greasy scale over mildly erythematous skin in the affected areas. Slight redness and scaling are seen on the anterior chest.

3. The most likely diagnosis is

A. seborrheic dermatitis
B. psoriasis
C. lupus erythematosus
D. tinea faciae
E. polymorphous light eruption

4. Therapy may include any of the following EXCEPT

A. shampoos containing salicylic acid
B. shampoos containing tar
C. warm oil soaks
D. systemic corticosteroids
E. topical corticosteroids

5. Which one of the following findings would be useful in differentiating between lupus erythematosus and pemphigoid?

A. Linear immunofluorescence at the dermal-epidermal junction in bullous lesions on direct immunofluorescence
B. Immunoglobulin and complement at the dermal-epidermal junction
C. Accumulation of circulating antigen-antibody complexes at the dermal-epidermal junction
D. Circulating antibody reactive to the basement membrane zone of the epidermis
E. Presence of mucosal lesions

6. A 17-year-old girl consults you because of an acute eruption of macules and papules on the trunk. She feels well except for the moderate pruritus caused by the lesions. Physical examination reveals small, oval, papular lesions with a fine scale arranged along skin lines. A similar, much larger lesion is seen on the left thigh. No mucosal, palmar, or plantar lesions are seen. Initial evaluation and treatment would include all the following EXCEPT

A. serologic test for syphilis (VDRL)
B. potassium hydroxide preparation of scale to detect fungi
C. inquiry as to the patient's use of medications
D. examination for hepatosplenomegaly and lymphadenopathy
E. benzathine penicillin G, 2.4 million units intramuscularly

7. Which of the following features would be LEAST helpful in distinguishing between pemphigoid and pemphigus vulgaris?

A. Oral ulcerations
B. Intraepidermal bullae
C. An underlying malignancy
D. Bullae arising in normal-appearing skin
E. Serum antibodies localized to the epidermal basement membrane zone

8. Which of the following is NOT an important complication of atopic dermatitis?

A. Cataract
B. Recurrent pyoderma
C. Pernicious anemia
D. Kaposi's varicelliform eruption
E. Eczema herpeticum

9. The spectrum of ultraviolet light reaching earth from the sun consists of two spectral ranges: UVB (290 to 320 nm) and UVA (320 to 400 nm). A common property of UVA and UVB is that they are both

A. responsible for sunburn
B. blocked by esters of aminobenzoic acid (PABA)
C. blocked by benzophenones
D. filtered out by window glass
E. involved in drug-induced photosensitivity

10. Squamous cell carcinomas arising in which one of the following situations tend to have the best prognosis?

A. Actinic keratosis
B. Burn scar
C. Area of previous x-ray therapy
D. After exposure to arsenic
E. In chronic granulomas such as lupus vulgaris

11. A 33-year old white man is referred to you because he has a tan-colored lesion on the abdomen as shown in the illustration. There is a similar lesion on the right thigh. The patient was treated with Fowler's solution for asthma many years ago. The skin lesions have not responded to topical antipsoriatic therapy prescribed by his physician. Which one of the following would you do?

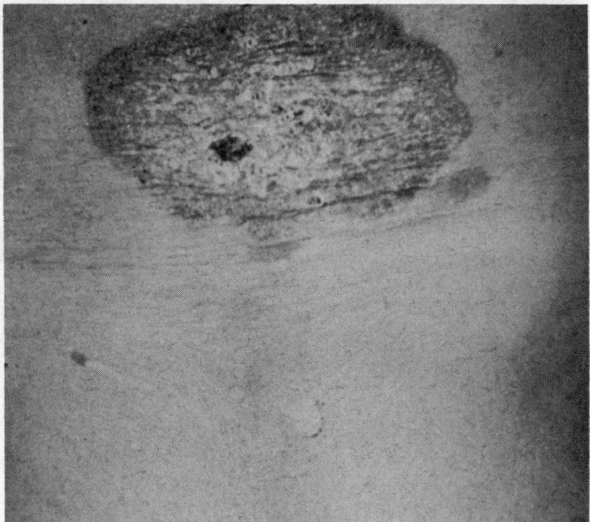

A. Reassure him and send him back to his physician for further similar therapy
B. Determine the HLA type
C. Administer methotrexate for resistant psoriasis
D. Recommend alternate-day systemic steroids
E. Take a biopsy of the lesion

QUESTIONS 12–15

A 20-year-old man consults you because of an acute exacerbation of a chronic recurrent dermatosis that he has had for his "entire life." It is extremely pruritic and interferes with sleep. The eruption is mainly confined to the flexural areas of the neck, antecubital and popliteal folds, and area behind the ears. It is an excoriated, weeping dermatitis superimposed on chronically thickened and hyperpigmented skin. Family history reveals that the mother has asthma and a sister has "hay fever."

12. The most likely diagnosis is

A. contact dermatitis
B. dyshidrotic eczema
C. atopic dermatitis
D. seborrheic dermatitis
E. nummular eczema

13. Treatment for this patient would include all the following EXCEPT

A. wet dressings for acute lesions
B. systemic antihistamines
C. systemic antibiotics for secondary infection
D. topical corticosteroids
E. cromolyn sodium

The patient's dermatologic disease is controlled well with your therapy, but he returns eight months later with a sudden, acute recurrence. He looks ill and has a low-grade fever. Examination shows numerous scattered, umbilicated vesicles in the dermatitic areas.

14. Which one of the following would you order first?

A. Tzanck smear
B. Potassium hydroxide examination of a skin scraping
C. Skin biopsy
D. Wood's light examination
E. A trial of systemic adenine arabinoside (ara-A)

15. Which of the following immunologic abnormalities is most likely in this patient?

A. Deficient T-lymphocyte function
B. Increased T-lymphocyte function
C. Decreased number of B lymphocytes
D. Increased number of B lymphocytes
E. Loss of immediate skin test reactivity to common antigens

QUESTIONS 16–17

A 46-year-old woman consults you for evaluation of a skin eruption. Examination reveals erythematous papules and plaques with surface scale on the knees and elbows. There is very little dermal infiltration in the lesions, which are distributed mainly over the knees, elbows, and presacral area. Erythema and fissuring in the intergluteal fold are noted. The scalp is scaly; the nails show pitting. Further questioning reveals that the patient has had the eruption for many years and that her father and one sibling have a similar eruption.

16. The most likely diagnosis is

A. psoriasis
B. pityriasis rosea
C. tinea corporis
D. lichen planus
E. seborrheic dermatitis

17. Which one of the following should NOT be used in the treatment of this disease?

A. Tar and ultraviolet light
B. Topical corticosteroids
C. Antimalarials
D. Methotrexate
E. Psoralen plus ultraviolet light A (PUVA)

QUESTIONS 18–20

A 47-year-old white man has had a slowly growing nodule on the left temple for three months. It bleeds occasionally with mild trauma. Examination shows a nodular, pearly, translucent 6-mm papule with telangiectasia.

18. The most likely diagnosis is

A. squamous cell carcinoma
B. basal cell epithelioma
C. granuloma annulare

D. lupus erythematosus
E. fungal infection

19. Conditions that predispose to these lesions include all the following EXCEPT

A. xeroderma pigmentosa
B. basal cell nevus syndrome
C. chronic arsenic intoxication
D. dyskeratosis congenita
E. chronic sun exposure

20. Acceptable treatment for the lesion includes any of the following EXCEPT

A. complete excision
B. electrodesiccation and curettage
C. topical 5-fluorouracil
D. cryosurgery
E. x-irradiation

QUESTIONS 21–22

A 22-year-old man consults you because he has had three small, moderately tender ulcers on the dorsum of the shaft of the penis for two days. He has been otherwise well. Examination reveals the penile ulcers and moderately tender inguinal lymph nodes.

21. Possible diagnoses include all the following EXCEPT

A. lymphogranuloma venereum
B. chancroid
C. herpes progenitalis
D. primary syphilis
E. granuloma inguinale

22. Which of the following diagnostic tests should be performed on these lesions first?

A. Frei test
B. Dark-field examination
C. Tzanck smear
D. Gram stain
E. Touch prep for Donovan bodies

QUESTIONS 23–26

Questions 23–26 pertain to cutaneous malignant melanoma.

23. The most common type of malignant melanoma is

A. lentigo maligna
B. nodular
C. acral-lentiginous
D. superficial spreading
E. mucosal

24. In order to assess the prognosis of a melanoma, the pathologist should be *particularly* careful to examine the

A. center of the nodule
B. thickness of the tumor
C. surface of the nodule
D. extent of the radial growth phase
E. intensity of the host's inflammatory response

25. Which of the following is NOT known to possess a potential for malignant transformation?

A. Lentigo maligna
B. Congenital melanocytic nevus
C. Halo nevus
D. Senile lentigo
E. Giant, "bathing-trunk" nevus

26. If a pigmented lesion arouses suspicion of being a melanoma, the most acceptable approach is

A. punch biopsy
B. incisional biopsy
C. excisional biopsy
D. wide excision
E. shave biopsy

QUESTIONS 27–28

A 33-year-old man has had urticaria and intermittent episodes of angioedema for eight weeks.

27. A work-up for an underlying cause in this patient is most likely to reveal

A. vasculitis
B. collagen-vascular disease
C. malignancy
D. no apparent cause
E. parasitic infestation

28. This patient should be cautioned to avoid intake of obligate histamine releasers. These include all the following EXCEPT

A. penicillin
B. acetaminophen
C. opiates
D. salicylates
E. polymyxins

DIRECTIONS: For questions 29 to 50, you are to decide whether EACH choice is true or false. Any combination of answers, from all true to all false, may be present. Mark the answer sheet "T" or "F" in the space provided.

29. Which of the following factors enhance(s) the absorption of most drugs across the stratum corneum?

A. Increased temperature
B. Increased lipid solubility
C. Increased skin occlusion
D. Increased thickness of the stratum corneum
E. Increased hydration of the stratum corneum

30. Which of the following features is/are useful in differentiating between pemphigoid and erythema multiforme?

A. Circulating anti–basement membrane antibodies
B. Immunoglobulins in the basement membrane
C. An association with herpes simplex virus
D. An underlying malignancy
E. Lesions in the scalp

31. Which of the following cells is/are found in the epidermis?

A. Merkel's cells
B. Mast cells
C. Langerhans' cells
D. Endothelial cells
E. Granular cells

32. Which of the following is/are true about acne rosacea?

A. Comedones form a major part of the eruption
B. It occurs more commonly in men than in women
C. It is occasionally complicated by ocular inflammation
D. Its distribution is similar to that of acne vulgaris
E. Telangiectasias are seen

33. Which of the following is/are true of guttate psoriasis?

A. It is precipitated by β-hemolytic streptococcal pharyngitis
B. It responds more quickly to standard antipsoriatic therapy than does plaque-type psoriasis
C. It is associated with arthritis more frequently than is plaque-type psoriasis
D. It develops into extensive plaque-type disease if untreated
E. It occurs more commonly in children than in adults

34. Which of the following statements is/are true with regard to sweating?

A. Sweat is formed by simple passive filtration
B. Lactate is exchanged for sodium in the secretory portion of the sweat gland
C. Profuse sweating results in very little loss of sodium
D. Repeated thermal stress reduces the loss of sodium in sweat
E. Dysfunction of the sweat glands (anhidrosis) is a common cause of heat stroke

35. Which of the following statements regarding intestinal polyps in Peutz-Jeghers syndrome is/are true?

A. They occur along the entire gastrointestinal tract
B. They are likely to be premalignant when present in large numbers in the large bowel
C. They are likely to be premalignant when present in the duodenum
D. They are frequently associated with acral melanosis
E. They secrete a variety of polypeptide hormones

36. Clinical conditions likely to be associated with patchy alopecia include

A. lupus erythematosus
B. status three months postpartum
C. secondary syphilis
D. convalescence after a febrile illness
E. systemic chemotherapy

37. Superficial dilated blood vessels (telangiectasias) are seen in which of the following conditions?

A. Solar damage
B. Scleroderma (acrosclerosis)
C. X-irradiation damage
D. Basal cell epithelioma
E. Fabry's disease

38. Erythropoietic protoporphyria

A. begins in childhood
B. can be diagnosed by fluorescent porphyrins in the urine
C. is characterized by redness, burning, and vesicle formation on sun-exposed areas of the body
D. is associated with increased protoporphyrin levels in erythrocytes
E. is associated with cirrhosis of the liver in adult life

39. Multinucleated giant cells are seen in scrapings of the blister base stained with Wright's or Giemsa's stain in which of the following disorders?

A. Contact dermatitis
B. Herpes zoster
C. Smallpox and vaccinia
D. Erythema multiforme
E. Varicella

40. Which of the following statements concerning porphyria cutanea tarda is/are true?

A. Bullae develop following exposure to sunlight
B. Urinary levels of uroporphyrins are increased
C. Estrogens and barbiturates exacerbate the disorder
D. Bullae are produced by trauma
E. Chloroquine is the treatment of choice

41. Wood's light examination is useful in the identification of which of the following conditions?

A. *Microsporum audouini* infections of the hair
B. Porphyrias
C. Tuberous sclerosis
D. *Pseudomonas* superinfection of burn wounds

42. Which of the following effects is/are obtained with open wet dressings applied to inflamed skin?

A. Reduction of heat and drying of lesion
B. Antimicrobial effect
C. Debridement
D. Maintenance of fluid and electrolyte balance

43. Which of the following is/are true concerning the adverse effects of topical corticosteroids?

A. Adverse effects occur almost exclusively with fluorinated compounds
B. Use on the face is associated with perioral dermatitis
C. Prolonged use around the eyes frequently causes glaucoma
D. Occlusion increases the chance of epidermal and dermal atrophy

44. A 36-year-old man has the axillary eruption illustrated below. The buccal fold, groin, and skin over the knuckles are also involved. The patient should be investigated for

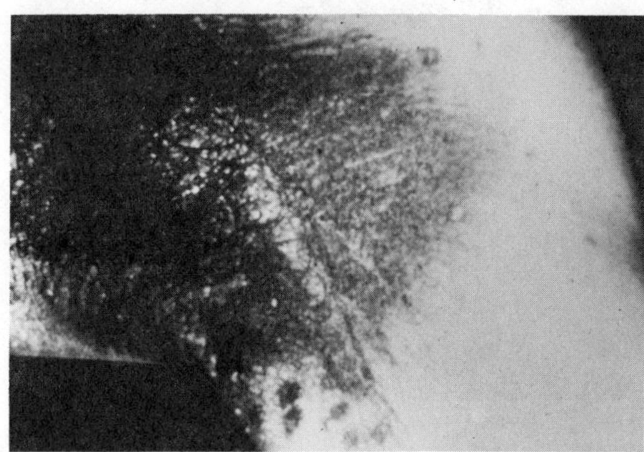

A. an underlying malignancy
B. a fungal infection
C. a metabolic disorder
D. contact dermatitis

45. Cutaneous stigmata of arsenic ingestion include which of the following?

A. Palmar and plantar keratoses
B. Seborrheic keratoses
C. "Rain drop" hyperpigmentation over the thorax
D. Melasma

46. A 6-year-old boy has had the lesions illustrated (see top of next column) since birth. He has eight other similar lesions scattered over his body. No other skin lesions are seen. Which of the following is/are associated with lesions of this type?

A. Raised blood pressure
B. Polyostotic fibrous dysplasia
C. Deafness
D. Precocious puberty

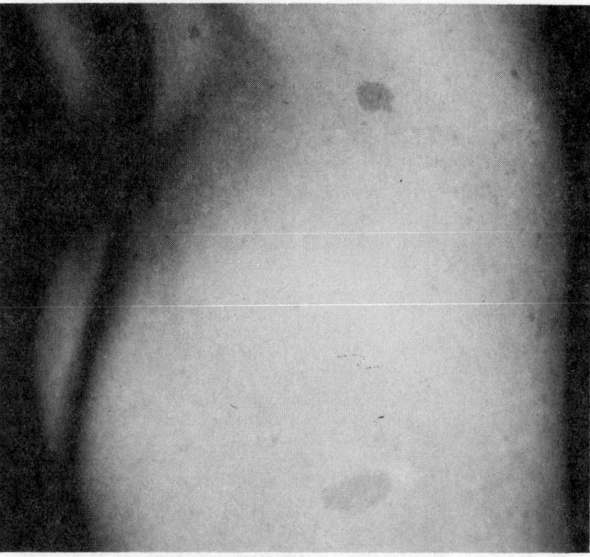

47. Which of the following is/are signals of an underlying malignancy?

A. Paget's disease of the breast
B. Appearance of nodules in a giant pigmented hairy nevus
C. Dusky papules in a persistently lymphedematous extremity
D. Necrolytic migratory erythema

48. A 62-year-old man has the lesions shown in the illustration below. Histopathologic examination of a lesion shows a heavy infiltrate of pleomorphic cells hugging the epidermis, and collections of abnormal cells in the epidermis (Pautrier microabscesses). The presence of which of the following would suggest a poor prognosis for this patient?

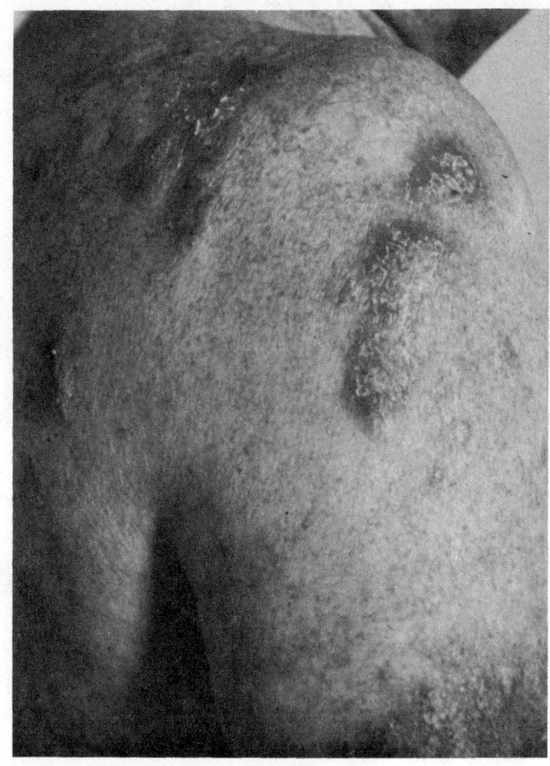

A. Skin tumor
B. Unremitting pruritus
C. Ulceration of the lesions
D. Clinical lymphadenopathy

49. A 60-year-old white man has had the pigmented lesion illustrated below for three months. There has been no recent change in the lesion. Which of the following clinical features suggest(s) that this is a malignant melanoma?

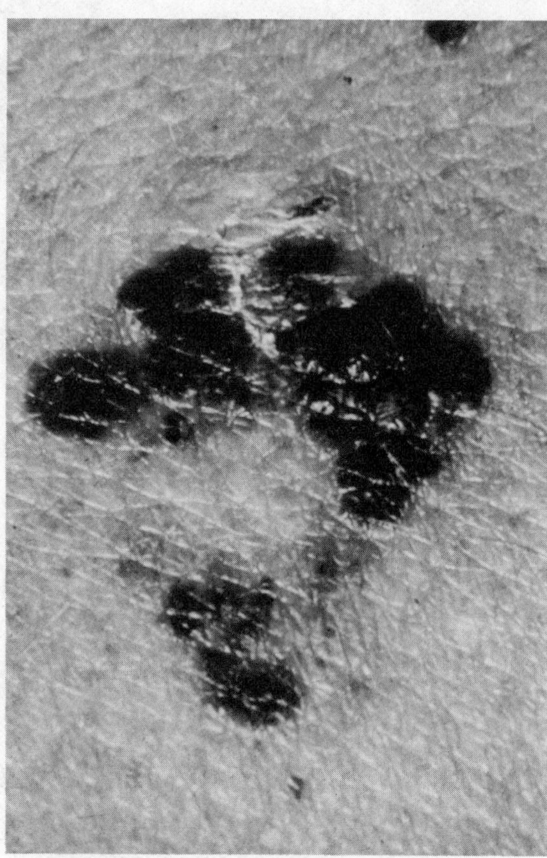

A. The gray-white area in the center
B. Notching in the border
C. Nodular areas in the lesion
D. The presence of hypopigmented "halo" around other pigmented lesions

50. A patient has the truncal eruption illustrated below. It does not involve the face. Which of the following tests would confirm your clinical diagnosis?

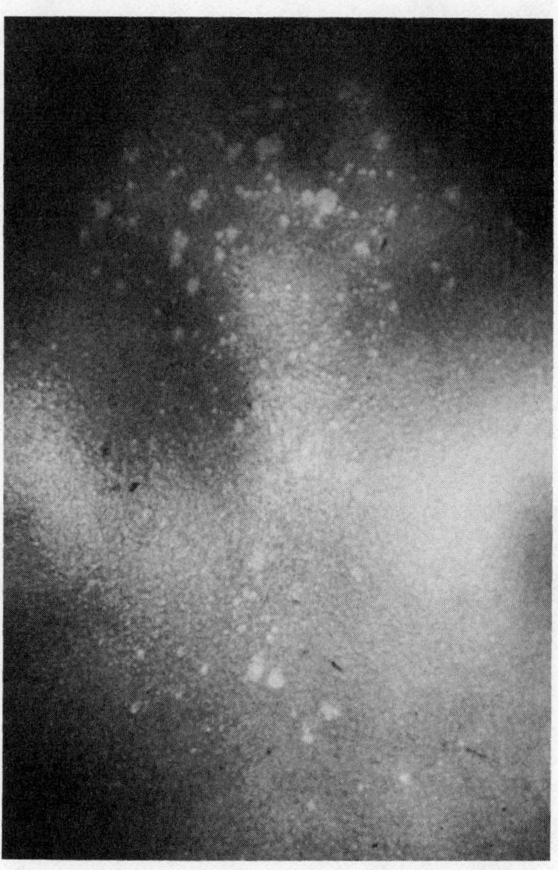

A. Cultures for superficial fungus
B. Skin biopsies for evidence of inflammation
C. Cultures for bacteria
D. Potassium hydroxide examination of scale

PART 11

DERMATOLOGY

ANSWERS

1. (C) Multiform skin lesions such as urticaria, tense blisters, crusts, and mucous membrane involvement are characteristic of erythema multiforme (EM). Iris or target lesions with dark, purpuric centers are pathognomonic of this disease. Pemphigus has flaccid blisters that spread easily on pressure. Bullous pemphigoid is a chronic disease in older patients and has little mucosal involvement. Both lupus erythematosus and vasculitis can exhibit bullous lesions, but not iris lesions, except in those rare instances in which EM is a manifestation of underlying SLE or vasculitis. *(Cecil, p. 2290)*

2. (E) Erythema multiforme is not a cutaneous manifestation of ulcerative colitis. The most common diagnosable cause of EM is recurrent herpes simplex infection. Drugs (especially long-acting sulfonamides), *Mycoplasma* infections, and x-ray therapy for malignancies all induce bouts of EM. *(Cecil, p. 2290)*

3. (A) The diagnosis of seborrheic dermatitis is based on the appearance of greasy scales in a typical distribution. In psoriasis, plaques have a thick white scale, and lesions are usually seen elsewhere on the body. Lupus erythematosus typically has atrophy, telangiectasia, and follicular plugging. Tinea faciae has inflammatory pustules. Polymorphous light eruption is limited to sun-exposed areas, and therefore spares the scalp and body folds. *(Cecil, pp. 2263–2264)*

4. (D) Various medicated shampoos are adequate to control most cases of seborrheic dermatitis. Warm oil soaks are useful in softening thick scale. Topical steroid lotions reduce inflammation. Systemic steroids are not indicated. *(Cecil, p. 2264)*

5. (D) Basement membrane deposition of immunoglobulin and complement is seen in both lupus erythematosus and bullous pemphigoid. Only in bullous pemphigoid is it possible to demonstrate *circulating* immunoglobulins and complement on indirect immunofluorescence. Mucosal lesions are uncommon in both disorders. *(Cecil, pp. 2228–2229)*

6. (E) Oval, scaly lesions along lines of skin cleavage preceded by a large "herald patch", are typical of pityriasis rosea. Secondary syphilis is in the differential diagnosis, but is less likely because of the absence of systemic symptoms, pharyngitis, and palmar or plantar lesions. Penicillin therefore is not indicated initially. Drug eruptions should always be considered, and a fungal infection can be ruled out by the potassium hydroxide preparation. *(Cecil, p. 2226)*

7. (C) The association of malignancy with either pemphigus or pemphigoid is tenuous. Both these diseases occur predominantly in older individuals, in whom coincidental associations occur frequently. Oral ulcerations are common in pemphigus and rare in pemphigoid. An intraepidermal cleft is suggestive of pemphigus; pemphigoid produces subepidermal bullae. Bullae arising in normal-appearing skin occur more frequently in pemphigoid than in pemphigus. Circulating antibodies that bind to the basement membrane on indirect immunofluorescence are found in pemphigoid, but not in pemphigus, in which intercellular binding in the epidermis is found instead. *(Cecil, pp. 2288–2289)*

8. (C) Complications of atopic dermatitis include cataracts, recurrent skin infections, and severe secondary viral infections, especially from herpes simplex and vaccinia viruses. *(Cecil, pp. 2270–2271)*

9. (C) Sunburn and skin cancer are caused principally by UVB, which is effectively filtered by window glass. UVA penetrates window glass and is responsible for most drug-induced photosensitivity, most skin lesions in the porphyrias, and some cases of polymorphous light reactions. The PABA sunscreens block UVB, but not UVA; the benzophenones block not only UVB and UVA, but also germicidal radiation (UVC). *(Fitzpatrick et al., pp. 983–985)*

10. (A) Squamous cell carcinomas arising in exposed areas in actinic keratoses tend to be less aggressive and metastasize rarely, except when they arise on the lip. Those from the other lesions listed tend to metastasize rapidly. *(Cecil, p. 2293)*

11. (E) Well-circumscribed, red-brown plaque with scale that is unresponsive to topical therapy should suggest the diagnosis of Bowen's disease. This is likely in a patient with a history of arsenic exposure. The correct method of evaluation is to take a biopsy of the lesion. Looking for HLA-B27 is not indicated because the patient has no history of Reiter's triad (urethritis, arthritis, and conjunctivitis). *(Cecil, p. 2273)*

12. (C) The typical morphology and distribution of a pruritic, chronic, recurrent dermatosis in a patient with a family history of atopy suggests the diagnosis of atopic dermatitis. Contact dermatitis presents as a localized eruption with linear erythema and vesicles. Seborrheic dermatitis is a red, greasy eruption that occurs in the scalp, eyebrows, and nasolabial folds. Dyshidrotic eczema is located on the palms and soles. Nummular eczema has coin-shaped lesions and is only occasionally associated with the atopic diathesis. *(Cecil, pp. 2270–2271)*

13. (E) Wet dressings reduce erythema and weeping, topical steroids reduce inflammation, and antihistamines suppress pruritus. Patients with atopic dermatitis are prone to secondary bacterial infections and should be treated with appropriate antibiotics. Although cromolyn sodium helps patients with other atopic diseases, it has never been shown to benefit atopic dermatitis. *(Cecil, pp. 2270–2271)*

14. (A) The presence of umbilicated vesicles in an acute flare of atopic dermatitis should suggest Kaposi's varicelliform eruption. This is a superinfection with herpes simplex or vaccinia. A Tzanck smear will show multinucleated giant cells in patients with herpes simplex infection. *(Cecil, pp. 2257, 2270–2271)*

15. (A) Immunoglobulin E levels are elevated in patients with atopic dermatitis, and T-lymphocyte function has been shown to be diminished. Immediate urticarial reactions to common antigens are very frequent in atopic patients. No other specific immunologic defects have been demonstrated *(Cecil, pp. 2270–2271)*

16. (A) The familial pattern of inheritance, the distribution and morphology of lesions, and the involvement of nail and scalp are characteristic of psoriasis. The other conditions listed do not have pitted nails. Pityriasis rosea has oval lesions along lines of cleavage; lichen planus has flat-topped, polygonal papules on the flexor surfaces; dermatophyte infections usually have spreading active borders. Severe seborrheic dermatitis can mimic psoriasis, particularly when the latter is confined to the scalp. However, psoriasis is more refractory to topical therapy, possesses a more tenacious, silvery scale, and is not usually limited to the scalp and body folds. *(Cecil, pp. 2267–2268)*

17. (C) Antimalarials are contraindicated in patients with psoriasis or a history of psoriasis, because they can stimulate severe exacerbation or even pustular flares of the disease. Topical corticosteroids and tar and ultraviolet light produce flattening and clearing of lesions by inhibiting cell division and reducing inflammation. Methotrexate is used in carefully selected patients, especially those with severe arthritis. PUVA is an effective, but still experimental, treatment for psoriasis. *(Cecil, pp. 2267–2268)*

18. (B) A tumor on an exposed area with a nodular, pearly border and telangiectasia is typical of basal cell epithelioma. Squamous cell carcinomas tend to be scaly and buffy red with indurated bases. Granuloma annulare has a nodular, enlarging border that is not pearly and has no telangiectasia. Lupus erythematosus shows atrophy and scaling. Fungal infection is not nodular and has an active, spreading, scaly, or vesicular border *(Cecil, pp. 2292–2293)*

19. (D) Patients with xeroderma pigmentosa develop not only basal cell carcinomas, but also squamous cell carcinomas and malignant melanomas. In basal cell nevus syndrome, numerous ectodermal abnormalities occur, but patients invariably develop scores of basal cell carcinomas. Both squamous cell and basal cell carcinomas occur in arsenicalism. Dyskeratosis congenita predisposes only to adenocarcinomas and squamous cell carcinomas. *(Cecil, pp. 2292–2293)*

20. (C) Complete removal by any of the surgical methods or x-irradiation is adequate. Topical 5-fluorouracil is not uniformly successful and should not be used routinely. *(Cecil, pp. 2292–2293)*

21. (A) Lymphogranuloma venerum (LGV) is the only venereal disease without a chronic chancriform lesion — the primary chancre is usually evanescent, and lymphadenopathy is the presenting sign. All the other diseases can present as one or more chancres. Tenderness is not a very useful clinical sign to help rule out syphilis. Nevertheless, the presence of multiple, small, tender chancriform lesions should alert one to herpes. *(Cecil, pp. 1571–1572)*

22. (C) A positive Tzanck preparation is diagnostic of herpes; however, secondary infections do occur, so additional laboratory studies should be performed when appropriate. For example, chancroid and syphilis can secondarily invade lesions of each other. Likewise, lesions of herpes progenitalis rarely can harbor syphilis also. *(Fitzpatrick et al., pp. 1669–1677)*

23. (D) Superficial spreading melanoma accounts for approximately two thirds of malignant melanoma, followed by nodular melanoma (15 to 20%); "unclassified" melanoma, including acral lentiginous (10%); and lentigo maligna melanoma (5%). *(Cecil, pp. 2294–2296; Fitzpatrick et al., pp. 629–654)*

24. (B) In recent years the principal criterion for establishing the prognosis in malignant melanoma has been tumor thickness as measured by ocular micrometer. This method has supplanted the method of Clark and McGovern, which was based on level of invasion. Evaluation of the host's inflammatory response is occasionally important when regression is evident — thickness then is not so useful for determining the prognosis. *(Cecil, pp. 2294–2296; Sober, Fitzpatrick, and Mihm)*

25. (D) Lentigo maligna represents the *in situ* stage of lentigo maligna melanoma, although it may not become invasive for many years. Both giant hairy nevi and smaller congenital nevi (greater than 1.5 cm in diameter) are currently thought to have a slightly greater chance of developing into melanoma. The halo nevus can be a sign either of melanoma regression or an altered immune response to melanoma elsewhere. Senile lentigo has no enhanced tendency for malignant transformation. *(Cecil, pp. 2294–2296; Fitzpatrick et al., pp. 629–654)*

26. (C) An excisional biopsy is preferred because it ensures sufficient material to gauge the thickness of the lesion accurately. Under certain circumstances a punch biopsy or incisional biopsy may be acceptable. A shave biopsy is never appropriate, and wide excision is reserved for a lesion with an established diagnosis. *(Cecil, pp. 2294–2296; Fitzpatrick et al., pp. 629–654)*

27. (D) In most cases of chronic urticaria no apparent cause is found, although a minority of patients have vasculitis, malignancy, collagen disease, or chronic infections. *(Cecil, pp. 1796–1800; Fitzpatrick et al., pp. 532–541)*

28. (B) Penicillin, opiates, salicylates, and polymyxins are obligate histamine releasers from mast cells. Use of these agents in patients with urticaria or angioedema can exacerbate the disease through nonimmunologic stimulation. Other agents, such as acetaminophen, can be safely substituted for obligate releasers in such patients. *(Cecil, pp. 1796–1800; Fitzpatrick et al., pp. 532–541)*

29. (A — True; B — True; C — True; D — False; E — True) The stratum corneum is the limiting membrane for passage of drug and water. All the factors listed enhance absorption of lipophilic agents except choice D. *(Cecil, pp. 48–49)*

30. A — True; B — True; C — True; D — False; E — False) Previous herpes infection is suggestive of erythema multiforme, and the finding of immunoglobulins in the basement membrane on direct or indirect immunofluorescence is indicative of pemphigoid. There is no known association of bullous pemphigoid or of EM with underlying malignancy. Neither commonly occurs in the scalp. *(Cecil, pp. 2289, 2290)*

31. (A — True; B — False; C — True; D — False; E — False) Langerhans' cells, recently thought to be involved in delayed hypersensitivity and contact dermatitis, are found in the epidermis. Merkel's cells, sensory receptor cells, are found in the epidermis in some locations, such as the palms and soles. The granular cell is found in the stratum granulosum, the outermost living layer of the epidermis. Mast cells and endothelial cells reside solely in the dermis. *(Cecil, pp. 2249–2250)*

32. (A — False; B — False; C — True; D — False; E — True) Acne rosacea is most common in 30- to 50-year-old women. It characteristically involves the central third of the face, whereas acne vulgaris more often occurs in the forehead, cheeks, and chin. Erythema and telangiectasia are prominent features, and comedones are usually absent. Keratitis, episcleritis, and conjunctivitis are serious complications. *(Cecil, p. 2265)*

33. (A — True; B — True; C — False; D — True; E — True) Guttate psoriasis frequently is precipitated by a pharyngeal infection with β-hemolytic streptococci. Generally, the disease occurs in children and young adults, is more responsive to topical therapy than is plaque-type psoriasis, and is considered a more benign variant. *(Cecil, pp. 2267–2268)*

34. (A — False; B — True; C — False; D — True; E — False) Sweat is formed by an active process. Lactate is formed in the secretory segment of the sweat gland, and sodium is reabsorbed in the duct. The capacity to reabsorb sodium is limited; therefore, significant sodium may be lost with profuse sweating. True adaptation to heat occurs with repeated thermal stress, and sodium is conserved by increased aldosterone secretion. Heat stroke secondary to anhidrosis occurs only rarely. *(Cecil, pp. 2251–2252)*

35. A — True; B — False; C — True; D — True; E — False) In the Peutz-Jeghers syndrome, polyps can occur along the entire gastrointestinal tract. Nevertheless, only those polyps that occur proximal to the ligament of Treitz are considered to be potentially premalignant. The polyps are associated with melanosis of the perioral and oral mucosa, as well as of the acral extremities. *(Cecil, pp. 725–726; Fitzpatrick et al., p. 1203)*

36. (A — True; B — False; C — True; D — False; E — False) Patchy or "moth-eaten" alopecia is a feature of discoid lupus erythematosus and of secondary syphilis. In contrast, the hair loss following febrile episodes, chemotherapy, or seizures, or that of the postpartum period, is diffuse. *(Cecil, pp. 2252–2254)*

37. (A — True; B — True; C — True; D — True; E — False) Fine, wiry telangiectasias are seen extensively in sun-damaged skin and on the surface of basal cell epitheliomas. Mat-like telangiectasias are characteristically seen in scleroderma. X-irradiation produces atrophy, pigment change, and telangiectasias. In Fabry's disease, papular lesions called angiokeratomas are seen, not telangiectasias. *(Cecil, pp. 2256–2257)*

38. (A — True; B — False; C — True; D — True; E — True) Erythropoietic protoporphyria (EPP) is an autosomal dominant disorder that begins in childhood as photosensitivity. The diagnosis depends on finding protoporphyrins in erythrocytes (the urine does not contain porphyrins). Some adults with EPP develop cirrhosis owing to intrahepatic deposition of porphyrin crystals. *(Cecil, p. 1123; Fitzpatrick et al., pp. 1072–1105)*

39. (A — False; B — True; C — False; D — False; E — True) The Tzanck smear shows multinucleated epidermal giant cells in the vesicles of herpes simplex, herpes zoster, and varicella, but not in other vesicular viral infections such as vaccinia, orf, or variola. *(Cecil, p. 2257)*

40. (A — True; B — True; C — True; D — True; E — False) Porphyria cutanea tarda is characterized by bullous lesions in sun-exposed areas, but patients often note fragility more than sun sensitivity. The diagnosis is made by measuring urinary uroporphyrins, and the disease can be exacerbated by the ingestion of estrogens, alcohol, or barbiturates. Chloroquine is unacceptably risky; phlebotomy is the treatment of choice. *(Cecil, p. 1125; Fitzpatrick et al., pp. 1072–1105)*

41. (A — False; B — True; C — True; D — True) The Wood's lamp, which emits long-wave ultraviolet light, detects fungi that fluoresce at 360 nm, such as in tinea versicolor and some, but not all, of the agents that cause tinea capitis. The urine of a patient with porphyria cutanea tarda shows a pink fluorescence with the Wood's light. The Wood's light is useful for the detection of ash-leaf hypopigmented macules in tuberous sclerosis. The urine of patients with *Pseudomonas* superinfection of burn wounds fluoresces blue-green. *(Cecil, p. 2258; Fitzpatrick et al., pp. 34–35)*

42. (A — True; B — True; C — True; D — False) Open wet dressings reduce heat in inflamed lesions by evaporation, and enhance drying of a weeping lesion by coagulation of serum. The wet dressings debride the wound and reduce bacterial contamination. Continuous wet dressings eventually lead to drying, cracking, and fissuring of the skin. Wet dressings provide no protection for the patient's fluid and electrolyte status. *(Cecil, p. 2261)*

43. (All are True) In addition, topical steroids produce telangiectasia, purpura, and striae. *(Cecil, pp. 2262–2263)*

44. (A — True; B — False; C — True; D — False) The brown-black, velvety change seen in the typical distribution is characteristic of acanthosis nigricans. This disease may be seen as an inherited disorder, in obesity, with malignancy, or with a variety of metabolic disturbances. Cutaneous fungal infections are scaly or pustular, and contact dermatitis is vesicular and inflamed. (*Cecil, pp. 2271–2272*)

45. (A — True; B — False; C — True; D — False) Discrete keratoses of palms and soles and a fine hyperpigmentation of the anterior thorax are characteristic of chronic arsenic exposure. Seborrheic keratoses are brown, verrucous lesions that have a "stuck-on" appearance and are benign. Melasma is a blotchy pigmentation of the face of women during and after pregnancy or as a result of taking oral contraceptives. *(Cecil, pp. 2221–2222)*

46. (All are True) The illustration shows café au lait lesions, which are most common in neurofibromatosis, but also can occur in Albright's disease. The former is associated with pheochromocytomas (hypertension) and acoustic neuromas (deafness); the latter is associated with fibrous dysplasia of bone and precocious puberty. *(Cecil, pp. 1264, 1351, 2043–2044, 2279)*

47. (All are True) Paget's disease is always associated with underlying breast carcinoma; nodules arising in a giant pigmented nevus should suggest melanoma. Lymphangiosarcoma, or the Stewart-Treves syndrome, presents as purple-red papules on a lymphedematous area. Necrolytic migratory erythema is associated with glucagonomas, which are glucagon-secreting alpha-cell tumors of the pancreas. *(Cecil, pp. 1029–1032)*

48. (A — True; B — False; C — True; D — True) The clinical appearance and the histology confirm the diagnosis of mycosis fungoides. The prognosis in this disease is highly variable, survival in some patients being as long as 15 to 20 years. The development of lymphadenopathy, tumors, or ulcers is associated with a decrease in survival to less than two years, and the presence of all three indicates survival of less than one year. Pruritus is an unreliable sign of prognosis, and may actually improve during the tumor stage of mycosis fungoides. *(Cecil, pp. 2293–2294; Epstein et al.)*

49. (All are True) Variants in color (red, white, and blue), notching of the border, and nodularity in the lesion are characteristic clinical features of malignant melanoma. "Halos" around the primary lesion or other pigmented lesions may signify changes in immunologic reactivity associated with the development of malignant melanoma. *(Cecil, pp. 2294–2296; Kopf, Bart, and Rodriguez-sains)*

50. (A — False; B — False; C — False; D — True) A scaly, macular eruption consisting of lesions of different sizes and shapes, varying in color from white to tan-brown, is characteristic of tinea versicolor infection. This is caused by infestation of the keratin layer of the skin by the fungal organism *Malassezia furfur*. Potassium hydroxide examination of scale shows the characteristic short hyphae and clusters of budding forms. The organism cannot usually be cultured nor does it cause skin inflammation, since it does not invade beneath the stratum corneum. *(Cecil, p. 2268)*

BIBLIOGRAPHY

Epstein, E. H., Jr., Levin, D. L., Croft, J. D., Jr., et al.: Mycosis fungoides. Survival, prognostic features, response to therapy, and autopsy findings. Medicine, *51*:61, 1971.

Fitzpatrick, T. B., Eisen, A. Z., Wolff, K., et al. (eds.): Dermatology in General Medicine. 2nd ed. New York, McGraw-Hill Book Company, 1979.

Kopf, A. W., Bart, R. S., and Rodriguez-sains, R. S.: Malignant melanoma: a review. J. Dermatol. Surg. Oncol., *3*:41, 1977.

Sober, A. J., Fitzpatrick, T. B., and Mihm, M. C., Jr.: Primary melanoma of the skin: recognition and management. J. Am. Acad. Dermatol., *2*:179, 1980.

INDEX TO QUESTIONS

NOTE: Some entries in this index may provide clues to correct answers. For self-assessment, therefore, it is recommended that use of the index be delayed until after the examination has been taken.

Numbers in parentheses are *Question* numbers.

ANSWERS

PART 1. CARDIOVASCULAR DISEASES

1. D
2. B
3. A
4. B
5. A
6. B
7. E
8. C
9. D
10. D
11. B
12. D
13. B
14. D
15. D
16. D
17. E
18. E
19. E
20. C
21. G
22. D
23. C
24. D
25. C
26. E
27. A
28. B
29. D
30. A
31. B
32. E
33. D
34. B
35. D
36. B
37. C
38. B
39. C
40. C
41. C
42. E
43. B
44. B
45. E
46. E
47. A–T; B–F; C–T; D–F; E–T
48. A–F; B–T; C–F; D–T; E–F
49. All are True
50. A–T; B–T; C–F; D–T; E–T; F–T; G–F
51. A–T; B–F; C–F; D–F; E–T
52. A–T; B–F; C–T; D–T; E–T; F–F; G–F
53. A–F; B–T; C–T; D–T; E–F; F–F
54. A–T; B–F; C–F; D–T; E–T; F–F
55. A–T; B–F; C–F; D–T; E–T
56. A–F; B–F; C–T; D–T; E–T
57. A–T; B–T; C–T; D–T; E–F
58. A–F; B–T; C–T; D–T; E–T
59. A–T; B–T; C–T; D–F; E–F
60. A–T; B–T; C–T; D–F; E–F
61. A–T; B–T; C–F; D–T; E–T
62. All are True
63. All are True
64. A–F; B–T; C–F; D–T; E–T
65. A–F; B–T; C–F; D–T; E–F
66. A–T; B–F; C–T; D–T; E–F
67. A–T; B–T; C–F; D–F; E–T
68. A–F; B–T; C–F; D–T; E–T; F–F
69. A–T; B–T; C–T; D–F; E–F; F–F
70. A–F; B–T; C–F; D–T; E–T
71. A–T; B–F; C–T; D–F; E–T; F–T
72. A–F; B–F; C–T; D–F; E–F
73. A–T; B–T; C–T; D–F; E–T
74. A–T; B–T; C–F; D–T; E–F
75. All are True
76. All are True
77. A–T; B–T; C–T; D–F; E–T
78. All are True
79. A–F; B–F; C–F; D–T; E–F
80. A–T; B–T; C–T; D–T; E–F
81. A–T; B–T; C–T; D–F; E–F
82. A–T; B–T; C–T; D–T; E–F
83. A–F; B–T; C–F; D–T; E–T
84. A–T; B–F; C–T; D–T; E–T
85. A–T; B–T; C–T; D–F; E–T
86. A–F; B–T; C–T; D–F
87. A–T; B–T; C–T; D–F; E–F
88. A–T; B–T; C–F; D–F; E–F
89. A–F; B–T; C–F; D–F; E–T; F–F
90. A–T; B–T; C–F; D–F; E–T; F–F
91. A–F; B–F; C–T; D–T; E–F
92. A–F; B–F; C–F; D–F; E–T
93. All are True
94. A–F; B–F; C–F; D–T; E–T; F–T
95. A–T; B–F; C–T; D–F; E–F
96. A–F; B–T; C–T; D–T; E–F
97. A–T; B–T; C–T; D–F; E–T
98. All are True
99. A–T; B–T; C–F; D–T; E–F
100. A–T; B–T; C–F; D–T; E–T
101. A–F; B–T; C–T; D–F; E–T
102. A–F; B–T; C–T; D–T; E–F
103. All are True
104. A–F; B–T; C–T; D–T; E–T
105. A–T; B–T; C–T; D–T; E–F; F–T
106. A–T; B–F; C–T; D–T; E–T; F–T
107. A–F; B–T; C–F; D–F; E–T
108. A–T; B–F; C–F; D–F; E–F
109. All are False

110. A
111. D
112. E
113. E
114. F
115. D
116. C
117. A
118. C
119. A
120. C
121. E
122. E
123. A
124. C
125. D
126. E
127. C
128. C
129. A
130. B
131. D
132. B
133. A
134. E
135. F
136. D
137. A
138. E
139. C
140. B
141. A
142. D
143. C
144. B
145. A
146. D
147. C
148. B
149. C
150. D
151. A
152. E
153. B
154. C
155. E
156. D
157. A
158. B
159. C
160. D
161. E
162. F
163. D
164. C
165. C
166. E
167. E
168. D
169. A
170. E
171. B
172. B
173. C
174. B
175. A
176. E
177. C
178. E
179. F
180. D
181. G
182. B
183. I
184. B
185. C
186. E
187. A
188. F
189. D
190. A
191. B
192. D
193. E
194. A
195. A
196. C
197. B
198. D
199. A
200. A
201. F
202. E
203. A
204. A
205. F
206. C
207. B
208. C
209. D
210. A
211. B
212. E
213. A
214. B
215. D
216. C
217. B
218. D
219. A
220. C
221. E
222. B
223. A
224. C
225. D
226. E
227. A
228. A
229. D
230. D
231. A

PART 2. RESPIRATORY DISEASE

1. E
2. D
3. B
4. E
5. B
6. D
7. D
8. D
9. C
10. C
11. A
12. E
13. E
14. C
15. C
16. D
17. D
18. D
19. B
20. A
21. D
22. D
23. E
24. D
25. E
26. D
27. D
28. C
29. C

30. A–F; B–F; C–T; D–F; E–F
31. A–T; B–T; C–T; D–F; E–T
32. A–F; B–F; C–F; D–T; E–T
33. A–T; B–T; C–T; D–T; E–F
34. A–T; B–F; C–F; D–T; E–T
35. A–F; B–T; C–F; D–F; E–F
36. A–F; B–F; C–F; D–F; E–T
37. A–F; B–T; C–F; D–F; E–T
38. A–F; B–T; C–F; D–F; E–T
39. A–F; B–T; C–T; D–T; E–T
40. A–T; B–F; C–T; D–T; E–T
41. All are True
42. A–T; B–T; C–F; D–T; E–T
43. A–T; B–F; C–F; D–T; E–T
44. A–F; B–F; C–T; D–T; E–T
45. A–T; B–F; C–T; D–F; E–F
46. All are True
47. A–F; B–T; C–F; D–F; E–F
48. A–T; B–F; C–F; D–F; E–F
49. A–F; B–F; C–T; D–F; E–T
50. A–F; B–T; C–F; D–T; E–F
51. A–T; B–F; C–T; D–F; E–T
52. A–T; B–T; C–T; D–F; E–T
53. A–T; B–T; C–F; D–F; E–T
54. A–F; B–T; C–F; D–T; E–F
55. A–T; B–F; C–F; D–T; E–F
56. A–T; B–T; C–T; D–F; E–T
57. A–T; B–F; C–T; D–F; E–T
58. A–T; B–F; C–T; D–F; E–T
59. A–T; B–T; C–T; D–F; E–F
60. A–T; B–T; C–F; D–F; E–F
61. A–F; B–F; C–F; D–T; E–F
62. All are False
63. A–T; B–T; C–T; D–F; E–T
64. A–F; B–F; C–T; D–T; E–T
65. A–T; B–F; C–T; D–F; E–F
66. All are True
67. A–F; B–T; C–F; D–F; E–T
68. A–F; B–F; C–F; D–T; E–T
69. A–F; B–T; C–F; D–T; E–F
70. A–T; B–F; C–F; D–T; E–F
71. A–F; B–F; C–F; D–F; E–T
72. A–F; B–T; C–F; D–T; E–F
73. A–T; B–T; C–F; D–F; E–F
74. A–F; B–F; C–F; D–T; E–F
75. A–F; B–T; C–F; D–F; E–F
76. A–F; B–T; C–T; D–T; E–T
77. A–T; B–F; C–T; D–F; E–F
78. A–F; B–T; C–F; D–T; E–T
79. A–T; B–F; C–T; D–F; E–T
80. A–F; B–T; C–F; D–F; E–F

81. B
82. E
83. A
84. C
85. D
86. A
87. D
88. E
89. C
90. B
91. C
92. D
93. B
94. A
95. E
96. B
97. C
98. A
99. D
100. D
101. A
102. C
103. E
104. A
105. C
106. B
107. D
108. B
109. C
110. A
111. D
112. E
113. C
114. D
115. B
116. A
117. D
118. A
119. E
120. B
121. C
122. B
123. A
124. D
125. C
126. E
127. D
128. C
129. E
130. B
131. A
132. C
133. B
134. A
135. D
136. E

PART 3. RENAL DISEASE

1. A
2. D
3. E
4. E
5. E
6. C
7. B
8. C
9. C
10. B
11. B

12. A–F; B–T; C–T; D–T; E–T
13. A–F; B–F; C–F; D–T; E–F
14. All are True
15. A–T; B–T; C–T; D–F; E–F
16. A–F; B–T; C–T; D–F; E–F
17. All are True
18. A–T; B–T; C–F; D–T; E–T
19. A–T; B–F; C–T; D–F
20. A–F; B–T; C–F; D–T
21. A–F; B–T; C–F; D–T; E–T
22. A–T; B–F; C–F; D–F; E–F
23. A–T; B–T; C–F; D–F; E–F
24. A–T; B–F; C–T; D–T; E–T
25. A–T; B–T; C–F; D–F; E–T
26. A–F; B–T; C–T; D–F; E–T
27. A–T; B–T; C–F; D–T; E–T
28. A–T; B–F; C–F; D–F; E–T
29. A–F; B–T; C–T; D–F
30. A–T; B–T; C–F; D–T
31. A–T; B–T; C–T; D–F
32. A–T; B–T; C–T; D–F
33. A–T; B–T; C–F; D–T; E–F
34. All are True
35. A–F; B–T; C–F; D–T
36. A–T; B–T; C–T; D–F
37. A–T; B–F; C–T; D–F
38. All are True
39. A–F; B–T; C–F; D–F; E–T
40. A–T; B–F; C–T; D–F
41. A–T; B–T; C–T; D–F
42. A–T; B–T; C–F; D–T
43. A–T; B–T; C–F; D–T
44. A–T; B–F; C–F; D–T
45. A–T; B–T; C–T; D–F
46. A–F; B–F; C–T; D–T
47. B and C are True
48. A is True
49. A and E are True
50. B and D are True
51. A and E are True

52. D
53. A
54. B
55. B
56. D
57. A
58. D
59. B
60. B
61. C
62. D
63. B
64. C
65. A
66. D
67. B
68. A
69. C
70. E
71. B
72. D
73. A
74. B
75. D
76. B
77. C
78. A
79. A
80. A
81. B
82. C
83. C
84. C
85. A
86. C
87. A
88. E
89. E

PART 4. GASTROINTESTINAL DISEASE

1. B
2. C
3. E
4. C
5. D
6. D
7. D
8. C
9. C
10. D
11. E
12. A
13. D
14. E
15. C
16. D
17. C
18. D
19. A
20. A
21. E
22. B
23. B
24. C
25. E
26. D
27. E
28. B
29. B
30. E
31. A
32. C
33. D
34. C
35. D
36. D
37. D
38. D
39. B
40. E
41. E
42. D
43. D
44. D
45. C
46. C
47. D
48. A
49. C
50. D
51. E
52. D
53. C
54. B
55. B
56. B
57. E
58. E
59. E
60. A
61. C
62. D
63. C
64. A
65. E
66. A
67. D
68. D

69. A–F; B–T; C–F; D–F; E–F
70. A–T; B–F; C–T; D–F; E–T
71. A–T; B–F; C–F; D–F; E–F
72. A–F; B–T; C–T; D–T; E–T
73. A–F; B–F; C–T; D–F; E–F
74. A–F; B–T; C–T; D–T; E–F
75. A–F; B–T; C–F; D–F; E–F
76. A–F; B–F; C–T; D–F; E–F
77. A–F; B–T; C–T; D–T; E–T
78. A–T; B–T; C–T; D–F; E–T
79. A–F; B–F; C–F; D–T; E–T
80. All are True
81. A–F; B–T; C–F; D–T; E–T
82. A–T; B–T; C–T; D–F; E–F
83. A–T; B–T; C–T; D–T; E–F
84. A–F; B–F; C–F; D–T; E–F
85. All are True
86. A–F; B–T; C–F; D–T; E–F
87. A–F; B–F; C–T; D–T; E–T
88. All are True
89. A–F; B–T; C–F; D–T; E–T
90. A–T; B–F; C–T; D–F; E–F
91. A–F; B–T; C–F; D–T; E–T
92. All are True
93. A–T; B–T; C–T; D–F; E–F
94. A–F; B–F; C–T; D–T; E–F
95. All are True

96. A–F; B–T; C–T; D–F; E–T
97. A–T; B–T; C–F; D–F; E–T
98. A–F; B–F; C–F; D–T; E–F
99. A–T; B–F; C–T; D–T; E–F
100. A–T; B–F; C–T; D–F; E–F
101. All are True
102. All are True
103. A–T; B–T; C–F; D–T; E–T
104. A–F; B–T; C–F; D–T; E–T
105. A–F; B–F; C–T; D–T; E–F
106. A–T; B–T; C–T; D–F; E–T
107. A–T; B–F; C–F; D–T; E–T
108. A–F; B–F; C–F; D–T; E–T
109. A–F; B–T; C–F; D–T; E–T
110. A–T; B–F; C–F; D–T; E–F
111. A–T; B–F; C–F; D–T; E–F
112. A–F; B–F; C–F; D–T; E–F
113. A–T; B–T; C–F; D–T; E–T
114. A–T; B–F; C–T; D–T; E–F
115. A–T; B–F; C–F; D–T; E–T
116. A–F; B–T; C–F; D–T; E–T
117. A–F; B–T; C–F; D–F; E–F
118. A–F; B–T; C–T; D–T; E–F
119. A–T; B–T; C–F; D–F; E–T

120. E
121. A
122. D
123. B
124. C
125. B
126. D
127. A
128. E
129. C
130. A
131. D
132. B
133. C
134. E
135. A
136. C
137. D
138. G
139. I
140. D
141. C
142. B
143. D
144. C
145. F
146. A
147. E
148. B
149. C
150. B
151. A
152. D
153. C
154. B
155. C
156. A
157. F
158. D
159. B
160. A
161. B
162. D
163. C
164. E
165. A
166. F
167. C
168. D
169. D
170. A
171. D
172. C
173. B
174. A
175. B
176. E
177. A
178. D
179. B
180. C
181. D
182. B
183. A
184. E
185. C
186. C
187. B
188. A
189. D
190. C
191. A
192. C
193. D
194. B
195. E
196. B
197. C
198. D
199. A
200. D
201. B
202. E
203. F
204. A
205. C
206. D
207. E
208. A
209. C
210. B

PART 5. HEMATOLOGY AND ONCOLOGY

1. D
2. C
3. D
4. D
5. C
6. A
7. B
8. D
9. C
10. C
11. C
12. A
13. D
14. C
15. B
16. B
17. D
18. A
19. B
20. B
21. A
22. D
23. C
24. B
25. C
26. E
27. B
28. B

29. A–F; B–F; C–T; D–F; E–F
30. A–F; B–T; C–F; D–T; E–F
31. A–T; B–T; C–F; D–F
32. A–T; B–F; C–F; D–T
33. A–T; B–T; C–F; D–T
34. All are True
35. A–F; B–F; C–T; D–F
36. A–F; B–F; C–T; D–T
37. All are True
38. A–T; B–T; C–F; D–F
39. A–T; B–T; C–T; D–F
40. A–T; B–F; C–T; D–F
41. A–T; B–T; C–T; D–F
42. A–F; B–F; C–F; D–T
43. A–T; B–F; C–T; D–F
44. A–T; B–T; C–T; D–F
45. All are True
46. A–T; B–F; C–T; D–T
47. A–T; B–T; C–T; D–F
48. A–T; B–T; C–T; D–F
49. A–T; B–T; C–F; D–F
50. A–T; B–F; C–T; D–T
51. A–F; B–T; C–T; D–T; E–T
52. All are True
53. A–T; B–T; C–T; D–F
54. A–T; B–F; C–T; D–F
55. A–T; B–T; C–F; D–T
56. All are True
57. A–T; B–F; C–T; D–T
58. A–T; B–T; C–T; D–F
59. A–T; B–T; C–T; D–F
60. A–F; B–F; C–F; D–T
61. A–T; B–T; C–T; D–F
62. A–F; B–T; C–F; D–T
63. A–T; B–T; C–T; D–F; E–T
64. A–F; B–T; C–T; D–T
65. All are True
66. A–T; B–F; C–F; D–F
67. A–T; B–T; C–F; D–F
68. A–T; B–T; C–T; D–F
69. A–F; B–T; C–T; D–T
70. A–F; B–T; C–F; D–T
71. A–T; B–T; C–F; D–F
72. A–F; B–T; C–F; D–T
73. A–F; B–T; C–F; D–T
74. A–T; B–T; C–T; D–F
75. A–T; B–F; C–T; D–T
76. A–F; B–T; C–F; D–T
77. A–F; B–T; C–F; D–T
78. A–F; B–T; C–T; D–F
79. A–F; B–T; C–F; D–T
80. A–F; B–T; C–F; D–T
81. A–F; B–T; C–F; D–T
82. A–F; B–T; C–F; D–T
83. A–T; B–T; C–T; D–F
84. A–T; B–T; C–F; D–F
85. A–T; B–F; C–F; D–T
86. A–F; B–F; C–T; D–F

87. E	97. A	107. A	117. A	127. B	137. B	147. D	157. C
88. G	98. A	108. D	118. A	128. A	138. B	148. B	158. D
89. F	99. A	109. C	119. A	129. A	139. C	149. B	159. E
90. H	100. B	110. E	120. A	130. B	140. F	150. D	160. G
91. H	101. A	111. E	121. B	131. C	141. E	151. B	161. I
92. D	102. B	112. A	122. B	132. B	142. D	152. C	162. F
93. C	103. A	113. B	123. B	133. C	143. A	153. C	163. B
94. A	104. B	114. D	124. C	134. B	144. C	154. A	164. F
95. A	105. B	115. B	125. D	135. A	145. C	155. B	165. C
96. B	106. C	116. C	126. D	136. C	146. B	156. B	166. A

PART 6. GENETICS AND METABOLIC DISEASE

1. C	6. E	11. D	16. D	21. A	26. C	31. A	36. D
2. E	7. D	12. D	17. A	22. C	27. D	32. C	37. A
3. B	8. C	13. B	18. B	23. C	28. C	33. C	
4. C	9. A	14. D	19. C	24. C	29. C	34. C	
5. A	10. C	15. C	20. B	25. A	30. A	35. B	

38. A–F; B–T; C–T; D–F
39. All are False
40. A–F; B–T; C–F; D–T
41. A–F; B–T; C–T; D–F
42. A–T; B–T; C–F; D–F
43. All are True
44. All are True
45. A–T; B–T; C–T; D–F
46. A–T; B–T; C–T; D–F
47. A–F; B–T; C–F; D–T
48. A–F; B–T; C–T; D–F
49. A–F; B–T; C–T; D–T
50. A–T; B–F; C–T; D–F
51. A–T; B–F; C–T; D–F
52. A–T; B–T; C–T; D–F
53. A–F; B–F; C–T; D–T
54. A–F; B–T; C–T; D–F
55. A–T; B–F; C–F; D–T
56. All are True
57. A–F; B–T; C–F; D–T

58. A	66. E	74. B	82. C	90. B	98. A	106. B	114. A
59. F	67. C	75. B	83. D	91. D	99. D	107. B	115. C
60. C	68. E	76. A	84. B	92. E	100. A	108. D	116. B
61. D	69. B	77. B	85. A	93. F	101. B	109. A	117. C
62. B	70. G	78. A	86. A	94. A	102. C	110. E	118. A
63. C	71. G	79. C	87. B	95. G	103. A	111. C	119. E
64. A	72. B	80. D	88. C	96. A	104. C	112. B	
65. D	73. A	81. E	89. D	97. B	105. B	113. D	

PART 7. ENDOCRINOLOGY AND DIABETES MELLITUS

1. A	11. D	21. E	31. D	41. C	51. A	61. D	71. C
2. A	12. A	22. D	32. B	42. A	52. A	62. B	72. D
3. D	13. B	23. D	33. A	43. B	53. C	63. C	73. B
4. B	14. B	24. C	34. D	44. B	54. A	64. E	74. A
5. B	15. B	25. C	35. C	45. B	55. B	65. C	75. D
6. A	16. E	26. C	36. B	46. D	56. B	66. B	76. E
7. A	17. B	27. B	37. D	47. B	57. A	67. D	77. A
8. E	18. B	28. A	38. B	48. E	58. C	68. C	78. D
9. D	19. B	29. B	39. D	49. D	59. D	69. B	79. E
10. D	20. A	30. B	40. E	50. C	60. B	70. D	80. A

81. A–T; B–T; C–T; D–F
82. A–F; B–T; C–F; D–T
83. A–T; B–F; C–T; D–F
84. A–F; B–T; C–T; D–T
85. A–F; B–F; C–T; D–T; E–T
86. A–F; B–T; C–F; D–T
87. A–T; B–F; C–T; D–T
88. A–T; B–F; C–F; D–T
89. A–T; B–T; C–F; D–T; E–T
90. All are True
91. A–F; B–T; C–F; D–T
92. All are True
93. A–T; B–F; C–F; D–T; E–T
94. A–T; B–F; C–F; D–F; E–T
95. A–F; B–T; C–T; D–T; E–F
96. A–T; B–T; C–F; D–T
97. All are True
98. All are True
99. A–T; B–T; C–T; D–F
100. A–T; B–T; C–T; D–F
101. A–F; B–F; C–T; D–T
102. A–T; B–T; C–F; D–T; E–T
103. A–T; B–F; C–T; D–T; E–T
104. A–F; B–F; C–F; D–T
105. A–T; B–T; C–T; D–F
106. All are True
107. A–T; B–F; C–T; D–F
108. A–F; B–F; C–T; D–T
109. A–T; B–T; C–T; D–F
110. All are True
111. All are False
112. A–T; B–T; C–F; D–T
113. A–T; B–T; C–F; D–T
114. A–T; B–T; C–T; D–F
115. A–T; B–T; C–F; D–T; E–T
116. A–T; B–F; C–T; D–F
117. A–F; B–T; C–F; D–T
118. All are True

119. B
120. D
121. A
122. C
123. A
124. B
125. D
126. C
127. D
128. C
129. B
130. A
131. E
132. D
133. F
134. A
135. E
136. C
137. B
138. E
139. B
140. A
141. E
142. C
143. E
144. B
145. C
146. A
147. D
148. E
149. E
150. B
151. A
152. C
153. A
154. E
155. B
156. A
157. D
158. B
159. D
160. C
161. A
162. D
163. B
164. A
165. C
166. E
167. B
168. E
169. C
170. A
171. D

PART 8. INFECTIOUS DISEASES

1. D
2. C
3. A
4. C
5. C
6. D
7. B
8. A
9. B
10. E
11. B
12. D
13. E
14. A
15. C
16. E
17. C
18. C
19. B
20. E
21. E
22. C
23. B
24. D
25. A
26. D
27. C
28. C
29. B
30. A
31. C
32. E
33. C
34. A
35. C
36. D
37. E
38. C
39. C
40. D
41. A
42. B
43. D
44. B

45. A–F; B–T; C–F; D–T; E–T
46. A–T; B–F; C–F; D–F
47. All are True
48. A–T; B–T; C–F; D–F
49. A–T; B–T; C–F; D–T; E–T
50. A–F; B–F; C–T; D–T; E–F
51. A–F; B–F; C–T; D–F
52. A–T; B–F; C–F; D–F
53. A–T; B–T; C–F; D–F; E–T
54. A–T; B–F; C–F; D–T
55. All are False
56. A–F; B–F; C–F; D–F; E–T
57. A–T; B–F; C–F; D–F; E–F
58. A–F; B–T; C–F; D–T; E–T
59. All are True
60. A–F; B–T; C–F; D–T; E–F
61. A–T; B–T; C–T; D–F
62. A–T; B–T; C–T; D–F
63. A–T; B–F; C–T; D–F
64. All are True
65. A–T; B–T; C–F; D–F
66. A–F; B–T; C–T; D–T
67. A–T; B–T; C–T; D–F
68. A–T; B–T; C–F; D–T
69. A–T; B–T; C–F; D–F
70. A–T; B–F; C–T; D–F
71. A–F; B–T; C–F; D–T
72. A–F; B–T; C–T; D–T
73. All are True
74. All are True
75. A–T; B–T; C–T; D–F
76. A–F; B–T; C–F; D–T
77. A–T; B–T; C–F; D–T
78. A–T; B–T; C–T; D–F
79. A–F; B–F; C–F; D–T
80. A–F; B–T; C–F; D–T
81. All are True
82. All are True
83. All are True
84. A–F; B–T; C–T; D–F
85. A–F; B–T; C–T; D–F
86. A–F; B–T; C–F; D–T
87. A–T; B–T; C–T; D–F
88. A–T; B–F; C–T; D–T
89. All are True
90. A–F; B–T; C–F; D–T
91. A–T; B–F; C–T; D–F
92. A–F; B–T; C–T; D–T
93. A–T; B–F; C–T; D–F
94. A–T; B–T; C–T; D–F
95. A–F; B–F; C–F; D–T
96. A–F; B–T; C–T; D–T
97. A–F; B–T; C–F; D–F
98. A–F; B–T; C–T; D–F
99. All are True
100. A–T; B–T; C–T; D–F
101. A–F; B–F; C–T; D–T
102. All are True
103. A–F; B–T; C–T; D–T
104. A–T; B–T; C–F; D–T
105. All are True
106. All are True

107. A
108. B
109. C
110. C
111. B
112. B
113. C
114. E
115. D
116. B
117. A
118. B
119. C
120. A
121. C
122. A
123. A
124. C
125. C
126. C
127. B
128. A
129. A
130. B
131. A
132. B
133. B
134. A
135. E
136. C
137. F
138. D
139. D
140. B
141. A
142. E
143. C
144. A
145. C
146. E
147. B
148. A
149. E
150. A
151. C
152. D
153. C
154. B
155. C
156. D
157. E
158. A
159. B
160. C
161. D
162. A
163. E
164. A
165. D
166. E
167. C
168. D
169. B
170. C
171. D
172. E
173. A
174. E
175. A
176. B
177. D
178. F
179. C
180. C
181. A
182. F
183. C
184. B
185. D
186. C
187. E
188. C
189. A
190. D
191. C
192. C
193. B
194. D
195. E
196. B
197. C
198. A
199. F
200. B
201. D
202. B

PART 9. CLINICAL IMMUNOLOGY AND RHEUMATOLOGY

1. A
2. E
3. E
4. A
5. C
6. C
7. B
8. E
9. C
10. D
11. B
12. D
13. C
14. B
15. C
16. A
17. C
18. E
19. B
20. B
21. C
22. E
23. A
24. A
25. B
26. D
27. A
28. E
29. E
30. D
31. D
32. D
33. D
34. C
35. A
36. D
37. D
38. B
39. A

40. A–F; B–F; C–T; D–F; E–F
41. A–T; B–F; C–T; D–T; E–F
42. A–F; B–F; C–F; D–F; E–T
43. A–T; B–F; C–F; D–T; E–T
44. A–F; B–F; C–F; D–T
45. A–T; B–F; C–F; D–T; E–T
46. A–T; B–F; C–F; D–T; E–F
47. A–F; B–T; C–T; D–T; E–F
48. A–T; B–T; C–T; D–F
49. A–F; B–F; C–T; D–F; E–F
50. A–F; B–T; C–F; D–F; E–F
51. A–F; B–F; C–T; D–T; E–F
52. A–T; B–F; C–T; D–F; E–F
53. A–T; B–T; C–T; D–T; E–F
54. A–F; B–T; C–T; D–T; E–T
55. A–F; B–T; C–F; D–T; E–T
56. A–F; B–F; C–F; D–T; E–F
57. A–T; B–F; C–T; D–F; E–T
58. A–F; B–T; C–F; D–T; E–F
59. A–F; B–F; C–T; D–T; E–T
60. A–F; B–F; C–T; D–T; E–F

61. B
62. D
63. D
64. C
65. C
66. D
67. A
68. B
69. E
70. C
71. C
72. A
73. A
74. D
75. B
76. C
77. E
78. A
79. D
80. B
81. C
82. C
83. B
84. E
85. D
86. A
87. B
88. C
89. E
90. A
91. D
92. C
93. A
94. B
95. D
96. E
97. C
98. A
99. B
100. D
101. D
102. A
103. E
104. B
105. C

PART 10. NEUROLOGIC DISEASE

1. C
2. C
3. E
4. D
5. D
6. C
7. D
8. E
9. B
10. A
11. E
12. C
13. B
14. D
15. A
16. D
17. E
18. D
19. A
20. E
21. E
22. B
23. D
24. D
25. C
26. B
27. C
28. B
29. D
30. E
31. A
32. E
33. D
34. B
35. C
36. E
37. C
38. D
39. C
40. E
41. E
42. A
43. C
44. A
45. D
46. A
47. A
48. C
49. A
50. B
51. A
52. A
53. A
54. A
55. B
56. A
57. B
58. D
59. D
60. D
61. A
62. D
63. B
64. A
65. A
66. D
67. D
68. D
69. D
70. A
71. C
72. A
73. D
74. D
75. C
76. D
77. A

78. A–T; B–F; C–T; D–T; E–T
79. A–T; B–F; C–F; D–T; E–T; F–T
80. A–F; B–T; C–F; D–T; E–F
81. A–T; B–F; C–T; D–T; E–T
82. A–F; B–F; C–F; D–T; E–F
83. All are True
84. A–T; B–F; C–T; D–F; E–F
85. A–T; B–F; C–T; D–F; E–T
86. A–T; B–T; C–T; D–T; E–F
87. A–F; B–F; C–F; D–F; E–T
88. A–T; B–F; C–T; D–T; E–F
89. A–T; B–T; C–T; D–F; E–T
90. All are True
91. A–T; B–T; C–F; D–T; E–F
92. A–T; B–T; C–T; D–F; E–F
93. A–F; B–T; C–T; D–T; E–F
94. All are True
95. A–F; B–T; C–F; D–T; E–F
96. A–F; B–T; C–T; D–T; E–T
97. A–F; B–T; C–F; D–T; E–T
98. A–F; B–F; C–F; D–T; E–T
99. A–T; B–T; C–T; D–F; E–T
100. A–T; B–F; C–T; D–T; E–F
101. A–T; B–T; C–T; D–F; E–F
102. A–T; B–T; C–T; D–F; E–T
103. A–T; B–F; C–F; D–F; E–T
104. A–T; B–T; C–T; D–F; E–F
105. A–F; B–F; C–T; D–T; E–F
106. A–T; B–F; C–T; D–F; E–T
107. A–T; B–T; C–T; D–T; E–F
108. All are True
109. A–F; B–F; C–T; D–T; E–T
110. A–T; B–T; C–T; D–T; E–F
111. A–F; B–T; C–T; D–T; E–T
112. All are True
113. A–F; B–T; C–T; D–T; E–T
114. All are True
115. All are True
116. A–F; B–F; C–F; D–T; E–T
117. A–T; B–T; C–T; D–T; E–F
118. All are True

119. D
120. A
121. B
122. C
123. E
124. B
125. E
126. A
127. D
128. C
129. D
130. C
131. A
132. E
133. F
134. B
135. A
136. F
137. E
138. C
139. B
140. D
141. D
142. A
143. E
144. C
145. B
146. C
147. D
148. B
149. E
150. A
151. B
152. D
153. C
154. A
155. E
156. B
157. D
158. A
159. C
160. E
161. C
162. A
163. B
164. D
165. A
166. C
167. B
168. D
169. E
170. B
171. D
172. C
173. A
174. A
175. C
176. B
177. E
178. D
179. A
180. C
181. D
182. F
183. D
184. A
185. C
186. B
187. E
188. C
189. E
190. D
191. A
192. B

PART 11. DERMATOLOGY

1. C
2. E
3. A
4. D
5. D
6. E
7. C
8. C
9. C
10. A
11. E
12. C
13. E
14. A
15. A
16. A
17. C
18. B
19. D
20. C
21. A
22. C
23. D
24. B
25. D
26. C
27. D
28. B

29. A–T; B–T; C–T; D–F; E–T
30. A–T; B–T; C–T; D–F; E–F
31. A–T; B–F; C–T; D–F; E–F
32. A–F; B–F; C–T; D–F; E–T
33. A–T; B–T; C–F; D–T; E–T
34. A–F; B–T; C–F; D–T; E–F
35. A–T; B–F; C–T; D–T; E–F
36. A–T; B–F; C–T; D–F; E–F
37. A–T; B–T; C–T; D–T; E–F
38. A–T; B–F; C–T; D–T; E–T
39. A–F; B–T; C–F; D–F; E–T
40. A–T; B–T; C–T; D–T; E–F
41. A–F; B–T; C–T; D–T
42. A–T; B–T; C–T; D–F
43. All are True
44. A–T; B–F; C–T; D–F
45. A–T; B–F; C–T; D–F
46. All are True
47. All are True
48. A–T; B–F; C–T; D–T
49. All are True
50. A–F; B–F; C–F; D–T

PART 1 CARDIOVASCULAR DISEASES

No.									
1	A	B	C	D	E	F	G	H	I
2	A	B	C	D	E	F	G	H	I
3	A	B	C	D	E	F	G	H	I
4	A	B	C	D	E	F	G	H	I
5	A	B	C	D	E	F	G	H	I
6	A	B	C	D	E	F	G	H	I
7	A	B	C	D	E	F	G	H	I
8	A	B	C	D	E	F	G	H	I
9	A	B	C	D	E	F	G	H	I
10	A	B	C	D	E	F	G	H	I
11	A	B	C	D	E	F	G	H	I
12	A	B	C	D	E	F	G	H	I
13	A	B	C	D	E	F	G	H	I
14	A	B	C	D	E	F	G	H	I
15	A	B	C	D	E	F	G	H	I
16	A	B	C	D	E	F	G	H	I
17	A	B	C	D	E	F	G	H	I
18	A	B	C	D	E	F	G	H	I
19	A	B	C	D	E	F	G	H	I
20	A	B	C	D	E	F	G	H	I
21	A	B	C	D	E	F	G	H	I
22	A	B	C	D	E	F	G	H	I
23	A	B	C	D	E	F	G	H	I
24	A	B	C	D	E	F	G	H	I
25	A	B	C	D	E	F	G	H	I
26	A	B	C	D	E	F	G	H	I
27	A	B	C	D	E	F	G	H	I
28	A	B	C	D	E	F	G	H	I
29	A	B	C	D	E	F	G	H	I
30	A	B	C	D	E	F	G	H	I
31	A	B	C	D	E	F	G	H	I
32	A	B	C	D	E	F	G	H	I
33	A	B	C	D	E	F	G	H	I
34	A	B	C	D	E	F	G	H	I
35	A	B	C	D	E	F	G	H	I
36	A	B	C	D	E	F	G	H	I
37	A	B	C	D	E	F	G	H	I
38	A	B	C	D	E	F	G	H	I
39	A	B	C	D	E	F	G	H	I
40	A	B	C	D	E	F	G	H	I
41	A	B	C	D	E	F	G	H	I
42	A	B	C	D	E	F	G	H	I
43	A	B	C	D	E	F	G	H	I
44	A	B	C	D	E	F	G	H	I
45	A	B	C	D	E	F	G	H	I
46	A	B	C	D	E	F	G	H	I
47	A	B	C	D	E	F	G	H	I
48	A	B	C	D	E	F	G	H	I
49	A	B	C	D	E	F	G	H	I
50	A	B	C	D	E	F	G	H	I
51	A	B	C	D	E	F	G	H	I
52	A	B	C	D	E	F	G	H	I
53	A	B	C	D	E	F	G	H	I
54	A	B	C	D	E	F	G	H	I
55	A	B	C	D	E	F	G	H	I
56	A	B	C	D	E	F	G	H	I
57	A	B	C	D	E	F	G	H	I
58	A	B	C	D	E	F	G	H	I
59	A	B	C	D	E	F	G	H	I
60	A	B	C	D	E	F	G	H	I
61	A	B	C	D	E	F	G	H	I
62	A	B	C	D	E	F	G	H	I
63	A	B	C	D	E	F	G	H	I
64	A	B	C	D	E	F	G	H	I
65	A	B	C	D	E	F	G	H	I
66	A	B	C	D	E	F	G	H	I
67	A	B	C	D	E	F	G	H	I
68	A	B	C	D	E	F	G	H	I
69	A	B	C	D	E	F	G	H	I
70	A	B	C	D	E	F	G	H	I
71	A	B	C	D	E	F	G	H	I
72	A	B	C	D	E	F	G	H	I
73	A	B	C	D	E	F	G	H	I
74	A	B	C	D	E	F	G	H	I
75	A	B	C	D	E	F	G	H	I
76	A	B	C	D	E	F	G	H	I
77	A	B	C	D	E	F	G	H	I
78	A	B	C	D	E	F	G	H	I
79	A	B	C	D	E	F	G	H	I
80	A	B	C	D	E	F	G	H	I
81	A	B	C	D	E	F	G	H	I
82	A	B	C	D	E	F	G	H	I
83	A	B	C	D	E	F	G	H	I
84	A	B	C	D	E	F	G	H	I
85	A	B	C	D	E	F	G	H	I
86	A	B	C	D	E	F	G	H	I
87	A	B	C	D	E	F	G	H	I
88	A	B	C	D	E	F	G	H	I
89	A	B	C	D	E	F	G	H	I
90	A	B	C	D	E	F	G	H	I
91	A	B	C	D	E	F	G	H	I
92	A	B	C	D	E	F	G	H	I
93	A	B	C	D	E	F	G	H	I
94	A	B	C	D	E	F	G	H	I
95	A	B	C	D	E	F	G	H	I
96	A	B	C	D	E	F	G	H	I
97	A	B	C	D	E	F	G	H	I
98	A	B	C	D	E	F	G	H	I
99	A	B	C	D	E	F	G	H	I
100	A	B	C	D	E	F	G	H	I
101	A	B	C	D	E	F	G	H	I
102	A	B	C	D	E	F	G	H	I
103	A	B	C	D	E	F	G	H	I
104	A	B	C	D	E	F	G	H	I
105	A	B	C	D	E	F	G	H	I

PART 1 CARDIOVASCULAR DISEASES

106 A B C D E F G H I
107 A B C D E F G H I
108 A B C D E F G H I
109 A B C D E F G H I
110 A B C D E F G H I
111 A B C D E F G H I
112 A B C D E F G H I
113 A B C D E F G H I
114 A B C D E F G H I
115 A B C D E F G H I
116 A B C D E F G H I
117 A B C D E F G H I
118 A B C D E F G H I
119 A B C D E F G H I
120 A B C D E F G H I
121 A B C D E F G H I
122 A B C D E F G H I
123 A B C D E F G H I
124 A B C D E F G H I
125 A B C D E F G H I
126 A B C D E F G H I
127 A B C D E F G H I
128 A B C D E F G H I
129 A B C D E F G H I
130 A B C D E F G H I
131 A B C D E F G H I
132 A B C D E F G H I
133 A B C D E F G H I
134 A B C D E F G H I
135 A B C D E F G H I
136 A B C D E F G H I
137 A B C D E F G H I
138 A B C D E F G H I
139 A B C D E F G H I
140 A B C D E F G H I
141 A B C D E F G H I
142 A B C D E F G H I
143 A B C D E F G H I
144 A B C D E F G H I
145 A B C D E F G H I
146 A B C D E F G H I
147 A B C D E F G H I
148 A B C D E F G H I
149 A B C D E F G H I
150 A B C D E F G H I
151 A B C D E F G H I
152 A B C D E F G H I
153 A B C D E F G H I
154 A B C D E F G H I
155 A B C D E F G H I
156 A B C D E F G H I
157 A B C D E F G H I
158 A B C D E F G H I
159 A B C D E F G H I
160 A B C D E F G H I
161 A B C D E F G H I
162 A B C D E F G H I
163 A B C D E F G H I
164 A B C D E F G H I
165 A B C D E F G H I
166 A B C D E F G H I
167 A B C D E F G H I
168 A B C D E F G H I
169 A B C D E F G H I
170 A B C D E F G H I
171 A B C D E F G H I
172 A B C D E F G H I
173 A B C D E F G H I
174 A B C D E F G H I
175 A B C D E F G H I
176 A B C D E F G H I
177 A B C D E F G H I
178 A B C D E F G H I
179 A B C D E F G H I
180 A B C D E F G H I
181 A B C D E F G H I
182 A B C D E F G H I
183 A B C D E F G H I
184 A B C D E F G H I
185 A B C D E F G H I
186 A B C D E F G H I
187 A B C D E F G H I
188 A B C D E F G H I
189 A B C D E F G H I
190 A B C D E F G H I
191 A B C D E F G H I
192 A B C D E F G H I
193 A B C D E F G H I
194 A B C D E F G H I
195 A B C D E F G H I
196 A B C D E F G H I
197 A B C D E F G H I
198 A B C D E F G H I
199 A B C D E F G H I
200 A B C D E F G H I
201 A B C D E F G H I
202 A B C D E F G H I
203 A B C D E F G H I
204 A B C D E F G H I
205 A B C D E F G H I
206 A B C D E F G H I
207 A B C D E F G H I
208 A B C D E F G H I
209 A B C D E F G H I
210 A B C D E F G H I

PART 1 CARDIOVASCULAR DISEASE

	A	B	C	D	E	F	G	H	I
211	A	B	C	D	E	F	G	H	I
212	A	B	C	D	E	F	G	H	I
213	A	B	C	D	E	F	G	H	I
214	A	B	C	D	E	F	G	H	I
215	A	B	C	D	E	F	G	H	I
216	A	B	C	D	E	F	G	H	I
217	A	B	C	D	E	F	G	H	I
218	A	B	C	D	E	F	G	H	I
219	A	B	C	D	E	F	G	H	I
220	A	B	C	D	E	F	G	H	I
221	A	B	C	D	E	F	G	H	I
222	A	B	C	D	E	F	G	H	I
223	A	B	C	D	E	F	G	H	I
224	A	B	C	D	E	F	G	H	I
225	A	B	C	D	E	F	G	H	I
226	A	B	C	D	E	F	G	H	I
227	A	B	C	D	E	F	G	H	I
228	A	B	C	D	E	F	G	H	I
229	A	B	C	D	E	F	G	H	I
230	A	B	C	D	E	F	G	H	I
231	A	B	C	D	E	F	G	H	I

PART 2 RESPIRATORY DISEASE

No.								
1	A	B	C	D	E	F	G	H
2	A	B	C	D	E	F	G	H
3	A	B	C	D	E	F	G	H
4	A	B	C	D	E	F	G	H
5	A	B	C	D	E	F	G	H
6	A	B	C	D	E	F	G	H
7	A	B	C	D	E	F	G	H
8	A	B	C	D	E	F	G	H
9	A	B	C	D	E	F	G	H
10	A	B	C	D	E	F	G	H
11	A	B	C	D	E	F	G	H
12	A	B	C	D	E	F	G	H
13	A	B	C	D	E	F	G	H
14	A	B	C	D	E	F	G	H
15	A	B	C	D	E	F	G	H
16	A	B	C	D	E	F	G	H
17	A	B	C	D	E	F	G	H
18	A	B	C	D	E	F	G	H
19	A	B	C	D	E	F	G	H
20	A	B	C	D	E	F	G	H
21	A	B	C	D	E	F	G	H
22	A	B	C	D	E	F	G	H
23	A	B	C	D	E	F	G	H
24	A	B	C	D	E	F	G	H
25	A	B	C	D	E	F	G	H
26	A	B	C	D	E	F	G	H
27	A	B	C	D	E	F	G	H
28	A	B	C	D	E	F	G	H
29	A	B	C	D	E	F	G	H
30	A	B	C	D	E	F	G	H
31	A	B	C	D	E	F	G	H
32	A	B	C	D	E	F	G	H
33	A	B	C	D	E	F	G	H
34	A	B	C	D	E	F	G	H
35	A	B	C	D	E	F	G	H
36	A	B	C	D	E	F	G	H
37	A	B	C	D	E	F	G	H
38	A	B	C	D	E	F	G	H
39	A	B	C	D	E	F	G	H
40	A	B	C	D	E	F	G	H
41	A	B	C	D	E	F	G	H
42	A	B	C	D	E	F	G	H
43	A	B	C	D	E	F	G	H
44	A	B	C	D	E	F	G	H
45	A	B	C	D	E	F	G	H
46	A	B	C	D	E	F	G	H
47	A	B	C	D	E	F	G	H
48	A	B	C	D	E	F	G	H
49	A	B	C	D	E	F	G	H
50	A	B	C	D	E	F	G	H
51	A	B	C	D	E	F	G	H
52	A	B	C	D	E	F	G	H
53	A	B	C	D	E	F	G	H
54	A	B	C	D	E	F	G	H
55	A	B	C	D	E	F	G	H
56	A	B	C	D	E	F	G	H
57	A	B	C	D	E	F	G	H
58	A	B	C	D	E	F	G	H
59	A	B	C	D	E	F	G	H
60	A	B	C	D	E	F	G	H
61	A	B	C	D	E	F	G	H
62	A	B	C	D	E	F	G	H
63	A	B	C	D	E	F	G	H
64	A	B	C	D	E	F	G	H
65	A	B	C	D	E	F	G	H
66	A	B	C	D	E	F	G	H
67	A	B	C	D	E	F	G	H
68	A	B	C	D	E	F	G	H
69	A	B	C	D	E	F	G	H
70	A	B	C	D	E	F	G	H
71	A	B	C	D	E	F	G	H
72	A	B	C	D	E	F	G	H
73	A	B	C	D	E	F	G	H
74	A	B	C	D	E	F	G	H
75	A	B	C	D	E	F	G	H
76	A	B	C	D	E	F	G	H
77	A	B	C	D	E	F	G	H
78	A	B	C	D	E	F	G	H
79	A	B	C	D	E	F	G	H
80	A	B	C	D	E	F	G	H
81	A	B	C	D	E	F	G	H
82	A	B	C	D	E	F	G	H
83	A	B	C	D	E	F	G	H
84	A	B	C	D	E	F	G	H
85	A	B	C	D	E	F	G	H
86	A	B	C	D	E	F	G	H
87	A	B	C	D	E	F	G	H
88	A	B	C	D	E	F	G	H
89	A	B	C	D	E	F	G	H
90	A	B	C	D	E	F	G	H
91	A	B	C	D	E	F	G	H
92	A	B	C	D	E	F	G	H
93	A	B	C	D	E	F	G	H
94	A	B	C	D	E	F	G	H
95	A	B	C	D	E	F	G	H
96	A	B	C	D	E	F	G	H
97	A	B	C	D	E	F	G	H
98	A	B	C	D	E	F	G	H
99	A	B	C	D	E	F	G	H
100	A	B	C	D	E	F	G	H
101	A	B	C	D	E	F	G	H
102	A	B	C	D	E	F	G	H
103	A	B	C	D	E	F	G	H
104	A	B	C	D	E	F	G	H
105	A	B	C	D	E	F	G	H

PART 2 PULMONARY DISEASE

106	A	B	C	D	E	F	G	H
107	A	B	C	D	E	F	G	H
108	A	B	C	D	E	F	G	H
109	A	B	C	D	E	F	G	H
110	A	B	C	D	E	F	G	H
111	A	B	C	D	E	F	G	H
112	A	B	C	D	E	F	G	H
113	A	B	C	D	E	F	G	H
114	A	B	C	D	E	F	G	H
115	A	B	C	D	E	F	G	H
116	A	B	C	D	E	F	G	H
117	A	B	C	D	E	F	G	H
118	A	B	C	D	E	F	G	H
119	A	B	C	D	E	F	G	H
120	A	B	C	D	E	F	G	H
121	A	B	C	D	E	F	G	H
122	A	B	C	D	E	F	G	H
123	A	B	C	D	E	F	G	H
124	A	B	C	D	E	F	G	H
125	A	B	C	D	E	F	G	H
126	A	B	C	D	E	F	G	H
127	A	B	C	D	E	F	G	H
128	A	B	C	D	E	F	G	H
129	A	B	C	D	E	F	G	H
130	A	B	C	D	E	F	G	H
131	A	B	C	D	E	F	G	H
132	A	B	C	D	E	F	G	H
133	A	B	C	D	E	F	G	H
134	A	B	C	D	E	F	G	H
135	A	B	C	D	E	F	G	H
136	A	B	C	D	E	F	G	H

PART 3 RENAL DISEASE

1 A B C D E F G H
2 A B C D E F G H
3 A B C D E F G H
4 A B C D E F G H
5 A B C D E F G H
6 A B C D E F G H
7 A B C D E F G H
8 A B C D E F G H
9 A B C D E F G H
10 A B C D E F G H
11 A B C D E F G H
12 A B C D E F G H
13 A B C D E F G H
14 A B C D E F G H
15 A B C D E F G H
16 A B C D E F G H
17 A B C D E F G H
18 A B C D E F G H
19 A B C D E F G H
20 A B C D E F G H
21 A B C D E F G H
22 A B C D E F G H
23 A B C D E F G H
24 A B C D E F G H
25 A B C D E F G H
26 A B C D E F G H
27 A B C D E F G H
28 A B C D E F G H
29 A B C D E F G H
30 A B C D E F G H
31 A B C D E F G H
32 A B C D E F G H
33 A B C D E F G H
34 A B C D E F G H
35 A B C D E F G H
36 A B C D E F G H
37 A B C D E F G H
38 A B C D E F G H
39 A B C D E F G H
40 A B C D E F G H
41 A B C D E F G H
42 A B C D E F G H
43 A B C D E F G H
44 A B C D E F G H
45 A B C D E F G H
46 A B C D E F G H
47 A B C D E F G H
48 A B C D E F G H
49 A B C D E F G H
50 A B C D E F G H
51 A B C D E F G H
52 A B C D E F G H
53 A B C D E F G H
54 A B C D E F G H
55 A B C D E F G H
56 A B C D E F G H
57 A B C D E F G H
58 A B C D E F G H
59 A B C D E F G H
60 A B C D E F G H
61 A B C D E F G H
62 A B C D E F G H
63 A B C D E F G H
64 A B C D E F G H
65 A B C D E F G H
66 A B C D E F G H
67 A B C D E F G H
68 A B C D E F G H
69 A B C D E F G H
70 A B C D E F G H
71 A B C D E F G H
72 A B C D E F G H
73 A B C D E F G H
74 A B C D E F G H
75 A B C D E F G H
76 A B C D E F G H
77 A B C D E F G H
78 A B C D E F G H
79 A B C D E F G H
80 A B C D E F G H
81 A B C D E F G H
82 A B C D E F G H
83 A B C D E F G H
84 A B C D E F G H
85 A B C D E F G H
86 A B C D E F G H
87 A B C D E F G H
88 A B C D E F G H
89 A B C D E F G H

PART 4 GASTROINTESTINAL DISEASE

No.	A	B	C	D	E	F	G	H	I	J
1	A	B	C	D	E	F	G	H	I	J
2	A	B	C	D	E	F	G	H	I	J
3	A	B	C	D	E	F	G	H	I	J
4	A	B	C	D	E	F	G	H	I	J
5	A	B	C	D	E	F	G	H	I	J
6	A	B	C	D	E	F	G	H	I	J
7	A	B	C	D	E	F	G	H	I	J
8	A	B	C	D	E	F	G	H	I	J
9	A	B	C	D	E	F	G	H	I	J
10	A	B	C	D	E	F	G	H	I	J
11	A	B	C	D	E	F	G	H	I	J
12	A	B	C	D	E	F	G	H	I	J
13	A	B	C	D	E	F	G	H	I	J
14	A	B	C	D	E	F	G	H	I	J
15	A	B	C	D	E	F	G	H	I	J
16	A	B	C	D	E	F	G	H	I	J
17	A	B	C	D	E	F	G	H	I	J
18	A	B	C	D	E	F	G	H	I	J
19	A	B	C	D	E	F	G	H	I	J
20	A	B	C	D	E	F	G	H	I	J
21	A	B	C	D	E	F	G	H	I	J
22	A	B	C	D	E	F	G	H	I	J
23	A	B	C	D	E	F	G	H	I	J
24	A	B	C	D	E	F	G	H	I	J
25	A	B	C	D	E	F	G	H	I	J
26	A	B	C	D	E	F	G	H	I	J
27	A	B	C	D	E	F	G	H	I	J
28	A	B	C	D	E	F	G	H	I	J
29	A	B	C	D	E	F	G	H	I	J
30	A	B	C	D	E	F	G	H	I	J
31	A	B	C	D	E	F	G	H	I	J
32	A	B	C	D	E	F	G	H	I	J
33	A	B	C	D	E	F	G	H	I	J
34	A	B	C	D	E	F	G	H	I	J
35	A	B	C	D	E	F	G	H	I	J
36	A	B	C	D	E	F	G	H	I	J
37	A	B	C	D	E	F	G	H	I	J
38	A	B	C	D	E	F	G	H	I	J
39	A	B	C	D	E	F	G	H	I	J
40	A	B	C	D	E	F	G	H	I	J
41	A	B	C	D	E	F	G	H	I	J
42	A	B	C	D	E	F	G	H	I	J
43	A	B	C	D	E	F	G	H	I	J
44	A	B	C	D	E	F	G	H	I	J
45	A	B	C	D	E	F	G	H	I	J
46	A	B	C	D	E	F	G	H	I	J
47	A	B	C	D	E	F	G	H	I	J
48	A	B	C	D	E	F	G	H	I	J
49	A	B	C	D	E	F	G	H	I	J
50	A	B	C	D	E	F	G	H	I	J
51	A	B	C	D	E	F	G	H	I	J
52	A	B	C	D	E	F	G	H	I	J
53	A	B	C	D	E	F	G	H	I	J
54	A	B	C	D	E	F	G	H	I	J
55	A	B	C	D	E	F	G	H	I	J
56	A	B	C	D	E	F	G	H	I	J
57	A	B	C	D	E	F	G	H	I	J
58	A	B	C	D	E	F	G	H	I	J
59	A	B	C	D	E	F	G	H	I	J
60	A	B	C	D	E	F	G	H	I	J
61	A	B	C	D	E	F	G	H	I	J
62	A	B	C	D	E	F	G	H	I	J
63	A	B	C	D	E	F	G	H	I	J
64	A	B	C	D	E	F	G	H	I	J
65	A	B	C	D	E	F	G	H	I	J
66	A	B	C	D	E	F	G	H	I	J
67	A	B	C	D	E	F	G	H	I	J
68	A	B	C	D	E	F	G	H	I	J
69	A	B	C	D	E	F	G	H	I	J
70	A	B	C	D	E	F	G	H	I	J
71	A	B	C	D	E	F	G	H	I	J
72	A	B	C	D	E	F	G	H	I	J
73	A	B	C	D	E	F	G	H	I	J
74	A	B	C	D	E	F	G	H	I	J
75	A	B	C	D	E	F	G	H	I	J
76	A	B	C	D	E	F	G	H	I	J
77	A	B	C	D	E	F	G	H	I	J
78	A	B	C	D	E	F	G	H	I	J
79	A	B	C	D	E	F	G	H	I	J
80	A	B	C	D	E	F	G	H	I	J
81	A	B	C	D	E	F	G	H	I	J
82	A	B	C	D	E	F	G	H	I	J
83	A	B	C	D	E	F	G	H	I	J
84	A	B	C	D	E	F	G	H	I	J
85	A	B	C	D	E	F	G	H	I	J
86	A	B	C	D	E	F	G	H	I	J
87	A	B	C	D	E	F	G	H	I	J
88	A	B	C	D	E	F	G	H	I	J
89	A	B	C	D	E	F	G	H	I	J
90	A	B	C	D	E	F	G	H	I	J
91	A	B	C	D	E	F	G	H	I	J
92	A	B	C	D	E	F	G	H	I	J
93	A	B	C	D	E	F	G	H	I	J
94	A	B	C	D	E	F	G	H	I	J
95	A	B	C	D	E	F	G	H	I	J
96	A	B	C	D	E	F	G	H	I	J
97	A	B	C	D	E	F	G	H	I	J
98	A	B	C	D	E	F	G	H	I	J
99	A	B	C	D	E	F	G	H	I	J
100	A	B	C	D	E	F	G	H	I	J
101	A	B	C	D	E	F	G	H	I	J
102	A	B	C	D	E	F	G	H	I	J
103	A	B	C	D	E	F	G	H	I	J
104	A	B	C	D	E	F	G	H	I	J
105	A	B	C	D	E	F	G	H	I	J

PART 4 GASTROINTESTINAL DISEASE

106 A B C D E F G H I J
107 A B C D E F G H I J
108 A B C D E F G H I J
109 A B C D E F G H I J
110 A B C D E F G H I J
111 A B C D E F G H I J
112 A B C D E F G H I J
113 A B C D E F G H I J
114 A B C D E F G H I J
115 A B C D E F G H I J
116 A B C D E F G H I J
117 A B C D E F G H I J
118 A B C D E F G H I J
119 A B C D E F G H I J
120 A B C D E F G H I J
121 A B C D E F G H I J
122 A B C D E F G H I J
123 A B C D E F G H I J
124 A B C D E F G H I J
125 A B C D E F G H I J
126 A B C D E F G H I J
127 A B C D E F G H I J
128 A B C D E F G H I J
129 A B C D E F G H I J
130 A B C D E F G H I J
131 A B C D E F G H I J
132 A B C D E F G H I J
133 A B C D E F G H I J
134 A B C D E F G H I J
135 A B C D E F G H I J
136 A B C D E F G H I J
137 A B C D E F G H I J
138 A B C D E F G H I J
139 A B C D E F G H I J
140 A B C D E F G H I J
141 A B C D E F G H I J
142 A B C D E F G H I J
143 A B C D E F G H I J
144 A B C D E F G H I J
145 A B C D E F G H I J
146 A B C D E F G H I J
147 A B C D E F G H I J
148 A B C D E F G H I J
149 A B C D E F G H I J
150 A B C D E F G H I J
151 A B C D E F G H I J
152 A B C D E F G H I J
153 A B C D E F G H I J
154 A B C D E F G H I J
155 A B C D E F G H I J
156 A B C D E F G H I J
157 A B C D E F G H I J
158 A B C D E F G H I J
159 A B C D E F G H I J
160 A B C D E F G H I J
161 A B C D E F G H I J
162 A B C D E F G H I J
163 A B C D E F G H I J
164 A B C D E F G H I J
165 A B C D E F G H I J
166 A B C D E F G H I J
167 A B C D E F G H I J
168 A B C D E F G H I J
169 A B C D E F G H I J
170 A B C D E F G H I J
171 A B C D E F G H I J
172 A B C D E F G H I J
173 A B C D E F G H I J
174 A B C D E F G H I J
175 A B C D E F G H I J
176 A B C D E F G H I J
177 A B C D E F G H I J
178 A B C D E F G H I J
179 A B C D E F G H I J
180 A B C D E F G H I J
181 A B C D E F G H I J
182 A B C D E F G H I J
183 A B C D E F G H I J
184 A B C D E F G H I J
185 A B C D E F G H I J
186 A B C D E F G H I J
187 A B C D E F G H I J
188 A B C D E F G H I J
189 A B C D E F G H I J
190 A B C D E F G H I J
191 A B C D E F G H I J
192 A B C D E F G H I J
193 A B C D E F G H I J
194 A B C D E F G H I J
195 A B C D E F G H I J
196 A B C D E F G H I J
197 A B C D E F G H I J
198 A B C D E F G H I J
199 A B C D E F G H I J
200 A B C D E F G H I J
201 A B C D E F G H I J
202 A B C D E F G H I J
203 A B C D E F G H I J
204 A B C D E F G H I J
205 A B C D E F G H I J
206 A B C D E F G H I J
207 A B C D E F G H I J
208 A B C D E F G H I J
209 A B C D E F G H I J
210 A B C D E F G H I J

PART 5 HEMATOLOGY AND ONCOLOGY

1 A B C D E F G H I
2 A B C D E F G H I
3 A B C D E F G H I
4 A B C D E F G H I
5 A B C D E F G H I
6 A B C D E F G H I
7 A B C D E F G H I
8 A B C D E F G H I
9 A B C D E F G H I
10 A B C D E F G H I
11 A B C D E F G H I
12 A B C D E F G H I
13 A B C D E F G H I
14 A B C D E F G H I
15 A B C D E F G H I
16 A B C D E F G H I
17 A B C D E F G H I
18 A B C D E F G H I
19 A B C D E F G H I
20 A B C D E F G H I
21 A B C D E F G H I
22 A B C D E F G H I
23 A B C D E F G H I
24 A B C D E F G H I
25 A B C D E F G H I
26 A B C D E F G H I
27 A B C D E F G H I
28 A B C D E F G H I
29 A B C D E F G H I
30 A B C D E F G H I
31 A B C D E F G H I
32 A B C D E F G H I
33 A B C D E F G H I
34 A B C D E F G H I
35 A B C D E F G H I
36 A B C D E F G H I
37 A B C D E F G H I
38 A B C D E F G H I
39 A B C D E F G H I
40 A B C D E F G H I
41 A B C D E F G H I
42 A B C D E F G H I
43 A B C D E F G H I
44 A B C D E F G H I
45 A B C D E F G H I
46 A B C D E F G H I
47 A B C D E F G H I
48 A B C D E F G H I
49 A B C D E F G H I
50 A B C D E F G H I
51 A B C D E F G H I
52 A B C D E F G H I
53 A B C D E F G H I
54 A B C D E F G H I
55 A B C D E F G H I
56 A B C D E F G H I
57 A B C D E F G H I
58 A B C D E F G H I
59 A B C D E F G H I
60 A B C D E F G H I
61 A B C D E F G H I
62 A B C D E F G H I
63 A B C D E F G H I
64 A B C D E F G H I
65 A B C D E F G H I
66 A B C D E F G H I
67 A B C D E F G H I
68 A B C D E F G H I
69 A B C D E F G H I
70 A B C D E F G H I
71 A B C D E F G H I
72 A B C D E F G H I
73 A B C D E F G H I
74 A B C D E F G H I
75 A B C D E F G H I
76 A B C D E F G H I
77 A B C D E F G H I
78 A B C D E F G H I
79 A B C D E F G H I
80 A B C D E F G H I
81 A B C D E F G H I
82 A B C D E F G H I
83 A B C D E F G H I
84 A B C D E F G H I
85 A B C D E F G H I
86 A B C D E F G H I
87 A B C D E F G H I
88 A B C D E F G H I
89 A B C D E F G H I
90 A B C D E F G H I
91 A B C D E F G H I
92 A B C D E F G H I
93 A B C D E F G H I
94 A B C D E F G H I
95 A B C D E F G H I
96 A B C D E F G H I
97 A B C D E F G H I
98 A B C D E F G H I
99 A B C D E F G H I
100 A B C D E F G H I
101 A B C D E F G H I
102 A B C D E F G H I
103 A B C D E F G H I
104 A B C D E F G H I
105 A B C D E F G H I

PART 5 HEMATOLOGY AND ONCOLOGY

106 A B C D E F G H I
107 A B C D E F G H I
108 A B C D E F G H I
109 A B C D E F G H I
110 A B C D E F G H I
111 A B C D E F G H I
112 A B C D E F G H I
113 A B C D E F G H I
114 A B C D E F G H I
115 A B C D E F G H I
116 A B C D E F G H I
117 A B C D E F G H I
118 A B C D E F G H I
119 A B C D E F G H I
120 A B C D E F G H I
121 A B C D E F G H I
122 A B C D E F G H I
123 A B C D E F G H I
124 A B C D E F G H I
125 A B C D E F G H I
126 A B C D E F G H I
127 A B C D E F G H I
128 A B C D E F G H I
129 A B C D E F G H I
130 A B C D E F G H I
131 A B C D E F G H I
132 A B C D E F G H I
133 A B C D E F G H I
134 A B C D E F G H I
135 A B C D E F G H I
136 A B C D E F G H I
137 A B C D E F G H I
138 A B C D E F G H I
139 A B C D E F G H I
140 A B C D E F G H I
141 A B C D E F G H I
142 A B C D E F G H I
143 A B C D E F G H I
144 A B C D E F G H I
145 A B C D E F G H I
146 A B C D E F G H I
147 A B C D E F G H I
148 A B C D E F G H I
149 A B C D E F G H I
150 A B C D E F G H I
151 A B C D E F G H I
152 A B C D E F G H I
153 A B C D E F G H I
154 A B C D E F G H I
155 A B C D E F G H I
156 A B C D E F G H I
157 A B C D E F G H I
158 A B C D E F G H I
159 A B C D E F G H I
160 A B C D E F G H I
161 A B C D E F G H I
162 A B C D E F G H I
163 A B C D E F G H I
164 A B C D E F G H I
165 A B C D E F G H I
166 A B C D E F G H I

PART 6 GENETICS AND METABOLIC DISEASE

1 A B C D E F G H
2 A B C D E F G H
3 A B C D E F G H
4 A B C D E F G H
5 A B C D E F G H
6 A B C D E F G H
7 A B C D E F G H
8 A B C D E F G H
9 A B C D E F G H
10 A B C D E F G H
11 A B C D E F G H
12 A B C D E F G H
13 A B C D E F G H
14 A B C D E F G H
15 A B C D E F G H
16 A B C D E F G H
17 A B C D E F G H
18 A B C D E F G H
19 A B C D E F G H
20 A B C D E F G H
21 A B C D E F G H
22 A B C D E F G H
23 A B C D E F G H
24 A B C D E F G H
25 A B C D E F G H
26 A B C D E F G H
27 A B C D E F G H
28 A B C D E F G H
29 A B C D E F G H
30 A B C D E F G H
31 A B C D E F G H
32 A B C D E F G H
33 A B C D E F G H
34 A B C D E F G H
35 A B C D E F G H
36 A B C D E F G H
37 A B C D E F G H
38 A B C D E F G H
39 A B C D E F G H
40 A B C D E F G H
41 A B C D E F G H
42 A B C D E F G H
43 A B C D E F G H
44 A B C D E F G H
45 A B C D E F G H
46 A B C D E F G H
47 A B C D E F G H
48 A B C D E F G H
49 A B C D E F G H
50 A B C D E F G H
51 A B C D E F G H
52 A B C D E F G H
53 A B C D E F G H
54 A B C D E F G H
55 A B C D E F G H
56 A B C D E F G H
57 A B C D E F G H
58 A B C D E F G H
59 A B C D E F G H
60 A B C D E F G H
61 A B C D E F G H
62 A B C D E F G H
63 A B C D E F G H
64 A B C D E F G H
65 A B C D E F G H
66 A B C D E F G H
67 A B C D E F G H
68 A B C D E F G H
69 A B C D E F G H
70 A B C D E F G H
71 A B C D E F G H
72 A B C D E F G H
73 A B C D E F G H
74 A B C D E F G H
75 A B C D E F G H
76 A B C D E F G H
77 A B C D E F G H
78 A B C D E F G H
79 A B C D E F G H
80 A B C D E F G H
81 A B C D E F G H
82 A B C D E F G H
83 A B C D E F G H
84 A B C D E F G H
85 A B C D E F G H
86 A B C D E F G H
87 A B C D E F G H
88 A B C D E F G H
89 A B C D E F G H
90 A B C D E F G H
91 A B C D E F G H
92 A B C D E F G H
93 A B C D E F G H
94 A B C D E F G H
95 A B C D E F G H
96 A B C D E F G H
97 A B C D E F G H
98 A B C D E F G H
99 A B C D E F G H
100 A B C D E F G H
101 A B C D E F G H
102 A B C D E F G H
103 A B C D E F G H
104 A B C D E F G H
105 A B C D E F G H

PART 6 GENETICS AND METABOLIC DISEASE

	A	B	C	D	E	F	G	H
106								
107								
108								
109								
110								
111								
112								
113								
114								
115								
116								
117								
118								
119								

PART 7 ENDOCRINOLOGY AND DIABETES MELLITUS

No.								
1	A	B	C	D	E	F	G	H
2	A	B	C	D	E	F	G	H
3	A	B	C	D	E	F	G	H
4	A	B	C	D	E	F	G	H
5	A	B	C	D	E	F	G	H
6	A	B	C	D	E	F	G	H
7	A	B	C	D	E	F	G	H
8	A	B	C	D	E	F	G	H
9	A	B	C	D	E	F	G	H
10	A	B	C	D	E	F	G	H
11	A	B	C	D	E	F	G	H
12	A	B	C	D	E	F	G	H
13	A	B	C	D	E	F	G	H
14	A	B	C	D	E	F	G	H
15	A	B	C	D	E	F	G	H
16	A	B	C	D	E	F	G	H
17	A	B	C	D	E	F	G	H
18	A	B	C	D	E	F	G	H
19	A	B	C	D	E	F	G	H
20	A	B	C	D	E	F	G	H
21	A	B	C	D	E	F	G	H
22	A	B	C	D	E	F	G	H
23	A	B	C	D	E	F	G	H
24	A	B	C	D	E	F	G	H
25	A	B	C	D	E	F	G	H
26	A	B	C	D	E	F	G	H
27	A	B	C	D	E	F	G	H
28	A	B	C	D	E	F	G	H
29	A	B	C	D	E	F	G	H
30	A	B	C	D	E	F	G	H
31	A	B	C	D	E	F	G	H
32	A	B	C	D	E	F	G	H
33	A	B	C	D	E	F	G	H
34	A	B	C	D	E	F	G	H
35	A	B	C	D	E	F	G	H
36	A	B	C	D	E	F	G	H
37	A	B	C	D	E	F	G	H
38	A	B	C	D	E	F	G	H
39	A	B	C	D	E	F	G	H
40	A	B	C	D	E	F	G	H
41	A	B	C	D	E	F	G	H
42	A	B	C	D	E	F	G	H
43	A	B	C	D	E	F	G	H
44	A	B	C	D	E	F	G	H
45	A	B	C	D	E	F	G	H
46	A	B	C	D	E	F	G	H
47	A	B	C	D	E	F	G	H
48	A	B	C	D	E	F	G	H
49	A	B	C	D	E	F	G	H
50	A	B	C	D	E	F	G	H
51	A	B	C	D	E	F	G	H
52	A	B	C	D	E	F	G	H
53	A	B	C	D	E	F	G	H
54	A	B	C	D	E	F	G	H
55	A	B	C	D	E	F	G	H
56	A	B	C	D	E	F	G	H
57	A	B	C	D	E	F	G	H
58	A	B	C	D	E	F	G	H
59	A	B	C	D	E	F	G	H
60	A	B	C	D	E	F	G	H
61	A	B	C	D	E	F	G	H
62	A	B	C	D	E	F	G	H
63	A	B	C	D	E	F	G	H
64	A	B	C	D	E	F	G	H
65	A	B	C	D	E	F	G	H
66	A	B	C	D	E	F	G	H
67	A	B	C	D	E	F	G	H
68	A	B	C	D	E	F	G	H
69	A	B	C	D	E	F	G	H
70	A	B	C	D	E	F	G	H
71	A	B	C	D	E	F	G	H
72	A	B	C	D	E	F	G	H
73	A	B	C	D	E	F	G	H
74	A	B	C	D	E	F	G	H
75	A	B	C	D	E	F	G	H
76	A	B	C	D	E	F	G	H
77	A	B	C	D	E	F	G	H
78	A	B	C	D	E	F	G	H
79	A	B	C	D	E	F	G	H
80	A	B	C	D	E	F	G	H
81	A	B	C	D	E	F	G	H
82	A	B	C	D	E	F	G	H
83	A	B	C	D	E	F	G	H
84	A	B	C	D	E	F	G	H
85	A	B	C	D	E	F	G	H
86	A	B	C	D	E	F	G	H
87	A	B	C	D	E	F	G	H
88	A	B	C	D	E	F	G	H
89	A	B	C	D	E	F	G	H
90	A	B	C	D	E	F	G	H
91	A	B	C	D	E	F	G	H
92	A	B	C	D	E	F	G	H
93	A	B	C	D	E	F	G	H
94	A	B	C	D	E	F	G	H
95	A	B	C	D	E	F	G	H
96	A	B	C	D	E	F	G	H
97	A	B	C	D	E	F	G	H
98	A	B	C	D	E	F	G	H
99	A	B	C	D	E	F	G	H
100	A	B	C	D	E	F	G	H
101	A	B	C	D	E	F	G	H
102	A	B	C	D	E	F	G	H
103	A	B	C	D	E	F	G	H
104	A	B	C	D	E	F	G	H
105	A	B	C	D	E	F	G	H

PART 7 ENDOCRINOLOGY AND DIABETES MELLITUS

106 A B C D E F G H
107 A B C D E F G H
108 A B C D E F G H
109 A B C D E F G H
110 A B C D E F G H
111 A B C D E F G H
112 A B C D E F G H
113 A B C D E F G H
114 A B C D E F G H
115 A B C D E F G H
116 A B C D E F G H
117 A B C D E F G H
118 A B C D E F G H
119 A B C D E F G H
120 A B C D E F G H
121 A B C D E F G H
122 A B C D E F G H
123 A B C D E F G H
124 A B C D E F G H
125 A B C D E F G H
126 A B C D E F G H
127 A B C D E F G H
128 A B C D E F G H
129 A B C D E F G H
130 A B C D E F G H
131 A B C D E F G H
132 A B C D E F G H
133 A B C D E F G H
134 A B C D E F G H
135 A B C D E F G H
136 A B C D E F G H
137 A B C D E F G H
138 A B C D E F G H
139 A B C D E F G H
140 A B C D E F G H
141 A B C D E F G H
142 A B C D E F G H
143 A B C D E F G H
144 A B C D E F G H
145 A B C D E F G H
146 A B C D E F G H
147 A B C D E F G H
148 A B C D E F G H
149 A B C D E F G H
150 A B C D E F G H
151 A B C D E F G H
152 A B C D E F G H
153 A B C D E F G H
154 A B C D E F G H
155 A B C D E F G H
156 A B C D E F G H
157 A B C D E F G H
158 A B C D E F G H
159 A B C D E F G H
160 A B C D E F G H
161 A B C D E F G H
162 A B C D E F G H
163 A B C D E F G H
164 A B C D E F G H
165 A B C D E F G H
166 A B C D E F G H
167 A B C D E F G H
168 A B C D E F G H
169 A B C D E F G H
170 A B C D E F G H
171 A B C D E F G H

PART 8 INFECTIOUS DISEASES

1 A B C D E F G H
2 A B C D E F G H
3 A B C D E F G H
4 A B C D E F G H
5 A B C D E F G H
6 A B C D E F G H
7 A B C D E F G H
8 A B C D E F G H
9 A B C D E F G H
10 A B C D E F G H
11 A B C D E F G H
12 A B C D E F G H
13 A B C D E F G H
14 A B C D E F G H
15 A B C D E F G H
16 A B C D E F G H
17 A B C D E F G H
18 A B C D E F G H
19 A B C D E F G H
20 A B C D E F G H
21 A B C D E F G H
22 A B C D E F G H
23 A B C D E F G H
24 A B C D E F G H
25 A B C D E F G H
26 A B C D E F G H
27 A B C D E F G H
28 A B C D E F G H
29 A B C D E F G H
30 A B C D E F G H
31 A B C D E F G H
32 A B C D E F G H
33 A B C D E F G H
34 A B C D E F G H
35 A B C D E F G H
36 A B C D E F G H
37 A B C D E F G H
38 A B C D E F G H
39 A B C D E F G H
40 A B C D E F G H
41 A B C D E F G H
42 A B C D E F G H
43 A B C D E F G H
44 A B C D E F G H
45 A B C D E F G H
46 A B C D E F G H
47 A B C D E F G H
48 A B C D E F G H
49 A B C D E F G H
50 A B C D E F G H
51 A B C D E F G H
52 A B C D E F G H
53 A B C D E F G H
54 A B C D E F G H
55 A B C D E F G H
56 A B C D E F G H
57 A B C D E F G H
58 A B C D E F G H
59 A B C D E F G H
60 A B C D E F G H
61 A B C D E F G H
62 A B C D E F G H
63 A B C D E F G H
64 A B C D E F G H
65 A B C D E F G H
66 A B C D E F G H
67 A B C D E F G H
68 A B C D E F G H
69 A B C D E F G H
70 A B C D E F G H
71 A B C D E F G H
72 A B C D E F G H
73 A B C D E F G H
74 A B C D E F G H
75 A B C D E F G H
76 A B C D E F G H
77 A B C D E F G H
78 A B C D E F G H
79 A B C D E F G H
80 A B C D E F G H
81 A B C D E F G H
82 A B C D E F G H
83 A B C D E F G H
84 A B C D E F G H
85 A B C D E F G H
86 A B C D E F G H
87 A B C D E F G H
88 A B C D E F G H
89 A B C D E F G H
90 A B C D E F G H
91 A B C D E F G H
92 A B C D E F G H
93 A B C D E F G H
94 A B C D E F G H
95 A B C D E F G H
96 A B C D E F G H
97 A B C D E F G H
98 A B C D E F G H
99 A B C D E F G H
100 A B C D E F G H
101 A B C D E F G H
102 A B C D E F G H
103 A B C D E F G H
104 A B C D E F G H
105 A B C D E F G H

PART 8 INFECTIOUS DISEASES

106 A B C D E F G H
107 A B C D E F G H
108 A B C D E F G H
109 A B C D E F G H
110 A B C D E F G H
111 A B C D E F G H
112 A B C D E F G H
113 A B C D E F G H
114 A B C D E F G H
115 A B C D E F G H
116 A B C D E F G H
117 A B C D E F G H
118 A B C D E F G H
119 A B C D E F G H
120 A B C D E F G H
121 A B C D E F G H
122 A B C D E F G H
123 A B C D E F G H
124 A B C D E F G H
125 A B C D E F G H
126 A B C D E F G H
127 A B C D E F G H
128 A B C D E F G H
129 A B C D E F G H
130 A B C D E F G H
131 A B C D E F G H
132 A B C D E F G H
133 A B C D E F G H
134 A B C D E F G H
135 A B C D E F G H
136 A B C D E F G H
137 A B C D E F G H
138 A B C D E F G H
139 A B C D E F G H
140 A B C D E F G H
141 A B C D E F G H
142 A B C D E F G H
143 A B C D E F G H
144 A B C D E F G H
145 A B C D E F G H
146 A B C D E F G H
147 A B C D E F G H
148 A B C D E F G H
149 A B C D E F G H
150 A B C D E F G H
151 A B C D E F G H
152 A B C D E F G H
153 A B C D E F G H
154 A B C D E F G H
155 A B C D E F G H
156 A B C D E F G H
157 A B C D E F G H
158 A B C D E F G H
159 A B C D E F G H
160 A B C D E F G H
161 A B C D E F G H
162 A B C D E F G H
163 A B C D E F G H
164 A B C D E F G H
165 A B C D E F G H
166 A B C D E F G H
167 A B C D E F G H
168 A B C D E F G H
169 A B C D E F G H
170 A B C D E F G H
171 A B C D E F G H
172 A B C D E F G H
173 A B C D E F G H
174 A B C D E F G H
175 A B C D E F G H
176 A B C D E F G H
177 A B C D E F G H
178 A B C D E F G H
179 A B C D E F G H
180 A B C D E F G H
181 A B C D E F G H
182 A B C D E F G H
183 A B C D E F G H
184 A B C D E F G H
185 A B C D E F G H
186 A B C D E F G H
187 A B C D E F G H
188 A B C D E F G H
189 A B C D E F G H
190 A B C D E F G H
191 A B C D E F G H
192 A B C D E F G H
193 A B C D E F G H
194 A B C D E F G H
195 A B C D E F G H
196 A B C D E F G H
197 A B C D E F G H
198 A B C D E F G H
199 A B C D E F G H
200 A B C D E F G H
201 A B C D E F G H
202 A B C D E F G H

PART 9 CLINICAL IMMUNOLOGY AND RHEUMATOLOGY

1 A B C D E F G H
2 A B C D E F G H
3 A B C D E F G H
4 A B C D E F G H
5 A B C D E F G H
6 A B C D E F G H
7 A B C D E F G H
8 A B C D E F G H
9 A B C D E F G H
10 A B C D E F G H
11 A B C D E F G H
12 A B C D E F G H
13 A B C D E F G H
14 A B C D E F G H
15 A B C D E F G H
16 A B C D E F G H
17 A B C D E F G H
18 A B C D E F G H
19 A B C D E F G H
20 A B C D E F G H
21 A B C D E F G H
22 A B C D E F G H
23 A B C D E F G H
24 A B C D E F G H
25 A B C D E F G H
26 A B C D E F G H
27 A B C D E F G H
28 A B C D E F G H
29 A B C D E F G H
30 A B C D E F G H
31 A B C D E F G H
32 A B C D E F G H
33 A B C D E F G H
34 A B C D E F G H
35 A B C D E F G H
36 A B C D E F G H
37 A B C D E F G H
38 A B C D E F G H
39 A B C D E F G H
40 A B C D E F G H
41 A B C D E F G H
42 A B C D E F G H
43 A B C D E F G H
44 A B C D E F G H
45 A B C D E F G H
46 A B C D E F G H
47 A B C D E F G H
48 A B C D E F G H
49 A B C D E F G H
50 A B C D E F G H
51 A B C D E F G H
52 A B C D E F G H
53 A B C D E F G H
54 A B C D E F G H
55 A B C D E F G H
56 A B C D E F G H
57 A B C D E F G H
58 A B C D E F G H
59 A B C D E F G H
60 A B C D E F G H
61 A B C D E F G H
62 A B C D E F G H
63 A B C D E F G H
64 A B C D E F G H
65 A B C D E F G H
66 A B C D E F G H
67 A B C D E F G H
68 A B C D E F G H
69 A B C D E F G H
70 A B C D E F G H
71 A B C D E F G H
72 A B C D E F G H
73 A B C D E F G H
74 A B C D E F G H
75 A B C D E F G H
76 A B C D E F G H
77 A B C D E F G H
78 A B C D E F G H
79 A B C D E F G H
80 A B C D E F G H
81 A B C D E F G H
82 A B C D E F G H
83 A B C D E F G H
84 A B C D E F G H
85 A B C D E F G H
86 A B C D E F G H
87 A B C D E F G H
88 A B C D E F G H
89 A B C D E F G H
90 A B C D E F G H
91 A B C D E F G H
92 A B C D E F G H
93 A B C D E F G H
94 A B C D E F G H
95 A B C D E F G H
96 A B C D E F G H
97 A B C D E F G H
98 A B C D E F G H
99 A B C D E F G H
100 A B C D E F G H
101 A B C D E F G H
102 A B C D E F G H
103 A B C D E F G H
104 A B C D E F G H
105 A B C D E F G H

PART 10 NEUROLOGIC DISEASE

1 A B C D E F G H
2 A B C D E F G H
3 A B C D E F G H
4 A B C D E F G H
5 A B C D E F G H
6 A B C D E F G H
7 A B C D E F G H
8 A B C D E F G H
9 A B C D E F G H
10 A B C D E F G H
11 A B C D E F G H
12 A B C D E F G H
13 A B C D E F G H
14 A B C D E F G H
15 A B C D E F G H
16 A B C D E F G H
17 A B C D E F G H
18 A B C D E F G H
19 A B C D E F G H
20 A B C D E F G H
21 A B C D E F G H
22 A B C D E F G H
23 A B C D E F G H
24 A B C D E F G H
25 A B C D E F G H
26 A B C D E F G H
27 A B C D E F G H
28 A B C D E F G H
29 A B C D E F G H
30 A B C D E F G H
31 A B C D E F G H
32 A B C D E F G H
33 A B C D E F G H
34 A B C D E F G H
35 A B C D E F G H
36 A B C D E F G H
37 A B C D E F G H
38 A B C D E F G H
39 A B C D E F G H
40 A B C D E F G H
41 A B C D E F G H
42 A B C D E F G H
43 A B C D E F G H
44 A B C D E F G H
45 A B C D E F G H
46 A B C D E F G H
47 A B C D E F G H
48 A B C D E F G H
49 A B C D E F G H
50 A B C D E F G H
51 A B C D E F G H
52 A B C D E F G H
53 A B C D E F G H
54 A B C D E F G H
55 A B C D E F G H
56 A B C D E F G H
57 A B C D E F G H
58 A B C D E F G H
59 A B C D E F G H
60 A B C D E F G H
61 A B C D E F G H
62 A B C D E F G H
63 A B C D E F G H
64 A B C D E F G H
65 A B C D E F G H
66 A B C D E F G H
67 A B C D E F G H
68 A B C D E F G H
69 A B C D E F G H
70 A B C D E F G H
71 A B C D E F G H
72 A B C D E F G H
73 A B C D E F G H
74 A B C D E F G H
75 A B C D E F G H
76 A B C D E F G H
77 A B C D E F G H
78 A B C D E F G H
79 A B C D E F G H
80 A B C D E F G H
81 A B C D E F G H
82 A B C D E F G H
83 A B C D E F G H
84 A B C D E F G H
85 A B C D E F G H
86 A B C D E F G H
87 A B C D E F G H
88 A B C D E F G H
89 A B C D E F G H
90 A B C D E F G H
91 A B C D E F G H
92 A B C D E F G H
93 A B C D E F G H
94 A B C D E F G H
95 A B C D E F G H
96 A B C D E F G H
97 A B C D E F G H
98 A B C D E F G H
99 A B C D E F G H
100 A B C D E F G H
101 A B C D E F G H
102 A B C D E F G H
103 A B C D E F G H
104 A B C D E F G H
105 A B C D E F G H

PART 10 NEUROLOGIC DISEASE

	A	B	C	D	E	F	G	H
106	A	B	C	D	E	F	G	H
107	A	B	C	D	E	F	G	H
108	A	B	C	D	E	F	G	H
109	A	B	C	D	E	F	G	H
110	A	B	C	D	E	F	G	H
111	A	B	C	D	E	F	G	H
112	A	B	C	D	E	F	G	H
113	A	B	C	D	E	F	G	H
114	A	B	C	D	E	F	G	H
115	A	B	C	D	E	F	G	H
116	A	B	C	D	E	F	G	H
117	A	B	C	D	E	F	G	H
118	A	B	C	D	E	F	G	H
119	A	B	C	D	E	F	G	H
120	A	B	C	D	E	F	G	H
121	A	B	C	D	E	F	G	H
122	A	B	C	D	E	F	G	H
123	A	B	C	D	E	F	G	H
124	A	B	C	D	E	F	G	H
125	A	B	C	D	E	F	G	H
126	A	B	C	D	E	F	G	H
127	A	B	C	D	E	F	G	H
128	A	B	C	D	E	F	G	H
129	A	B	C	D	E	F	G	H
130	A	B	C	D	E	F	G	H
131	A	B	C	D	E	F	G	H
132	A	B	C	D	E	F	G	H
133	A	B	C	D	E	F	G	H
134	A	B	C	D	E	F	G	H
135	A	B	C	D	E	F	G	H
136	A	B	C	D	E	F	G	H
137	A	B	C	D	E	F	G	H
138	A	B	C	D	E	F	G	H
139	A	B	C	D	E	F	G	H
140	A	B	C	D	E	F	G	H
141	A	B	C	D	E	F	G	H
142	A	B	C	D	E	F	G	H
143	A	B	C	D	E	F	G	H
144	A	B	C	D	E	F	G	H
145	A	B	C	D	E	F	G	H
146	A	B	C	D	E	F	G	H
147	A	B	C	D	E	F	G	H
148	A	B	C	D	E	F	G	H
149	A	B	C	D	E	F	G	H
150	A	B	C	D	E	F	G	H
151	A	B	C	D	E	F	G	H
152	A	B	C	D	E	F	G	H
153	A	B	C	D	E	F	G	H
154	A	B	C	D	E	F	G	H
155	A	B	C	D	E	F	G	H
156	A	B	C	D	E	F	G	H
157	A	B	C	D	E	F	G	H
158	A	B	C	D	E	F	G	H
159	A	B	C	D	E	F	G	H
160	A	B	C	D	E	F	G	H
161	A	B	C	D	E	F	G	H
162	A	B	C	D	E	F	G	H
163	A	B	C	D	E	F	G	H
164	A	B	C	D	E	F	G	H
165	A	B	C	D	E	F	G	H
166	A	B	C	D	E	F	G	H
167	A	B	C	D	E	F	G	H
168	A	B	C	D	E	F	G	H
169	A	B	C	D	E	F	G	H
170	A	B	C	D	E	F	G	H
171	A	B	C	D	E	F	G	H
172	A	B	C	D	E	F	G	H
173	A	B	C	D	E	F	G	H
174	A	B	C	D	E	F	G	H
175	A	B	C	D	E	F	G	H
176	A	B	C	D	E	F	G	H
177	A	B	C	D	E	F	G	H
178	A	B	C	D	E	F	G	H
179	A	B	C	D	E	F	G	H
180	A	B	C	D	E	F	G	H
181	A	B	C	D	E	F	G	H
182	A	B	C	D	E	F	G	H
183	A	B	C	D	E	F	G	H
184	A	B	C	D	E	F	G	H
185	A	B	C	D	E	F	G	H
186	A	B	C	D	E	F	G	H
187	A	B	C	D	E	F	G	H
188	A	B	C	D	E	F	G	H
189	A	B	C	D	E	F	G	H
190	A	B	C	D	E	F	G	H
191	A	B	C	D	E	F	G	H
192	A	B	C	D	E	F	G	H

PART 11 DERMATOLOGY

	A	B	C	D	E	F	G	H
1								
2								
3								
4								
5								
6								
7								
8								
9								
10								
11								
12								
13								
14								
15								
16								
17								
18								
19								
20								
21								
22								
23								
24								
25								
26								
27								
28								
29								
30								
31								
32								
33								
34								
35								
36								
37								
38								
39								
40								
41								
42								
43								
44								
45								
46								
47								
48								
49								
50